Survival of Cancer Patients in Europe:

The EUROCARE-2 Study

INTERNATIONAL AGENCY FOR RESEARCH ON CANCER

The International Agency for Research on Cancer (IARC) was established in 1965 by the World Health Assembly, as an independently financed organization within the framework of the World Health Organization. The headquarters of the Agency are at Lyon, France.

The Agency conducts a programme of research concentrating particularly on the epidemiology of cancer and the study of potential carcinogens in the human environment. Its field studies are supplemented by biological and chemical research carried out in the Agency's laboratories in Lyon, and, through collaborative research agreements, in national research institutions in many countries. The Agency also conducts a programme for the education and training of personnel for cancer research.

The publications of the Agency are intended to contribute to the dissemination of authoritative information on different aspects of cancer research. Information about IARC publications and how to order them, is also available via the Internet at: **http://www.iarc.fr/**

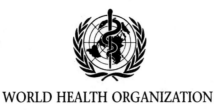

WORLD HEALTH ORGANIZATION

INTERNATIONAL AGENCY FOR RESEARCH ON CANCER

EUROPEAN COMMISSION

Survival of Cancer Patients in Europe:
the EUROCARE-2 Study

Edited by

F. Berrino, R. Capocaccia, J. Estève, G. Gatta, T. Hakulinen, A. Micheli,

M. Sant and A. Verdecchia

IARC Scientific Publications No. 151

International Agency for Research on Cancer

Lyon, France

1999

Published by the International Agency for Research on Cancer,
150 cours Albert Thomas, 69372 Lyon cédex 08, France

© International Agency for Research on Cancer, 1999

Distributed by Oxford University Press, Walton Street, Oxford OX2 6DP, UK
(fax: +44 1865 267782) and in the USA by Oxford University Press, 2001 Evans Road, Carey,
NC 27513 (fax: +1 919 677 1303). All IARC publications can also be ordered directly from IARCPress
(fax: +33 04 72 73 83 02; E-mail: press@iarc.fr).

IARC Library Cataloguing in Publication Data

Survival of cancer patients in Europe: the EUROCARE-2 study / editors, F. Berrino ... [et al.]

(IARC scientific publications ; 151)

1. Neoplasms – Europe 2. Neoplasms – mortality 3. Survival Rate – Europe
I. Berrino, F.   II. Series

ISBN 92 832 2151 6   (NLM Classification W1)
ISSN 0300-5085

Printed in France

Contents

Foreword

Reliable data on the magnitude of the cancer problem are essential for monitoring the health of the community and the performance of the health-care system, and allow health authorities to make informed decisions regarding the most effective investment of resources. For three decades, IARC has been gathering and disseminating to scientists and decision-makers information on cancer incidence and mortality in populations covered by cancer registration systems across the world. The EUROCARE project complements these data, by analysing systematically the survival of cancer patients, on the basis of information provided by European cancer registries. EUROCARE (European Cancer Registry-based Study on Survival and Care of Cancer Patients) is a Concerted Action supported by the European Union since 1990. The EUROCARE-2 study, the results of which are presented in this volume, analyses data on patients diagnosed during the late 1980s, and was financed by the Biomed II program of the European Union. It involved the collaboration of 50 oncological or public health institutions in 17 European countries.

The survival of patients is a basic parameter by which the effectiveness of medical treatment for cancer can be judged. The interpretation of survival differences between populations and of time trends in survival, however, is not straightforward and must take into consideration several factors. A major predictor of the survival of cancer patients, as well as of certain other health indicators, is the level of material well-being of the population. Accordingly, differences in material well-being are likely to obscure differences between health care systems. Moreover, increases in survival may be due either to earlier diagnosis or later death, or to both. Early diagnosis is a major determinant of the likelihood of cure, but may not confer any advantage for patients who eventually die of the cancer or for those who would have been cured anyway. The next phase of the EUROCARE project will try to determine the extent to which improvements in survival are the result of better treatment, and to what extent more effective treatment is due to early diagnosis. This will require the collection of information not only on diagnosis and survival, but also on disease stage at diagnosis and on diagnostic procedures that may affect stage definition.

The EUROCARE survival analyses, however, have already identified several public-health priorities and have suggested ways in which health authorities can improve cancer care. Future research should include measurement of the effectiveness of different interventions and estimation of the potential impact of future actions.

P. Kleihues, M.D.
Director, IARC

Preface

F. Berrino

Since the earliest days of scientific medicine, the proportion of patients who are cured of a disease has been considered the basic parameter by which to assess the effectiveness of health care practices (Berrino *et al.*, 1995). The study of the survival rates of patients treated in any given hospital, however, may be heavily biased because of different selection practices by different hospitals or physicians. Population-based survival data (i.e., survival figures computed on all the cases occurring in a given period in defined populations, as provided by cancer registries), in contrast, provide prognostic information on unselected sets of patients, suitable for estimating the overall effectiveness of cancer control and for comparing different populations.

The aims of population-based studies of cancer patients' survival include: quantifying the challenge facing those who work in the field of cancer care, establishing priorities for health care investment as well as for health care research, monitoring the global effect of improvements in diagnosis and treatment, estimating the potential for further improvement (e.g., through comparisons between populations over time), planning clinical trials, discovering inequalities between and within health systems, and estimating prevalence, i.e., the number of subjects requiring either treatment or some form of clinical surveillance because of a past diagnosis of cancer. A knowledge of prevalence, along with information on incidence and survival, helps those who have responsibility for planning and financing health services to quantify the resources needed.

In countries where population-based cancer registries have been established for several decades, survival of cancer patients has increased dramatically for many cancer sites (Miller *et al.*,1992; Dickman *et al.*, 1999). Cancer, however, is still a highly lethal disease. In the present monograph, the relative survival at five years from diagnosis for cancer patients diagnosed in Europe between 1985 and 1989, for all sites combined (except non-melanoma skin cancer), has been estimated at 43%, with 35% for male patients and 50% for females. But five-year survival does not mean cure: even 10 years after diagnosis some excess mortality due to cancer is still present for several cancer sites, notably breast and prostate, but also lung, brain, non-Hodgkin's lymphoma, multiple myeloma and leukaemia (Dickman *et al.*, 1999). Theoretically, the proportion of cured patients can be estimated by extending the relative survival curves up to the point where the population of patients does not show any further excess mortality compared with the general population. Such an exercise has been carried out only for a few cancer sites (Verdecchia *et al.*, 1998).

One may speculate, however, that today the proportion of European cancer patients who are cured from their cancer (excluding non-melanoma skin cancers) is unlikely to be much higher than one third.

Since 1990, the European Union has funded a concerted action of European population-based cancer registries (the EUROCARE project), of which the major aim is to establish the extent of survival differences between European populations and reasons for them (Berrino *et al.*, 1995). The present monograph analyses the most recent available data with complete five-year follow-up, concerning patients diagnosed between 1985 and 1989 in 47 populations covered by cancer registration in 17 European countries. It presents age- and sex-specific survival rates by country as well as estimates for the whole of Europe (defined as the sum of the 17 countries contributing to this monograph). The latter estimates have been computed assuming that where cancer registration covers only a fraction of the country, survival rates measured in that fraction hold true for the whole national population. To distinguish between cancer-specific deaths and deaths from other causes, for which the frequencies are fairly different between countries, both observed and relative survival rates are given, i.e. the actual survival and an estimate of the survival that cancer patients would experience in the absence of other causes of death. As survival is heavily dependent on age and the age distribution of cancer cases is different in males and females and in different countries, age-standardized relative survival figures are also provided for comparisons between countries and sexes. The latter data are given in the bottom table of the European summary pages. They express the theoretical survival figures that one would observe if the age distribution of patients with a given cancer were the same in every country and in both sexes. In contrast, the figures provided in the country-specific tables, as well as those in the central table of the European pages, are not age-standardized. As they express the actual survival in each country (and the estimated actual average survival in Europe), they are useful for public health and planning purposes but neither for comparing different countries nor for examining the effect of gender on survival.

The results show that survival is still uniformly low for several frequent cancers such as those of the lung, pancreas and oesophagus. For other frequent cancers, survival is much lower in eastern European countries than in western Europe, where, however, the overall pattern suggests that there is still room for improvement. For many tumours, in fact, survival is clearly higher than the European average in certain countries, e.g., Sweden for several head and neck sites, colon, rectum, melanoma, breast, cervix and corpus uteri, ovary, prostate and bladder cancer, Switzerland for melanoma, breast, ovary, prostate and bladder, the Netherlands for colon, rectum and corpus uteri, Finland for breast, prostate and bladder, France for lung, prostate and breast cancer, and Italy for stomach and breast cancer. All these are cancer sites for which the extent of disease at the time of first diagnosis is the major prognostic determinant. Where highly effective medical treatment is available, e.g. for testicular cancer and Hodgkin's disease, the intercountry variability in western Europe is lower.

The interpretation of survival differences, however, is not straightforward. Fairly large differences, in fact, may be explained by reasons other than early diagnosis and better treatment. Detailed analyses of the various factors that may affect survival and of the difficulties encountered in estimating and comparing relative survival in different populations are given elsewhere (Berrino et al., 1995, 1997). To avoid misinterpretation, some potential sources of bias, as well as a few inevitable simplifications required to summarize such a huge amount of data, need some discussion here.

First, the quality of cancer registry data is not the same all over Europe, in terms both of completeness of cancer registration and of reliability of the diagnosis provided by the health system. Some overestimation of survival, in particular, may be due to the exclusion from survival estimates of cases known to the registry from death certificate only (DCO). Among such cases, short-term survivors are likely to be over-represented. When the information system of a cancer registry is not exhaustive, however, long-term survivors may also be missed. A low diagnostic specificity for highly lethal visceral cancers such as pancreatic and liver cancer is also likely to have entailed a substantial overestimation of survival in some eastern countries. Further errors may derive from incomplete follow-up. The size of the biases deriving from a high proportion of DCO cases or from loss to follow-up has been shown to be small compared with genuine inter-country differences and time trends observed in the EUROCARE data-set (Berrino et al., 1995; Sant & Gatta, 1995; Raymond et al., 1996). We are confident that the overall pattern of cancer survival differences between populations reported in this monograph largely depends on differences in access to effective health care, rather than on methodological biases. When interest is focused on the difference between two specific countries or registries, however, we recommend that the indicators of data quality presented in Chapter 1 should be borne in mind.

Second, the same cancer sites in different countries are not necessarily comparable. The case mix of different subsites and histologies grouped under the same heading, as defined by the three-digit code of the International Classification of Diseases, may actually be quite different. In southern Europe, for instance, head and neck cancers include a higher proportion of subsites with a bad prognosis, such as hypopharynx versus oropharynx, and supraglottic versus glottic cancer. In contrast, in some countries the rapid decrease of stomach cancer incidence may have left a higher proportion of more malignant histotypes and/or subsites (e.g., cardia versus antrum) compared with, for instance, southern Europe, where the incidence of stomach cancer is still fairly high. A similar phenomenon is likely to have occurred for cervical cancer, for which organized screening programmes may lead to the selective prevention of the less aggressive biotypes.

Third, the present monograph shows survival rates by country, but in many of the countries included in the analysis, cancer registration covers only a small fraction of the national population, often less than 20%. The oncological equipment and access to modern treatment may be more advanced in those areas where cancer registration has been implemented than in the rest of the country. The actual survival for the whole country, therefore, could be lower. Nevertheless these are population-based data, suggesting that, with proper investment, the same rates are achievable.

Fourth, longer survival does not necessarily imply later death. Theoretically, it might just reflect earlier diagnosis, without any advantage for the patients. In most cases, however, earlier diagnosis is expected to increase the effectiveness of treatment, thus contributing to the postponement of death. In observational studies, distinguishing how much increasing survival is due to earlier diagnosis, to more effective treatment because of a more favourable stage distribution at diagnosis, or to more effective stage-specific treatment, may be very difficult. A knowledge of survival by stage of the disease at diagnosis could help to clarify the issue, but this information is either not available from cancer registries or not easily comparable between registries, because the rules for establishing and registering the extent of disease are far from standardized. Even if properly recorded according to standard rules, however, the information on stage would not provide an unambiguous interpretation of survival differences. Examples from registries that can provide stage-specific survival data over time may help to illustrate this difficulty. When survival increases both in the overall series and in stage-specific analyses, one would conclude that treatment is improving, but the lead-time due to early diagnosis still cannot easily be estimated. If the overall increase in survival is steeper than the stage-specific trends, one could speculate that most of the effect is due to the shift to early stages. If, on the other hand, stage-specific survival rates increase more steeply than overall survival, one should suspect a stage migration over time. This depends on the evolution of diagnostic practices and on the increasing availability of diagnostic techniques to discover metastatic dissemination that is not clinically overt. As a consequence, the present 'localized' cases are more localized than the previous ones, because several cases with silent metastatic spread are now properly classified as advanced. The present 'advanced' stages, on the other hand, will also perform better because of the inclusion of less advanced metastatic cases that in the previous period were still classified as localized (Feinstein *et al.*, 1985). Frequently, however, an increase in survival is mostly confined to localized tumours, the overall survival increase is less steep, and that for locally advanced or metastatic cases is even less marked (Dickman *et al.*, 1999). Such a pattern is compatible with a complex mixture of the effects of improved treatment effectiveness, especially increased access to adequate care facilities, earlier diagnosis, and stage migration.

A proper interpretation of these differences and trends would be facilitated by the availability of standardized information not only on stage but also on the staging procedures actually performed in individual cases, and by simultaneous consideration of trends in incidence, stage-specific incidence, survival and mortality rates.

Through an unprecedented effort of gathering together, standardizing and analysing cancer registry survival data, the EUROCARE project has unequivocally demonstrated that there are differences in survival between European countries and that for several cancer sites and countries the differences are substantial. In many cases, survival is increasing. The issue today is to understand what can be done to further improve these trends and to reduce the gaps between populations: whether we need more screening programmes, more educational programmes for the recognition of early symptoms, more qualified general practitioners, more efficient referral systems, less economic barriers to access to advanced cancer clinics, more modern diagnostic and treatment equipment, more oncologists, more specialized cancer centres, more qualified nurses and other health professionals, or more efficient palliative treatment.

The basic question that remains to be answered is: how much of the improved average survival is due to better treatment (or to access of a larger proportion of patients to conventional treatment), to more effective treatment because of earlier diagnosis, or just to earlier diagnosis? A major EUROCARE endeavour for the future will be to proceed to a proper comparison of stage-specific survival, taking into account the intercountry differences in staging procedures, which will help in distinguishing the role of more effective stage-specific treatment from that of diagnosis at earlier stages of disease ('downstaging'). Preliminary results already available for colorectal cancer suggest that most of the difference between western European populations is due to early versus late diagnosis, but that the low survival performance of some eastern countries is a result largely of insufficient access to proper treatment.

Further relevant questions are: how much postponement of death is due to an increased proportion of cured patients, or to increased survival of incurable patients? How much of the apparent increasing proportion of cured patients is due to the increased detection of cases that would not have occurred as clinical cancer in the absence of screening programmes or intense clinical case-finding of asymptomatic lesions? Survival, in fact, has several components: the proportion of patients who are cured of a disease that eventually would have killed them, the proportion of patients who are still alive but will eventually die of it and the proportion of patients who would have not died from it even in the absence of any treatment. Distinguishing these components and their evolution over time remains a major challenge for future studies.

References

Berrino, F., Estève, J. & Coleman, M.P. (1995) Basic issues in estimating and comparing the survival of cancer patients. In: Berrino, F., Sant, M., Verdecchia, A., Capocaccia, R., Hakulinen, T. & Estève, J., eds, *Survival of Cancer Patients in Europe. The Eurocare Study* (IARC Scientific Publications No.132), Lyon, IARC, pp. 1–14

Berrino, F., Sant, M., Verdecchia, A., Capocaccia, R., Hakulinen, T. & Estève, J., eds (1995) *Survival of Cancer Patients in Europe. The Eurocare Study* (IARC Scientific Publications No.132), Lyon, IARC

Berrino, F., Micheli, A., Sant, M. & Capocaccia, R. (1997) Interpreting survival differences and trends. In: Verdecchia, A., Micheli, A. & Gatta, G., eds, Survival of Cancer Patients in Italy. The Itacare Study. *Tumori*, **83**, 9–16

Dickman, P.W., Hakulinen, T., Luostarinen, T., Pukkala, E., Sankila, R., Söderman, B. & Teppo, L. (1999) Survival of Cancer Patients in Finland, 1955–1994. *Acta Oncol.*, **38** (Suppl. 12), 1–103

Feinstein, A.R., Sosin, D.M. & Wells, C.K. (1985) The Will Rogers phenomenon: stage migration and new diagnostic techniques as a source of misleading statistics for survival in cancer. *New Engl. J. Med.*, **312**, 1604–1608

Gatta, G., Capocaccia, R., Sant, M., Bell, C.M.J., Coebergh, J.W.W., Damhuis, R., Faivre, J., Martinez-Garcia, C., Pawlega, J., Ponz de Leon, M., Pottier, D., Raverdy, N., Williams, E.M.I. & Berrino, F. (1999) Understanding variations in survival for colorectal cancer in Europe. a EUROCARE high resolution study (submitted for publication)

Miller, B.A., Ries, L.A.G., Hankey, B.F., Kosary, C.L., & Edwards, B.K. (1992) *Cancer Statistics Review: 1973–1989* (NIH Publication No. 92-2789), Bethesda, National Cancer Institute

Raymond, L., Fisher, B., Fioretta, G. & Bouchardy, C. (1996) Migration bias in cancer survival rates. *J. Epidemiol. Biostat.*, **1**, 167–173

Sant M. & Gatta G. (1995) The EUROCARE database. In: Berrino, F., Sant, M., Verdecchia, A., Capocaccia, R., Hakulinen, T. & Estève, J., eds, *Survival of Cancer Patients in Europe. The Eurocare Study* (IARC Scientific Publications No.132), Lyon, IARC, pp. 15–31

Verdecchia, A., De Angelis, R., Capocaccia, R., Sant, M., Micheli, A, Gatta, G. & Berrino, F. (1998) The cure for colon cancer: results from the EUROCARE study. *Int. J. Cancer*, **77**, 322–329

Contributors

Aareleid, T.
Department of Epidemiology and
Biostatistics
Institute of Experimental and Clinical
Medicine
Hiiu Street, 42
EE 11619 Tallinn, Estonia
Tel. +372 6 504 337,
Fax +372 6 706 814
E-mail: tiiu@onkoloogia.estpak.ee

Ardanaz, E.
Navarra Cancer Registry
Instituto de Salud Publica
Servicio Navarra de Salud-Osasunbidea
C). Leyre, 15
E-31003 Pamplona, Spain
Tel. +34 948 423440/64,
Fax +34 948 423474
E-mail: ispepi01@cfnavarra.es

Arveux, P.
Doubs Cancer Registry
Centre Hospitalier Universitaire de
Besançon
F-25030 Besançon cedex, France
Tel. +33 (03) 81 21 83 14/12,
Fax +33 (03) 81 21 83 11
*E-mail: patrick.arveux@ufc-chu.univ-
fcomte.fr*

Barchielli, A.
Tuscany Cancer Registry
Unità Operativa di Epidemiologia
Presidio per la Prevenzione Oncologica
Azienda Ospedaliera Careggi
Via S. Salvi, 12
I-50135 Firenze, Italy
Tel. +39 (055) 6263694,
Fax +39 (055) 679954
E-mail: md0632@mclink.it

Bell, J.
Thames Cancer Registry
1st Floor, Capital House
Weston Street
London SE1 3QD, UK
Tel. +44 (171) 378 7688,
Fax +44 (171) 378 9510
E-mail: j.bell@umds.ac.uk

Berrino, F.
Lombardy Cancer Registry
Division of Epidemiology
Istituto Nazionale per lo Studio e la
Cura dei Tumori
Via Venezian, 1
I-20133 Milano, Italy
Tel. +39 (02) 70601853, 2390460/501/502,
Fax +39 (02) 2390762
E-mail: berrino@istitutotumori.mi.it

Bielska-Lasota, M.
Warsaw Cancer Registry
M. Sklodowska-Curie Cancer Center &
Institute of Oncology
Dept of Mass Screening Organization
5, W.K. Roentgena Street
02-781 Warsaw, Poland
Tel. +48 22-64450-24 Ext. 2889,
Fax +48 22 6480219
E-mail: mbielskalasota@coi.waw.pl

Borràs, J.
Tarragona Cancer Registry
Registre del Cancer de Tarragona
Lliga Contra el Cancer de les
Comarques de Tarragona
C/ Reina Maria Cristina, 54
E-43002 Tarragona, Spain
Tel. +34 (977) 232423,
Fax +34 (977) 211111
E-mail: jgalceran@lccct.org.es

Bouchardy C.
Geneva Cancer Registry
Bd. de la Cluse, 55
CH-1205 Geneva, Switzerland
Tel. +41 (22) 329 10 11,
Fax +41 (22) 328 29 33
E-mail:bouchardy-c@ge-dass.etat-ge.ch

Capocaccia, R.
Istituto Superiore di Sanità
Department of Epidemiology and
Biostatistics
Viale Elena Regina, 299
I-00161 Rome, Italy
Tel. +39 06 49902230,
Fax +39 06 49387069
E-mail: rcap@iss.it

Carli, P.M.
Côte d'Or Haematological Malignancies
Registry
Faculté de Médecine
7 Boulevard Jeanne d'Arc
F-21034 Dijon cedex, France
Tel./Fax +33 (03) 80 39 33 93
E-mail: mmaynadie@chu-dijon.fr

Carrani E.
Istituto Superiore di Sanità
Electronic Data Processing Services
Viale Elena Regina, 299
I-00161 Rome, Italy
Tel. +39 06 49903763
E-mail: carrani@iss.it

Chaplain, G.
Côte d'Or Breast and Gynaecologic
Cancer Registry
Centre Georges-François Leclerc
1 rue du Professeur Marion
F-21034 Dijon cedex, France
Tel. +33 (03) 80 73 75 33,
Fax +33 (03) 80 73 77 06
E-mail: gchaplain@dijon.fnclcc.fr

Coebergh, J.W.W.
Eindhoven Cancer Registry
Comprehensive Cancer Centre South
PO Box 231
NL-5600 AE Eindhoven,
The Netherlands
Tel. +31 402971616,
Fax +31 402971610
E-mail: jw.coebergh@ikz.nl

Coleman, M.P.
Cancer and Public Health Unit
London School of Hygiene and Tropical
Medicine
Keppel Street
London WC1E 7HT, UK
Tel. +44 171 636 8636;
Fax +44 171 436 4230
E-mail: m.coleman@lshtm.ac.uk

Conti, E.M.S.
Latina Cancer Registry
Istituto Regina Elena per lo Studio e la
Cura dei Tumori
Viale Regina Elena, 291
I-00161 Rome, Italy
Tel. +39(06) 49852016,
Fax +39(06) 499852388

Crosignani, P.
Lombardy Cancer Registry
Division of Epidemiology
Istituto Nazionale per lo studio e la
Cura dei Tumori
Via Venezian, 1
I-20133 Milano, Italy
Tel. +39 (02) 2390460/501/502,
Fax +39 (02) 2390762
E-mail: canreg@istitutotumori.mi.it

Damhuis, R.A.M.
Rotterdam Cancer Registry
Comprehensive Cancer Center
Rotterdam
P.O. Box 289
NL-3000 AG Rotterdam,
The Netherlands
Tel. +31 (10) 4405803,
Fax +31 (10) 4364784
E-mail: canreg@ikr.nl

Davies, T.W.
East Anglian Cancer Registry
Institute of Public Health
University Forvie Site
Robinson Way
Cambridge CB2 2SR, UK
Tel. +44 (1223) 330318,
Fax +44 (1223) 330330
E-mail: twd10@medschl.cam.ac.uk

De Angelis, G.
Istituto Superiore di Sanità
Department of Epidemiology and
   Biostatistics
Viale Elena Regina, 299
I-00161 Rome, Italy
Tel. +39 06 49902230,
Fax +39 06 49387069

De Lisi, V.
Parma Cancer Registry
Via Gramsci, 14
I-43100 Parma, Italy
Tel. +39 (0521) 259571/991094,
Fax +39 (0521) 995448
E-mail: oncolog@ipruniv.cce.unipr.it

Edwards, S.
Oxford Cancer Intelligence Unit
Institute of Health Sciences
Old Road
Headington, Oxford OX3 7LF, UK
Tel. +44 1865 227040,
Fax +44 1865 226809
E-mail:ociu@cix.compulink.co.uk

Estève, J.
Service de Biostatistique
Pavillon 1M
Centre Hospitalier Lyon Sud
165, chemin du Grand Revoyet
F-69495 Pierre Bénite, France
Tel. +33 (04) 78.86.57.75,
Fax +33 (04) 78 86 57 74
E-mail: esteve@iarc.fr

Exbrayat, C.
Isère Cancer Registry
21 Chemin des Sources
F-38240 Meylan, France
Tel. +33 (04) 76 90 76 10,
Fax +33 (04) 76 41 87 00
E-mail: registre.cancer.isere@wanadoo.fr

Faivre, J.
Côte-d'Or Digestive Cancer Registry
Faculté de Médecine
CRI INSERM 9505
7 Bld Jeanne d'Arc
F-21033 Dijon cedex, France
Tel.+33 (03) 80 39 33 40,
Fax +33 (03) 80 66 82 51
E-mail: jean.faivre@u-bourgogne.fr

Falcini, F.
Romagna Cancer Registry
Ospedale G.B. Morgagni-L. Pierantoni
Via Forlanini, 11
47100 Forlí, Italy
Tel. +39 (0543) 731583,
Fax +39 (0543) 731736
E-mail: i.o.r.@fo.nettuno.it

Federico, M.
Modena Cancer Registry
University of Modena
Via del Pozzo, 71
I-41100 Modena, Italy
Tel. +39 (059) 424151/ 424150,
Fax +39 (059) 424152
E-mail:federico@unimo.it

Forman, D.
Northern and Yorkshire Cancer Registry
   & Information Service (NYCRIS)
Cookridge Hospital
Arthington House
Hospital Lane
Leeds LS16 6QB, UK
Tel. +44 113 292 4309,
Fax +44 113 292 4178
E-mail: d.forman@leeds.ac.uk

Gafà, L.
Ragusa Cancer Registry
Via Dante n. 109
I-97100 Ragusa, Italy
Tel. +39 (0932) 600468/654018
Fax +39 (0932) 682169

Galceran, J.
Tarragona Cancer Registry
Registre del Cancer de Tarragona
Lliga Contra el Cancer de les
   Comarques de Tarragona
C/ Reina Maria Cristina, 54
E-43002 Tarragona, Spain
Tel. +34 (977) 232423,
Fax +34 (977) 211111
E-mail: jgalceran@lccct.org.es

Garau, I.
Mallorca Cancer Registry
Unitat d'Epidemiologia i Registre de
   Cancer de Mallorca
Universitat de les Illes Balears. Edifici Sa
   Riera
Miquel dels Sants Oliver n 2
E-07012 Palma de Mallorca, Spain
Tel. +34 (971) 172714,
Fax +34 (971) 172715

Gatta, G.
Division of Epidemiology
Istituto Nazionale per lo Studio e la
   Cura dei Tumori
Via Venezian, 1
I-20133 Milano, Italy
Tel. +39 (02) 70601853,
2390460/501/502,
Fax +39 (02) 2390762
E-mail: gatta@istitutotumori.mi.it

Gould, A.
Scottish Cancer Intelligence Unit
NHS in Scotland
Information and Statistics Division
Trinity Park House
Edinburgh EH5 3SQ, Scotland
Tel. +44 (131) 551 8903,
Fax +44 (131) 551 1392

Hakulinen, T.
Finnish Cancer Registry
Liisankatu, 21 B
00170 Helsinki, Finland
Tel. +358 (9) 135.331,
Fax +358 (9) 1355378
E-mail: timo.hakulinen@cancer.fi

Izarzugaza, I.
Basque Country Cancer Registry
Departamento de Sanidad
Gobierno Vasco
Duque de Wellington, 2
E-01010 Vitoria-Gasteiz, Spain
Tel. +34 (945) 189235
Fax +34 (945) 189192
E-mail:info-san@ej-gv.es

Kaatsch, P.
German Childhood Cancer Registry
IMSD – University of Mainz
Langenbeckstrasse,1
D-55101 Mainz, Germany
Tel. +49 (6131) 173252/3111,
Fax +49 (6131) 172968
E-mail: kaatsch@imsd.uni-mainz.de

Lawrence, G.
West Midlands Cancer Intelligence Unit
Public Health Building
Birmingham University
Birmingham, B15 2TT, UK
Tel. +44 121 414 7711,
Fax +44 121 414 7712
E-mail:yvette.styler@wmciu.thenhs.com

Littler, J.
Merseyside and Cheshire Cancer Registry
Muspratt Building
University of Liverpool
Liverpool L69 3GB, UK
Tel. +44 151 794 5691,
Fax + 44 151 794 5700

Mace-Lesec'h, J.
Calvados General Cancer Registry
Centre François Baclesse
Route de Lion-sur-Mer
F-14076 Caen cedex, France
Tel. +33 (02) 31 45 50 98,
Fax +33 (02) 31 45 50 97
E-mail: j.mace.lesech@baclesse.fr

Magnani, C.
Childhood Cancer Registry of Piedmont
Cancer Epidemiology Unit
Ospedale S. Giovanni Battista
Via Santena, 7
I-10126 Torino, Italy
Tel. +39 (011) 6706531,
Fax +39 (011) 6706692
E-mail:magnani@ipsnet.it

Mangone L.
Modena Cancer Registry
University of Modena
Via del Pozzo, 71
I-41100 Modena, Italy
Tel. +39 (059) 42 4151/ 424150,
Fax +39 (059) 42 41 52
E-mail: mangone@unimo.it

Martinez-Garcia, C.
Granada Cancer Registry
Escuela Andaluza de Salud Publica
ap correos 2070
E-18080 Granada, Spain
Tel. +34 (958) 161044,
Fax +34(958)161142
E-mail:carmen@easp.es

Michaelis, J.
Institut für Med. Statistik und
Dokumentation der Johannes
   Gutenberg-Universität Mainz
German Childhood Cancer Registry
Obere Zahlbacher Str.69
D-55131 Mainz, Germany
Tel. +49 (6131) 17 73 2 52,
Fax +49 (6131) 17 29 68
E-mail: michael@imsd.uni-mainz.de

Micheli, A.
Division of Epidemiology
Istituto Nazionale per lo Studio e la
   Cura dei Tumori
Via Venezian, 1
I-20133 Milano, Italy
Tel. +39 (02) 2390820/821,
Fax +39 (02) 70638101
E-mail: epi4@icil64.cilea.it

Möller, T.
Southern Swedish Regional Tumour
   Registry
University Hospital
S-221 85 Lund, Sweden
Tel. +46 46 17 75 50,
Fax +46 46 18 81 43
E-mail:torgil.moller@cancerepid.lu.se

Moreno, C.
Navarra Cancer Registry
Instituto de Salud Publica
Servicio Navarro de Salud-Osasunbidea
C). Leyre,15
E-31003 Pamplona, Spain
Tel. +34 948 423440/70,
Fax +34 948 423474
E-mail: ispepi01@cfnavarra.es

Oberaigner, W.
Cancer Registry of Tyrol
Nachsorgeregister Tyrol
Anichstrabe, 35
A-6020 Innsbruck, Austria
Tel. +43 512 504 2310,
Fax +43 512 504 315
E-mail: wilhelm.oberaigner@uibk.ac.at

Obradovic, M.
Geneva Cancer Registry
Bd de la Cluse, 55
CH-1205 Geneva, Switzerland
Tel. +41 (22) 3291011,
Fax +41 22 3282933
E-mail: bouchardy-c@ge-dass.etat-ge.ch

Obsitnikova A.,
National Cancer Registry of Slovakia
National Cancer Institute
Klenova' 1
SV-83310 Bratislava, Slovak Republic
Tel. +421758378531 or 554,
Fax +421 7 54776598

Pawlega J.
Department of Oncology
Collegium Medicum
Jagiellonian University
Sniadeckich 10
31 531 Krakow, Poland
Tel. +48 12 4213592/4214065,
Fax +48 12 4213592
E-mail: pharmanet@com.pl

Plesko, I.
National Cancer Registry of Slovakia
National Cancer Institute
Klenova' 1
SV-83310 Bratislava, Slovak Republic
Tel. +421 7 58378531 or 554,
Fax +421 7 54776598

Pompe-Kirn, V.
Cancer Registry of Slovenia
Insitute of Oncology
Zaloska 2
SI-1001 Ljubljana, Slovenia
Tel. +386-61-1324-113,
Fax +386-61-1321-076
E-mail:vpompe@onko-i.si

Ponz de Leon, M.
Modena Colorectal Cancer Registry
Istituto di Patologia Medica, Policlinico
Via del Pozzo,71
I-41100 Modena, Italy
Tel. +39 (059) 42 22 69,
Fax +39 (059) 363114
E-mail: deleon@unimo.it

Pottier, D.
Calvados Digestive Cancer Registry
Faculté de Médecine
Niveau 03, Pièce 703 C.H.U.
Côte de Nacre
F-14044 Caen cedex, France
Tel. +33 (02) 31 06 44 64,
Fax +33 (02) 31 53 08 52
E-mail: pottier@medecine.unicaen.fr

Quaglia, A.
Liguria Cancer Registry
Istituto Nazionale per la Ricerca sul Cancro
Largo R. Benzi, 10
I-16132 Genova, Italy
Tel. +39 (010) 5600961,
Fax +39 (010) 5600501
E-mail: vercelli@hp380.ist.unige.it

Quinn, M.J.
Office for National Statistics
Bessborough Tower
1 Drummond Gate
London SW1V 2QQ, UK
Tel. +44 171 533 5257,
Fax +44 171 533 5252,
E-mail: mike.quinn@ons.gov.uk

Rachtan, J.
Kracow Cancer Registry
Unit of Epidemiology
Centre of Oncology M.Sklodowski-Curie
Memorial Institute
ul. Garncarska, 11
31-115 Krakow, Poland
Tel. +48 (12) 422 99 00,
Fax +48 (12) 422 66 80

Raverdy, N.
Somme Cancer Registry
CHR Nord
Bât. de Santé Publique
F-80054 Amiens cedex1, France
Tel. +33 (03) 22 66 82 26,
Fax +33 (03) 22 66 82 25
E-mail: nraverdy@europost.org

Raymond L.
Geneva Cancer Registry
Bd de la Cluse,55
CH-1205 Geneva, Switzerland
Tel. +41 (22) 3291011,
Fax +41 (22) 3282933
E-mail: bouchardy-c@ge-dass.etat-ge.ch

Roazzi, P.
Istituto Superiore di Sanità
Electronic Data Processing Centre
Viale Elena Regina, 299
I-00161 Rome, Italy
Tel. +39 06 49903370,
Fax +39 06 49387069
E-mail: roazzi@iss.it

Roche, M.
Oxford Cancer Intelligence Unit
Institute of Health Sciences
Old Road
Headington, Oxford OX3 7LF, UK
Tel. +44 1865 227040,
Fax +44 1865 226809
E-mail:ociu@cix.compulink.co.uk

Sant, M.
Division of Epidemiology
Istituto Nazionale per lo Studio e la
Cura dei Tumori
Via Venezian, 1
I-20133 Milano, Italy
Tel. +39 (02) 2390460/501/502,
Fax +39 (02) 2390762
E-mail: eurocare@istitutotumori.mi.it

Santaquilani M.
Istituto Superiore di Sanità
Department of Epidemiology and
Biostatistics
Viale Elena Regina, 299
I-00161 Rome, Italy
Tel. +39 (06) 49902230,
Fax +39 (06) 49387069
E-mail: verdeck@iss.it

Serventi, L.
Parma Cancer Registry
Via Gramsci, 14
I-43100 Parma, Italy
Tel. +39 (0521) 259571
Fax +39 (0521) 995448
E-mail: oncolog@ipruniv.cce.unipr.it

Smith, J.
South and West Cancer Intelligence Unit
Highcroft
Ramsey Road
Winchester SO22 5DH, UK
Tel. +44 1962 863511,
Fax +44 1962 878360
E-mail: jenifer@clu.clara.net

Stockton, D.
East Anglian Cancer Registry
Department of Community Medicine
University Forvie Site
Robinson Way
Cambridge CB2 2SR, UK
Tel. +44 (1223) 330318,
Fax +44 (1223) 330330
E-mail: twd10@medschl.cam.ac.uk

Storm, H.H.
Danish Cancer Society
Research Department IV
Strandboulevarden 49
DK 21000 Copenhagen, Denmark
Tel. +45 (35) 257625,
Fax +45 (35)25 7731
E-mail: hans@cancer.dk

Torhorst, J.
Basel Cancer Registry
Krebsregister Basel-Stadt und Basel-
Landschaft
Department of Pathology,
University of Basel
Schonbeinstrasse 40
CH-4003 Basel, Switzerland
Tel. +41 (61) 265 2525,
Fax +41 (61) 265 3194

Tryggvadottir, L.
Icelandic Cancer Registry
Skogarhlid 8
PO Box 5420
IS 125 Reykjavik, Iceland
Tel. +354 562 1414 or 562 2612,
Fax +354 562 1417
E-mail: laufeyt@krabb.is

Tulinius, H.
Icelandic Cancer Registry
Skogarhlid 8
PO Box 5420
IS 125 Reykjavik, Iceland
Tel. +354 562 1519,
Fax +354 562 1417
E-mail: hrafnt@krabb.is

Tumino R.
Ragusa Cancer Registry
Via Dante n. 109
I-97100 Ragusa, Italy
Tel. +39(0932) 600468/652200,
Fax +39 (0932) 682169

Vercelli, M.
Liguria Cancer Registry
Istituto Nazionale per la Ricerca sul Cancro
Largo R. Benzi, 10
I-16132 Genova, Italy
Tel. +39 (010) 5600961,
Fax +39 (010) 5600501
E-mail: vercelli@hp380.ist.unige.it

Verdecchia, A.
Istituto Superiore di Sanità
Department of Epidemiology and
Biostatistics
Viale Elena Regina, 299
I-00161 Rome, Italy
Tel. +39 (06) 49902230,
Fax +39 (06) 49387069
E-mail:verdeck@iss.it

Viladiu Quemada, P.
Girona Cancer Registry (UERCG)
Placa Hospital 5
E-17001 Girona, Spain
Tel. +34 (972) 20 74 06,
Fax +34 (972) 20 61 80
E-mail: izfo@ene.es

Williams, E.M.I.
Merseyside and Cheshire Cancer Registry
Muspratt Building
University of Liverpool
Liverpool L69 3GB, UK
Tel. +44 151 794 5691,
Fax + 44 151 794 5700

Wronkowski, Z.
Warsaw Cancer Registry
M. Sklodowska-Curie Cancer Center &
Institute of Oncology
Dept of Mass Screening Org.
5, W.K. Roentgena Street
02-781 Warsaw, Poland
Tel. +48-22-643-93-79,
Fax +48 22 6480219
E-mail: mbielskalasota@coi.waw.pl

Zanetti, R.
Piedmont Cancer Registry
Unità di Epidemiologia, CPO,
Ospedale S.Giovanni
Via S. Francesco da Paola, 31
I-10123 Torino, Italy
Tel. +39 (011) 5662006/7
Fax +39 (011) 5662005

Ziegler, H.
Saarland Cancer Registry
Statistisches Landesamt-Krebsregister
Virchowstrabe, 7
Postfach 1003044
D-66119 Saarbrucken, Germany
Tel. +49(681) 5015969,
Fax +49 (681) 5015998
E-mail: ziegler@stala.saarland.de

Acknowledgements

The Editors wish to thank the following people who collaborated in the preparation of this volume:

Technical support, preparation of figures and tables:

Livio Dell'Era [1]
Chiara Mancina [1]
Sara Oldani [1]
Maria Rosa Ruzza [1]
Daniele Speciale [1]

English revision, secretarial support of the Eurocare project:

Emily Taussig [1]
Suzanne Hartley [2]
Donald Ward [3]

Support for statistical analysis:

Dr Erminio Bonizzoni [3]

[1] Division of Epidemiology, Istituto Nazionale per lo Studio e la Cura dei Tumori, Via Venezian, 1, 20133 Milano, Italy, Tel. +39 (02) 2390460/501/502, Fax +39 (02) 2390762
E-mail: taussig@istitutotumori.mi.it

[2] Department of Epidemiology and Biostatistics, Viale Elena Regina, 299, 00161 Rome, Italy, Tel. +39 (06) 49902230, Fax +39 (06) 49387069 E-mail:Verdeck@iss.it

[3] Consultants

Chapter 1

The EUROCARE-2 Study

R. Capocaccia, G. Gatta, E. Chessa, F. Valente and the
EUROCARE Working Group

Introduction

In the EUROCARE project, a common methodology was used for the first time to collect and analyse population-based data on survival of cancer patients from a large number of European countries. In view of this standardization of the data collection, checking and analysis procedures, it may be deduced that the wide inter-country differences in relative survival rates observed for many cancers are real (Coebergh, 1995). The extension of the study in the EUROCARE-2 project, and continuing in the forthcoming EUROCARE-3 project, has two principal aims. The first is to update the survival database of European cancer registries in order to study variation in survival in more recent incidence periods. The second is to interpret the differences in survival observed over time and between populations in terms of earlier diagnosis or effectiveness of treatment, or an interaction of both factors.

In the first stage of the EUROCARE project, data were not collected for cancers at a number of sites (Sant et al., 1995), because of possible variations between registries in disease definition and coding criteria. The experience gained in this first stage of the project, the process of increasing standardization of practices among registries, and the realization that detailed data examination in turn leads to an increase in the level of standardization, convinced us to remove this limitation in the subsequent stages of the study. A second change introduced in the EUROCARE-2 protocol was to collect data for all cancer patients, including those lost to follow-up, those known to the registries through death certificate only (DCO) and those detected at autopsy. This decision was based on the belief that detailed ad hoc analyses of data on lost, DCO and autopsy cases could help in assessing the comparability of survival statistics.

The survival data collected in the EUROCARE project now cover cancers at all sites diagnosed during the 12-year period 1978–89. They were provided by 47 cancer registries from 17 European countries, a total of 14 registries and 5 countries more than were involved during the first stage of the study. The present volume reports in a detailed and systematic way survival data for about 1 300 000 patients for 45 cancer sites or aggregations of cancer sites, diagnosed during the period 1985–89. In

addition, survival trends in the period 1978–89 are presented and analysed, for those registries that provided incident cases for the whole period considered.

This chapter describes the general EUROCARE database and the methods and the procedures used for the collection, checking and validation of the data. Further details, in particular for those aspects that remained unchanged, can be found in the first EUROCARE monograph (Sant et al., 1995). Chapter 2 provides a brief description of the statistical methodology used, and the detailed results for each cancer site and country, by age and sex and for the period of diagnosis 1985–89, are presented in a standard format in Chapter 4. An overview of the results and conclusions that may be drawn from them are given in Chapter 5. Chapter 6 presents the main results of survival trend analysis for the period 1978–89. More detailed comments and discussion, including the analysis of trends, for most of the cancer sites have been reported in a special issue of the European Journal of Cancer (Coebergh et al., 1998).

Registries and proportion of population covered

The 47 population-based cancer registries that sent data for the second stage of the EUROCARE project cover six countries completely (Denmark, Estonia, Finland, Iceland, Slovakia and Slovenia) and several major regions in the UK. Forty-one of the areas involved in the study are covered by general registries. Two registries (Calvados, Côte d'Or) specialize in digestive tract cancers, two (Côte d'Or, Girona) in gynaecological cancers, one (Côte d'Or) in haematological cancers, and two (Mainz and Piedmont) are childhood cancer registries. There is not a one-to-one correspondence between areas and cancer registries. The region of Calvados is covered by two different registries (general and digestive), while in the region of Côte d'Or three different specialized registries (digestive, gynaecological and haematological) operate. Overall, forty-four populations are involved in the study. Figure 1 shows the geographical distribution of the participating registries.

The list of cancer registries, the average size of population covered during the study period, and the

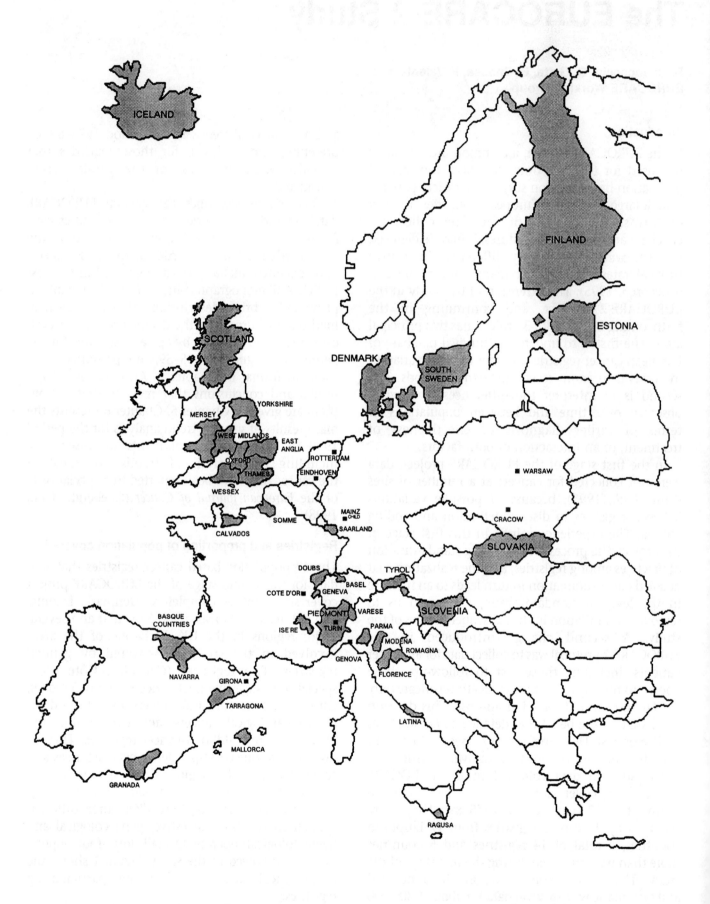

Figure 1. Map showing coverage of the cancer registries participating in the EUROCARE-2 project

Table 1. Population covered (in thousands) and percentage coverage of the national population of each participating registry

Country/Registry	Population	% coverage	Notes
Iceland	**255**	**100**	
Finland	**4986**	**100**	
South Sweden	1474	17.5	
Sweden	**8414**	**17.5**	
Denmark	**5140**	**100**	
East Anglia	2059	4.0	
Mersey	2423	4.7	
Oxford	2437	4.8	
South Thames	6564	12.9	
Wessex	2935	5.8	
West Midlands	5182	10.2	
Yorkshire	3662	7.2	
England	**51000**	**49.6**	
Scotland	**5100**	**100**	
Eindhoven	850	5.7	
Rotterdam	2216	14.8	Only stomach, colon and rectum
Netherlands	**14951**	**5.7–20.5**	
Calvados	607	1.1	
Côte d'Or	494	0.9	Digestive, gynaecological and haematological
Doubs	490	0.9	
Isère	1000	1.8	Only breast
Somme	545	1.0	
France	**56735**	**3.0–5.7**	
Basque Country	2139	5.5	
Girona	509	1.3	Gynaecological
Granada	767	2.0	Only stomach, lung and breast
Mallorca	577	1.5	
Navarra	515	1.3	
Tarragona	523	1.3	
Spain	**38959**	**9.6–12.9**	
Florence	1174	2.0	
Genoa	725	1.3	
Latina	447	0.8	
Modena	260	0.5	
Parma	396	0.7	
Piedmont	4297	7.5	Regional childhood registry
Ragusa	285	0.5	
Romagna	432	0.7	
Turin	1033	1.8	
Varese	790	1.4	
Italy	**57661**	**9.7**	

Table 1. Population covered (in thousands) and percentage coverage of the national population of each participating registry (contd)

Country/Registry	Population	% coverage	Notes
Basel	424	6.3	
Geneva	370	5.5	
Switzerland	**6712**	**11.8**	
Mainz	62702	100	National childhood registry
Saarland	1051	1.7	
Germany (West)	**62702**	**1.7**	
Tyrol	629	7.8	
Austria	**8030**	**7.8**	
Slovenia	**2000**	**100**	
Slovakia	**5325**	**100**	
Cracow	740	1.9	
Warsaw	1626	4.3	
Poland	**38119**	**6.2**	
Estonia	**1571**	**100**	

proportion of coverage of the corresponding national population are reported in Table 1. Due to the presence of specialized registries or of registries contributing data for few sites, the proportion of coverage differs for some countries according to site. Low proportions of coverage (well below 10%) were obtained for Austria, France, the Netherlands (for most cancer sites), Poland and Germany. An intermediate proportion (10–20%) was achieved for Italy, Spain, Sweden and Switzerland. A high proportion of coverage (about 50%) was obtained for United Kingdom, which contributed more than half of the whole database. The survival data from England and from Scotland were analysed separately (no Welsh cancer registry participated in the study). Therefore England and Scotland are presented in the analysis as individual countries.

The following paragraphs provide brief descriptions of the cancer registries newly participating in the EUROCARE-2 project and of the main aspects of the health care system covering the respective populations. Similar information about the other registries can be found in the first EUROCARE monograph (Berrino et al., 1995).

Tyrol (Austria). The cancer registry which covers the Austrian province of Tyrol, with an area of 12 648 km^2 and population of 630 000 (1991 census), was founded at the end of 1986, and since 1988 has been population-based. It is independent and responsible for cancer registration, but works in close collaboration with the Austrian Cancer Registry, to which the law obliges hospitals to report every cancer case. The information collected includes incidence date, most valid basis of diagnosis, topography, histology, staging and summary of first treatment. For reporting purposes, the IARC definition of multiple cancers is followed strictly. Follow-up is passive, by record linkage established annually with the mortality files of the region of Tyrol and through agreements with hospitals, some of which send information regularly, others only on demand by the registry. Health care is essentially public, with medical facilities offered by the University Hospital in Innsbruck, nine local hospitals and two semi-private hospitals in Innsbruck; most pathological diagnoses are performed by one institute in Innsbruck. For all cases, the date of the next check-up is stored and the hospital contacted if no notification is received.

Oxford (England). Cancer registration data have been collected on a regional basis since 1952. The population covered is about 2.6 million inhabitants (2.4 million in 1989). The registry collects data on patients who are resident in or treated within the region. Information on non-residents treated within the Oxford Region is passed to the appropriate regional registry. Cases are notified by histopathology and cytopathology laboratories and medical records departments. There is collaboration with specialized registers (e.g., Childhood Cancer Research Group, Oxford Regional Leukaemia Register) and directly with clinicians to collect certain types of data. As for the other UK registries, with the exception of East Anglia, the follow-up of cases is passive. Death certificates relating to the region's resident population, on which cancer is mentioned, are passed to the registry from the Office of National Statistics. In addition, all registered cancer patients are flagged on the National Health Service Central Register to ensure that the local registry is informed of deaths among the registered population, including those from causes other than cancer and those occurring outside the region. All UK residents have access to free health service from general practitioners and hospitals within the National Health Service (for more detailed information regarding the UK health care system, see Berrino *et al.* (1995)).

Iceland. The Icelandic Cancer Registry has been in operation since 1 January 1954 and covers the entire area and population of Iceland (approx. 250 000 inhabitants). It is a part of the Icelandic Cancer Society and it keeps updated files on all malignant neoplastic diseases diagnosed in the population of Iceland since 1 January 1955. The sources of information are the Department of Pathology of the University of Iceland, other pathology laboratories, all hospitals and health centres, all medical doctors and death certificates. Health care is public in Iceland, with some private specialists. Hospitals and doctors are encouraged to send repeated registrations of cancer patients. Follow-up as to vital status is passive, being effected through the Icelandic National Roster, which is updated regularly.

Rotterdam (The Netherlands). The Rotterdam Cancer Registry is run by the Comprehensive Cancer Centre Rotterdam and covers the south-western part of the Netherlands, an area with a population of about 2.3 million inhabitants. The registry started in 1982 and registration is considered to have been complete in the central part of the region since 1987. Case ascertainment is accomplished by routine notification from pathology laboratories and a check of hospital discharge diagnoses. The index date for computing survival is the date of histological verification. Because death certificates are not available to the registry due to privacy regulations, follow-up is performed by active data collection, but only for specific research projects, in this case for

stomach and colorectal cancer. In the Netherlands, 40% of the population has private insurance and 60% of the population is covered by the Sickness Benefit Fund, a compulsory social insurance policy for people with lower incomes and those on welfare. Less than 1% of the population is uninsured.

Italian cancer registries. The cancer registries newly included in the EUROCARE study are Torino, Genoa, Modena and Romagna, located in northern–central Italy. These registries cover about 2.5 million inhabitants and increase the coverage of the country up to 10%. They started to operate in the 1980s. All these registries search for cases actively, using various information sources, but mainly hospital clinical records and pathology department records. Follow-up is mixed active and passive, the latter through linkage of regional mortality data with the registry's files. For all people not thus identified as dead, an active search in the municipalities' population files is performed. The Italian National Health Service (NHS) provides health assistance for all citizens. Most health care services are public. Private facilities are also partially supported by the NHS.

Isère (France). The Isère Cancer Registry was established in 1978 and published its first cancer incidence report in 1979. The population covered is about 1 million. In 1989, the department of Isère had 15 hospitals, one of which is a regional and university hospital, and 9 private clinics. Data are obtained from 80 sources of information in Isère and the surrounding departments. These include pathology and cytology laboratories, health insurance companies, public and private clinics, as well as the administrative departments of several hospitals. There is no follow-up of the registered cases, except for specific survival studies. This is why only breast cancer cases were sent for analysis in the EUROCARE study. For these, follow-up of cases is both active and passive. The active follow-up is carried out by letters to the location of birth and from medical files. Passive follow-up comes from anonymous death certificates and from information about certain events such as metastasis.

The French national health system provides health assistance for all citizens. Expenses in relation to diagnosis, treatment and surveillance of cancer are paid in full directly by the health system. Patients may be treated in either public or private health facilities under the same conditions.

Warsaw (Poland). The Warsaw Cancer Registry is an active, population-based registry. It collects data on cancer incidence and mortality in the area of Warsaw city, with a population of 1 600 000 (1980s) and in Warsaw Selected Rural areas, population 615 000 (not included in EUROCARE 2). The registry, founded in 1963, was organized in collaboration with the United States National Cancer Institute and is located in the Maria Sklodowska-Curie Memorial Centre and Institute of Oncology in Warsaw. It is funded by the Ministry of Health and Social Welfare. Information is derived from cancer reporting cards submitted obligatorily since 1952 by all health service institutions and individual physicians, and from death certificates. Cancer incidence data collected since the 1960s can be considered almost complete. The Warsaw Cancer Registry carries out active follow-up of cancer patients. Poland is divided into 11 regions with regional oncological centres located in each. In Warsaw, specialized care of cancer patients is provided by the Maria Sklodowska-Curie Memorial Cancer Centre and Institute of Oncology and other specialized hospitals, as well as by all other hospital wards in Warsaw, district outpatient clinics and specialist centres (both private and state-run), together with cooperatives and foundations.

Slovakia. The population-based national cancer registry of Slovakia (population approx. 5 300 000), covering the whole territory of Slovakia, was established in 1980 at the National Cancer Institute in Bratislava. It consists of two independent institutes: the Cancer Research Institute of the Slovak Academy of Sciences and the Institute of Clinical Oncology of the Ministry of Health. The system of notification is based on a network of outpatient clinics for clinical oncology established during 1976–85 in the districts of Slovakia. Cases notified by physicians are reviewed and completed at the district oncological clinics, where active follow-up is performed. Revision at a more central level is oriented mainly to evaluation of diagnostic and treatment details in the different hospitals. All medical institutions form an administrative organization called the 'Institute of National Health'. Medical care is free of charge for all of the population, paid for by obligatory health insurance for employers and self-employed, and by the state for the unemployed.

Slovenia. The Cancer Registry of Slovenia was founded in 1950 in Ljubljana at the Institute of Oncology. It covers the entire population (approx. 2 000 000) and territory of Slovenia. Each resident of Slovenia has his/her personal identification number,

which through linkage with the cancer registry provides information on the vital status of each cancer patient. Liaison between the registry and health centres is satisfactory. Follow-up is both passive through linkage with the Central Registry of the Population, and partly active through reports on long-term follow-up of cancer patients on re-admission to hospital. Basic health services are provided in Slovenia by 22 outpatient establishments. Private practice was virtually non-existent in the Republic before 1991. The public health service is provided by nine regional institutes for social medicine and hygiene, and by the Public Health Institute of the Republic of Slovenia.

Basque Country (Spain). The Basque Country Cancer Registry was founded in 1986 by the Department of Health of the Autonomous Basque Government. The area covered by the registry is 7235 km² and is located in the north of Spain. The total population (1996 municipal census) was 2 100 000 inhabitants, with a life expectancy of 72.8 years for men and 81.5 years for women. The Basque Public Health Service (Osakidetza) has since 1988 provided health service coverage for 95% of the population. There are 4.3 doctors and 4.6 hospital beds per 1000 inhabitants. Data are collected from public and private centres, among them the Oncological Institute of Gipuzkoa, both actively and passively. Follow-up of cases is passive, by use of only those death certificates which mention cancer as cause of death. This may lead to a certain degree of underestimation of patients' mortality.

Navarra (Spain). The population-based Cancer Registry of Navarra was established in 1970, through a collaboration between the Association for the Fight against Cancer and the Institute of Public Health of the Government of Navarra. It covers the region of Navarra (population about 523 000, 1991 census), one of the 17 autonomous regions of Spain. The public health system provides health care for all citizens, covering practically the whole population. The principal data sources for the registry are the anatomical pathology, haematology, radiotherapy and oncology services, together with the archive services of all hospitals, both public and private which perform active follow-up of cases. The cancer registry has access to the mortality registry. Follow-up is carried out largely through the Bulletins of Death Statistics of the Institute of Statistics of the Government of Navarra, which collects the death data in this Autonomous Community.

South Sweden. Cancer registration in Sweden started on a nationwide basis in 1958, when a central cancer registry for the entire country was established. Regional tumour registries in each of the six health care regions of the country were instituted in the late 1970s. The Southern Swedish Tumour Registry covers a population of about 1.5 million inhabitants. The registration of incident cases is based upon reports from hospitals, both public or private. No case with a diagnosis of cancer based on a death certificate alone is accepted. The only follow-up undertaken by the registry is passive through the regularly updated population registries on vital status, with no cases lost to follow-up.

A fundamental principle of the health care system in Sweden is that it is a public-sector responsibility to provide and finance health services for the entire population, with equal access to health services for everyone. Responsibility for these services rests primarily with the county councils, which levy taxes to cover the costs and also operate almost all the services provided. There are 26 such geographical areas within Sweden, making up a total of six health care regions. The care of cancer patients is organized within six oncological centres, each corresponding to a health care region. The oncological centres perform population-based cancer registration and epidemiological research, initiate cancer care programmes (management protocols, 'gold standards') and evaluate their effect by means of specialized site-specific registers. The oncological centres also have a responsibility for organizing multidisciplinary teams, consulting and counselling, to ensure a suitable psycho-social orientation of cancer care, and to assist in setting up and evaluating screening activities and preventive activities.

Sites

Survival data have been collected for all malignant neoplasms. The present monograph includes data for twelve cancer sites that were not represented in the first EUROCARE publication, namely, cancers of the lip, small intestine, biliary tract, liver, nasal cavities, pleura, soft tissues, melanoma, male breast, prostate, bladder, thyroid, choroid (melanoma), multiple myeloma and non-Hodgkin lymphoma. Furthermore, the category of all malignant neoplasms has been added. Table 2 lists the ICD-9 codes, the short name used in the tables, and the exact denomination (if different from the short name) of all cancer sites for which a separate analysis has been made.

The total numbers of patients considered in the present study, by cancer site and area, and the corresponding incidence periods, are presented in Table 3.

The numbers appearing in this table include patients of all ages and include DCO and autopsy-derived cases. However, these cases, as well as patients aged less than 15 years, were excluded from the analyses.

The general registries of Basel, Granada, Isère and Rotterdam contributed a subset of cancer sites for which follow-up was complete. The majority of registries contributed cases diagnosed during the whole study period, 1985–89, but those of Genoa, Isère, Latina, Parma, Romagna and Rotterdam contributed only three years of incidence data, and the registries of Tyrol and Warsaw only two years. All the registries had, for most of their cases, a potential follow-up of at least five years.

Information collected, inclusion criteria, data-checking

For each patient, information was requested on sex, date of birth, date of diagnosis, date of end of follow-up, vital status, tumour site (as ICD-9 code), microscopic verification, morphology and behaviour codes. When available, additional dates, such as those of first hospital admission and first treatment recorded as alternative index dates, and broad stage category were collected. For confidentiality reasons, only anonymous data were collected, and the day of the month was omitted from all dates to prevent identification of patients. A registry-specific identification code for each record was requested to facilitate quality control and updating operations.

Only multiple tumours were *a priori* excluded at the data collection stage. Each registry was asked to send data regarding only the first diagnosed tumour, in cases of multiple metachronous tumours, and the most advanced one, in cases of multiple synchronous tumours. Bilateral tumours of symmetric organs were treated as a single disease. No exclusion was made regarding cancer site or vital status. Non-malignant, autopsy-derived and DCO cases were excluded at a later stage of the analysis. Due to the lack of standardized rules for inclusion of papillomas and non-invasive carcinomas, tumours with non-malignant behaviour were also included in the analysis of bladder cancer.

In order to evaluate the completeness of the survival data files, the number of cases collected from each registry was compared with the corresponding number of incident cases from the registry reported in Volume 7 of *Cancer Incidence in Five Continents* (Parkin *et al.*, 1997). The two data-sets were not expected to coincide because, firstly, multiple tumours were excluded from the survival data, while they are considered in incidence statistics and, secondly, many registries contributed cases

Table 2. ICD-9 codes for cancer sites, with short description of cancer site adopted in this monograph

ICD-9 code	Short description	Full description
140	Lip	Lip (excluding skin of lip)
141	Tongue	Tongue
142	Salivary gland	Major salivary glands
143–145	Oral cavity	Gum, floor of mouth, other and unspecified parts of mouth
146	Oropharynx	Oropharynx
147	Nasopharynx	Nasopharynx
148	Hypopharynx	Hypopharynx
141, 143–148	Head and neck	Tongue, gum, floor of mouth, other and unspecified of mouth, oropharynx, nasopharynx, hypopharynx
150	Oesophagus	
151	Stomach	
152	Small intestine	Small intestine (excluding ileocaecal valve)
153	Colon	
154	Rectum	Rectum, rectosigmoid junction, anal canal and anus
155	Liver, primary	Liver and intrahepatic bile ducts
156	Biliary tract	Gallbladder, ampulla of Vater and extrahepatic bile ducts
157	Pancreas	
160	Nasal cavities	Nasal cavity, accessory sinuses, middle and inner ear
161	Larynx	
162	Lung	Trachea, bronchus and lung
163	Pleura	
170	Bone	Bone, joints and articular cartilage
171	Soft tissues	Connective, subcutaneous and other soft tissues
172	Melanoma of skin	
174, 175	Breast	Breast
180	Cervix uteri	
182	Corpus uteri	
183	Ovary	Ovary and other uterine adnexa
184	Vagina and vulva	Vagina, vulva and other and unspecified female genital organs
185	Prostate	
186	Testis	
187	Penis	Penis and other male genital organs
188	Bladder	Urinary bladder (including benign neoplasms)
189	Kidney	Kidney and other and unspecified urinary organs (excluding urinary bladder)
190.6	Choroid (melanoma)	
191	Brain	
193	Thyroid gland	
200, 202	Non-Hodgkin's lymphomas	
201	Hodgkin's disease	
203	Multiple myeloma	
204.0	Acute lymphatic leukaemia	
204.1	Chronic lymphatic leukaemia	
205.0	Acute myeloid leukaemia	
205.1	Chronic myeloid leukaemia	
204–208	Leukaemia	
140–208	Malignant neoplasms (excluding non-melanoma skin tumours, 173)	

diagnosed in a period that did not fully cover the incidence period for *Cancer Incidence in Five Continents*. For these registries, comparisons were made on the basis of the average number of cases per year. The results of this check are reported, in terms of the ratio between the number of incident cases and the number of cases in the survival analysis, in Appendix 1A. The registries of Côte d'Or, Rotterdam and South Sweden were not included in these tables because their data do not appear in Volume 7 of *Cancer Incidence in Five Continents*. The registry of Romagna was not included because the population covered changed between the periods considered in the present study and in *Cancer Incidence in Five Continents*. The data for the Eindhoven registry should be considered with caution because the population followed up for survival is not exactly the same as that covered for incidence, and about 7% of cases were previously discarded from the database (see Table 4). For Parma, Latina and Torino, the comparison was not possible because the study periods did not overlap.

In general, a ratio close to 1 indicates complete recruitment of incident cases into the survival analysis. Ratios lower than 1 may indicate inclusion of non-malignant or borderline cases, whereas ratios above 1 indicate loss of cases in the survival file. Furthermore, ratios ranging between 1.2 and 1.0 can be explained by the exclusion from the survival data of multiple tumours, which were considered in the incidence statistics. In this last case, the magnitude of the difference is expected to depend on the time since establishment of the registry: the older the registry, the lower the likelihood of having missed possible earlier tumours in cases diagnosed during the study period. A certain difference could also arise when the periods on which the numerator and the denominator are based do not exactly overlap, due to both random variability and time trends of incidence.

Topography codes for extra-nodal lymphomas attributed to a specific organ were re-coded as lymphomas, as appropriate.

For the Finnish and Swedish cancer registries, morphology was transformed from the particular codes used in these registries to the standard morphology codes. Since their morphology codes are generally less detailed than the standard classification, information on morphology for these two registries is in some cases not fully comparable with that of the other registries.

After this preliminary stage of checking for completeness, the data underwent validity and consistency checks. All the records sent to the data analysis centre were checked, irrespective of their potential inclusion in the EUROCARE-2 analysis. Individual records in which some fields contained invalid code values, and records with impossible, or even improbable, sex–site–morphology combinations were sent back to the registries for checking and, when appropriate and possible, for correction. Data resubmitted by the registries were again subjected to the same validation procedure. Records still presenting invalid fields were definitively excluded from the database. For records with an unusual sex–site–morphology combination, however, the final judgement of the registry responsible was accepted. Table 4 reports the results of the validation procedure, which was applied to the whole data-set sent by each registry.

A total of 41 516 records were sent back to the registries. These represent 1.2% of the total number received, a percentage that varied between registries from 0 to 10%. For 18 287 of these records, it was possible to recover the correct information and to include them in the database, while the remaining 23 229 records (0.66%) were rejected. At the end of this process, the EUROCARE database was based on a total of 3 473 659 individual records. The corresponding incidence period varies between the registries.

Indicators of data quality

The quality of population-based survival data depends mainly on two factors: the accuracy of diagnosis and the validity of vital status assessment. No independent source able to give a direct external check of the quality of such information is generally available in this type of study. Here we have therefore used indirect indicators, based on cross-validation analysis of consistency of the relevant variables.

In Table 5, some data related to the completeness and quality of data are reported. The number of cases lost to follow-up, the number of cases known from death certificate only (DCO), and the number of cases discovered by autopsy, as well as the corresponding percentages of the total number of cases are given for the period 1985–89.

The proportion of cases lost to follow-up is below 1% in 27, and over 5% in only 3, out of 42 registry areas for which we have this information. The proportion of cases known to the registry only from a death certificate is more variable, ranging from a maximum of 17.6% in South Thames to below 5% in 24 registries. A variable proportion of DCO cases may substantially affect survival comparisons, as a high proportion of DCO usually tends to lead to overestimation of survival. Survival estimates can be considered unbiased only if the survival time of cases

Table 3. Cancer registry areas participating in the EUROCARE-2 study: period of incidence, date of closure of follow-up and number of cases included by cancer site and registry

Registry	Country	Period (year)	End of follow-up	ICD-9 code 140	141	142	143–145	146	147	148	150	151
Basel	CH	1985–88	12/94	–	34	–	35	28	–	23	70	301
Basque Country	E	1986–88	12/91	177	210	43	231	151	64	138	438	1682
Calvados	F	1985–89	06/96	64	148	20	195	217	12	251	481	441
Côte d'Or	F	1985–89	12/95	–	–	–	–	–	–	–	192	351
Cracow	PL	1985–89	09/94	33	41	27	41	40	14	9	113	730
Denmark	DK	1985–89	12/94	629	323	231	684	360	116	173	1129	3549
Doubs	F	1985–89	12/94	7	98	17	104	148	13	124	200	302
East Anglia	ENG	1985–89	01/95	161	104	60	139	59	30	82	913	1884
Eindhoven	NL	1985–89	04/94	49	46	27	66	26	12	19	105	777
Estonia	EST	1985–89	12/94	124	87	52	154	121	36	61	262	2663
Finland	FIN	1985–89	12/95	703	237	177	262	74	66	93	956	4986
Florence	I	1985–89	12/94	58	97	47	144	73	55	52	243	3527
Geneva	CH	1985–89	12/94	23	68	15	65	69	8	52	105	288
Genoa	I	1986–88	12/94	12	54	19	73	39	29	27	95	739
Girona	E	1985–89	11/93	–	–	–	–	–	–	–	–	–
Granada	E	1985–89	12/95	–	–	–	–	–	–	–	–	370
Iceland	ICE	1985–89	05/96	23	6	2	20	3	4	1	48	258
Isère	F	1987–89	05/96	–	–	–	–	–	–	–	–	–
Latina	I	1985–87	12/95	22	16	16	12	10	3	1	20	226
Mainz childhood	D	1985–89	12/94	1	1	2	6	2	22	0	0	2
Mallorca	E	1985–89	12/93	58	25	3	37	18	14	21	48	139
Mersey	ENG	1985–89	04/97	14	188	73	267	106	57	144	1287	2899
Modena	I	1985–89	07/95	3	16	9	21	14	7	18	33	499
Navarra	E	1985–89	12/94	143	37	17	72	33	19	20	138	819
Oxford	ENG	1985–89	12/94	145	142	84	159	68	49	62	840	2231
Parma	I	1985–87	07/95	5	30	11	34	18	10	19	50	749
Piedmont childhood	I	1985–89	12/95	0	0	1	0	1	0	0	0	0
Ragusa	I	1985–89	05/95	55	14	15	14	3	13	2	18	291
Romagna	I	1986–88	12/93	4	18	17	17	9	16	7	32	854
Rotterdam	NL	1987–89	12/92	–	–	–	–	–	–	–	–	253
Saarland	D	1985–89	12/92	53	183	50	219	118	34	96	269	1439
Scotland	SCO	1985–89	12/94	322	416	267	670	180	96	204	2746	5903
Slovakia	SK	1985–89	12/92	836	630	166	692	623	123	458	946	6080
Slovenia	SLO	1985–89	12/94	160	218	28	313	369	44	208	445	2661
Somme	F	1985–89	12/92	29	136	11	168	226	13	150	381	406
Sweden, South	S	1985–89	12/96	179	91	86	157	53	36	60	324	1366
Tarragona	E	1985–89	01/94	117	40	18	56	38	21	22	99	458
Thames, South	ENG	1985–89	12/94	112	335	225	421	199	123	207	3029	6412
Turin	I	1985–87	04/93	57	69	29	89	74	18	18	124	793
Tyrol	A	1988–89	12/95	2	16	8	44	12	5	12	40	439
Varese	I	1985–89	05/97	28	92	34	92	108	29	60	215	1333
Warsaw	PL	1988–89	06/97	27	48	7	19	57	10	8	124	570
Wessex	ENG	1985–89	12/95	84	189	112	199	65	56	85	1656	3082
West Midlands	ENG	1985–89	12/95	62	303	145	404	167	90	187	2336	6142
Yorkshire	ENG	1985–89	12/95	92	200	101	323	93	44	133	1466	3976
TOTAL				**4673**	**5006**	**2272**	**6718**	**4072**	**1411**	**3307**	**22016**	**72870**

152	153	154	155	156	157	160	161	162	163	170	171	172	174	175	180
–	547	356	112	72	169	–	67	843	–	–	–	253	984	–	77
31	1231	924	447	300	472	52	772	2266	26	59	119	269	2053	18	239
15	732	547	165	81	168	37	230	942	33	28	56	209	1414	16	498
24	782	461	149	92	191	–	–	–	–	–	–	–	1104	–	154
15	444	433	224	260	368	23	228	1853	15	28	50	162	1111	8	48
284	9544	6239	2042	1110	3261	276	1225	15422	428	350	536	3236	14346	87	2791
20	586	432	101	59	107	8	189	845	23	16	42	152	977	4	134
85	3387	2154	119	293	1128	86	301	6428	123	65	218	830	5447	46	768
29	1127	728	44	182	294	24	181	2333	29	34	81	288	2119	9	166
35	1240	1008	279	176	817	49	323	3352	35	66	169	337	1955	14	806
234	4251	2883	1324	1300	3070	135	580	9994	247	184	551	2143	10584	42	686
61	2506	1513	548	403	738	42	719	3700	40	79	126	421	3362	32	327
20	616	298	136	69	232	7	123	884	16	15	47	273	1139	2	467
13	937	486	264	189	314	21	261	1811	110	19	51	141	1382	8	168
–	–	–	–	–	–	–	–	–	–	–	–	–	730	–	99
–	–	–	–	–	–	–	–	604	–	–	–	–	496	–	–
16	286	91	36	28	126	13	19	407	7	12	20	50	521	3	65
–	–	–	–	–	–	–	–	–	–	–	–	–	1561	–	–
6	211	145	75	52	65	3	64	489	4	13	39	41	361	5	79
0	1	0	77	1	1	17	2	7	0	333	253	7	0	0	1
3	637	491	81	60	86	5	92	501	6	6	18	65	414	2	310
69	3882	2587	291	275	1516	87	541	10549	236	81	214	579	6107	30	1323
13	681	386	156	62	177	3	134	840	10	6	29	82	661	3	86
12	582	404	247	195	208	13	272	779	21	29	38	118	886	6	156
98	3801	2112	226	222	1349	93	353	7413	135	104	246	993	6212	48	851
16	532	288	157	74	183	9	149	780	19	4	37	73	739	2	108
0	0	0	6	0	1	0	0	2	0	40	29	0	0	0	0
7	221	187	143	95	125	4	76	400	5	25	14	55	468	5	101
15	549	264	115	65	176	6	129	939	12	14	34	90	731	8	105
–	1387	728	–	–	–	–	–	–	–	–	–	–	–	–	–
68	2103	1285	245	533	616	21	321	3111	40	50	134	459	2668	15	434
218	9184	4518	798	669	2976	141	1148	22298	529	200	466	2162	12571	60	2109
148	4908	4785	1275	1793	2512	137	1557	12681	81	235	483	1272	6018	67	2462
32	1485	1672	197	506	776	71	495	4016	69	73	131	533	3160	22	807
15	678	461	109	90	166	29	231	1067	31	17	35	103	1090	11	381
152	2699	1561	442	561	1048	60	223	2439	98	67	211	1225	3952	33	438
19	614	410	138	109	165	13	211	859	9	35	71	102	917	10	159
186	10478	5952	785	705	4225	231	1060	23531	517	331	519	2207	17278	143	2291
28	1057	548	357	173	337	25	335	1827	41	36	63	174	1683	18	213
9	345	210	50	72	140	8	62	584	6	12	47	211	583	1	175
26	1333	670	411	224	410	27	337	2260	24	55	63	226	2210	9	196
9	559	420	153	344	344	6	203	1654	12	34	59	152	983	9	354
119	6063	3010	340	304	1942	124	518	10534	367	153	373	1516	8638	66	1292
244	8406	5294	446	730	2771	171	926	17499	186	192	480	1602	12426	91	2247
144	5530	3787	411	400	2018	107	724	13264	259	132	380	1103	8644	65	1862
2538	96142	60728	13721	12928	35788	2184	15381	192007	3849	3232	6532	23914	150685	1018	26471

Table 3 (contd)

Registry	Country	Period (year)	End of follow-up	ICD-9 code								
				182	183	184	185	186	187	188	189	190
Basel	CH	1985–88	12/94	221	174	–	669	86	–	200	205	–
Basque Country	E	1986–88	12/91	394	277	117	857	59	56	1264	449	45
Calvados	F	1985–89	06/96	229	197	50	841	57	20	417	243	24
Côte d'Or	F	1985–89	12/95	182	178	14	–	–	–	–	–	–
Cracow	PL	1985–89	09/94	303	343	61	242	50	10	275	321	26
Denmark	DK	1985–89	12/94	3093	2937	549	6940	1269	214	7485	3153	293
Doubs	F	1985–89	12/94	147	142	41	558	50	15	233	176	14
East Anglia	ENG	1985–89	01/95	867	1019	207	2951	277	67	1924	721	67
Eindhoven	NL	1985–89	04/94	300	261	44	819	86	26	549	344	19
Estonia	EST	1985–89	12/94	763	764	139	751	60	35	569	665	81
Finland	FIN	1985–89	12/95	2330	1911	346	5724	296	68	2645	2849	218
Florence	I	1985–89	12/94	670	473	137	1352	117	41	2154	766	42
Geneva	CH	1985–89	12/94	228	187	49	555	72	19	405	208	18
Genoa	I	1986–88	12/94	216	215	48	460	33	15	680	253	7
Girona	E	1985–89	11/93	171	121	28	–	–	–	–	–	–
Granada	E	1985–89	12/95	–	–	–	–	–	–	–	–	–
Iceland	IS	1985–89	05/96	78	115	9	459	36	7	182	152	12
Isère	F	1987–89	05/96	–	–	–	–	–	–	–	–	–
Latina	I	1985–87	12/95	86	51	20	109	11	6	212	62	9
Mainz childhood	D	1985–89	12/94	0	31	8	6	62	1	11	391	207
Mallorca	E	1985–89	12/93	109	54	35	240	5	10	306	75	11
Mersey	ENG	1985–89	04/97	872	1129	234	2488	316	103	2707	814	66
Modena	I	1985–89	07/95	131	129	35	282	19	4	385	169	14
Navarra	E	1985–89	12/94	210	157	51	593	21	22	531	198	17
Oxford	ENG	1985–89	12/94	1021	1171	222	2820	355	92	2468	834	67
Parma	I	1985–87	07/95	152	137	30	248	15	3	302	161	9
Piedmont childhood	I	1985–89	12/95	0	4	0	1	3	2	1	16	8
Ragusa	I	1985–89	05/95	145	76	15	179	10	2	180	59	2
Romagna	I	1986–88	12/93	143	113	37	295	26	11	419	206	21
Rotterdam	NL	1987–89	12/92	–	–	–	–	–	–	–	–	–
Saarland	D	1985–89	12/92	658	460	140	1117	176	25	1055	618	26
Scotland	SCO	1985–89	12/94	1569	2547	472	5606	700	192	5764	2090	310
Slovakia	SK	1985–89	12/92	2497	1690	368	3201	584	143	2738	2103	239
Slovenia	SL	1985–89	12/94	933	714	162	1122	200	42	758	553	70
Somme	F	1985–89	12/92	197	191	54	771	53	14	511	195	26
Sweden, South	S	1985–89	12/96	715	864	134	3896	179	53	1580	1008	77
Tarragona	E	1985–89	01/94	233	141	51	441	27	20	575	121	13
Thames, South	ENG	1985–89	12/94	2550	3522	615	7712	823	191	7085	2174	308
Turin	I	1985–87	04/93	298	244	50	506	45	21	912	305	21
Tyrol	A	1988–89	12/95	121	138	25	413	39	5	295	201	15
Varese	I	1985–89	05/97	438	299	59	716	95	24	1001	458	16
Warsaw	PL	1988–89	06/97	307	297	57	227	76	10	309	369	14
Wessex	ENG	1985–89	12/95	1202	1590	336	4499	413	117	3792	1215	147
West Midlands	ENG	1985–89	12/95	1829	2544	493	5432	441	186	4919	1723	148
Yorkshire	ENG	1985–89	12/95	1170	1578	396	3954	402	132	3802	1262	143
TOTAL				27778	29185	5938	70052	7644	2024	61600	27885	2870

191	193	195, 199	196	200, 202	201	203	204.0	204.1	205.0	205.1	204–208	140–208 [a]
106	–	–	–	229	51	54	11	72	46	23	205	6176
385	120	16	1184	452	169	204	87	130	77	59	455	19391
107	96	12	183	298	76	90	24	63	24	34	182	11235
–	–	–	–	247	63	89	33	127	94	118	393	4676
182	75	8	234	158	93	80	46	48	47	20	218	10184
2423	489	121	1297	2906	619	1239	310	1273	974	342	3084	127084
96	67	11	23	227	54	77	29	65	72	26	206	8450
690	165	43	0	1295	285	542	89	307	292	133	918	44921
156	96	17	703	401	92	152	45	92	81	46	306	13231
367	195	24	370	294	192	149	59	306	100	83	661	20407
1396	1202	116	1023	2479	562	1213	353	649	564	219	2025	73434
471	269	41	793	649	222	369	64	200	135	111	671	28527
115	66	6	169	258	60	82	23	65	42	43	192	10111
166	111	15	328	280	81	148	29	82	64	43	266	11531
–	–	–	–	1	–	–	–	–	–	–	–	1150
–	–	–	–	–	–	–	–	–	–	–	–	1470
94	95	9	109	81	18	58	15	24	27	10	93	3819
–	–	–	–	1	–	–	–	–	–	–	–	1562
65	22	10	78	103	42	29	17	32	36	14	107	3488
772	16	190	9	415	234	0	1604	0	257	56	1987	5387
89	25	5	200	112	26	48	13	25	31	13	97	5838
722	154	47	114	1266	274	503	127	271	313	142	1002	55375
73	58	21	140	245	30	85	6	56	25	23	125	5951
226	144	11	210	212	71	85	19	73	46	30	210	9664
880	242	77	2470	1255	332	583	151	250	311	180	1055	52462
69	72	3	163	146	56	85	16	36	46	20	168	6039
104	3	25	0	36	18	0	113	0	21	5	144	466
82	28	4	84	83	24	69	25	18	27	21	115	4234
117	89	4	120	256	45	83	19	67	45	32	186	7406
–	–	–	–	–	–	–	–	–	–	–	–	2368
318	200	48	1013	429	131	209	61	171	115	102	578	25653
1420	481	113	5447	2985	652	1236	285	764	685	277	2364	105920
1260	564	107	1769	1302	538	761	314	912	443	400	2280	74523
372	247	39	1231	573	167	225	106	328	148	125	759	27215
130	68	12	324	239	66	90	22	137	60	41	281	9802
527	547	549	748	968	163	469	93	341	204	78	848	33199
156	72	14	432	165	57	112	30	77	42	40	224	9351
1976	513	154	7266	3888	813	1737	315	1051	945	426	3220	145016
216	108	19	388	288	97	115	33	46	71	38	237	13835
64	77	14	105	140	28	53	18	52	32	17	136	5297
243	200	18	435	589	150	166	50	119	112	83	408	17993
156	63	16	1	198	69	80	26	39	52	27	173	8690
1009	276	77	3010	2166	379	1025	211	608	509	324	1866	71532
1350	427	151	6224	2250	576	1168	287	729	654	341	2332	111989
1036	271	61	4718	1836	449	951	189	664	454	276	1761	80011
20186	8013	2228	43115	32401	8124	14513	5367	10369	8323	4441	32538	1296063

[a] Including 173.

Table 4. Process of data validation and consistency check for the EUROCARE database: incidence period and numbers of records submitted, corrected and accepted. Registries marked with an asterisk are those contributing to the analysis of time trends.

Registry	Period	Received and checked	Sent to the registry	Rejected	Accepted
Basel	1981–88	11946	201	0	11946
Basque Country	1986–88	19448	57	57	19391
Calvados*	1978–89	26641	920	800	25841
Côte d'Or*	1976–95	15197	456	112	15085
Cracow*	1978–92	30570	1617	805	29765
Denmark*	1978–94	424451	2633	6	424445
Doubs*	1978–92	24993	546	454	24539
East Anglia*	1979–92	134482	316	204	134278
Eindhoven*	1978–92	40187	2455	2449	37738
Estonia*	1978–92	58624	85	0	58624
Finland*	1978–94	246203	209	82	246121
Florence	1985–89	29157	1311	0	29157
Geneva*	1978–89	21599	5	0	21599
Genoa	1986–88	12030	864	1	12029
Girona	1980–89	2073	2	0	2073
Granada	1985–89	1472	2	2	1470
Iceland*	1955–92	20363	4	0	20363
Isère	1987–89	1563	1	1	1562
Latina	1983–87	5600	199	1	5599
Mainz childhood	1980–92	13962	268	259	13703
Mallorca	1982–90	9271	247	181	9090
Mersey	1985–89	62707	33	12	62695
Modena	1985–90	8469	556	29	8440
Navarra	1985–89	9691	48	27	9664
Oxford*	1979–90	132358	352	202	132156
Parma*	1978–87	18668	293	4	18664
Piedmont childhood	1975–89	1596	500	6	1590
Ragusa	1981–89	7591	445	8	7583
Romagna	1986–88	7721	330	0	7721
Rotterdam	1987–90	3012	3	0	3012
Saarland*	1970–92	109815	13	2	109813
Scotland*	1978–93	337902	1223	331	337571
Slovakia	1972–91	214388	3208	168	214220
Slovenia	1985–91	39320	788	90	39230
Somme	1982–89	15946	948	277	15669
Sweden, South*	1978–95	118488	922	33	118455
Tarragona	1985–92	16597	1708	372	16225
Thames, South*	1978–92	414351	6983	6799	407552
Turin	1985–87	13948	413	111	13837
Tyrol	1988–92	13903	0	0	13903
Varese*	1976–92	51401	538	52	51349
Warsaw[a]	1988–89	9673	983	983	8690
Warsaw[a]	1989–93	31081	2389	2346	28735
Wessex*	1979–92	214755	2053	2053	212702
West Midlands*	1978–89	272789	4003	3905	268884
Yorkshire*	1978–90	220886	386	5	220881
Total		**3496888**	**41516**	**23229**	**3473659**

[a] The Warsaw Cancer Registry contributed two partially overlapping data-sets that were checked separately.

Table 5. Numbers and percentages of cases lost to follow-up, death certificate only (DCO) cases and autopsy-derived cases, by registry 1985–89

Registry	Country	Lost to follow-up		DCO		Autopsy	
		No. of cases	%	No. of cases	%	No. of cases	%
Basel	CH	82	1.1	0	0	327	5.3
Basque Country	E	0	0	2419	12.4	0	0
Calvados	F	159	1.4	n.a.	–	9	0.1
Côte d'Or	F	31	0.6	n.a.	–	6	0.1
Cracow	PL	488	2.2	1089	10.4	66	0.6
Denmark	DK	n.a.	–	n.a.	–	n.a.	–
Doubs	F	n.a.	–	n.a.	–	n.a.	–
East Anglia	ENG	1881	3.6	299	0.6	663	1.3
Eindhoven	NL	252	1.9	n.a.	–	n.a.	–
Estonia	EST	166	0.8	23	0.1	1016	5.0
Finland	FIN	12	0.0	507	0.7	1864	2.5
Florence	I	249	0.9	1355	4.6	69	0.2
Geneva	CH	468	4.7	123	1.2	145	1.4
Genoa	I	50	0.4	622	5.2	0	0
Girona	E	85	7.4	0	0	0	0
Granada	E	98	6.6	192	13.1	2	0.1
Iceland	ICE	0	0	7	0.2	122	3.2
Isère	F	n.a.	–	n.a.	–	n.a.	–
Latina	I	57	1.6	18	0.5	0	0
Mainz childhood	D	0	0	0	0	0	0
Mallorca	E	36	0.7	226	3.9	1	0.0
Mersey	ENG	0	0	2087	3.3	1355	2.2
Modena	I	90	1.5	211	3.5	15	0.3
Navarra	E	0	0	663	6.9	90	0.9
Oxford	ENG	0	0	861	1.5	0	0
Parma	I	18	0.3	264	4.4	17	0.3
Piedmont childhood	I	26	5.6	29	5.7	0	0
Ragusa	I	0	0	4	0	0	0
Romagna	I	2	0.0	150	1.9	24	0.3
Rotterdam	NL	52	2.2	n.a.	–	17	0.7
Saarland	D	0	0	2151	8.0	179	0.7
Scotland	SCO	37	0.0	3863	3.6	0	0
Slovakia	SK	0	0	5414	7.0	4209	5.4
Slovenia	SLO	157	0.6	1071	3.9	577	2.1
Somme	F	282	2.9	n.a.	–	n.a.	–
Sweden, South	S	0	0	n.a.	–	2060	6.2
Tarragona	E	36	0.4	407	4.3	38	0.4
Thames, South	ENG	249	0.1	25585	17.6	0	0
Turin	I	287	2.1	611	4.4	0	0
Tyrol	A	0	0	595	10.8	67	1.2
Varese	I	126	0.7	451	2.5	72	0.4
Warsaw	PL	190	2.2	605	7.0	39	0.4
Wessex	ENG	0	0	6827	8.6	0	0
West Midlands	ENG	34	0.0	2319	1.9	1307	1.1
Yorkshire	ENG	0	0	3454	3.8	0	0

n.a.: not available

excluded as not notified to the registry or notified through death certificates is equal, on average, to that of all cases in the analysis. A method to take into account DCO cases in survival analysis has been presented in a recent paper (Verdecchia *et al.*, 1998), based on experience from the EUROCARE project. The shape of the relative survival curve is analysed in order to estimate the proportion of 'cured' cases, with no excess of mortality with respect to the general population, the complementary proportion of fatal cases, and their corresponding relative survival curve. The overall survival of the whole sample of patients is then corrected, attributing to DCO cases the same relative survival levels estimated for the fatal cases. The application of this method was beyond the purpose of the present analysis. However, the detailed distribution of DCO cases by site, sex, age and country is reported in Appendix 1B. The proportion of autopsy-derived cases is generally lower, and less variable across registries, than that of either cases lost to follow-up or of DCO cases. Autopsy-derived cases are therefore not expected to constitute a problem in interpreting the data in this monograph.

Some cancers are known to have a very poor prognosis, with little room for therapeutic efforts. An unexpectedly high survival level for such cancers therefore indicates inaccurate diagnosis, the existence of deaths not known to the registry, or both. Table 6 reports the five-year relative survival rates estimated, by country, in both sexes and all ages, for the seven most fatal cancer sites. Clearly outlying values are found in Austria for acute myeloid leukaemia, and pancreas, biliary tract and liver cancers, in Iceland for oesophagus and biliary tract cancers, and in Spain for pleura and biliary tract cancers. All these cases are from countries with very small populations covered by cancer registries, and the survival rates are therefore characterized by large random variability. Some concern may derive from the data of the Austrian registry of Tyrol, which presents surprisingly high survival rates for four of the highly lethal cancer sites out of seven.

Table 7 reports the percentage of deaths occurring within one month after diagnosis, by site and registry. The proportion of short-term survivors is very variable between sites, being higher, as expected, for highly lethal cancers, such as those of the pancreas, oesophagus, biliary tract and liver. For each site, the proportion of very early deaths is also variable between registries. A high proportion is generally observed in the data from east European and UK registries. This finding is consistent with the low survival level often estimated in these areas, and can be explained by a high proportion of cases diagnosed at a very advanced stage. In other cases, a high proportion of deaths in the first month is observed in cancer registries where five-year survival rates are average to high. In these cases, the high proportion of sudden deaths may indicate problems in quality of follow-up or inclusion of prevalent cases.

Table 8 presents the percentage of cases with histological or cytological confirmation for some selected tumours characterized by different frequencies of these diagnostic procedures. In the table, histological and cytological confirmation are considered together, as 'microscopic' confirmation, because some cancer registries cannot distinguish between the two procedures.

Three registries (Basel, East Anglia and Mainz) show a 100% proportion of cases microscopically verified for all the cancer sites considered.

The proportion of microscopically verified (MV) cases varies considerably across registries and cancer sites. It is higher for patients surviving for five years or more than for those surviving for less than five years. This can be explained by the fact that many short-term survivors are not operated upon and therefore are less likely to undergo histologically- or cytologically-based diagnosis. A high proportion of MV cases is present in the data from the northern and western European countries, while the UK, Italian, and eastern European registries have low proportions. The proportion of MV cases is relatively low for cancers of lung, stomach, colon and prostate. It is intermediate for breast, and high for melanoma and non-Hodgkin lymphoma. For long-term survivors, most registries present a proportion of MV of 90% or greater.

Conclusions

When comparing survival of cancer patients in different countries, various aspects of the validity of cancer registry data must be taken into account. First of all, one must be confident that cancer registration was fairly exhaustive, as indicated by a low proportion of DCO cases, that diagnoses were reliable, as indicated by a high proportion of cases confirmed by a microscopic examination, and that follow-up was complete. The proportions of DCO cases, microscopically verified cases and cases lost to follow-up are therefore reported, by registry country, in this chapter. The size of the biases introduced by different proportions of DCO and of cases lost to follow-up is discussed elsewhere (Sant *et al.*, 1995); in the vast majority of cases, however, the bias is small with respect to the wide inter-country differences. Similarly, different definitions of the date of diagnosis (e.g., date of first hospital admission, date of first histological confirmation or date of first treatment) have been

Table 6. Five-year relative survival rates (%) for cancer sites with high lethality

Country	Acute myeloid leukaemia	Pleura	Lung	Pancreas	Biliary tract	Liver	Oesophagus
Austria	25	0	12	9	20	11	14
Denmark	11	2	6	2	5	1	5
England	11	5	7	3	11	4	9
Estonia	9	11	8	1	4	2	3
Finland	14	7	11	3	8	4	8
France	18	12	14	8	16	8	9
Germany	13	8	11	4	16	6	8
Iceland	5	0	12	3	19	9	25
Italy	9	3	10	4	9	4	8
Netherlands	9	n.e.	13	2	8	0	12
Poland	1	14	8	4	6	3	3
Scotland	9	2	6	4	8	2	7
Slovakia	6	8	13	8	11	5	8
Slovenia	7	6	8	3	5	0	3
Spain	15	16	13	5	17	10	9
Sweden	10	8	10	3	8	4	14
Switzerland	13	0	12	2	12	3	15
Europe	12	7	10	4	12	5	9

n.e.: not estimable

shown to affect survival rates to only a very minor extent (Sant *et al.*, 1995). In some cases, however, problems may arise from the capacity of the registry to trace the relevant date. This is notably the case for cancer registries with a very high proportion of cases dying in the first month (Table 7). Finally, a further comparability problem derives from the different coverage of cancer registration between countries, from 100% in Nordic countries and some eastern European countries to less than 10% in some central and southern European countries. In the latter, the areas covered by registries may not be representative of the whole nation. Registries are perhaps more likely to be established in areas where the local medical community has above-average interest in oncology, and this could positively influence the standard and availability of care in those areas. This issue does not affect the validity of comparison between populations, but only the extrapolation of data from one or a set of regional registries to the whole country. All the comparisons made here are between geographically defined populations, without the risk of patient selection that affects the comparison of clinical series. Nevertheless, in this EUROCARE-2 study the number of registries increased and some countries were better represented than in the EUROCARE-1 study. This is the case for France, the Netherlands, Spain, Italy, Poland and England, for which the general position

for cancer survival did not change between these studies.

References

Berrino, F., Sant, M., Verdecchia, A., Capocaccia, R., Hakulinen, T. & Estève, J., eds (1995) *Survival of Cancer Patients in Europe. The EUROCARE Study* (IARC Scientific Publications No. 132), Lyon, IARC

Coebergh, J.W.W. (1995) Summary and discussion of results. In: Berrino, F., Sant, M., Verdecchia, A., Capocaccia, R., Hakulinen, T. & Estève, J., eds, *Survival of Cancer Patients in Europe. The EUROCARE Study* (IARC Scientific Publications No. 132), Lyon IARC, pp. 444–463

Coebergh, J.W.W., Sant, M., Berrino, F. & Verdecchia, A., eds (1998) Special issue: *Survival of adult cancer patients in Europe diagnosed from 1978–1989*: The EUROCARE II Study. *Eur. J. Cancer*, **34**, No. 14

Parkin, D.M., Whelan, S.L., Ferlay, J., Raymond, L. & Young, J., eds (1997) *Cancer Incidence in Five Continents*, Vol VII (IARC Scientific Publications No. 143), Lyon, IARC

Sant, M. & Gatta, G. (1995) The EUROCARE database. In: Berrino, F., Sant, M., Verdecchia, A., Capocaccia, R., Hakulinen, T. & Estève, J., eds (1995) *Survival of Cancer Patients in Europe. The EUROCARE Study* (IARC Scientific Publications No. 132), Lyon, IARC, pp. 15–31

Verdecchia, A., De Angelis, R., Capocaccia, R., Sant, M., Micheli, A., Gatta, G. & Berrino, F. (1998) The cure for colon cancer: results from the EUROCARE study. *Int. J. Cancer*, **77**, 322–329

Table 7. Percentage of deaths within one month of diagnosis, by cancer site and registry

Registry	Country	ICD-9 code 140	141	142	143–145	146	147	148	150	151	152	153	154	155	156	157
Basel	CH	–	0.0	–	0.0	0.0	–	4.3	9.1	6.9	_	3.7	3.2	24.1	8.8	11.5
Basque Country	E	0.6	2.0	0.0	0.4	0.7	4.8	1.5	5.7	9.1	11.1	9.1	4.3	39.5	15.1	24.4
Calvados	F	1.6	0.7	0.0	1.5	0.9	8.3	1.2	2.9	6.1	6.7	6.0	2.6	17.3	16.0	12.7
Côte d'Or	F	–	–	–	–	–	–	–	4.2	10.9	12.5	4.0	3.0	18.7	19.6	16.2
Cracow	PL	0.0	7.7	11.1	7.3	12.8	0.0	25.0	23.1	27.4	15.4	23.2	14.3	38.5	30.8	38.9
Denmark	DK	0.3	3.4	0.9	1.9	1.4	3.4	3.5	9.9	9.9	9.2	7.4	4.9	21.6	13.7	16.2
Doubs	F	0.0	13.3	17.6	8.6	2.7	15.4	4.8	5.5	8.6	20.0	15.2	10.9	23.8	18.6	23.4
East Anglia	ENG	2.5	1.0	6.7	2.9	5.1	10.0	3.7	12.5	15.5	9.5	10.0	6.3	18.6	12.3	20.1
Eindhoven	NL	0.0	2.2	0.0	0.0	3.8	0.0	5.3	3.8	6.9	6.9	4.9	2.6	11.4	11.0	11.2
Estonia	EST	0.0	1.2	0.0	1.3	0.8	0.0	0.0	5.8	7.7	23.1	11.5	6.2	25.9	20.3	17.0
Finland	FIN	0.4	2.1	0.0	0.7	1.4	0.0	0.0	6.3	7.5	5.9	5.8	3.3	19.3	14.1	14.2
Florence	I	0.0	2.1	2.3	1.4	0.0	1.9	0.0	6.8	6.6	5.1	4.1	3.4	18.5	8.0	7.0
Geneva	CH	4.3	0.0	0.0	0.0	0.0	0.0	3.9	4.9	4.7	5.3	4.4	2.1	13.6	9.4	8.3
Genoa	I	0.0	5.7	0.0	2.7	0.0	3.6	0.0	2.2	7.2	0.0	4.2	3.7	11.6	6.7	8.0
Girona	E	–	–	–	–	–	–	–	–	–	–	–	–	–	–	–
Granada	E	–	–	–	–	–	–	–	–	8.2	–	–	–	–	–	–
Iceland	ICE	0.0	0.0	0.0	5.0	0.0	0.0	0.0	4.3	6.0	0.0	5.4	2.2	9.1	14.3	20.3
Isère	F	–	–	–	–	–	–	–	–	–	–	–	–	–	–	–
Latina	I	4.5	0.0	0.0	0.0	0.0	0.0	0.0	5.0	6.6	0.0	7.1	2.8	16.2	15.4	12.5
Mainz childhood	D	0.0	0.0	0.0	0.0	0.0	0.0	–	–	0.0	–	0.0	–	1.3	0.0	0.0
Mallorca	E	0.0	0.0	0.0	0.0	0.0	0.0	4.8	2.3	7.7	0.0	8.1	6.4	27.9	17.9	29.9
Mersey	ENG	7.1	1.1	2.9	1.2	1.0	1.8	5.6	12.0	13.5	9.2	9.1	6.5	23.9	15.8	20.3
Modena	I	0.0	0.0	0.0	5.0	0.0	0.0	0.0	9.7	9.3	15.4	6.2	3.1	18.4	12.1	15.3
Navarra	E	0.7	0.0	7.1	0.0	3.1	0.0	0.0	5.6	3.0	8.3	3.8	4.7	18.6	9.8	7.9
Oxford	ENG	0.0	2.1	3.6	2.5	1.5	2.0	4.9	13.5	14.2	14.6	10.5	7.1	26.8	16.8	20.2
Parma	I	0.0	0.0	0.0	0.0	0.0	0.0	10.5	6.2	6.9	0.0	5.0	3.2	17.4	12.5	9.4
Piedmont childhood	I	–	–	0.0	–	0.0	–	–	–	–	–	–	–	0.0	–	0.0
Ragusa	I	0.0	7.1	0.0	0.0	0.0	0.0	0.0	5.6	7.3	14.3	7.2	5.3	14.8	6.5	8.2
Romagna	I	0.0	0.0	0.0	0.0	0.0	0.0	0.0	9.7	4.7	7.7	1.7	3.1	8.4	4.7	5.5
Rotterdam	NL	–	–	–	–	–	–	–	6.8	–	–	5.1	3.5	–	–	–
Saarland	D	0.0	0.6	2.0	0.5	0.9	0.0	0.0	7.0	8.4	18.2	5.3	2.8	19.6	9.7	14.9
Scotland	SCO	0.3	2.0	1.9	1.8	2.2	3.2	3.0	11.7	15.7	10.9	9.6	7.6	29.8	23.0	23.6
Slovakia	SK	1.5	1.7	3.9	2.2	3.4	5.1	4.3	11.4	12.1	14.3	12.2	7.6	31.2	18.7	17.1
Slovenia	SLO	0.6	2.8	14.3	1.3	0.8	2.3	3.9	10.4	11.0	7.1	10.9	6.0	26.0	17.7	18.9
Somme	F	0.0	2.9	0.0	0.6	0.9	0.0	2.0	7.6	9.9	0.0	6.2	3.3	20.2	16.7	21.7
Sweden, South	S	0.6	0.0	1.2	1.3	0.0	0.0	0.0	3.0	4.5	4.0	3.7	2.3	17.7	13.9	11.2
Tarragona	E	0.0	2.6	5.6	1.7	0.0	0.0	0.0	12.2	9.4	5.6	6.5	4.2	19.2	24.5	15.4
Thames, South	ENG	0.9	2.3	1.5	2.0	3.2	4.6	4.6	12.2	16.8	13.7	10.5	6.7	33.2	23.7	23.7
Turin	I	0.0	2.9	7.7	3.4	5.6	0.0	0.0	23.1	23.9	14.3	16.0	11.5	51.9	42.8	35.4
Tyrol	A	0.0	0.0	0.0	0.0	25.0	0.0	0.0	12.5	11.6	12.5	9.1	9.2	31.2	14.5	17.0
Varese	I	3.6	2.2	5.9	0.0	0.9	0.0	1.7	7.0	4.7	3.8	3.6	2.1	11.7	9.4	6.6
Warsaw	PL	7.4	10.4	0.0	0.0	1.8	0.0	25.0	12.9	16.5	12.5	15.3	7.7	31.7	19.3	19.2
Wessex	ENG	2.4	3.3	3.6	4.3	6.5	1.8	4.9	10.0	13.0	12.5	9.0	6.4	35.0	15.3	19.9
West Midlands	ENG	1.6	3.0	2.1	1.2	2.4	4.4	8.0	14.9	19.3	15.8	12.6	8.4	31.7	21.8	25.6
Yorkshire	ENG	1.1	3.1	2.0	1.9	5.6	2.3	4.5	16.2	15.2	15.3	9.8	6.7	25.1	14.6	19.6

158	160	161	162	163	170	171	172	174	175	180	182	183	184	185	186	187	188	189	190	191
–	–	0.0	8.6	_	–	–	0.0	0.4	–	0.0	1.8	4.1	–	1.1	0.0	–	2.6	6.1	–	3.9
15.4	6.1	1.0	11.0	13.0	0.0	2.6	0.8	0.9	0.0	1.3	0.8	5.4	1.0	3.7	3.4	0.0	2.5	5.5	0.0	13.4
0.0	0.0	0.4	5.4	6.1	0.0	3.6	0.0	0.4	0.0	0.2	0.4	4.1	2.0	1.5	0.0	0.0	0.5	3.3	0.0	1.9
0.0	–	–	–	–	–	–	–	2.4	–	0.0	1.6	7.9	0.0	–	–	–	–	–	–	–
30.4	0.0	5.5	16.7	7.1	19.0	10.6	4.5	4.8	14.3	4.0	3.4	13.5	15.4	19.0	4.0	11.1	14.8	12.7	3.8	22.0
12.9	1.4	1.1	12.6	9.6	4.0	0.9	0.3	1.7	0.0	1.5	1.2	5.3	3.1	3.2	0.6	3.3	2.1	6.3	0.0	7.7
15.8	0.0	3.2	5.4	26.1	0.0	19.0	12.5	6.1	0.0	3.7	12.9	9.2	24.4	17.2	10.0	13.3	9.9	19.3	21.4	10.4
14.3	1.2	3.3	13.1	5.3	1.6	4.1	1.8	2.2	0.0	2.1	3.9	7.7	3.4	3.5	1.8	1.5	3.9	7.0	6.1	8.5
7.1	0.0	0.6	5.4	0.0	0.0	0.0	0.3	0.6	0.0	0.0	0.7	4.6	2.3	2.1	0.0	0.0	1.1	3.8	0.0	5.1
9.7	2.1	0.3	8.2	8.8	8.2	4.3	0.6	1.3	0.0	0.8	1.9	3.9	2.9	3.8	3.4	0.0	5.7	6.0	1.2	13.5
17.2	1.5	1.2	7.1	5.5	1.1	4.2	0.2	0.6	2.4	1.3	1.4	4.6	1.7	1.7	1.0	0.0	2.2	4.4	0.0	5.1
11.1	2.4	2.6	6.0	0.0	8.2	2.4	0.7	1.2	9.4	2.2	0.9	4.5	3.0	3.1	0.9	2.4	1.8	3.4	9.8	7.6
0.0	0.0	0.0	4.7	6.2	0.0	0.0	0.0	0.5	0.0	0.9	0.0	1.6	2.1	1.6	0.0	0.0	0.7	2.1	5.6	1.8
0.0	0.0	0.4	6.2	2.9	5.6	0.0	0.7	0.7	0.0	0.0	0.5	4.3	2.1	1.7	0.0	0.0	1.1	0.8	0.0	2.0
–	–	–	–	–	–	–	–	0.1	–	0.0	0.6	0.0	0.0	–	–	–	–	–	–	–
–	–	–	6.7	–	–	–	–	1.1	–	–	–	–	–	–	–	–	–	–	–	–
18.2	0.0	0.0	5.4	0.0	0.0	5.0	0.0	0.6	0.0	0.0	0.0	3.5	0.0	0.7	0.0	16.7	1.1	0.7	0.0	7.8
–	–	–	–	–	–	–	–	5.4	–	–	–	–	–	–	–	–	–	–	–	–
0.0	0.0	3.1	6.3	25.0	0.0	0.0	0.0	0.6	0.0	1.3	1.2	3.9	0.0	1.8	0.0	0.0	3.8	6.5	0.0	4.6
6.5	0.0	0.0	0.0	–	0.9	1.2	14.3	–	–	0.0	–	3.2	0.0	0.0	1.6	0.0	0.0	4.3	4.8	3.0
12.5	0.0	1.1	8.7	0.0	0.0	5.6	1.5	1.2	0.0	0.0	0.9	0.0	6.1	3.6	0.0	10.0	1.7	4.2	0.0	7.4
6.4	0.0	1.9	13.7	5.2	2.5	2.9	0.5	2.6	6.7	2.6	2.1	7.6	3.4	4.4	1.0	0.0	2.4	5.8	0.0	8.9
0.0	0.0	2.4	6.2	10.0	0.0	3.6	1.2	1.1	0.0	1.2	0.0	5.5	0.0	0.7	0.0	0.0	1.8	3.6	0.0	4.3
12.0	0.0	0.4	6.6	0.0	4.3	0.0	0.0	0.4	0.0	0.0	1.0	3.3	4.3	1.1	0.0	0.0	0.8	3.3	0.0	2.6
20.3	4.3	2.0	16.2	11.9	4.9	4.9	0.8	2.2	2.1	1.4	1.9	7.0	2.7	4.7	0.8	3.3	3.2	10.2	3.0	9.7
15.4	0.0	0.0	8.2	0.0	0.0	0.0	0.0	0.4	0.0	0.0	0.7	3.8	3.4	2.1	0.0	0.0	2.7	5.8	0.0	6.2
0.0	–	–	0.0	–	0.0	3.4	–	–	–	–	–	0.0	–	0.0	0.0	0.0	0.0	0.0	0.0	6.7
0.0	0.0	0.0	8.0	0.0	4.0	0.0	0.0	0.6	0.0	2.0	0.7	2.6	0.0	4.5	0.0	0.0	3.4	1.7	0.0	7.5
10.0	0.0	0.0	2.4	0.0	0.0	0.0	0.0	0.3	0.0	0.0	0.0	2.7	0.0	1.8	0.0	0.0	0.5	2.5	0.0	8.0
–	–	–	–	–	–	–	–	–	–	–	–	–	–	–	–	–	–	–	–	–
8.3	0.0	1.3	9.5	5.6	0.0	2.4	0.7	0.9	0.0	0.7	1.5	7.6	0.9	1.9	0.0	0.0	1.4	4.4	0.0	5.0
16.4	2.1	2.2	16.3	12.0	5.1	3.3	0.5	2.5	1.8	2.7	2.9	8.3	2.6	5.2	0.4	1.1	3.5	11.3	0.3	9.8
12.5	3.1	2.7	10.9	18.7	6.0	3.1	1.9	2.4	7.6	1.4	2.1	6.8	4.5	6.8	1.2	3.7	4.9	6.2	0.4	12.1
4.4	2.9	0.4	7.6	11.3	1.5	2.3	0.4	1.4	5.0	1.0	1.4	5.1	5.1	5.9	1.0	5.0	3.6	6.0	2.9	6.8
14.3	0.0	2.6	6.6	9.7	5.9	8.6	0.0	0.9	0.0	0.3	1.5	4.2	0.0	3.1	1.9	0.0	2.0	6.7	3.8	4.6
3.7	0.0	0.5	8.1	3.3	0.0	1.9	0.3	0.5	0.0	1.4	0.4	2.9	0.8	1.6	0.0	0.0	1.2	3.4	0.0	2.1
21.4	7.7	1.5	9.1	11.1	3.3	2.9	2.0	1.1	0.0	0.6	0.4	7.1	0.0	2.7	3.8	0.0	1.1	6.2	0.0	4.5
14.4	2.9	2.0	16.1	9.9	4.3	5.1	0.9	2.2	5.9	2.2	2.8	8.5	3.0	4.2	0.5	3.3	3.5	9.5	0.7	8.5
18.4	4.2	3.3	23.1	21.1	8.8	4.9	1.2	1.7	0.0	1.9	2.0	14.8	9.1	6.7	4.4	0.0	3.2	12.8	4.8	22.8
25.0	25.0	9.4	14.0	20.0	25.0	2.3	0.5	5.8	100.0	5.5	1.8	10.1	4.2	6.0	2.6	0.0	1.8	4.8	0.0	12.5
6.2	0.0	1.2	4.9	0.0	1.8	3.2	1.3	1.2	0.0	0.5	0.7	3.7	3.4	2.7	1.1	0.0	1.8	1.5	0.0	4.1
12.5	0.0	1.5	13.5	0.0	5.9	3.4	3.9	2.9	0.0	1.4	3.3	6.8	10.5	7.1	1.3	10.0	5.8	7.1	0.0	13.5
18.8	2.6	3.1	17.1	19.8	7.4	9.4	0.7	2.9	9.1	1.8	2.1	7.6	1.9	5.0	0.5	1.8	2.6	13.6	0.0	18.4
10.6	4.1	3.0	19.4	11.1	2.1	4.0	0.2	2.9	0.0	2.2	3.0	10.1	3.3	5.5	1.8	1.1	4.7	12.8	0.7	10.6
8.8	0.9	2.0	16.5	9.8	2.3	2.2	0.6	2.0	0.0	2.2	1.7	7.6	3.4	3.4	1.0	4.6	3.4	8.9	2.1	10.8

Registry	Country	ICD-9 code 192	193	194	195	196–199	200–202	201	203	204.0	204.1	205.0	205.1
Basel	CH	–	–	–	–	–	4.9	0.0	5.6	9.1	1.4	11.9	8.7
Basque Country	E	0.0	6.2	7.7	23.1	24.8	5.6	7.3	4.4	8.2	2.5	21.1	8.3
Calvados	F	0.0	0.0	8.3	0.0	6.5	4.0	0.0	0.0	0.0	0.0	12.5	0.0
Côte d'Or	F	–	–	–	–	–	3.2	3.2	3.4	3.0	0.8	13.8	1.7
Cracow	PL	37.5	18.1	33.3	29.3	45.5	9.9	3.4	13.2	2.4	30.4	23.1	15.0
Denmark	DK	3.3	5.1	4.1	20.6	17.9	5.1	2.4	6.1	5.2	5.3	15.6	7.3
Doubs	F	0.0	20.9	0.0	33.3	39.1	14.5	9.3	10.3	0.0	4.6	8.3	19.2
East Anglia	ENG	0.0	2.5	12.8	24.4	–	5.4	2.1	10.7	10.1	4.0	19.3	7.6
Eindhoven	NL	0.0	1.0	5.9	7.7	11.7	3.5	0.0	0.7	8.9	2.2	9.9	8.7
Estonia	EST	22.2	5.4	38.5	12.5	11.7	9.3	3.3	6.3	14.0	4.3	26.9	7.5
Finland	FIN	0.0	2.2	9.7	17.3	10.7	4.9	2.2	5.8	6.0	3.4	12.7	3.3
Florence	I	6.7	3.4	5.1	20.0	15.4	4.1	1.9	5.8	7.9	3.2	8.5	5.9
Geneva	CH	0.0	3.1	0.0	16.7	9.3	2.4	0.0	2.4	13.0	4.8	22.0	9.3
Genoa	I	0.0	2.8	0.0	27.7	11.1	1.5	1.3	2.8	10.3	1.2	7.9	4.7
Girona	E	–	–	–	–	–	0.0	–	–	–	–	–	–
Granada	E	–	–	–	–	–	–	–	–	–	–	–	–
Iceland	ICE	2.9	0.0	0.0	0.0	12.5	2.6	0.0	3.5	0.0	9.1	20.0	0.0
Isère	F	–	–	–	–	–	0.0	–	–	–	–	–	–
Latina	I	0.0	4.5	0.0	9.1	15.8	4.8	0.0	3.4	5.9	6.2	16.7	0.0
Mainz childhood	D	0.0	12.5	2.6	0.0	0.0	0.9	0.0	–	1.2	–	4.7	3.6
Mallorca	E	0.0	4.0	20.0	33.3	19.9	4.5	0.0	4.3	0.0	0.0	22.6	0.0
Mersey	ENG	2.7	4.7	15.0	23.2	7.3	5.6	0.7	9.6	5.2	6.3	17.7	11.1
Modena	I	–	0.0	0.0	16.7	17.0	4.5	3.3	1.2	0.0	5.4	20.8	8.7
Navarra	E	0.0	0.7	0.0	19.2	17.4	1.5	0.0	5.3	0.0	1.4	17.1	3.7
Oxford	ENG	4.1	4.6	9.5	0.0	27.4	9.2	1.5	11.9	4.0	12.8	24.1	13.3
Parma	I	0.0	1.4	0.0	22.2	16.2	5.6	1.8	1.3	6.2	8.3	17.4	15.0
Piedmont childhood	I	0.0	0.0	0.0	–	–	2.8	0.0	_	0.9	–	0.0	0.0
Ragusa	I	0.0	0.0	0.0	0.0	14.3	4.8	4.2	4.3	16.0	0.0	18.5	4.8
Romagna	I	0.0	1.1	0.0	30.0	8.9	3.2	0.0	3.7	11.1	1.5	17.1	0.0
Rotterdam	NL	–	–	–	–	–	–	–	–	–	–	–	–
Saarland	D	4.3	4.7	4.3	26.9	18.8	3.2	1.6	7.1	1.8	3.3	19.8	7.6
Scotland	SCO	6.1	4.8	6.3	35.9	26.5	8.2	3.1	11.2	7.4	6.8	20.8	7.8
Slovakia	SK	10.9	9.7	5.7	35.1	14.9	7.8	3.2	8.9	10.0	7.0	22.8	9.6
Slovenia	SLO	3.0	7.1	11.4	21.4	13.8	2.8	0.6	5.9	4.7	8.1	22.1	4.8
Somme	F	20.0	7.4	8.3	15.8	23.8	3.3	3.0	4.4	9.1	2.2	18.3	2.4
Sweden, South	S	3.0	2.4	0.8	12.1	8.8	3.6	0.6	2.4	5.4	6.0	13.0	3.8
Tarragona	E	0.0	4.3	7.7	18.6	19.8	8.1	1.9	3.8	13.8	2.6	26.2	5.0
Thames, South	ENG	3.7	7.0	8.9	18.2	29.5	8.2	1.7	9.7	6.2	7.2	14.8	9.0
Turin	I	0.0	7.7	11.1	41.7	45.5	13.7	8.3	14.6	21.9	15.4	47.1	16.7
Tyrol	A	100.0	4.1	7.7	66.7	34.3	8.4	0.0	2.4	5.6	4.4	27.6	13.3
Varese	I	0.0	2.5	0.0	38.5	9.6	2.7	0.0	1.2	6.0	5.0	21.4	2.4
Warsaw	PL	7.7	6.3	0.0	30.8	0.0	6.1	4.3	18.7	7.7	5.1	32.7	11.1
Wessex	ENG	15.1	5.5	9.3	16.0	43.5	5.7	2.7	9.6	4.5	8.0	17.8	9.3
West Midlands	ENG	3.0	9.2	10.3	0.0	28.9	10.2	3.0	14.3	5.6	8.3	20.6	9.6
Yorkshire	ENG	7.1	3.8	5.3	23.9	25.5	7.5	1.6	10.7	7.0	4.1	19.9	8.1

Table 8. Proportion of microscopic verification for some cancer sites stratified by short-term (S < 5) and long-term (S>5) survival, by registry

Registry	Country	Lung		Stomach		Breast	
		S < 5	S > 5	S < 5	S > 5	S < 5	S > 5
Basel	CH	100.0	100.0	100.0	100.0	100.0	100.0
Basque Country	E	79.2	98.0	78.3	100.0	85.7	99.2
Calvados	F	95.6	97.2	93.4	98.7	94.5	99.5
Côte d'Or	F	–	–	100.0	100.0	97.8	100.0
Cracow	PL	61.1	74.1	40.1	67.4	72.5	92.2
Denmark	DK	n.a.	n.a.	n.a.	n.a.	n.a.	n.a.
Doubs	F	96.4	98.9	97.5	100.0	96.7	97.2
East Anglia	ENG	100.0	100.0	99.9	100.0	99.9	99.9
Eindhoven	NL	94.2	98.9	97.2	100.0	96.5	98.9
Estonia	EST	68.2	80.2	78.1	94.2	87.1	98.9
Finland	FIN	90.6	98.8	92.6	99.2	97.1	99.8
Florence	I	61.8	64.8	64.9	86.3	72.6	95.6
Geneva	CH	99.1	–	98.6	–	98.6	–
Genoa	I	69.3	78.9	69.4	88.1	76.0	96.8
Girona	E	–	–	–	–	100.0	100.0
Granada	E	74.8	100.0	73.8	100.0	75.0	99.2
Iceland	ICE	84.1	95.2	91.9	100.0	97.3	100.0
Isère	F	–	–	–	–	91.2	97.2
Latina	I	84.0	87.0	83.6	93.9	92.7	98.7
Mainz childhood	D	100.0	100.0	100.0	–	–	–
Mersey	ENG	51.2	88.1	68.0	96.2	68.0	95.5
Mallorca	E	80.5	100.0	86.2	100.0	96.0	100.0
Modena	I	64.4	87.0	78.0	95.6	86.0	98.7
Navarra	E	84.9	98.4	82.0	98.3	84.5	98.9
Oxford	ENG	56.3	81.3	72.2	89.8	75.0	95.7
Parma	I	73.8	91.5	77.0	99.1	88.3	99.8
Piedmont childhood	I	–	100.0	–	–	–	–
Ragusa	I	47.6	100.0	54.3	97.0	74.5	93.7
Romagna	I	80.9	90.7	81.1	96.9	85.9	97.7
Rotterdam	NL	–	–	96.7	100.0	–	–
Saarland	D	68.6	96.1	83.7	97.0	91.0	100.0
Scotland	SCO	56.3	79.4	74.1	94.7	72.2	95.0
Slovakia	SK	71.5	81.2	67.2	81.9	78.6	94.8
Slovenia	SLO	86.5	93.3	73.8	97.5	86.9	99.2
Somme	F	91.8	95.3	94.9	98.0	93.3	97.9
Sweden, South	S	99.0	100.0	97.7	99.4	99.1	100.0
Tarragona	E	83.4	100.0	82.2	100.0	88.4	99.1
Thames, South	ENG	50.4	83.9	53.5	94.8	53.7	89.0
Turin	I	72.7	90.2	79.2	99.2	81.1	98.6
Tyrol	A	72.0	98.0	75.5	100.0	73.5	99.7
Varese	I	85.8	85.2	90.0	98.5	91.1	98.8
Warsaw	PL	66.9	68.0	65.7	77.5	83.9	95.9
Wessex	ENG	41.3	58.7	51.7	66.3	46.9	80.6
West Midlands	ENG	29.4	40.6	36.5	45.2	54.0	71.9
Yorkshire	ENG	55.6	90.5	69.6	97.2	66.3	96.0

n.a.: not available

Table 8. (Contd)

Colon		Melanoma		Non-Hodgkin lymphoma		Prostate	
S < 5	S > 5	S < 5	S > 5	S < 5	S > 5	S < 5	S > 5
100.0	100.0	100.0	100.0	100.0	100.0	100.0	100.0
77.7	99.2	94.7	100.0	92.6	98.6	62.0	93.5
94.8	99.7	100.0	100.0	99.4	100.0	97.0	100.0
100.0	100.0	–	–	100.0	100.0	–	–
35.8	71.2	87.6	97.3	86.2	94.3	42.1	83.0
n.a.	n.a.	n.a	n.a.	n.a.	n.a.	n.a.	n.a.
96.7	97.9	100.0	98.8	98.0	92.3	99.2	98.4
100.0	100.0	100.0	100.0	99.9	100.0	100.0	99.9
95.7	99.3	100.0	99.4	99.6	99.2	97.9	99.6
75.0	96.9	98.1	99.5	99.6	95.6	63.4	76.6
90.9	99.4	99.1	99.9	98.2	99.7	95.7	99.4
65.6	90.7	88.1	92.0	78.3	87.4	57.9	81.8
98.1	–	100.0	–	99.2	–	98.0	–
68.6	92.3	81.0	100.0	88.3	91.7	63.2	92.8
–	–	–	–	–	100.0	–	–
–	–	–	–	–	–	–	–
89.5	100.0	100.0	100.0	88.6	100.0	86.2	100.0
–	–	–	–	–	100.0	–	–
91.5	97.5	87.5	100.0	98.3	97.8	91.5	92.6
100.0	–	100.0	100.0	100.0	100.0	100.0	100.0
66.4	97.7	93.0	98.0	80.8	95.9	70.5	94.8
82.1	99.3	100.0	100.0	98.9	100.0	84.8	95.2
83.4	98.0	95.1	100.0	97.3	100.0	81.7	96.9
77.8	98.3	100.0	100.0	96.7	97.8	78.1	99.6
71.7	96.6	99.6	99.5	98.8	99.4	72.7	90.3
72.2	97.4	100.0	100.0	100.0	100.0	80.3	98.5
–	–	–	–	93.3	100.0	–	100.0
64.1	100.0	95.0	100.0	92.3	100.0	32.2	81.8
77.9	98.3	100.0	100.0	97.2	98.2	71.6	92.6
96.4	100.0	–	–	–	–	–	–
85.7	100.0	96.1	100.0	88.7	98.9	85.2	100.0
75.7	96.9	97.5	99.3	89.2	95.3	76.5	95.5
69.7	93.2	94.1	97.4	95.4	100.0	70.4	89.3
75.8	96.4	96.9	99.6	99.7	100.0	73.5	94.0
89.4	98.0	100.0	100.0	97.6	98.6	90.7	98.1
95.1	100.0	100.0	100.0	100.0	100.0	98.7	99.8
81.6	100.0	98.0	100.0	98.2	100.0	75.2	96.3
56.2	97.1	79.3	97.8	70.4	90.3	60.1	93.0
75.6	96.5	97.0	99.1	94.7	94.9	74.1	96.2
72.1	100.0	83.8	100.0	82.9	98.6	71.8	99.4
82.3	98.1	100.0	98.6	98.5	100.0	87.3	96.5
52.8	81.0	93.9	96.3	91.2	95.1	59.4	94.7
52.6	74.6	67.9	77.3	72.7	83.6	51.7	80.7
32.8	41.2	97.7	99.3	46.9	55.2	34.6	42.7
71.7	99.1	93.3	99.2	88.2	97.8	76.6	96.6

Appendix 1A

Ratio between the number of incidence cases reported in *Cancer Incidence in Five Continents,* Vol. VII and the corresponding number of cases available to the Eurocare II database, diagnosed in the period reported within brackets.

| Registry | ICD-9 code | | | | | | | | | | | |
	140	141	142	143–145	146	147	148	150	151	152	153	154
Basel (1988–88)	1.45			0.92	1.47		4.10	0.90	1.15		1.26	1.22
Basque Country (1988–88)	1.15	1.02	1.15	0.96	1.01	1.08	0.99	1.01	1.00	1.42	1.03	1.08
Cracow (1988–92)	1.05	1.00	1.16	1.07	1.02	1.00	1.09	1.06	1.01	1.00	1.02	1.03
Denmark (1988–92)	0.97	1.01	0.88	0.99	1.00	0.99	0.99	1.03	1.04	0.98	1.03	1.01
Doubs (1988–92)	1.00	1.05	1.08	1.01	1.03	1.11	1.02	1.03	0.99	1.07	1.01	1.00
East Anglia (1988–92)	0.99	1.17	1.02	1.06	1.00	1.10	1.09	1.08	1.08	1.15	1.08	1.06
Eindhoven (1988–92)	1.08	1.11	1.05	1.09	1.28	1.04	1.11	1.15	1.09	1.21	1.11	1.08
Estonia (1988–92)	1.02	1.06	1.02	1.06	1.04	1.03	1.06	1.05	1.04	1.13	1.06	1.07
Finland (1989–92)	0.95	0.82	0.92	0.85	0.83	0.87	0.91	0.90	0.93	0.95	0.91	0.90
Florence (1988–89)	1.10	1.42	0.91	0.98	1.11	0.89	1.07	1.06	1.06	1.14	1.09	1.04
Geneva (1988–89)	1.25	1.17	0.90	1.06	1.23	3.20	1.42	0.96	1.01	1.27	1.17	1.03
Genoa (1988–88)	1.70	1.15	2.25	1.05	0.85	0.80	1.69	1.17	0.91	1.33	1.21	1.11
Granada (1988–89)									1.02			
Iceland (1988–92)	1.13	1.00	1.50	1.14	1.00	1.00	0.67	1.23	1.06	1.15	1.11	1.10
Isère (1988–92)												
Mallorca (1988–90)	0.94	0.89	1.07	1.06	1.24	0.77	1.12	1.08	1.11	1.44	1.04	1.00
Mersey (1988–89)	0.96	0.93	1.37	1.04	1.25	0.95	1.08	1.00	0.97	1.15	0.94	0.91
Modena (1988–90)	1.20	1.56	1.15	0.99	1.12	1.32	1.14	1.07	0.96	1.23	1.16	1.14
Navarra (1988–89)	0.83	1.54	1.33	1.29	1.07	1.07	1.17	0.96	0.94	1.12	1.14	0.98
Oxford (1988–90)	0.74	1.08	1.21	1.07	1.09	0.79	0.91	1.15	0.97	1.16	1.06	1.05
Ragusa (1988–89)	1.14	1.36	0.80	0.76		1.20	0.40	1.20	0.88	1.20	1.39	1.02
Saarland (1988–92)	1.13	1.07	1.14	1.06	1.04	1.08	1.05	1.09	1.10	1.10	1.10	1.08
Scotland (1988–92)	1.08	1.06	1.09	1.08	1.09	1.03	1.05	1.07	1.06	1.12	1.07	1.06
Slovakia (1988–91)	0.98	1.05	1.08	1.01	1.02	0.96	1.00	1.01	1.00	1.02	1.01	1.01
Slovenia (1988–91)	1.06	1.03	1.17	1.07	1.06	1.01	1.03	1.04	0.99	1.03	1.04	1.02
Somme (1988–92)	2.09	1.00	1.50	0.94	0.88	0.96	1.23	1.02	0.91	1.15	1.04	1.07
Tarragona (1988–92)	1.03	1.13	1.05	1.09	1.03	1.00	1.17	1.06	1.06	1.07	1.04	1.03
Thames, South (1988–92)	1.01	1.12	1.12	1.13	1.10	1.10	1.13	1.10	1.10	1.12	1.11	1.09
Tyrol (1988–92)	1.00	1.00	1.00	1.00	1.04	1.07	1.07	1.05	1.01	1.00	1.01	1.02
Varese (1988–92)	1.16	1.30	1.12	1.33	1.23	1.06	1.19	1.21	1.11	1.25	1.14	1.10
Warsaw (1988–92)	0.72	0.70	0.88	0.87	0.68	0.80	0.80	0.70	0.69	0.89	0.71	0.70
Wessex (1988–92)	0.97	0.95	0.95	0.93	0.93	0.98	0.96	0.97	0.96	0.99	0.97	0.96
West Midlands (1988–89)	0.84	1.13	0.96	1.25	1.19	1.31	1.34	1.14	1.05	1.02	1.13	1.14
Yorkshire (1988–90)	0.99	1.11	1.30	1.08	1.13	1.26	0.86	1.08	1.03	1.14	1.08	1.04

Appendix 1A (contd)

Registry	ICD-9 code 155	156	157	160	161	162	170	171	172	174	175	180	182	183	184
Basel (1988–88)	0.86	0.77	1.12		0.90	1.03			1.07	1.08		1.40	1.04	0.95	
Basque Country (1988–88)	1.16	0.91	1.09	1.00	1.03	1.02	1.29	1.14	0.93	1.07	0.82	1.15	1.19	1.32	0.90
Cracow (1988–92)	1.03	1.01	1.03	1.00	1.03	1.02	1.02	1.52	1.03	1.03	1.00	1.03	1.03	1.06	1.02
Denmark (1988–92)	0.58	1.06	1.08	0.99	1.01	1.04	0.69	0.99	0.97	0.97	0.95	1.01	1.00	1.01	1.00
Doubs (1988–92)	1.09	1.00	0.98	1.00	1.00	1.01	1.09	1.22	1.05	1.01	1.00	0.98	1.02	1.02	1.00
East Anglia (1988–92)	1.08	1.09	1.10	1.10	1.05	1.07	1.27	1.00	1.05	1.07	1.11	1.06	1.09	1.09	1.05
Eindhoven (1988–92)	1.25	1.13	1.15	1.10	1.09	1.11	1.36	1.27	1.11	1.05	1.00	1.05	1.10	1.19	1.07
Estonia (1988–92)	1.04	1.04	1.03	1.07	1.05	1.05	1.02	1.05	1.07	1.06	1.11	1.03	1.06	1.05	1.06
Finland (1989–92)	0.89	0.90	0.90	0.85	0.90	0.90	1.49	1.56	0.89	0.86	0.80	0.94	0.87	0.86	0.96
Florence (1988–89)	1.05	1.04	1.06	0.93	0.98	1.06	1.19	1.64	1.17	1.05	1.04	1.05	1.04	1.12	0.88
Geneva (1988–89)	1.27	1.10	1.07	7.60	0.79	1.08	1.28	0.82	0.99	1.01	3.20	0.17	1.02	1.07	0.83
Genoa (1988–88)	1.12	0.86	1.17	0.84	1.01	0.96	1.00	1.46	1.16	1.17	1.80	0.85	1.01	1.00	1.11
Granada (1988–89)						1.29				1.18					
Iceland (1988–92)	1.06	1.12	0.97	1.08	1.07	1.09	1.10	1.50	1.16	1.12	1.17	1.05	1.11	0.75	1.40
Isère (1988–92)										1.11					
Mallorca (1988–90)	1.13	1.16	1.08	1.04	1.13	1.07	1.00	1.14	0.95	1.01	1.50	0.31	0.99	1.28	0.86
Mersey (1988–89)	1.04	0.90	0.89	0.89	0.93	0.96	1.33	1.01	1.01	0.98	1.55	0.81	0.93	1.00	0.91
Modena (1988–90)	0.98	1.06	0.95	1.80	1.06	1.03	0.90	1.09	1.05	1.17	1.08	0.74	1.27	1.06	1.10
Navarra (1988–89)	1.09	1.03	1.21	2.13	1.18	1.20	1.65	1.54	0.95	1.21	1.10	0.44	0.88	0.95	1.23
Oxford (1988–90)	0.95	1.13	1.07	1.05	1.05	1.04	1.05	1.13	1.13	1.12	1.08	1.01	1.03	1.09	1.05
Ragusa (1988–89)	1.09	1.24	1.02	1.60	0.84	1.10	0.97	1.00	0.95	1.06	0.60	0.79	0.87	1.16	1.12
Saarland (1988–92)	1.04	1.04	1.04	1.15	1.07	1.06	0.94	1.07	1.09	1.06	1.06	1.07	1.09	1.08	1.09
Scotland (1988–92)	1.05	1.05	1.05	1.09	1.06	1.07	1.11	1.06	1.05	1.07	1.04	1.04	1.07	1.08	1.08
Slovakia (1988–91)	1.29	1.00	1.01	1.04	1.01	1.01	1.58	1.10	1.01	1.02	1.15	1.03	1.03	1.01	0.98
Slovenia (1988–91)	1.08	1.01	1.04	1.08	1.01	1.02	1.05	1.26	1.06	1.01	1.02	1.02	0.97	0.98	1.02
Somme (1988–92)	1.24	1.03	1.09	0.78	1.00	1.04	1.00	2.60	1.17	1.13	1.73	0.49	1.04	1.13	0.91
Tarragona (1988–92)	1.08	1.10	1.05	1.11	1.03	1.08	1.00	1.11	1.08	1.03	1.00	0.94	1.06	1.07	1.07
Thames, South (1988–92)	1.08	1.09	1.10	1.14	1.12	1.11	1.11	1.37	1.17	1.09	1.11	1.02	1.10	1.09	1.13
Tyrol (1988–92)	1.00	1.01	1.00	1.00	1.01	1.01	1.05	1.00	1.01	1.01	1.00	1.01	1.04	1.02	1.01
Varese (1988–92)	1.18	1.10	1.18	1.20	1.19	1.13	1.00	1.23	1.08	1.06	1.08	1.07	1.10	1.10	1.13
Warsaw (1988–92)	0.75	0.67	0.64	0.87	0.69	0.70	0.68	0.67	0.72	0.72	0.93	0.68	0.70	0.69	0.69
Wessex (1988–92)	0.98	0.95	0.95	0.94	0.93	0.96	0.89	0.97	0.97	0.96	0.96	0.99	0.96	0.97	0.95
West Midlands (1988–89)	1.16	1.29	1.15	1.21	1.19	1.12	2.28	1.39	1.12	1.26	1.07	1.06	1.23	1.13	1.13
Yorkshire (1988–90)	1.06	1.11	1.04	1.23	1.05	1.06	1.06	0.98	1.13	1.08	1.29	0.97	1.08	1.07	1.06

Appendix 1A (contd)

Registry	ICD-9 code														
	185	186	187	188	189	191	193	200, 202	201	203	204.0	204.1	205.0	205.1	Total
Basel (1988–88)	1.37	1.06		1.37	1.28	0.97		1.55	0.98	1.98	0.88	1.02	1.36	0.77	1.20
Basque Country (1988–88)	0.97	1.47	1.00	1.00	1.13	1.02	1.03	1.20	0.92	0.90	0.71	0.94	1.21	1.13	1.04
Cracow (1988–92)	1.02	1.00	1.11	1.04	1.02	0.99	1.04	1.03	0.99	1.05	1.03	1.10	1.01	1.05	1.02
Denmark (1988–92)	1.02	1.00	0.97	1.00	1.01	0.68	1.05	1.04	1.03	0.96	0.96	0.99	1.02	1.03	0.98
Doubs (1988–92)	1.00	1.01	0.95	1.69	1.05	0.99	1.01	1.04	1.02	1.07	1.00	0.98	0.97	1.03	1.04
East Anglia (1988–92)	1.08	1.00	1.05	1.08	1.08	1.04	1.05	1.06	1.00	1.11					1.04
Eindhoven (1988–92)	1.11	1.08	1.09	1.95	1.16	1.46	1.05	1.14	1.07	1.06	1.02	1.09	1.09	1.03	1.13
Estonia (1988–92)	1.07	1.05	1.00	1.06	1.06	1.02	1.07	1.07	1.01	1.02	1.03	1.05	1.07	1.02	1.05
Finland (1989–92)	0.89	0.80	0.88	0.91	0.90	0.95	0.84	0.93	0.85	0.94					0.87
Florence (1988–89)	1.11	0.98	1.13	1.06	1.20	0.98	1.01	1.21	0.89	1.16	1.04	0.97	1.13	1.01	1.06
Geneva (1988–89)	1.19	1.20	1.10	1.28	1.00	0.96	1.04	1.12	0.85	1.13	1.93	0.96	1.43	1.23	1.02
Genoa (1988–88)	1.17	1.32	1.50	1.25	1.20	1.03	1.03	1.36	1.50	1.09	1.03	0.86	0.72	1.16	1.09
Granada (1988–89)															
Iceland (1988–92)	1.09	1.02	1.29	1.08	1.19	1.01	1.21	1.19	1.04	1.00	1.00	0.91	1.04	0.78	1.06
Isère (1988–92)															
Mallorca (1988–90)	1.08	1.68	1.01	1.17	0.96	0.99	1.08	0.99	1.00	1.19	0.99	1.34	0.84	0.98	0.99
Mersey (1988–89)	1.03	0.93	0.78	0.95	1.00	0.95	1.15	0.90	0.86	0.94	0.90	0.92	0.87	0.92	0.95
Modena (1988–90)	1.12	1.13	0.82	1.13	1.25	1.18	1.22	1.11	1.33	1.03	1.80	1.10	1.26	1.07	1.08
Navarra (1988–89)	1.06	1.55	1.09	1.10	0.97	1.09	0.88	1.20	1.15	1.05	0.93	1.12	1.17	1.16	1.06
Oxford (1988–90)	1.13	1.08	1.16	1.07	1.09	1.08	1.04	1.12	1.09	1.28	1.09	1.31	1.18	1.18	1.08
Ragusa (1988–89)	1.11	0.80	2.80	0.89	1.33	0.95	0.88	1.68	1.69	1.20	1.26	1.77	1.29	1.03	1.06
Saarland (1988–92)	1.12	1.02	1.06	1.12	1.07	1.02	1.07	1.08	1.05	1.06	1.02	1.11	1.12	1.08	1.07
Scotland (1988–92)	1.07	1.02	1.04	1.06	1.09	1.04	1.06	1.06	1.01	1.06	1.05	1.08	1.06	1.02	1.06
Slovakia (1988–91)	1.00	0.88	0.97	1.02	1.02	1.11	1.08	1.01	0.98	0.97	1.02	0.97	1.00	0.97	1.01
Slovenia (1988–91)	1.02	1.03	1.04	1.03	1.00	1.00	1.03	1.06	0.96	1.03	1.08	1.05	0.91	1.03	1.01
Somme (1988–92)	1.05	1.05	0.60	0.97	1.32	0.96	1.02	1.23	1.12	0.82	1.45	0.92	0.68	0.78	1.03
Tarragona (1988–92)	1.03	1.04	0.97	1.10	1.10	1.02	1.04	1.05	1.04	1.07	1.10	1.11	1.10	1.18	1.05
Thames, South (1988–92)	1.14	1.04	1.07	1.12	1.10	1.05	1.11	1.10	1.04	1.12	1.27	1.21	1.12	1.15	1.10
Tyrol (1988–92)	1.02	1.02	0.93	1.03	1.04	1.01	1.01	1.01	1.03	1.00	1.02	0.96	0.97	0.97	1.01
Varese (1988–92)	1.19	1.01	0.88	1.15	1.15	1.09	1.13	1.09	1.05	1.11	1.06	1.17	1.12	1.12	1.12
Warsaw (1988–92)	0.76	0.66	0.91	0.72	0.71	0.75	0.70	0.66	0.66	0.71	0.66	0.73	0.70	0.72	0.70
Wessex (1988–92)	0.97	1.00	0.94	1.01	0.96	0.95	0.97	0.98	0.95	0.97	0.95	0.98	0.98	0.96	0.96
West Midlands (1988–89)	1.25	1.67	1.12	1.21	1.27	1.17	1.18	1.29	1.18	1.18	1.24	1.06	1.19	1.19	1.17
Yorkshire (1988–90)	1.11	1.16	1.02	1.40	1.15	1.09	1.03	1.12	1.06	1.08	1.09	0.93	1.11	1.12	1.09

Appendix 1B

The following tables report the numbers of cases known to the registries only from a death certificate (DCO), by cancer site, country, age and sex. DCO cases cannot be considered in survival calculation and their proportion is considered mainly as an indicator of the completeness of cancer registration. However, a variable proportion may affect inter-country comparisons, because the actual survival rates are different from those of the other incident cases.

MALIGNANT NEOPLASMS

| Country | Males | | | | | | Females | | | | | |
	15–44	45–54	55–64	65–74	75–99	15–99	15–44	45–54	55–64	65–74	75–99	15–99
Austria	4	10	40	60	154	268	5	12	30	65	215	327
Denmark	(not available)											
England	365	665	2637	6033	10692	20392	332	686	2020	4496	13066	20600
Estonia	1	0	2	4	5	12	0	0	1	2	8	11
Finland	4	6	25	57	139	231	5	5	10	36	220	276
France	(not available)											
Germany	16	63	174	258	529	1040	13	32	90	186	661	982
Iceland	0	0	0	0	4	4	0	1	0	0	2	3
Italy	21	58	234	447	1094	1854	27	48	133	293	1338	1839
Netherlands	(not available)											
Poland	22	50	212	211	309	804	20	38	133	207	458	856
Scotland	9	74	301	625	929	1938	7	58	241	483	1133	1922
Slovakia	73	226	604	869	1183	2955	93	111	322	522	1267	2315
Slovenia	3	28	69	103	311	514	4	6	35	72	439	556
Spain	51	97	291	569	1091	2099	53	72	159	286	1033	1603
Sweden	(not available)											
Switzerland	1	0	6	6	40	53	1	0	7	5	54	67
Pool	570	1277	4595	9242	16480	32164	560	1069	3181	6653	19894	31357

TONGUE

| Country | Males | | | | | | Females | | | | | |
	15–44	45–54	55–64	65–74	75–99	15–99	15–44	45–54	55–64	65–74	75–99	15–99
Austria	1	0	2	0	0	3	0	0	0	0	0	0
England	0	9	6	9	10	34	1	2	2	3	8	16
Estonia	0	0	0	0	0	0	0	0	0	0	0	0
Finland	0	0	0	0	0	0	0	0	0	0	1	1
Germany	0	1	0	1	0	2	0	0	0	0	0	0
Iceland	0	0	0	0	0	0	0	0	0	0	0	0
Italy	0	0	1	2	1	4	0	0	0	0	3	3
Poland	0	1	0	0	1	2	0	0	1	0	0	1
Scotland	1	0	2	1	4	8	0	0	0	0	1	1
Slovakia	3	3	2	5	2	15	0	0	0	2	0	2
Slovenia	0	1	0	1	3	5	0	0	0	0	0	0
Spain	0	2	4	1	4	11	0	0	1	0	2	3
Switzerland	0	0	0	0	0	0	0	0	0	0	0	0
Pool	5	17	17	20	25	84	1	2	4	5	15	27

SALIVARY GLAND

Country	Males						Females					
	15–44	45–54	55–64	65–74	75–99	15–99	15–44	45–54	55–64	65–74	75–99	15–99
Austria	0	0	0	0	0	0	0	0	1	0	0	1
England	0	0	0	4	3	7	0	0	3	0	16	19
Estonia	0	0	0	0	0	0	0	0	0	0	0	0
Finland	0	0	0	0	0	0	0	0	0	0	0	0
Germany	0	0	0	0	0	0	0	0	0	0	0	0
Iceland	0	0	0	0	0	0	0	0	0	0	0	0
Italy	0	0	1	1	3	5	1	0	0	0	1	2
Poland	0	0	0	0	0	0	0	0	0	0	1	1
Scotland	0	0	1	1	1	3	0	0	1	0	4	5
Slovakia	0	0	0	3	1	4	0	0	2	1	1	4
Slovenia	0	0	0	0	0	0	0	0	0	0	0	0
Spain	0	2	0	1	2	5	0	0	0	0	2	2
Switzerland	0	0	0	0	0	0	0	0	0	0	0	0
Pool	0	2	2	10	10	24	1	0	7	1	25	34

ORAL CAVITY

Country	Males						Females					
	15–44	45–54	55–64	65–74	75–99	15–99	15–44	45–54	55–64	65–74	75–99	15–99
Austria	0	0	0	0	1	1	0	0	0	0	0	0
England	0	3	10	9	7	29	0	0	2	9	12	23
Estonia	0	0	0	0	0	0	0	0	0	0	0	0
Finland	0	0	0	0	0	0	0	0	0	0	1	1
Germany	0	1	0	0	0	1	0	0	0	0	0	0
Iceland	0	0	0	0	0	0	0	0	0	0	0	0
Italy	0	0	0	1	1	2	0	1	0	0	2	3
Poland	0	0	0	0	0	0	0	0	0	0	1	1
Scotland	0	0	2	1	2	5	0	0	0	1	2	3
Slovakia	1	1	6	1	1	10	0	0	0	0	4	4
Slovenia	0	0	0	0	1	1	0	0	0	1	0	1
Spain	0	1	3	2	1	7	0	0	0	1	1	2
Switzerland	0	0	0	0	0	0	0	0	0	0	1	1
Pool	1	6	21	14	14	56	0	1	2	12	24	39

OROPHARYNX

Country	Males						Females					
	15–44	45–54	55–64	65–74	75–99	15–99	15–44	45–54	55–64	65–74	75–99	15–99
Austria	0	0	0	0	0	0	0	0	0	0	0	0
England	0	1	1	0	5	7	0	0	3	4	6	13
Estonia	0	0	0	0	0	0	0	0	0	0	0	0
Finland	0	0	0	0	0	0	0	0	0	0	0	0
Germany	0	1	1	0	0	2	0	0	0	0	0	0
Iceland	0	0	0	0	0	0	0	0	0	0	0	0
Italy	0	0	0	3	1	4	0	0	0	0	1	1
Poland	0	0	1	0	1	2	0	0	0	0	0	0
Scotland	0	0	0	1	1	2	0	0	0	0	0	0
Slovakia	0	1	2	0	2	5	0	0	0	2	3	5
Slovenia	0	0	3	1	1	5	0	0	0	0	0	0
Spain	0	1	0	0	1	2	0	0	0	1	0	1
Switzerland	0	0	0	0	1	1	0	0	0	0	0	0
Pool	0	4	8	5	13	30	0	0	3	7	10	20

NASOPHARYNX

Country	Males						Females					
	15–44	45–54	55–64	65–74	75–99	15–99	15–44	45–54	55–64	65–74	75–99	15–99
Austria	0	0	0	0	0	0	0	0	0	0	0	0
England	0	2	5	2	3	12	0	0	0	1	3	4
Estonia	0	0	0	0	0	0	0	0	0	0	0	0
Finland	0	0	0	0	0	0	0	0	0	0	0	0
Germany	0	0	0	0	0	0	0	0	0	0	0	0
Iceland	0	0	0	0	0	0	0	0	0	0	0	0
Italy	0	0	1	0	1	2	0	0	0	0	1	1
Poland	0	0	0	0	0	0	0	0	0	0	0	0
Scotland	0	0	0	1	1	2	0	0	0	0	1	1
Slovakia	0	0	1	1	0	2	0	0	0	2	0	2
Slovenia	0	0	0	0	0	0	0	0	0	0	0	0
Spain	0	1	0	1	0	2	0	0	1	0	0	1
Switzerland	0	0	0	0	0	0	0	0	0	0	0	0
Pool	0	3	7	5	5	20	0	0	1	3	5	9

HYPOPHARYNX

Country	Males						Females					
	15–44	45–54	55–64	65–74	75–99	15–99	15–44	45–54	55–64	65–74	75–99	15–99
Austria	0	1	0	0	0	1	0	0	0	0	0	0
England	0	1	3	6	4	14	0	0	0	0	4	4
Estonia	0	0	0	0	0	0	0	0	0	0	0	0
Finland	0	0	0	0	0	0	0	0	0	0	0	0
Germany	1	1	0	0	0	2	0	0	0	0	0	0
Iceland	0	0	0	0	0	0	0	0	0	0	0	0
Italy	0	0	2	1	0	3	0	0	1	0	1	2
Poland	0	0	0	0	0	0	0	0	0	0	1	1
Scotland	0	0	0	1	1	2	0	0	1	1	1	3
Slovakia	0	1	4	2	5	12	0	0	1	0	4	5
Slovenia	0	0	0	1	1	2	0	0	0	0	2	2
Spain	0	0	1	0	0	1	0	0	0	0	0	0
Switzerland	0	0	0	0	0	0	0	0	0	0	0	0
Pool	1	4	10	11	11	37	0	0	3	1	13	17

HEAD & NECK

Country	Males						Females					
	15–44	45–54	55–64	65–74	75–99	15–99	15–44	45–54	55–64	65–74	75–99	15–99
Austria	1	1	2	0	1	5	0	0	0	0	0	0
England	0	16	25	26	29	96	1	2	7	17	33	60
Estonia	0	0	0	0	0	0	0	0	0	0	0	0
Finland	0	0	0	0	0	0	0	0	0	0	2	2
Germany	1	4	1	1	0	7	0	0	0	0	0	0
Iceland	0	0	0	0	0	0	0	0	0	0	0	0
Italy	0	0	4	6	5	15	0	1	1	0	8	10
Poland	0	1	1	0	2	4	0	0	1	0	3	4
Scotland	1	0	4	5	9	19	0	0	1	2	5	8
Slovakia	4	6	15	9	10	44	0	0	1	6	11	18
Slovenia	0	1	3	3	6	13	0	0	0	1	2	3
Spain	0	5	8	4	6	23	0	0	2	2	3	7
Switzerland	0	0	0	0	1	1	0	0	0	0	1	1
Pool	7	34	63	55	68	227	1	3	13	28	68	113

OESOPHAGUS

Country	Males						Females					
	15–44	45–54	55–64	65–74	75–99	15–99	15–44	45–54	55–64	65–74	75–99	15–99
Austria	0	2	2	0	2	6	0	0	0	0	0	0
England	17	20	108	182	270	597	4	7	44	103	325	483
Estonia	0	0	0	1	0	1	0	0	0	0	1	1
Finland	0	1	1	2	5	9	0	0	0	1	4	5
Germany	0	3	5	6	3	17	0	0	1	0	6	7
Iceland	0	0	0	0	0	0	0	0	0	0	0	0
Italy	0	1	4	6	24	35	0	0	0	2	14	16
Poland	1	0	8	8	5	22	0	0	0	4	8	12
Scotland	2	2	15	17	16	52	0	2	5	7	30	44
Slovakia	1	4	14	22	19	60	2	1	0	4	5	12
Slovenia	0	0	5	3	13	21	0	0	1	0	10	11
Spain	2	2	10	14	28	56	0	0	0	2	17	19
Switzerland	0	0	0	0	1	1	0	0	0	0	1	1
Pool	23	35	172	261	386	877	6	10	51	123	421	611

STOMACH

Country	Males						Females					
	15–44	45–54	55–64	65–74	75–99	15–99	15–44	45–54	55–64	65–74	75–99	15–99
Austria	0	1	4	8	14	27	0	1	2	11	22	36
England	18	62	196	484	873	1633	8	16	86	252	1066	1428
Estonia	0	0	0	0	0	0	0	0	0	0	0	0
Finland	0	0	0	2	9	11	0	0	0	2	18	20
Germany	0	5	2	10	30	47	0	1	3	7	69	80
Iceland	0	0	0	0	1	1	0	0	0	0	1	1
Italy	2	5	17	56	158	238	0	5	9	23	260	297
Poland	1	4	33	25	42	105	1	4	9	16	47	77
Scotland	1	2	20	58	69	150	1	2	16	32	103	154
Slovakia	6	13	49	70	154	292	1	5	22	49	188	265
Slovenia	1	6	16	19	65	107	0	0	6	13	95	114
Spain	8	9	28	66	112	223	5	3	18	16	169	211
Switzerland	0	0	1	0	1	2	0	0	0	0	1	1
Pool	37	107	366	798	1528	2836	16	37	171	421	2039	2684

SMALL INTESTINE

Country	Males						Females					
	15–44	45–54	55–64	65–74	75–99	15–99	15–44	45–54	55–64	65–74	75–99	15–99
Austria	0	0	1	0	0	1	0	0	0	0	0	0
England	3	3	5	10	8	29	1	0	6	2	26	35
Estonia	0	0	0	0	0	0	0	0	0	0	0	0
Finland	0	0	0	0	0	0	0	0	0	2	2	4
Germany	0	0	0	0	0	0	0	1	0	0	0	1
Iceland	0	0	0	0	0	0	0	0	0	0	0	0
Italy	0	0	0	1	3	4	0	0	0	0	1	1
Poland	0	0	1	0	0	1	0	0	0	0	1	1
Scotland	0	0	0	3	1	4	0	0	1	0	2	3
Slovakia	0	0	2	4	5	11	0	0	0	3	7	10
Slovenia	0	1	0	0	0	1	0	0	0	0	0	0
Spain	0	0	0	2	1	3	0	0	0	0	2	2
Switzerland	0	0	0	0	0	0	0	0	0	0	0	0
Pool	3	4	9	20	18	54	1	1	7	7	41	57

COLON

Country	Males						Females					
	15–44	45–54	55–64	65–74	75–99	15–99	15–44	45–54	55–64	65–74	75–99	15–99
Austria	0	0	2	2	8	12	0	0	2	6	25	33
England	22	53	205	413	772	1465	13	67	175	401	1673	2329
Estonia	0	0	0	0	0	0	0	0	0	1	2	3
Finland	0	1	1	1	2	5	0	0	1	2	12	15
Germany	0	0	3	11	33	47	0	3	7	13	75	98
Iceland	0	0	0	0	0	0	0	0	0	0	0	0
Italy	2	3	7	24	64	100	0	8	11	24	106	149
Poland	2	3	14	10	25	54	0	7	16	10	32	55
Scotland	0	5	17	28	56	106	0	4	23	43	151	221
Slovakia	1	9	25	45	58	138	2	2	16	41	134	195
Slovenia	0	1	2	4	11	18	0	0	0	3	26	29
Spain	1	3	16	43	72	135	1	4	7	27	94	133
Switzerland	0	0	0	0	5	5	0	0	0	1	6	7
Pool	28	78	292	582	1109	2089	16	95	258	572	2337	3278

RECTUM

Country	Males						Females					
	15–44	45–54	55–64	65–74	75–99	15–99	15–44	45–54	55–64	65–74	75–99	15–99
Austria	0	1	3	2	6	12	1	0	1	3	6	11
England	13	31	87	197	361	689	6	18	48	149	559	780
Estonia	0	0	0	0	0	0	0	0	0	0	1	1
Finland	0	0	2	0	0	2	0	0	1	0	6	7
Germany	1	1	1	3	11	17	0	0	2	1	17	20
Iceland	0	0	0	0	0	0	0	0	0	0	0	0
Italy	3	1	8	9	30	51	0	0	4	6	39	49
Poland	0	3	4	17	20	44	1	1	6	11	27	46
Scotland	0	8	7	15	23	53	0	1	8	10	41	60
Slovakia	1	3	17	41	57	119	3	2	7	26	84	122
Slovenia	0	1	4	10	19	34	0	1	1	5	32	39
Spain	1	2	7	10	31	51	0	1	4	8	48	61
Switzerland	0	0	0	0	1	1	0	0	0	0	0	0
Pool	19	51	140	304	560	1074	11	24	82	219	860	1196

LIVER

Country	Males						Females					
	15–44	45–54	55–64	65–74	75–99	15–99	15–44	45–54	55–64	65–74	75–99	15–99
Austria	0	0	2	0	3	5	0	0	0	2	7	9
England	12	13	49	85	88	247	6	7	26	49	110	198
Estonia	0	0	0	2	0	2	0	0	0	0	1	1
Finland	0	1	3	0	7	11	0	1	0	2	6	9
Germany	0	5	3	12	17	37	1	0	2	6	22	31
Iceland	0	0	0	0	0	0	0	0	0	0	0	0
Italy	2	7	20	45	77	151	1	0	8	23	111	143
Poland	1	3	13	13	12	42	2	1	8	20	61	92
Scotland	1	2	8	16	5	32	1	2	9	7	8	27
Slovakia	5	12	44	36	49	146	2	2	15	27	64	110
Slovenia	0	0	0	0	0	0	0	0	0	0	0	0
Spain	1	11	27	66	72	177	1	4	14	20	88	127
Switzerland	1	0	0	0	3	4	1	0	0	0	0	1
Pool	23	54	169	275	333	854	15	17	82	156	478	748

BILIARY TRACT

Country	Males						Females					
	15–44	45–54	55–64	65–74	75–99	15–99	15–44	45–54	55–64	65–74	75–99	15–99
Austria	0	0	0	0	2	2	0	0	2	1	10	13
England	0	4	17	33	37	91	2	7	19	47	98	173
Estonia	0	0	0	0	0	0	0	0	0	0	0	0
Finland	0	0	0	1	2	3	0	0	1	1	6	8
Germany	1	0	2	3	5	11	0	0	3	10	38	51
Iceland	0	0	0	0	0	0	0	0	0	0	0	0
Italy	0	0	2	4	16	22	0	2	2	2	29	35
Poland	2	2	4	2	7	17	0	1	9	16	26	52
Scotland	1	0	1	2	3	7	0	1	2	4	8	15
Slovakia	1	2	6	18	22	49	0	1	12	18	46	77
Slovenia	0	1	2	4	7	14	0	0	4	2	19	25
Spain	0	1	5	5	13	24	0	0	2	13	36	51
Switzerland	0	0	0	1	1	2	0	0	0	0	1	1
Pool	5	10	39	73	115	242	2	12	56	114	317	501

PANCREAS

Country	Males						Females					
	15–44	45–54	55–64	65–74	75–99	15–99	15–44	45–54	55–64	65–74	75–99	15–99
Austria	0	0	4	1	8	13	0	0	1	5	16	22
England	16	54	164	335	466	1035	13	34	121	307	714	1189
Estonia	0	0	0	1	0	1	0	0	0	0	0	0
Finland	0	1	1	4	9	15	0	1	0	5	14	20
Germany	1	6	12	16	33	68	0	2	10	22	48	82
Iceland	0	0	0	0	1	1	0	0	0	0	0	0
Italy	0	6	9	23	39	77	1	0	8	20	77	106
Poland	2	5	10	9	12	38	1	1	7	13	27	49
Scotland	0	6	19	33	33	91	0	4	18	27	56	105
Slovakia	6	12	28	44	40	130	4	7	15	34	67	127
Slovenia	0	2	1	7	6	16	0	0	1	5	23	29
Spain	0	7	22	27	42	98	1	2	9	20	79	111
Switzerland	0	0	0	1	1	2	0	0	1	1	3	5
Pool	25	97	272	501	690	1585	20	51	191	459	1124	1845

NASAL CAVITIES

Country	Males						Females					
	15–44	45–54	55–64	65–74	75–99	15–99	15–44	45–54	55–64	65–74	75–99	15–99
Austria	0	0	0	0	0	0	0	0	0	0	0	0
England	0	2	1	6	11	20	0	0	0	1	10	11
Estonia	0	0	0	0	0	0	0	0	0	0	0	0
Finland	0	0	0	0	0	0	0	0	0	0	0	0
Germany	0	0	0	0	0	0	0	0	0	1	0	1
Iceland	0	0	0	0	0	0	0	0	0	0	0	0
Italy	0	0	0	0	0	0	0	0	0	0	2	2
Poland	0	0	0	0	0	0	0	0	0	0	0	0
Scotland	0	0	0	0	0	0	0	0	0	0	1	1
Slovakia	1	0	0	0	2	3	1	0	0	1	1	3
Slovenia	0	0	0	0	0	0	0	1	0	1	0	2
Spain	1	0	1	0	1	3	0	0	0	0	0	0
Switzerland	0	0	0	0	0	0	0	0	0	0	0	0
Pool	2	2	2	6	14	26	1	1	0	4	14	20

LARYNX

Country	Males						Females					
	15–44	45–54	55–64	65–74	75–99	15–99	15–44	45–54	55–64	65–74	75–99	15–99
Austria	1	0	0	3	3	7	0	0	0	0	0	0
England	1	5	14	39	48	107	0	1	5	16	18	40
Estonia	0	0	0	0	0	0	0	0	0	0	0	0
Finland	0	0	0	0	0	0	0	0	0	0	0	0
Germany	0	1	1	2	1	5	0	0	0	0	0	0
Iceland	0	0	0	0	0	0	0	0	0	0	0	0
Italy	0	3	6	6	22	37	0	0	0	1	9	10
Poland	0	0	3	1	3	8	0	1	0	4	0	5
Scotland	0	1	1	4	7	13	0	0	0	2	1	3
Slovakia	2	12	22	15	21	72	0	1	0	1	5	7
Slovenia	0	3	2	2	2	9	0	0	0	0	0	0
Spain	1	3	17	13	8	42	0	0	0	0	2	2
Switzerland	0	0	1	1	0	2	0	0	0	0	0	0
Pool	5	28	67	87	115	302	0	3	5	24	35	67

LUNG

Country	Males						Females					
	15–44	45–54	55–64	65–74	75–99	15–99	15–44	45–54	55–64	65–74	75–99	15–99
Austria	2	1	12	18	40	73	1	0	1	5	11	18
England	31	147	929	2309	3776	7192	15	71	449	1022	1876	3433
Estonia	1	0	2	0	3	6	0	0	0	0	0	0
Finland	0	0	7	18	35	60	1	0	1	5	14	21
Germany	4	19	83	116	167	389	0	3	8	16	57	84
Iceland	0	0	0	0	0	0	0	0	0	0	0	0
Italy	2	15	91	148	233	489	2	3	14	36	71	126
Poland	5	11	62	62	83	223	0	3	8	11	16	38
Scotland	2	27	144	289	426	888	0	14	77	169	167	427
Slovakia	16	91	221	283	298	909	7	8	24	48	86	173
Slovenia	2	2	15	24	50	93	0	0	2	7	23	32
Spain	4	24	77	120	202	427	6	1	4	22	49	82
Switzerland	0	0	1	1	4	6	0	0	0	0	2	2
Pool	69	337	1644	3888	5317	10755	32	104	589	1339	2372	4436

PLEURA

Country	Males						Females					
	15–44	45–54	55–64	65–74	75–99	15–99	15–44	45–54	55–64	65–74	75–99	15–99
Austria	0	0	0	0	0	0	0	0	0	0	1	1
England	5	6	28	52	35	126	0	1	6	7	10	24
Estonia	0	0	0	0	0	0	0	0	0	0	0	0
Finland	0	0	0	0	1	1	0	0	0	0	2	2
Germany	0	0	1	0	0	1	0	0	0	1	0	1
Iceland	0	0	0	0	0	0	0	0	0	0	0	0
Italy	0	1	0	4	5	10	1	0	0	1	2	4
Poland	0	0	1	0	0	1	0	0	0	0	0	0
Scotland	0	0	1	2	0	3	0	0	0	0	0	0
Slovakia	0	1	3	1	5	10	1	0	0	1	2	4
Slovenia	0	0	0	0	0	0	0	0	1	0	2	3
Spain	0	0	1	0	2	3	0	1	0	0	0	1
Switzerland	0	0	0	0	0	0	0	0	0	0	0	0
Pool	5	8	35	59	48	155	2	2	7	10	19	40

BONE

Country	Males						Females					
	15–44	45–54	55–64	65–74	75–99	15–99	15–44	45–54	55–64	65–74	75–99	15–99
Austria	0	0	0	1	2	3	0	0	0	0	1	1
England	6	2	2	3	8	21	4	1	2	4	12	23
Estonia	0	0	0	0	0	0	0	0	0	0	0	0
Finland	0	0	0	0	0	0	0	0	0	0	0	0
Germany	0	0	0	0	1	1	0	0	0	3	1	4
Iceland	0	0	0	0	0	0	0	0	0	0	0	0
Italy	0	0	0	0	5	5	0	0	1	3	5	9
Poland	0	2	4	5	0	11	0	0	0	0	3	3
Scotland	0	0	0	2	1	3	0	0	0	0	0	0
Slovakia	2	2	2	4	8	18	1	2	4	1	4	12
Slovenia	0	1	0	0	1	2	0	0	1	0	2	3
Spain	2	0	1	3	3	9	3	0	0	2	4	9
Switzerland	0	0	0	0	0	0	0	0	0	0	0	0
Pool	10	7	9	18	29	73	8	3	8	13	32	64

SOFT TISSUES

Country	Males						Females					
	15–44	45–54	55–64	65–74	75–99	15–99	15–44	45–54	55–64	65–74	75–99	15–99
Austria	0	0	0	1	0	1	0	0	0	1	2	3
England	0	5	2	10	10	27	2	0	2	5	26	35
Estonia	0	0	0	0	0	0	0	0	0	0	0	0
Finland	0	0	0	0	0	0	0	0	0	0	2	2
Germany	2	0	1	0	1	4	0	1	0	0	0	1
Iceland	0	0	0	0	0	0	0	0	0	0	0	0
Italy	0	0	1	0	1	2	1	0	1	0	3	5
Poland	1	0	1	1	0	3	0	0	0	0	0	0
Scotland	0	0	1	1	1	3	0	1	0	1	3	5
Slovakia	0	1	2	1	3	7	1	0	1	2	4	8
Slovenia	0	0	0	0	0	0	0	0	0	0	1	1
Spain	1	0	1	1	0	3	0	0	0	0	1	1
Switzerland	0	0	0	0	0	0	0	0	0	0	0	0
Pool	4	6	9	15	16	50	4	2	4	9	42	61

MELANOMA OF SKIN

Country	Males						Females					
	15–44	45–54	55–64	65–74	75–99	15–99	15–44	45–54	55–64	65–74	75–99	15–99
Austria	0	0	2	1	0	3	0	0	0	0	3	3
England	15	10	14	12	21	72	12	12	21	18	44	107
Estonia	0	0	0	0	0	0	0	0	0	0	0	0
Finland	0	0	0	0	0	0	0	0	0	0	2	2
Germany	0	2	0	2	1	5	0	0	1	1	3	5
Iceland	0	0	0	0	0	0	0	0	0	0	0	0
Italy	1	1	0	0	6	8	0	0	1	1	4	6
Poland	1	0	3	0	0	4	0	2	1	0	4	7
Scotland	0	1	0	0	0	1	0	1	0	0	1	2
Slovakia	5	0	2	2	0	9	1	0	0	3	11	15
Slovenia	0	0	0	1	1	2	0	0	0	0	4	4
Spain	1	2	2	0	0	5	1	1	0	1	5	8
Switzerland	0	0	0	0	0	0	0	0	0	0	0	0
Pool	23	16	23	18	29	109	14	16	24	24	81	159

BREAST

Country	Males						Females					
	15–44	45–54	55–64	65–74	75–99	15–99	15–44	45–54	55–64	65–74	75–99	15–99
Austria	0	0	0	0	0	0	2	6	14	8	29	59
England	0	0	3	3	4	10	66	163	328	618	2246	3421
Estonia	0	0	0	0	0	0	0	0	0	0	1	1
Finland	0	0	0	0	0	0	0	1	0	3	8	12
Germany	0	0	0	0	4	4	1	7	6	15	59	88
Iceland	0	0	0	0	0	0	0	0	0	0	0	0
Italy	0	0	0	1	3	4	4	18	24	34	150	230
Poland	0	1	1	0	1	3	4	3	19	23	39	88
Scotland	0	0	0	3	0	3	2	11	24	58	210	305
Slovakia	0	0	0	0	1	1	6	16	71	67	127	287
Slovenia	0	0	0	0	2	2	2	3	5	15	59	84
Spain	0	0	0	0	1	1	15	32	53	58	132	290
Switzerland	0	0	0	0	0	0	0	0	3	1	12	16
Pool	0	1	4	7	16	28	102	260	547	900	3072	4881

CERVIX UTERI

Country	Males						Females					
	15–44	45–54	55–64	65–74	75–99	15–99	15–44	45–54	55–64	65–74	75–99	15–99
Austria	0	0	0	0	0	0	1	0	0	4	3	8
England	0	0	0	0	0	0	38	28	36	71	122	295
Estonia	0	0	0	0	0	0	0	0	0	0	0	0
Finland	0	0	0	0	0	0	0	0	0	0	1	1
Germany	0	0	0	0	0	0	0	0	1	0	3	4
Iceland	0	0	0	0	0	0	0	0	0	0	0	0
Italy	0	0	0	0	0	0	0	1	1	2	1	5
Poland	0	0	0	0	0	0	1	0	2	8	5	16
Scotland	0	0	0	0	0	0	0	2	0	5	9	16
Slovakia	0	0	0	0	0	0	6	6	11	14	18	55
Slovenia	0	0	0	0	0	0	0	0	0	1	0	1
Spain	0	0	0	0	0	0	3	3	2	1	2	11
Switzerland	0	0	0	0	0	0	0	0	0	0	1	1
Pool	0	0	0	0	0	0	49	40	53	106	165	413

CORPUS UTERI

Country	Males						Females					
	15–44	45–54	55–64	65–74	75–99	15–99	15–44	45–54	55–64	65–74	75–99	15–99
Austria	0	0	0	0	0	0	0	1	0	0	6	7
England	0	0	0	0	0	0	2	7	28	60	244	341
Estonia	0	0	0	0	0	0	0	0	0	0	1	1
Finland	0	0	0	0	0	0	0	0	0	0	2	2
Germany	0	0	0	0	0	0	0	0	2	3	5	10
Iceland	0	0	0	0	0	0	0	0	0	0	0	0
Italy	0	0	0	0	0	0	0	0	0	1	2	3
Poland	0	0	0	0	0	0	0	0	2	1	5	8
Scotland	0	0	0	0	0	0	0	2	2	4	12	20
Slovakia	0	0	0	0	0	0	3	1	11	23	39	77
Slovenia	0	0	0	0	0	0	0	0	3	2	5	10
Spain	0	0	0	0	0	0	0	0	3	3	8	14
Switzerland	0	0	0	0	0	0	0	0	1	0	0	1
Pool	0	0	0	0	0	0	5	11	52	97	329	494

OVARY

Country	Males						Females					
	15–44	45–54	55–64	65–74	75–99	15–99	15–44	45–54	55–64	65–74	75–99	15–99
Austria	0	0	0	0	0	0	0	1	3	5	5	14
England	0	0	0	0	0	0	19	81	169	222	469	960
Estonia	0	0	0	0	0	0	0	0	0	0	0	0
Finland	0	0	0	0	0	0	0	0	2	0	4	6
Germany	0	0	0	0	0	0	1	1	7	15	27	51
Iceland	0	0	0	0	0	0	0	0	0	0	0	0
Italy	0	0	0	0	0	0	1	1	8	11	28	49
Poland	0	0	0	0	0	0	2	4	8	4	13	31
Scotland	0	0	0	0	0	0	1	3	18	23	27	72
Slovakia	0	0	0	0	0	0	5	6	20	20	25	76
Slovenia	0	0	0	0	0	0	0	0	3	1	10	14
Spain	0	0	0	0	0	0	6	2	3	4	12	27
Switzerland	0	0	0	0	0	0	0	0	0	1	2	3
Pool	0	0	0	0	0	0	35	99	241	306	622	1303

VAGINA AND VULVA

Country	Males						Females					
	15–44	45–54	55–64	65–74	75–99	15–99	15–44	45–54	55–64	65–74	75–99	15–99
Austria	0	0	0	0	0	0	0	0	0	0	1	1
England	0	0	0	0	0	0	0	0	4	22	98	124
Estonia	0	0	0	0	0	0	0	0	0	0	0	0
Finland	0	0	0	0	0	0	0	0	0	0	3	3
Germany	0	0	0	0	0	0	0	3	0	3	17	23
Iceland	0	0	0	0	0	0	0	0	0	0	0	0
Italy	0	0	0	0	0	0	0	0	1	2	14	17
Poland	0	0	0	0	0	0	1	1	0	3	11	16
Scotland	0	0	0	0	0	0	0	1	1	1	8	11
Slovakia	0	0	0	0	0	0	1	1	3	5	18	28
Slovenia	0	0	0	0	0	0	0	0	0	0	3	3
Spain	0	0	0	0	0	0	0	0	1	3	19	23
Switzerland	0	0	0	0	0	0	0	0	0	0	2	2
Pool	0	0	0	0	0	0	2	6	10	39	194	251

PROSTATE

Country	Males						Females					
	15–44	45–54	55–64	65–74	75–99	15–99	15–44	45–54	55–64	65–74	75–99	15–99
Austria	0	1	3	10	33	47	0	0	0	0	0	0
England	1	5	90	441	1584	2121	0	0	0	0	0	0
Estonia	0	0	0	0	1	1	0	0	0	0	0	0
Finland	0	0	0	5	23	28	0	0	0	0	0	0
Germany	0	0	2	8	67	77	0	0	0	0	0	0
Iceland	0	0	0	0	1	1	0	0	0	0	0	0
Italy	0	0	8	24	140	172	0	0	0	0	0	0
Poland	0	1	2	19	31	63	0	0	0	0	0	0
Scotland	0	0	5	26	98	129	0	0	0	0	0	0
Slovakia	0	5	9	76	173	263	0	0	0	0	0	0
Slovenia	0	0	2	8	65	75	0	0	0	0	0	0
Spain	0	1	9	66	238	314	0	0	0	0	0	0
Switzerland	0	0	0	0	10	10	0	0	0	0	0	0
Pool	1	13	130	683	2474	3301	0	0	0	0	0	0

TESTIS

Country	Males						Females					
	15–44	45–54	55–64	65–74	75–99	15–99	15–44	45–54	55–64	65–74	75–99	15–99
Austria	0	0	0	0	0	0	0	0	0	0	0	0
England	13	2	3	4	9	31	0	0	0	0	0	0
Estonia	0	0	0	0	0	0	0	0	0	0	0	0
Finland	0	0	0	0	0	0	0	0	0	0	0	0
Germany	1	0	0	0	0	1	0	0	0	0	0	0
Iceland	0	0	0	0	0	0	0	0	0	0	0	0
Italy	0	0	0	0	2	2	0	0	0	0	0	0
Poland	0	0	0	0	0	0	0	0	0	0	0	0
Scotland	0	0	0	0	0	0	0	0	0	0	0	0
Slovakia	1	0	0	1	4	6	0	0	0	0	0	0
Slovenia	0	0	0	0	0	0	0	0	0	0	0	0
Spain	0	0	0	1	1	2	0	0	0	0	0	0
Switzerland	0	0	0	0	0	0	0	0	0	0	0	0
Pool	15	2	3	6	16	42	0	0	0	0	0	0

PENIS

Country	Males						Females					
	15–44	45–54	55–64	65–74	75–99	15–99	15–44	45–54	55–64	65–74	75–99	15–99
Austria	0	0	0	0	0	0	0	0	0	0	0	0
England	0	0	1	6	12	19	0	0	0	0	0	0
Estonia	0	0	0	0	0	0	0	0	0	0	0	0
Finland	0	0	0	0	0	0	0	0	0	0	0	0
Germany	0	0	0	0	1	1	0	0	0	0	0	0
Iceland	0	0	0	0	0	0	0	0	0	0	0	0
Italy	0	0	0	0	0	0	0	0	0	0	0	0
Poland	0	0	1	0	0	1	0	0	0	0	0	0
Scotland	0	0	1	1	1	3	0	0	0	0	0	0
Slovakia	0	1	1	2	2	6	0	0	0	0	0	0
Slovenia	0	0	1	0	1	2	0	0	0	0	0	0
Spain	1	0	0	0	3	4	0	0	0	0	0	0
Switzerland	0	0	0	0	0	0	0	0	0	0	0	0
Pool	1	1	5	9	20	36	0	0	0	0	0	0

BLADDER

Country	Males						Females					
	15–44	45–54	55–64	65–74	75–99	15–99	15–44	45–54	55–64	65–74	75–99	15–99
Austria	0	0	0	1	7	8	0	0	1	4	3	8
England	1	9	47	148	380	585	2	10	23	63	297	395
Estonia	0	0	0	0	1	1	0	0	0	0	0	0
Finland	0	0	0	1	4	5	0	0	0	0	0	0
Germany	0	1	4	7	18	30	0	0	0	5	11	16
Iceland	0	0	0	0	0	0	0	0	0	0	0	0
Italy	0	0	6	15	52	73	0	0	1	3	26	30
Poland	0	2	7	3	13	25	0	2	0	1	9	12
Scotland	0	0	3	6	19	28	0	0	0	3	17	20
Slovakia	0	4	9	29	57	99	0	1	5	6	22	34
Slovenia	0	2	1	2	8	13	0	0	1	0	9	10
Spain	0	0	6	23	69	98	1	0	2	3	20	26
Switzerland	0	0	0	0	1	1	0	0	1	0	0	1
Pool	1	18	83	235	629	966	3	13	34	88	414	552

KIDNEY

Country	Males						Females					
	15–44	45–54	55–64	65–74	75–99	15–99	15–44	45–54	55–64	65–74	75–99	15–99
Austria	0	0	0	2	4	6	0	1	0	1	6	8
England	11	20	91	124	181	427	2	9	36	66	173	286
Estonia	0	0	0	0	0	0	0	0	1	1	0	2
Finland	0	0	2	4	3	9	1	0	1	1	7	10
Germany	0	3	7	5	6	21	0	3	4	6	12	25
Iceland	0	0	0	0	0	0	0	0	0	0	0	0
Italy	1	1	8	5	17	32	0	0	3	8	18	29
Poland	2	2	9	5	8	26	0	1	4	5	13	23
Scotland	0	1	4	10	14	29	0	2	5	6	10	23
Slovakia	1	5	21	17	28	72	3	3	4	16	37	63
Slovenia	0	1	1	0	3	5	0	0	0	1	4	5
Spain	0	1	4	13	23	41	0	0	1	3	12	16
Switzerland	0	0	0	0	1	1	0	0	0	0	2	2
Pool	15	34	147	185	288	669	6	19	59	114	294	492

CHOROID (MELANOMA)

Country	Males						Females					
	15–44	45–54	55–64	65–74	75–99	15–99	15–44	45–54	55–64	65–74	75–99	15–99
Austria	0	0	0	0	0	0	0	0	0	0	0	0
England	0	0	0	0	0	0	0	1	0	0	4	5
Estonia	0	0	0	0	0	0	0	0	0	0	0	0
Finland	0	0	0	0	0	0	0	0	0	0	0	0
Germany	0	0	0	0	0	0	0	0	0	0	0	0
Iceland	0	0	0	0	0	0	0	0	0	0	0	0
Italy	0	0	0	0	0	0	0	0	0	0	1	1
Poland	0	0	0	0	0	0	0	0	0	0	0	0
Scotland	0	0	0	0	0	0	0	0	0	0	0	0
Slovakia	0	0	0	0	0	0	0	0	0	0	0	0
Slovenia	0	0	0	0	0	0	0	0	0	0	0	0
Spain	0	0	0	0	0	0	0	0	0	0	0	0
Switzerland	0	0	0	0	0	0	0	0	0	0	0	0
Pool	0	0	0	0	0	0	0	1	0	0	5	6

BRAIN

Country	Males						Females					
	15–44	45–54	55–64	65–74	75–99	15–99	15–44	45–54	55–64	65–74	75–99	15–99
Austria	0	0	1	1	0	2	0	2	1	0	1	4
England	25	27	53	61	33	199	16	21	39	63	58	197
Estonia	0	0	0	0	0	0	0	0	0	0	0	0
Finland	0	0	3	2	3	8	1	0	0	4	10	15
Germany	3	1	7	6	2	19	2	1	4	4	0	11
Iceland	0	0	0	0	1	1	0	1	0	0	0	1
Italy	5	3	11	11	9	39	4	2	3	12	15	36
Poland	2	1	5	3	2	13	3	2	9	2	6	22
Scotland	0	7	3	6	2	18	1	0	0	2	3	6
Slovakia	4	11	18	21	8	62	14	20	18	7	11	70
Slovenia	0	3	3	2	0	8	2	1	2	1	1	7
Spain	5	9	12	11	30	67	4	5	13	15	12	49
Switzerland	0	0	0	1	1	2	0	0	0	0	0	0
Pool	44	62	116	125	91	438	47	55	89	110	117	418

THYROID GLAND

Country	Males						Females					
	15–44	45–54	55–64	65–74	75–99	15–99	15–44	45–54	55–64	65–74	75–99	15–99
Austria	0	0	0	0	0	0	0	0	0	0	0	0
England	0	1	5	2	11	19	1	1	5	19	38	64
Estonia	0	0	0	0	0	0	0	0	0	0	1	1
Finland	0	0	0	0	0	0	0	0	0	0	1	1
Germany	0	0	0	0	1	1	0	1	1	0	5	7
Iceland	0	0	0	0	0	0	0	0	0	0	0	0
Italy	0	0	0	0	0	0	0	0	0	1	0	1
Poland	0	0	1	0	0	1	0	0	1	1	3	5
Scotland	0	0	2	2	0	4	0	0	1	0	1	2
Slovakia	0	0	0	0	0	0	0	0	0	0	0	0
Slovenia	0	0	0	0	0	0	0	0	0	0	0	0
Spain	0	0	0	0	0	0	0	0	0	0	0	0
Switzerland	0	0	0	0	0	0	0	0	0	0	0	0
Pool	0	1	8	4	12	25	1	2	8	21	49	81

NON-HODGKIN'S LYMPHOMA

Country	Males						Females					
	15–44	45–54	55–64	65–74	75–99	15–99	15–44	45–54	55–64	65–74	75–99	15–99
Austria	0	0	0	0	3	3	0	0	0	1	4	5
England	26	27	77	113	153	396	12	20	35	99	222	388
Estonia	0	0	0	0	0	0	0	0	0	0	0	0
Finland	1	0	1	1	2	5	0	0	0	0	2	2
Germany	1	0	3	3	3	10	1	1	3	2	8	15
Iceland	0	0	0	0	0	0	0	0	0	0	0	0
Italy	0	1	1	3	5	10	1	1	1	2	12	17
Poland	1	0	0	1	3	5	0	1	1	3	0	5
Scotland	1	0	3	4	6	14	0	0	1	7	19	27
Slovakia	1	5	10	10	8	34	1	0	4	8	16	29
Slovenia	0	0	0	0	0	0	0	0	0	0	0	0
Spain	3	3	1	4	6	17	0	2	1	2	9	14
Switzerland	0	0	0	0	1	1	0	0	0	0	1	1
Pool	34	36	96	139	190	495	15	25	46	124	293	503

HODGKIN'S DISEASE

Country	Males						Females					
	15–44	45–54	55–64	65–74	75–99	15–99	15–44	45–54	55–64	65–74	75–99	15–99
Austria	0	0	0	0	0	0	0	0	0	0	0	0
England	8	2	3	10	7	30	4	0	6	8	13	31
Estonia	0	0	0	0	0	0	0	0	0	0	0	0
Finland	1	0	0	0	0	1	0	0	0	0	1	1
Germany	0	0	1	2	1	4	0	0	1	1	0	2
Iceland	0	0	0	0	0	0	0	0	0	0	0	0
Italy	0	2	1	1	0	4	0	0	1	1	3	5
Poland	0	0	1	0	0	1	2	0	0	0	1	3
Scotland	0	0	0	0	0	0	0	0	1	0	0	1
Slovakia	4	3	2	2	1	12	5	1	1	0	3	10
Slovenia	0	0	0	0	0	0	0	0	0	0	0	0
Spain	2	0	0	0	0	2	1	1	0	2	1	5
Switzerland	0	0	0	0	0	0	0	0	0	0	0	0
Pool	15	7	8	15	9	54	12	2	10	12	22	58

MULTIPLE MYELOMA

	Males						Females					
Country	15–44	45–54	55–64	65–74	75–99	15–99	15–44	45–54	55–64	65–74	75–99	15–99
Austria	0	0	0	3	0	3	0	0	0	1	6	7
England	2	18	49	122	187	378	2	13	28	97	249	389
Estonia	0	0	0	0	0	0	0	0	0	0	0	0
Finland	0	2	1	4	3	10	0	0	1	1	14	16
Germany	0	1	1	0	11	13	0	1	2	7	13	23
Iceland	0	0	0	0	0	0	0	0	0	0	0	0
Italy	0	0	4	5	13	22	0	1	2	8	26	37
Poland	0	0	1	1	1	3	0	0	0	1	4	5
Scotland	0	0	5	7	10	22	0	0	1	6	15	22
Slovakia	0	5	8	7	8	28	0	2	3	6	9	20
Slovenia	0	0	0	0	1	1	0	0	0	0	0	0
Spain	0	2	3	5	12	22	0	0	0	5	12	17
Switzerland	0	0	0	0	0	0	0	0	0	0	0	0
Pool	2	28	72	154	246	502	2	17	37	132	348	536

LEUKAEMIA

	Males						Females					
Country	15–44	45–54	55–64	65–74	75–99	15–99	15–44	45–54	55–64	65–74	75–99	15–99
Austria	0	0	0	2	2	4	0	0	0	2	7	9
England	52	42	87	193	356	730	48	35	70	144	515	812
Estonia	0	0	0	0	0	0	0	0	0	0	0	0
Finland	2	0	2	7	9	20	1	2	1	3	19	26
Germany	0	1	8	5	21	35	3	1	5	15	27	51
Iceland	0	0	0	0	0	0	0	0	0	0	0	0
Italy	2	3	5	10	26	46	2	0	4	7	41	54
Poland	0	1	6	6	7	20	0	1	1	7	13	22
Scotland	0	1	6	14	19	40	1	1	3	8	37	50
Slovakia	8	7	28	33	40	116	11	13	16	25	45	110
Slovenia	0	0	0	0	1	1	0	0	1	0	6	7
Spain	8	2	14	10	26	60	4	1	2	8	16	31
Switzerland	0	0	2	1	3	6	0	0	0	0	2	2
Pool	72	57	158	281	510	1078	70	54	103	219	728	1174

ACUTE LYMPHATIC LEUKAEMIA

	Males						Females					
Country	15–44	45–54	55–64	65–74	75–99	15–99	15–44	45–54	55–64	65–74	75–99	15–99
Austria	0	0	0	0	0	0	0	0	0	0	0	0
England	9	4	3	6	7	29	3	2	3	7	11	26
Estonia	0	0	0	0	0	0	0	0	0	0	0	0
Finland	0	0	0	1	0	1	0	0	0	0	0	0
Germany	0	0	1	0	1	2	0	0	0	0	2	2
Iceland	0	0	0	0	0	0	0	0	0	0	0	0
Italy	0	0	0	0	2	2	0	0	0	0	1	1
Poland	0	0	2	0	1	3	0	0	0	1	1	2
Scotland	0	0	0	0	0	0	0	0	0	0	1	1
Slovakia	1	0	1	1	0	3	0	2	0	0	0	2
Slovenia	0	0	0	0	0	0	0	0	0	0	0	0
Spain	0	0	0	0	1	1	0	0	0	0	0	0
Switzerland	0	0	0	0	0	0	0	0	0	0	0	0
Pool	10	4	7	8	12	41	3	4	3	8	16	34

CHRONIC LYMPHATIC LEUKAEMIA

Country	Males						Females					
	15–44	45–54	55–64	65–74	75–99	15–99	15–44	45–54	55–64	65–74	75–99	15–99
Austria	0	0	0	1	2	3	0	0	0	0	3	3
England	1	5	24	51	145	226	3	1	13	29	215	261
Estonia	0	0	0	0	0	0	0	0	0	0	0	0
Finland	0	0	1	5	4	10	0	0	0	1	11	12
Germany	0	0	1	0	3	4	0	0	0	4	8	12
Iceland	0	0	0	0	0	0	0	0	0	0	0	0
Italy	0	0	1	2	6	9	1	0	1	0	10	12
Poland	0	0	0	1	2	2	0	0	0	1	3	4
Scotland	0	0	1	7	12	20	0	0	0	2	19	21
Slovakia	0	3	11	14	17	45	1	2	4	10	14	31
Slovenia	0	0	0	0	0	0	0	0	1	0	4	5
Spain	1	0	1	0	4	6	0	0	1	2	4	7
Switzerland	0	0	0	1	0	1	0	0	0	0	0	0
Pool	2	8	40	82	195	327	5	3	20	49	291	368

ACUTE MYELOID LEUKAEMIA

Country	Males						Females					
	15–44	45–54	55–64	65–74	75–99	15–99	15–44	45–54	55–64	65–74	75–99	15–99
Austria	0	0	0	1	0	1	0	0	0	1	0	1
England	23	18	34	69	74	218	27	22	33	45	95	222
Estonia	0	0	0	0	0	0	0	0	0	0	0	0
Finland	2	0	0	1	1	4	0	2	1	0	1	4
Germany	0	0	2	1	4	7	2	0	1	3	0	6
Iceland	0	0	0	0	0	0	0	0	0	0	0	0
Italy	0	0	4	2	0	6	1	0	1	2	2	6
Poland	0	0	2	1	1	4	0	1	0	1	6	8
Scotland	0	1	1	4	3	9	0	1	1	3	6	11
Slovakia	2	2	2	1	3	10	2	5	1	1	6	15
Slovenia	0	0	0	0	0	0	0	0	0	0	0	0
Spain	1	0	3	3	3	10	1	0	0	0	0	1
Switzerland	0	0	1	0	0	1	0	0	0	0	0	0
Pool	28	21	49	83	89	270	33	31	38	56	116	274

CHRONIC MYELOID LEUKAEMIA

Country	Males						Females					
	15–44	45–54	55–64	65–74	75–99	15–99	15–44	45–54	55–64	65–74	75–99	15–99
Austria	0	0	0	0	0	0	0	0	0	0	1	1
England	10	5	8	24	40	87	6	6	9	30	79	130
Estonia	0	0	0	0	0	0	0	0	0	0	0	0
Finland	0	0	1	0	1	2	0	0	0	1	1	2
Germany	0	0	1	1	3	5	0	0	1	0	2	3
Iceland	0	0	0	0	0	0	0	0	0	0	0	0
Italy	0	0	0	0	4	4	0	0	0	1	7	8
Poland	0	0	0	0	0	0	0	0	0	0	0	0
Scotland	0	0	1	0	0	1	0	0	0	0	6	6
Slovakia	3	1	5	8	4	21	5	0	1	5	6	17
Slovenia	0	0	0	0	0	0	0	0	0	0	1	1
Spain	2	0	2	1	5	10	0	1	1	0	2	4
Switzerland	0	0	0	0	0	0	0	0	0	0	0	0
Pool	15	6	18	34	57	130	11	7	12	37	105	172

Chapter 2

Methods of survival data analysis and presentation issues

A. Verdecchia, R. Capocaccia, M. Santaquilani and T. Hakulinen

Introduction

Basic methods for estimation of relative survival, for weighting country-specific survival in the European pool and for computing age-standardized relative survival rates for inter-country comparisons were described in the previous EUROCARE monograph (Verdecchia et al., 1995) and are briefly recalled here. Additional methodology used in the EUROCARE-2 analysis is then presented along with a description of the major choices made for presenting the results in Chapter 4.

Direct comparison of survival figures between the previous EUROCARE monograph (Berrino et al., 1995) and the present analysis for the 1985–89 period is strongly discouraged, as the cases refer to different countries and cancer registries (see Chapter 1) and a different standard population is assumed. In Chapter 6 of this monograph, survival time trend analysis for the 1978–89 study period is described, that was carried out for a selection of cancer registries which provided data for the whole period (see Table 4 in Chapter 1).

Methods

Relative survival, defined as the ratio of the observed survival rate in the group of patients to the survival rate expected in a group of people in the general population, who are similar to the patients with respect to all possible factors affecting survival at the beginning of the follow-up period, except for the disease of interest, was computed by using the Hakulinen method (Hakulinen, 1982; Hakulinen et al., 1985).

Relative survival from the beginning of follow-up to the end of the ith subinterval (one of those into which the entire follow-up period is divided, e.g., six months or one year), is expressed as:

$$R_i = \frac{S_i}{S_i^*}$$

where S_i represents the observed survival rate and S_i^* the corresponding expected survival rate.

Selection of patients occurs during follow-up simply because death hazard is usually lower for younger patients than for elderly patients. Expected survival can be biased by this selection of patients.

Expected survival rates are then computed by taking into account the potential follow-up of the patients. As explained in detail in the previous monograph (Verdecchia et al., 1995), the expected interval-specific survival rate is then derived as:

$$p_i^* = 1 - \frac{(d_i + \delta_i)}{\left(l_i - \frac{\omega_i}{2}\right)}$$

where d_i is the expected number of deaths among patients with potentially complete follow-up during the ith subinterval, i.e. $[i, i+1]$, δ_i the expected number of deaths with potential follow-up ending within the interval, l_i the expected number of patients at the start of each interval and ω_i the expected number of patients withdrawing alive during the interval.

The expected survival rate from 0 to i is obtained by calculating:

$$S_i^* = \prod_{m=0}^{i-1} p_m^*$$

The standard error of the estimated survival rate S_i is obtained using Greenwood's formula (Greenwood, 1926). Confidence intervals for R_i are computed as the roots of the second-degree equation in ϕ:

$$(S_i - S_i^* \phi)^2 = \frac{(1.96)^2 \, S_i^* \phi \, (1 - S_i^* \phi)}{n_i^*}$$

where n_i^* is the effective sample size at the start of the ith subinterval, estimated as:

$$n_i^* = \frac{S_i(1 - S_i)}{[SE(S_i)]^2}$$

Confidence intervals for R_i computed in this way are constrained within the range between 0 and $1/S_i^*$, since the observed survival rate S_i must be in the range 0–1.

European pooled survival figures and their standard errors have been computed as follows:

$$PR_{ij} = \sum_k \left(\frac{w_{jk}}{W_j} \right) R_{ijk}; \quad W_j = \sum_k w_{jk}$$

and

$$SE\ (PR_{ij}) = \left[\sum_k \left(\frac{w_{jk}}{W_j} \right)^2 [SE\ (R_{ijk})]^2 \right]^{1/2}$$

where R_{ijk} indicates the relative survival up to subinterval i estimated for age class j ($j = 1,..., a$) and population k ($k = 1,..., c$) and w_{jk} is a set of weights. Confidence intervals for pooled survival probabilities have been computed by assuming the Normal approximation on the logarithmic scale. Pooled probabilities and their confidence intervals are then always positive but not limited to being less than unity, although this rarely happens in practice. Weights consist of annual sex- and site-specific numbers of cases observed or estimated at national level in each country. The choice to use age-independent weights was made for both practical (availability of data, ease of presentation) and theoretical (comparability of results, stability of estimates) reasons. Pooled survival figures obtained in this way can be interpreted as estimates of the relative survival of the totality of cases diagnosed in all the countries considered.

Comparing relative survival between different populations requires either age-specific or age-adjusted survival rates to be considered. Comparisons between countries are presented in terms of age-adjusted survival, computed by the direct method, using the population of cases from the whole EUROCARE-2 database, for a given site, as a standard. Formally we have

$$ASR_{ik} = \sum_j \left(\frac{M_j}{M} \right) R_{ijk}$$

where

$$M = \sum_{jk} m_{jk}; \qquad M_j = \sum_k m_{jk};$$

and

$$SE(ASR_{ik}) = \left[\sum_j \left(\frac{M_j}{M} \right)^2 [SE\ (R_{ijk})]^2 \right]^{1/2}$$

where m_{jk} indicates the number of patients at the beginning of follow-up for age class j and population k. Confidence intervals for age-adjusted relative survival probabilities, similarly to the case of pooled relative survival probabilities, have been computed by assuming the Normal approximation on the logarithmic scale. Age-adjusted survival rates cannot be computed when there are no cases in one or more age classes.

This standard population differs from the one used in the previous monograph (Berrino et al., 1995), which was the whole EUROCARE-1 database. Although the age structures of these two standard populations do not differ greatly and the standardized figures obtained by using them also do not differ substantially, this is another reason why direct comparison of figures between the two EUROCARE monographs could be biased.

Table 1 reports site-specific values of M_j and M used for computing age-adjusted relative survival figures. Relative survival figures for males and females were adjusted using the same standard population in order to allow the reader to assess sex differences in addition to differences between countries.

Presentation of the results

Period of diagnosis was limited to the five-year interval 1985–89, so that all potential cases could have follow-up of at least five years (the closing date for follow-up of patients was December 1994 or later). Country was chosen as the statistical unit for the analysis. For countries with several cancer registries, data were combined to represent the country, thus assuming homogeneity in survival within countries. In order to allow the reader to gain an idea of possible within-country variation and of the appropriateness of this assumption, registry area- and sex-specific five-year crude relative survival rates are graphically presented as a bar chart, including 95% confidence intervals, and are reported in Appendix 2A. No further analysis of registry-specific data was performed, as this was beyond the aims of the EUROCARE project. Ad hoc studies, such as those recently carried out in Italy (Verdecchia et al., 1997) and in the United Kingdom (Coleman et al., 1999) are appropriate for exploring within-country variation in cancer survival. In order to facilitate the inspection of cancer registry area- and sex-specific five-year relative survival figures and their 95% confidence intervals, the data used to prepare the bar charts are reported in Appendix 2A, for the countries that contributed data from multiple cancer registries.

Table 1. Total number of cases by cancer site and age class, 1985–89. The EUROCARE-2 standard population.

Cases from specialized cancer registries are included here only for relevant sites, and do not contribute to all cancers combined.

Site	Age					
	15–44	45–54	55–64	65–74	75–99	All ages
Lip	189	495	1104	1379	1449	4616
Tongue	528	954	1359	1131	895	4867
Salivary glands	331	286	452	542	579	2190
Oral cavity	580	1336	1920	1563	1192	6591
Oropharynx	409	982	1305	861	450	4007
Nasopharynx	284	269	343	283	145	1324
Hypopharynx	228	694	1088	766	461	3237
Head and neck	2029	4235	6015	4604	3143	20026
Oesophagus	518	2047	4777	6093	6875	20310
Stomach	2203	4904	12923	20284	26021	66335
Small intestine	157	269	541	673	667	2307
Colon	3212	6657	16821	27334	35475	89499
Rectum	1945	4964	12527	18276	20335	58047
Liver	403	836	2592	3682	3587	11100
Gallbladder	226	653	2320	3662	4811	11672
Pancreas	834	2287	6487	9963	11651	31222
Nasal cavities	170	266	515	607	533	2091
Larynx	797	2519	5195	4278	2137	14926
Lung	3860	15128	47813	62363	44243	173407
Pleura	178	465	985	1096	821	3545
Bone [a]	646	226	362	400	384	2018
Soft tissues	1486	732	1089	1186	1212	5705
Melanoma	6984	4173	4609	4150	3419	23335
Breast	20239	28457	33924	32277	31097	145994
Cervix uteri	9090	4226	4704	4084	2763	24867
Corpus uteri	1083	4251	8662	7691	5423	27110
Ovary	3235	4655	7072	6917	5548	27427
Vagina	284	382	796	1498	2665	5625
Prostate [b]	1042	8501	24474	26471	5240	65728
Testis	6045	746	343	169	123	7426
Penis	182	237	428	540	568	1955
Bladder	1567	4045	12289	18928	19460	56289
Kidney	1448	3183	6716	7641	5684	24672
Choroid (melanoma)	153	205	301	261	197	1117
Brain	4065	2728	4188	3715	1572	16268
Thyroid gland	2619	1217	1256	1298	1111	7501
Hodgkin's disease	4439	763	817	766	578	7363
Non-Hodgkin's lymphomas	4221	3709	6141	8145	7733	29949
Multiple myeloma	332	1075	2834	4409	4735	13385
Acute lymphatic leukaemia	830	142	234	252	247	1705
Chronic lymphatic leukaemia	195	688	1893	3043	3778	9597
Acute myeloid leukaemia	1265	750	1304	1810	1961	7090
Chronic myeloid leukaemia	678	429	698	883	1293	3981
Leukaemia	3249	2235	4593	6803	8589	25469
All cancers	90902	116692	237672	311269	312069	1068604

[a] The first age class is 20–44 years
[b] Age classes are 15–54, 55–64, 65–74. 75–84, 85–99 years.

Death certificate only (DCO) cases and those cases identified from autopsy findings were excluded from the analysis. Cases lost to follow-up were included in the analysis up to the last information about their vital status.

Analyses by cancer site, country, sex and age were performed based on 45 cancer sites, 17 countries, two sexes and five age classes plus all ages combined, for cases diagnosed during the period 1985–89. Lists of the cancer sites and countries are presented in Tables 1 and 2 of Chapter 1. As in the EUROCARE-1 analysis (Gatta *et al.*, 1995), the data were classified in five age classes: 15–44, 45–54, 55–64, 65–74 and 75–99 years. Somewhat different age classes were used for bone and prostatic cancers in order to adapt the analysis to the particular incidence patterns for these two cancer sites.

Presentation of the results basically follows the layout used in the previous EUROCARE monograph, with survival figures presented for each cancer site at single country level and at the European level.

For each country- and site-specific presentation, a list of cancer registries including the number of cases, mean age of the patients and the period of collection of the diagnoses of cases is provided. Cancer registry-specific relative survival rates are presented as a bar chart, with 95% confidence intervals, to allow evaluation of potential within-country variation. Observed and relative survival figures are given by sex and age class, at one, three and five years since diagnosis. Crude observed and relative survival rates are also given for all ages combined (ALL).

Following the country-specific presentations, weighted survival figures for each cancer site are presented for the pool of European cancer registries. Mean European survival figures were obtained by weighting age- and country-specific survival figures, using the expected number of cases in each country as weight. Weights used for each country are presented in a table in terms of the percentage coverage by cancer registration and annual average number of cases reported by actual cancer registries in order to distinguish countries with national cancer registration and countries with multiple local cancer registries. The weights w_k used can be computed, for each country k, simply as follows:

$$w_k = \frac{100 \times (\text{average annual number of cancer patients registered by the actual cancer registeries})}{\text{percentage coverage by cancer registration}}$$

Observed and relative weighted mean European survival figures are presented by sex and by age class as well as for all ages combined, in a table similar to the one in each country-specific presentation.

Age-standardized relative survival rates and their 95% confidence intervals are presented in an additional table, at the foot of the page, and in a bar chart at the top right, by country and sex, at one year and five years. Age-standardized relative weighted mean European survival figures by sex at one year and five years are also reported. The standard population used was the EUROCARE-2 population of cases for 1985–89 (see Table 1). The figures for males and females were standardized by using the same standard population in order to allow comparisons by sex. For countries with no available cases in one or more age classes, age-adjusted survival rates cannot be computed and are presented in neither the table nor the bar chart.

Two weighted analyses are actually reported on this page, the first giving observed and relative weighted mean European survival figures age-specifically and for all ages combined and the second giving the age-standardized country-specific survival figures and the age-standardized relative weighted mean European survival figures as a reference. The two mean European survival figures provide different information. For comparison of survival between countries, only age-standardized figures should be used. If desired, figures for males and females can be combined weighting them by the sex-specific number of cases given in the top table of the same European page. Age-standardized figures for both sexes are provided on the compact disk, in the corresponding section.

Being based on the expected numbers of cases in each country and including 17 European countries, representing more than 75% of the European Union as well as some eastern European countries, we attributed the label of Europe to this pooled estimate. Survival figures reported here for Europe represent the average probability of surviving cancer for people living in Europe.

All cancer sites combined (except non-melanoma skin cancers) were analysed as an additional cancer site including all the cases, irrespective of the individual cancer site. Specialized cancer registries or those providing data for only a selection of cancer sites were excluded from this analysis (this applied to Côte d'Or and Isère in France, Rotterdam in the Netherlands, and Girona, Mallorca and Granada in Spain). When comparing results for all cancers combined (all malignant neoplasms) between countries, it is important to note that differences in the distribution of site of cancer can explain a major part of the differences in survival.

Survival for all cancers combined is highly relevant from the public health point of view, but less so for oncologists or epidemiologists, who much prefer to refer to specific cancer sites. There are two alternative possibilities with different interpretation for combining all cancers together: a crude pool and a pool adjusted by cancer site. The site-unadjusted pool ignores the site distribution, which may differ between countries and this may limit the interpretation of differences. Nevertheless, the survival for the crude pool, as a sort of picture of the country, represents an average level of cancer survival for that country. The site-adjusted pool of all cancers allows survival to represent an index that is more appropriate for inter-country comparison and can be used in interpreting differences in survival as due to the quality and effectiveness of the health care systems. However, in line with the descriptive character of the present analysis, we chose to present results for the crude pool of all cancers.

References

Berrino, F., Sant, M., Verdecchia, A., Capocaccia, R., Hakulinen, T., Estève, J., eds (1995) *Survival of Cancer Patients in Europe: the EUROCARE Study* (IARC Scientific Publications No. 132), Lyon, IARC

Coleman, M.P., Babb, P., Damiecki, P., Grosclaude, P., Honjo, S., Jones, J., Gerhardt, K., Pitard, A., Quinn, M., Sloggett, A. & De Stavola, B. (1999) *Cancer Survival Trends in England and Wales, 1971–1995: Deprivation and NHS Region* (Studies in Medical and Population Subjects No. 60), London, Stationery Office

Gatta, G. & Sant, M. (1995) Guide to tables. In: Berrino, F., Sant, M., Verdecchia, A., Capocaccia, R., Hakulinen, T. & Estève, J., eds, *Survival of Cancer Patients in Europe: the EUROCARE Study* (IARC Scientific Publications No. 132), Lyon, IARC, pp. 75–91

Greenwood, M. (1926) *The Natural Duration of Cancer* (Reports on Public Health and Medical Subjects No. 33), London, His Majesty's Stationery Office

Hakulinen, T. (1982) Cancer survival corrected for heterogeneity in patient withdrawal. *Biometrics, 39,* 93–942

Hakulinen, T. & Abeywickrama, K.H. (1985) A computer program package for relative survival analysis. *Computer Prog. Biomed.*, 19, 197–207

Verdecchia, A., Micheli, A. & Gatta, G., eds (1997) Special issue: Survival of cancer patients in Italy: the ITACARE Study. *Tumori,* 83

Verdecchia, A., Capocaccia, R. & Hakulinen, T. (1995) Methods of data analysis. In: Berrino, F., Sant, M., Verdecchia, A., Capocaccia, R., Hakulinen, T. & Estève, J., eds, *Survival of Cancer Patients in Europe: the EUROCARE Study* (IARC Scientific Publications No. 132), Lyon, IARC, pp. 32–37

Appendix 2A

Five-year relative survival (%), with 95% confidence interval (95% CI), by cancer registry and sex for countries with multiple local cancer registries				

Site	Males		Females		Site	Males		Females	
Registry area	R_{5y}	95% CI	R_{5y}	95% CI	Registry area	R_{5y}	95% CI	R_{5y}	95% CI
Lip					Genoa	43.2	31.0–57.0	81.8	59.1–98.6
England					Latina	26.2	9.3–57.1	61.1	11.6–110.7
East Anglia	99.5	88.5–108.6	100.0	100.0–100.0	Modena	19.6	5.5–52.7	100.0	100.0–100.0
Mersey	100.0	100.0–100.0	52.2	15.3–100.4	Parma	29.6	14.2–52.7	33.6	9.7–75.4
Oxford	94.4	82.5–104.4	100.0	100.0–100.0	Ragusa	45.5	19.0–80.8	35.3	6.5–83.8
Thames	89.3	75.5–100.6	88.3	63.8–107.9	Romagna	39.7	18.2–68.1	0.0	0.0–0.0
Wessex	79.9	62.5–96.1	85.5	56.4–109.4	Turin	39.4	25.7–55.9	14.9	5.2–36.5
West Midlands	91.6	74.1–104.8	99.2	66.2–116.7	Varese	37.8	26.7–51.0	55.5	30.7–82.8
Yorkshire	84.5	68.6–98.5	95.9	70.5–112.6	Poland				
France					Cracow	16.7	7.3–34.3	53.1	19.9–86.3
Amiens	67.4	41.4–93.4	58.2	17.1–111.9	Warsaw	14.0	5.6–31.8	43.1	18.0–76.2
Calvados	91.3	72.8–105.8	64.8	27.0–115.2	Spain				
Doubs	61.7	19.9–97.3	–		Basque Country	42.3	34.4–50.8	43.6	24.6–66.3
Italy					Mallorca	20.1	7.6–44.5	100.0	100.0–100.0
Florence	76.7	59.5–91.4	94.7	56.5–117.5	Navarra	45.5	27.4–65.6	85.4	48.4–108.9
Genoa	100.0	100.0–100.0	100.0	100.0–100.0	Tarragona	20.2	9.4–38.7	79.8	35.9–108.1
Latina	83.1	55.9–102.8	88.8	27.7–125.0	Switzerland				
Modena	100.0	100.0–100.0	–		Basel	38.5	21.6–59.7	40.7	14.9–75.3
Parma	75.4	29.0–110.8	–		Geneva	55.2	40.4–70.1	26.1	9.2–58.4
Ragusa	77.3	59.8–92.7	100.0	100.0–100.0					
Romagna	82.0	32.9–104.3	–						
Turin	88.4	70.6–101.5	84.1	55.1–102.2	***Salivary glands***				
Varese	92.4	68.2–109.1	100.0	100.0–100.0	England				
Poland					East Anglia	68.8	45.5–92.2	60.1	39.1–80.7
Cracow	73.0	48.4–97.0	100.0	100.0–100.0	Mersey	35.0	18.6–58.4	61.7	43.0–80.4
Warsaw	70.2	44.6–94.1	–		Oxford	54.0	37.0–72.5	66.2	47.7–83.2
Spain					Thames	58.4	46.6–70.5	69.0	56.9–80.7
Basque Country	100.0	100.0–100.0	100.0	100.0–100.0	Wessex	43.3	29.2–60.4	71.9	55.5–86.4
Mallorca	100.0	100.0–100.0	100.0	100.0–100.0	West Midlands	66.5	52.9–79.6	61.9	48.1–75.5
Navarra	95.6	86.4–102.8	100.0	100.0–100.0	Yorkshire	51.0	35.5–68.5	61.3	43.3–79.7
Tarragona	87.6	76.2–97.2	90.0	56.7–111.6	France				
					Amiens	53.9	19.9–94.3	100.0	100.0–100.0
Tongue					Calvados	83.9	53.3–103.7	62.4	23.4–101.3
England					Doubs	46.3	12.8–93.4	37.0	7.0–95.7
East Anglia	47.8	32.5–65.2	58.7	42.6–75.3	Italy				
Mersey	36.8	27.5–47.7	50.1	36.3–65.4	Florence	66.5	43.6–86.3	68.6	45.4–87.6
Oxford	50.2	38.1–63.1	55.2	40.4–70.6	Genoa	55.2	23.7–86.6	86.4	49.0–110.1
Thames	41.1	33.0–50.1	50.5	40.6–61.1	Latina	53.0	24.8–83.9	64.9	24.9–95.4
Wessex	42.1	31.2–54.6	43.4	32.0–56.4	Modena	34.6	9.9–77.6	56.8	10.7–102.8
West Midlands	36.0	28.8–44.2	42.6	32.6–53.8	Parma	47.1	17.2–87.1	82.0	25.5–115.4
Yorkshire	28.6	20.4–38.9	42.4	30.4–56.0	Ragusa	36.7	10.5–86.8	58.4	17.5–99.2
France					Romagna	38.6	11.1–86.6	62.5	32.6–86.7
Amiens	26.2	18.4–36.1	32.9	13.5–62.9	Turin	48.2	24.0–75.7	62.8	32.2–90.6
Calvados	33.3	25.2–42.8	77.2	51.3–94.9	Varese	69.4	43.9–90.6	95.8	67.8–106.9
Doubs	43.9	30.5–58.9	65.2	34.4–89.1	Poland				
Italy					Cracow	35.5	14.6–66.4	52.3	26.7–80.5
Florence	43.2	31.0–57.0	81.8	59.1–98.6	Warsaw	0.0	0.0–0.0	34.6	6.4–82.3

Five-year relative survival (%), with 95% confidence interval (95% CI), by cancer registry and sex for countries with multiple local cancer registries (Contd)

Site Registry area	Males R_{5y}	95% CI	Females R_{5y}	95% CI	Site Registry area	Males R_{5y}	95% CI	Females R_{5y}	95% CI
Spain					**France**				
Basque Country	47.2	25.7–72.8	80.4	52.9–100.5	Amiens	33.0	26.3–40.7	43.4	21.5–69.7
Mallorca	0.0	0.0–0.0	53.1	10.0–96.1	Calvados	29.7	23.2–37.1	51.1	28.4–74.9
Navarra	49.5	20.8–85.1	61.2	18.4–104.1	Doubs	35.6	25.1–48.2	0.0	0.0–0.0
Tarragona	68.4	32.8–99.8	48.8	20.7–80.6	**Italy**				
					Florence	34.3	21.5–50.7	52.6	32.9–72.9
Oral cavity					Genoa	26.1	13.2–45.7	47.6	20.2–78.6
England					Latina	25.5	7.2–62.7	0.0	0.0–0.0
East Anglia	51.2	38.4–64.9	55.1	40.3–70.7	Modena	21.2	6.0–55.6	35.4	6.5–84.1
Mersey	47.5	39.1–56.5	62.5	49.7–75.0	Parma	48.7	24.3–76.6	38.1	7.0–90.5
Oxford	54.9	43.1–67.2	70.7	55.7–84.5	Ragusa	34.5	6.4–82.0	–	
Thames	41.5	34.2–49.5	47.8	39.2–57.1	Romagna	14.8	2.7–55.8	0.0	0.0–0.0
Wessex	41.9	31.3–54.1	50.9	39.0–63.7	Turin	26.1	15.5–41.1	38.3	18.7–64.7
West Midlands	41.8	34.9–49.2	56.0	46.9–65.3	Varese	26.9	18.3–37.9	38.1	17.3–66.5
Yorkshire	41.4	33.8–49.8	55.3	44.7–66.4	**Poland**				
France					Cracow	19.0	9.0–36.5	73.7	37.0–94.7
Amiens	38.7	29.5–48.9	62.4	40.1–84.1	Warsaw	17.4	8.3–33.7	32.2	13.2–61.6
Calvados	38.8	31.2–47.2	58.4	33.9–82.9	**Spain**				
Doubs	67.1	52.2–80.4	78.4	51.5–94.9	Basque Country	28.8	21.3–37.8	59.3	27.2–90.2
Italy					Mallorca	22.0	7.7–49.6	40.7	7.5–96.7
Florence	38.0	28.0–49.5	52.2	35.8–70.1	Navarra	26.2	13.2–45.6	0.0	0.0–0.0
Genoa	34.8	21.8–51.5	41.8	22.5–67.3	Tarragona	14.0	5.6–31.4	61.7	23.2–100.3
Latina	35.9	13.0–69.5	49.4	9.1–117.5	**Switzerland**				
Modena	34.9	14.4–65.4	35.9	10.3–80.5	Basel	47.2	26.8–70.6	59.0	17.7–100.3
Parma	30.0	15.2–51.7	73.1	32.0–107.7	Geneva	31.5	19.6–47.1	57.9	31.0–84.7
Ragusa	48.2	20.3–82.9	99.2	39.8–126.2					
Romagna	38.9	16.1–71.1	0.0	0.0–0.0	***Nasopharynx***				
Turin	56.8	43.9–69.8	26.8	10.9–54.5	**England**				
Varese	47.4	35.0–60.8	47.1	26.8–70.5	East Anglia	22.8	8.6–49.9	28.9	9.0–64.3
Poland					Mersey	33.0	18.3–53.2	30.4	14.6–53.6
Cracow	48.1	30.3–68.0	44.1	18.6–75.9	Oxford	49.5	31.3–69.5	44.1	23.0–69.7
Warsaw	46.6	21.6–76.1	17.8	3.2–63.9	Thames	36.9	26.2–49.5	36.4	20.3–56.9
Spain					Wessex	25.5	12.9–45.0	60.9	39.4–81.0
Basque Country	44.5	36.4–53.2	60.6	42.2–79.0	West Midlands	31.1	20.0–45.6	25.1	12.0–46.0
Mallorca	43.6	26.7–63.2	61.4	21.5–103.8	Yorkshire	37.9	20.4–61.2	33.4	16.2–57.1
Navarra	45.8	33.2–59.6	19.1	3.4–64.4	**France**				
Tarragona	30.8	18.9–46.8	44.9	16.6–78.5	Amiens	57.1	27.0–87.1	100.0	100.0–100.0
Switzerland					Calvados	33.2	9.8–71.3	0.0	0.0–0.0
Basel	41.1	23.3–62.2	60.2	30.6–89.9	Doubs	0.0	0.0–0.0	–	
Geneva	48.2	32.7–64.9	53.2	31.5–76.4	**Italy**				
					Florence	34.4	20.8–51.6	16.4	4.6–45.1
Oropharynx					Genoa	37.2	18.2–62.8	68.0	35.4–94.2
England					Latina	34.0	6.3–80.9	–	
East Anglia	20.7	9.6–40.3	39.4	19.2–67.5	Modena	41.9	12.3–80.6	0.0	0.0–0.0
Mersey	35.0	24.3–47.8	48.9	28.6–72.4	Parma	46.7	13.7–89.7	100.0	100.0–100.0
Oxford	64.1	47.0–80.6	41.2	22.3–64.6	Ragusa	26.8	7.7–63.4	41.3	12.2–79.5
Thames	36.8	28.0–46.8	40.9	28.3–55.4	Romagna	50.2	25.3–77.1	0.0	0.0–0.0
Wessex	44.3	28.1–63.4	34.2	17.5–57.7	Turin	28.6	11.7–55.8	66.9	20.9–94.2
West Midlands	25.9	18.2–35.6	37.4	23.9–54.2	Varese	40.8	21.2–65.2	62.5	32.5–86.6
Yorkshire	26.6	16.8–40.0	24.8	11.0–48.2					

Five-year relative survival (%), with 95% confidence interval (95% CI), by cancer registry and sex for countries with multiple local cancer registries (Contd)

Site / Registry area	Males R_{5y}	Males 95% CI	Females R_{5y}	Females 95% CI	Site / Registry area	Males R_{5y}	Males 95% CI	Females R_{5y}	Females 95% CI
Poland					Wessex	36.2	30.3–42.6	43.9	37.0–51.3
Cracow	31.8	9.1–75.2	0.0	0.0–0.0	West Midlands	33.3	29.5–37.3	43.6	38.2–49.3
Warsaw	32.0	9.1–75.6	0.0	0.0–0.0	Yorkshire	32.6	28.1–37.6	40.5	34.2–47.3
Spain					**France**				
Basque Country	22.4	12.1–38.0	45.3	24.1–69.3	Amiens	31.3	27.3–35.6	47.6	34.6–61.7
Mallorca	36.5	13.2–70.8	34.9	6.4–83.0	Calvados	30.7	27.2–34.5	59.5	45.4–73.1
Navarra	30.1	12.4–57.6	0.0	0.0–0.0	Doubs	42.3	35.8–49.3	68.2	49.0–83.8
Tarragona	50.4	28.0–73.9	100.0	100.0–100.0	**Italy**				
					Florence	36.1	30.3–42.4	52.7	42.4–63.3
Hypopharynx					Genoa	30.3	23.0–39.0	47.7	34.8–61.9
England					Latina	28.5	15.7–46.6	43.4	12.6–91.2
East Anglia	13.8	6.0–29.3	19.6	8.7–39.4	Modena	26.6	16.2–40.9	40.2	19.7–66.8
Mersey	28.2	19.1–40.1	17.4	8.6–32.5	Parma	31.0	21.4–42.9	61.3	37.9–83.9
Oxford	28.2	14.2–50.3	18.4	7.3–40.2	Ragusa	41.1	25.0–60.6	56.1	28.5–83.7
Thames	32.1	23.3–42.8	24.0	15.3–36.2	Romagna	37.5	24.7–53.0	0.0	0.0–0.0
Wessex	14.7	6.9–29.3	16.8	6.7–37.6	Turin	41.1	33.9–49.0	29.3	18.8–43.0
West Midlands	20.1	13.3–29.4	28.6	18.3–42.2	Varese	35.5	29.9–41.6	45.5	33.3–58.9
Yorkshire	20.2	12.1–32.2	14.2	6.6–28.2	**Poland**				
France					Cracow	27.3	19.4–37.2	41.2	25.0–60.3
Amiens	24.0	17.1–32.7	17.3	3.1–58.4	Warsaw	20.9	13.6–31.0	32.2	17.8–51.9
Calvados	24.4	19.1–30.7	54.5	16.4–92.7	**Spain**				
Doubs	33.1	21.6–47.6	100.0	100.0–100.0	Basque Country	35.6	31.7–39.8	51.2	38.9–64.2
Italy					Mallorca	28.0	19.5–38.7	65.5	38.1–90.3
Florence	25.2	14.2–41.0	18.6	3.3–66.7	Navarra	36.9	29.1–45.5	41.6	22.5–65.9
Genoa	10.5	2.9–32.0	18.3	3.3–62.0	Tarragona	26.1	19.3–34.4	65.1	41.6–86.1
Latina	0.0	0.0–0.0	–		**Switzerland**				
Modena	23.1	8.2–51.3	0.0	0.0–0.0	Basel	34.4	25.0–45.5	53.2	32.4–75.3
Parma	14.3	4.0–42.6	–		Geneva	41.4	34.1–49.2	46.4	32.8–61.6
Ragusa	56.5	10.7–102.3	–						
Romagna	26.9	4.9–75.4	0.0	0.0–0.0	***Oesophagus***				
Turin	38.3	17.4–68.2	100.0	100.0–100.0	**England**				
Varese	29.6	18.4–44.4	0.0	0.0–0.0	East Anglia	6.2	4.2–9.0	8.4	5.6–12.6
Poland					Mersey	9.5	7.2–12.5	12.1	9.2–15.8
Cracow	23.1	4.2–72.1	0.0	0.0–0.0	Oxford	9.5	6.8–13.2	15.1	11.3–20.0
Warsaw	16.1	2.9–60.5	–		Thames	6.4	5.0–8.1	11.6	9.5–14.1
Spain					Wessex	8.8	6.9–11.2	11.7	9.0–15.2
Basque Country	26.1	18.9–35.0	68.1	21.2–95.9	West Midlands	8.1	6.6–10.0	9.6	7.6–12.1
Mallorca	15.3	5.3–37.2	–		Yorkshire	5.4	3.8–7.5	7.7	5.5–10.6
Navarra	17.2	6.0–40.9	0.0	0.0–0.0	**France**				
Tarragona	24.1	10.8–46.1	–		Amiens	7.9	5.3–11.7	16.6	6.6–37.1
Switzerland					Calvados	9.9	7.2–13.5	17.8	7.8–36.4
Basel	10.0	2.8–30.9	–		Côte d'Or	5.3	2.7–10.2	0.0	0.0–0.0
Geneva	27.0	15.7–42.7	39.9	11.6–83.7	Doubs	11.1	5.7–20.4	0.0	0.0–0.0
					Italy				
Head and neck					Florence	6.3	3.2–12.0	14.9	7.4–28.3
England					Genoa	5.8	2.0–16.0	10.3	2.9–31.9
East Anglia	35.9	29.0–43.6	46.0	37.6–55.1	Latina	6.9	1.2–31.6	42.0	7.7–99.8
Mersey	38.5	33.7–43.7	45.6	38.5–53.2	Modena	5.9	1.0–27.9	12.4	2.2–51.6
Oxford	51.5	44.7–58.6	52.4	44.1–60.9	Parma	3.1	0.5–15.8	15.7	2.8–59.2
Thames	38.5	34.5–42.8	42.8	37.7–48.2	Ragusa	0.0	0.0–0.0	0.0	0.0–0.0

Five-year relative survival (%), with 95% confidence interval (95% CI), by cancer registry and sex for countries with multiple local cancer registries (Contd)

Site Registry area	Males R_{5y}	95% CI	Females R_{5y}	95% CI	Site Registry area	Males R_{5y}	95% CI	Females R_{5y}	95% CI
Romagna	11.3	3.1–34.5	12.5	2.2–49.1	**Small intestine**				
Turin	2.7	0.8–9.5	15.5	6.2–34.8	England				
Varese	10.8	6.8–16.7	4.7	0.8–23.4	East Anglia	28.3	14.9–48.6	26.5	15.0–43.0
Poland					Mersey	15.6	6.8–32.5	15.6	5.4–39.2
Cracow	5.2	1.8–14.4	5.7	1.0–27.3	Oxford	29.5	17.5–46.1	32.6	19.5–49.9
Warsaw	1.4	0.2–7.6	4.0	0.7–20.0	Thames	29.9	19.4–43.8	18.9	11.3–30.0
Spain					Wessex	42.2	27.8–59.7	32.8	20.4–49.0
Basque Country	7.7	5.1–11.6	18.5	8.1–37.7	West Midlands	31.9	23.4–42.2	38.0	28.3–49.2
Mallorca	20.9	10.4–38.0	0.0	0.0–0.0	Yorkshire	34.0	23.2–47.5	31.0	19.9–45.3
Navarra	8.5	4.3–16.0	23.9	8.4–54.9	France				
Tarragona	2.8	0.8–9.8	0.0	0.0–0.0	Amiens	55.9	21.0–90.8	0.0	0.0–0.0
					Calvados	52.4	19.1–97.1	0.0	0.0–0.0
Stomach					Côte d'Or	21.1	6.0–55.3	59.1	27.3–96.4
England					Doubs	–		47.1	9.6–109.6
East Anglia	8.0	6.3–10.1	9.0	6.7–12.1	Italy				
Mersey	12.4	10.6–14.5	12.3	10.1–14.9	Florence	36.9	19.7–60.3	30.8	16.3–51.8
Oxford	11.7	9.9–13.9	12.1	9.6–15.0	Genoa	0.0	0.0–0.0	0.0	0.0–0.0
Thames	10.3	9.1–11.7	12.5	10.8–14.5	Latina	0.0	0.0–0.0	33.0	6.0–92.3
Wessex	14.1	12.3–16.2	14.7	12.2–17.7	Modena	29.5	8.4–69.7	23.2	4.2–72.5
West Midlands	12.0	10.8–13.3	10.7	9.2–12.3	Parma	44.7	18.6–79.4	42.2	12.4–81.2
Yorkshire	11.5	10.1–13.2	12.0	10.1–14.1	Ragusa	0.0	0.0–0.0	0.0	0.0–0.0
France					Romagna	12.3	2.2–49.6	70.3	21.9–99.0
Amiens	25.1	19.0–32.5	18.2	11.9–27.1	Turin	18.2	5.1–50.9	8.0	1.4–35.3
Calvados	26.0	20.2–33.0	28.1	20.5–37.6	Varese	46.4	21.4–77.8	44.5	20.5–74.6
Côte d'Or	21.4	15.6–28.9	24.0	16.5–33.9	Poland				
Doubs	30.9	23.5–39.6	34.4	24.3–46.9	Cracow	17.4	3.1–62.5	35.3	10.1–79.1
Italy					Warsaw	0.0	0.0–0.0	0.0	0.0–0.0
Florence	21.1	19.0–23.3	28.3	25.6–31.3	Spain				
Genoa	19.7	15.4–24.9	28.1	22.5–34.6	Basque Country	–		33.0	13.5–63.1
Latina	27.9	20.2–37.5	25.8	17.0–37.5	Mallorca	0.0	0.0–0.0	100.0	100.0–100.0
Modena	21.6	16.4–27.9	29.1	22.2–37.2	Navarra	34.3	9.9–76.9	45.2	13.3–86.9
Parma	19.0	15.0–23.8	22.1	17.0–28.3	Tarragona	29.0	10.3–61.7	0.0	0.0–0.0
Ragusa	17.7	12.0–25.6	12.3	6.8–21.6					
Romagna	23.3	19.2–28.1	30.2	24.9–36.3	**Colon**				
Turin	21.1	17.0–25.8	24.6	19.4–30.8	England				
Varese	26.0	22.5–29.9	27.6	23.5–32.2	East Anglia	41.9	38.7–45.1	40.6	37.9–43.4
Poland					Mersey	40.7	37.7–43.8	40.0	37.3–42.8
Cracow	9.5	6.6–13.5	13.3	8.9–19.5	Oxford	40.3	37.5–43.3	42.4	39.8–45.1
Warsaw	10.7	7.4–15.3	9.6	5.9–15.3	Thames	41.6	39.6–43.6	41.7	40.0–43.5
Spain					Wessex	44.8	42.4–47.4	44.2	42.0–46.4
Basque Country	33.6	30.1–37.4	31.9	27.4–36.9	West Midlands	40.1	38.2–42.1	40.7	38.9–42.5
Granada	13.7	8.7–21.0	13.5	7.9–22.3	Yorkshire	40.1	37.6–42.7	39.9	37.7–42.2
Mallorca	25.2	15.6–38.7	23.3	12.7–39.6	France				
Navarra	27.7	23.3–32.7	31.6	25.7–38.3	Amiens	45.5	38.6–52.9	45.6	38.9–52.8
Tarragona	21.0	16.0–27.2	26.5	19.4–35.3	Calvados	53.5	46.6–60.6	59.2	52.4–66.1
Switzerland					Côte d'Or	50.2	44.3–56.3	54.6	48.2–61.2
Basel	23.3	16.8–31.7	27.9	19.2–39.2	Doubs	62.7	51.1–74.4	61.1	51.8–70.5
Geneva	23.6	16.6–32.7	22.5	14.3–34.2					

Five-year relative survival (%), with 95% confidence interval (95% CI), by cancer registry and sex for countries with multiple local cancer registries (Contd)

Site Registry area	Males R_{5y}	95% CI	Females R_{5y}	95% CI	Site Registry area	Males R_{5y}	95% CI	Females R_{5y}	95% CI
Italy					**Poland**				
Florence	48.2	44.7–51.9	48.2	45.0–51.5	Cracow	23.3	16.9–31.5	22.1	16.3–29.4
Genoa	48.0	42.2–54.0	43.1	37.8–48.6	Warsaw	29.7	22.6–38.1	25.7	19.6–33.1
Latina	52.2	41.0–64.1	45.6	35.2–57.0	**Spain**				
Modena	50.4	43.8–57.3	47.1	40.9–53.6	Basque Country	45.5	40.3–51.0	46.1	39.6–52.9
Parma	47.7	40.3–55.5	49.9	42.5–57.7	Mallorca	36.4	29.7–43.9	31.9	24.7–40.2
Ragusa	30.4	20.6–43.2	42.4	33.1–52.8	Navarra	44.6	37.4–52.4	57.3	47.8–66.9
Romagna	57.0	49.5–64.6	50.4	43.7–57.4	Tarragona	44.5	37.1–52.5	40.8	32.7–49.7
Turin	44.8	39.6–50.4	46.0	41.1–51.1					
Varese	47.1	42.4–52.1	52.5	48.1–57.1	***Liver***				
Poland					**England**				
Cracow	18.1	12.1–26.5	23.7	17.8–30.8	East Anglia	6.6	2.3–18.0	0.0	0.0–0.0
Warsaw	33.2	26.5–40.9	24.7	19.5–30.9	Mersey	3.5	1.4–8.8	1.6	0.3–8.6
Spain					Oxford	3.0	1.0–8.6	3.1	0.8–10.7
Basque Country	52.2	46.7–57.8	53.4	48.2–58.8	Thames	4.8	2.7–8.4	6.3	3.3–11.5
Mallorca	49.2	41.9–56.9	44.3	37.9–51.0	Wessex	1.3	0.4–4.8	4.2	1.6–10.4
Navarra	53.7	46.2–61.6	52.7	45.9–59.6	West Midlands	6.9	4.1–11.6	3.7	1.5–9.3
Tarragona	42.9	36.4–49.8	48.6	41.9–55.5	Yorkshire	2.4	0.9–6.0	1.9	0.5–6.7
Switzerland					**France**				
Basel	57.4	49.4–65.7	47.7	40.5–55.3	Amiens	10.4	5.1–20.3	0.0	0.0–0.0
Geneva	50.7	43.4–58.4	51.5	44.2–59.1	Calvados	7.6	3.9–14.1	11.4	3.2–34.5
					Côte d'Or	2.1	0.6–7.5	8.9	2.5–28.3
Rectum					Doubs	21.1	10.6–38.5	18.5	5.4–49.1
England					**Italy**				
East Anglia	40.7	37.3–44.2	43.5	39.7–47.5	Florence	2.5	1.1–5.8	3.6	1.6–8.2
Mersey	37.6	34.5–40.8	39.3	35.8–43.0	Genoa	0.9	0.2–4.7	5.3	1.8–14.7
Oxford	43.4	39.9–47.1	44.9	41.1–48.9	Latina	9.5	3.3–25.2	3.8	0.7–19.2
Thames	39.3	37.1–41.7	39.0	36.7–41.4	Modena	2.9	0.8–9.9	2.4	0.4–12.7
Wessex	46.7	43.5–50.0	43.8	40.5–47.1	Parma	0.0	0.0–0.0	2.9	0.5–14.9
West Midlands	41.1	39.0–43.2	39.2	36.7–41.8	Ragusa	0.0	0.0–0.0	0.0	0.0–0.0
Yorkshire	38.8	36.2–41.4	41.8	39.0–44.8	Romagna	6.1	2.4–14.9	9.0	2.5–28.6
France					Turin	4.6	2.4–8.9	6.4	2.8–14.3
Amiens	45.1	37.5–53.5	40.2	32.3–48.9	Varese	6.3	3.8–10.4	2.9	1.0–8.3
Calvados	51.5	44.3–58.9	50.8	43.1–58.9	**Poland**				
Côte d'Or	46.0	38.9–53.7	54.9	46.1–64.1	Cracow	0.0	0.0–0.0	6.3	2.5–15.3
Doubs	56.9	44.8–69.5	46.0	33.9–59.6	Warsaw	3.6	1.0–12.5	0.0	0.0–0.0
Italy					**Spain**				
Florence	49.1	44.9–53.4	50.8	46.3–55.5	Basque Country	12.1	8.0–18.1	12.5	6.1–23.9
Genoa	35.2	28.4–42.9	36.9	30.1–44.4	Mallorca	26.1	14.3–43.8	–	
Latina	60.2	46.1–74.4	52.0	39.7–64.8	Navarra	6.9	3.4–13.6	8.0	2.7–21.3
Modena	46.4	38.8–54.5	37.0	29.1–46.1	Tarragona	5.4	1.8–14.9	0.0	0.0–0.0
Parma	40.8	31.8–51.1	43.0	33.8–53.2	**Switzerland**				
Ragusa	42.3	32.3–53.6	40.3	28.5–54.2	Basel	2.0	0.3–10.5	6.6	1.2–31.2
Romagna	45.1	35.9–55.3	56.0	45.0–67.2	Geneva	2.8	0.8–9.9	4.7	0.8–23.0
Turin	40.8	34.3–48.0	36.7	30.0–44.1					
Varese	44.5	38.6–50.8	46.1	39.6–52.8	***Gallbladder***				
Netherlands					**England**				
Eindhoven	49.6	43.8–55.7	50.3	43.8–56.9	East Anglia	7.6	3.7–15.2	4.9	2.2–10.3
Rotterdam	57.9	51.0–65.0	60.2	52.3–68.1	Mersey	10.9	5.6–20.4	8.3	4.2–15.7

Five-year relative survival (%), with 95% confidence interval (95% CI), by cancer registry and sex for countries with multiple local cancer registries (Contd)

Site Registry area	Males R_{5y}	95% CI	Females R_{5y}	95% CI
Oxford	9.3	4.3–19.1	14.9	9.2–23.5
Thames	16.7	11.7–23.5	9.2	6.2–13.5
Wessex	9.7	4.7–19.0	11.1	6.6–18.3
West Midlands	11.4	7.7–16.7	11.2	8.2–15.1
Yorkshire	13.1	7.8–21.6	12.5	8.4–18.2
France				
Amiens	0.0	0.0–0.0	20.5	11.5–34.6
Calvados	9.8	2.7–30.7	18.3	8.3–36.9
Côte d'Or	17.9	7.2–39.9	11.8	5.1–25.5
Doubs	14.0	2.6–53.4	29.6	14.6–52.5
Italy				
Florence	6.0	2.8–12.7	11.8	7.9–17.4
Genoa	2.2	0.4–11.8	7.4	3.6–14.7
Latina	44.2	20.1–78.7	29.0	15.3–49.4
Modena	8.4	1.5–38.0	12.5	5.0–28.8
Parma	14.2	4.9–36.1	5.3	1.5–17.7
Ragusa	0.0	0.0–0.0	7.0	2.4–19.0
Romagna	0.0	0.0–0.0	13.3	5.3–30.6
Turin	7.1	2.4–19.4	8.1	4.0–15.9
Varese	12.0	5.6–24.4	9.5	5.5–16.1
Poland				
Cracow	2.8	0.5–14.8	7.7	4.2–13.7
Warsaw	9.4	4.1–20.7	4.0	2.1–7.8
Spain				
Basque Country	35.9	24.4–50.0	11.7	7.2–18.7
Mallorca	27.9	7.9–69.7	18.8	8.8–36.9
Navarra	20.1	11.2–33.9	12.8	7.3–21.7
Tarragona	9.8	2.7–30.9	12.7	6.3–24.4

Pancreas

Site Registry area	Males R_{5y}	95% CI	Females R_{5y}	95% CI
England				
East Anglia	2.2	1.1–4.2	1.9	1.0–3.7
Mersey	2.5	1.4–4.4	1.8	1.0–3.5
Oxford	3.6	2.2–5.7	3.5	2.2–5.5
Thames	4.7	3.6–6.2	4.0	3.0–5.4
Wessex	5.2	3.7–7.5	4.2	2.9–6.1
West Midlands	1.5	0.9–2.5	2.0	1.3–3.1
Yorkshire	3.7	2.5–5.5	2.8	1.8–4.3
France				
Amiens	10.4	5.3–19.7	5.5	1.9–15.2
Calvados	7.4	3.0–17.2	4.3	1.2–14.2
Côte d'Or	4.9	1.9–12.0	10.1	5.0–19.8
Doubs	8.8	2.7–25.4	–	
Italy				
Florence	4.7	2.8–8.0	6.0	3.7–9.5
Genoa	4.4	1.9–10.0	1.0	0.2–5.4
Latina	15.6	6.2–35.0	8.7	2.4–27.6
Modena	2.9	0.8–10.2	1.6	0.3–8.8
Parma	1.2	0.2–6.3	1.9	0.3–10.3

Site Registry area	Males R_{5y}	95% CI	Females R_{5y}	95% CI
Ragusa	0.0	0.0–0.0	0.0	0.0–0.0
Romagna	3.2	0.9–10.9	2.8	0.8–9.9
Turin	8.6	4.7–15.3	1.6	0.4–5.8
Varese	2.5	1.0–6.2	2.4	1.0–6.2
Poland				
Cracow	4.9	2.2–10.3	7.4	3.7–14.1
Warsaw	3.1	1.2–7.8	2.3	0.8–6.6
Spain				
Basque Country	4.7	2.2–9.7	–	
Mallorca	2.6	0.5–13.6	12.3	4.2–31.4
Navarra	6.2	2.7–13.8	4.7	1.6–13.1
Tarragona	2.0	0.4–10.2	4.9	1.4–16.0
Switzerland				
Basel	3.4	0.9–11.7	6.2	2.4–15.1
Geneva	0.0	0.0–0.0	1.1	0.2–6.2

Nasal cavities

Site Registry area	Males R_{5y}	95% CI	Females R_{5y}	95% CI
England				
East Anglia	39.0	25.7–55.4	37.7	20.1–62.5
Mersey	39.0	24.5–57.3	40.6	24.5–61.2
Oxford	46.7	32.6–63.1	40.4	23.3–62.0
Thames	55.7	45.2–66.6	44.9	33.5–57.6
Wessex	47.9	34.8–62.3	39.8	25.9–56.6
West Midlands	39.6	28.9–52.0	38.1	26.6–52.1
Yorkshire	32.4	21.4–46.6	47.3	30.2–67.1
France				
Amiens	48.5	26.6–73.4	47.9	19.2–85.2
Calvados	31.9	17.0–53.2	64.2	28.1–94.5
Doubs	100.0	100.0–100.0	100.0	100.0–100.0
Italy				
Florence	43.4	25.9–64.4	71.1	39.5–94.8
Genoa	77.8	43.2–103.7	57.5	24.7–90.2
Latina	73.6	22.9–103.6	–	
Modena	69.4	13.1–125.6	0.0	0.0–0.0
Parma	41.6	15.2–76.9	100.0	100.0–100.0
Ragusa	0.0	0.0–0.0	53.7	10.2–97.3
Romagna	0.0	0.0–0.0	0.0	0.0–0.0
Turin	44.4	23.2–70.0	51.5	19.3–83.7
Varese	59.2	35.5–83.0	35.3	10.2–79.3
Poland				
Cracow	33.1	14.9–60.6	77.6	34.9–105.2
Warsaw	31.1	5.6–97.1	0.0	0.0–0.0
Spain				
Basque Country	52.4	33.4–73.2	42.8	21.1–70.0
Mallorca	53.6	16.1–91.2	100.0	100.0–100.0
Navarra	13.0	2.3–51.1	83.8	33.6–106.6
Tarragona	63.9	32.0–93.6	0.0	0.0–0.0

Five-year relative survival (%), with 95% confidence interval (95% CI), by cancer registry and sex for countries with multiple local cancer registries (Contd)

Site Registry area	Males R_{5y}	95% CI	Females R_{5y}	95% CI	Site Registry area	Males R_{5y}	95% CI	Females R_{5y}	95% CI
Larynx					Italy				
England					Florence	11.5	10.3–12.9	11.9	9.3–15.1
East Anglia	73.8	65.7–81.5	63.0	47.3–78.2	Genoa	9.4	7.8–11.2	10.5	7.0–15.5
Mersey	72.2	66.2–78.0	69.1	58.5–79.0	Latina	14.0	10.7–18.1	18.3	9.6–32.5
Oxford	74.2	66.9–81.1	63.6	49.4–77.5	Modena	11.7	9.2–14.6	12.4	7.0–21.0
Thames	66.7	62.4–71.0	51.6	43.2–60.4	Parma	8.3	6.2–11.1	7.1	3.5–13.9
Wessex	59.9	53.9–65.9	63.2	50.1–75.9	Ragusa	5.4	3.3–8.6	6.0	1.6–19.8
West Midlands	62.4	58.1–66.8	61.2	52.2–70.0	Romagna	10.3	8.1–12.9	10.7	6.3–17.6
Yorkshire	61.7	56.7–66.7	65.4	55.6–74.7	Turin	7.5	6.1–9.2	8.6	5.9–12.5
France					Varese	8.3	7.1–9.8	11.4	8.0–16.1
Amiens	48.2	40.3–56.6	32.6	10.8–68.2	Poland				
Calvados	51.7	44.1–59.5	39.3	14.4–75.2	Cracow	7.5	6.0–9.3	14.6	11.1–19.1
Doubs	56.1	45.3–66.9	97.1	67.5–104.7	Warsaw	6.7	5.2–8.5	5.9	3.9–8.9
Italy					Spain				
Florence	68.3	63.9–72.7	55.8	42.2–69.3	Basque Country	15.8	14.0–17.8	17.2	11.4–25.3
Genoa	65.4	57.9–72.7	45.1	24.8–68.3	Granada	6.5	4.4–9.4	16.8	7.4–34.4
Latina	46.1	33.0–60.7	86.1	34.5–109.6	Mallorca	12.0	9.0–15.9	14.5	6.3–30.2
Modena	73.1	62.6–82.8	90.5	51.4–102.9	Navarra	10.7	8.3–13.6	13.0	6.4–24.7
Parma	72.8	62.7–82.1	100.0	100.0–100.0	Tarragona	10.9	8.7–13.7	8.7	3.4–20.6
Ragusa	65.5	52.2–78.1	0.0	0.0–0.0					
Romagna	72.2	62.0–81.5	86.3	50.2–104.0	**Pleura**				
Turin	64.8	58.5–71.0	62.9	35.5–88.6	England				
Varese	70.8	64.4–76.8	65.4	40.7–88.2	East Anglia	3.9	1.3–11.0	12.3	3.4–36.7
Poland					Mersey	3.9	1.7–8.8	8.0	2.2–25.5
Cracow	40.1	32.7–48.2	65.6	41.1–87.1	Oxford	8.3	4.3–15.7	5.2	0.9–24.9
Warsaw	52.7	44.1–61.6	57.8	38.5–76.6	Thames	5.0	3.0–8.2	6.3	2.5–15.3
Spain					Wessex	4.2	2.4–7.4	3.2	0.6–16.3
Basque Country	64.4	60.0–68.6	76.8	45.0–99.3	West Midlands	2.6	0.9–7.5	11.0	3.8–28.5
Mallorca	64.7	52.7–76.0	–		Yorkshire	3.4	1.5–7.8	2.3	0.4–12.1
Navarra	68.2	61.4–74.6	43.3	12.7–83.3	France				
Tarragona	63.4	55.5–71.1	64.0	24.6–94.2	Amiens	15.0	5.2–37.3	45.8	16.9–80.2
Switzerland					Calvados	4.8	0.8–23.4	0.0	0.0–0.0
Basel	50.8	36.8–66.0	77.5	31.1–98.7	Doubs	0.0	0.0–0.0	–	
Geneva	67.0	56.1–77.3	76.3	45.0–95.2	Italy				
					Florence	4.5	0.8–22.1	0.0	0.0–0.0
					Genoa	1.7	0.3–9.1	0.0	0.0–0.0
Lung					Latina	0.0	0.0–0.0	0.0	0.0–0.0
England					Modena	0.0	0.0–0.0	0.0	0.0–0.0
East Anglia	6.6	5.8–7.6	5.9	4.7–7.2	Parma	11.3	2.0–46.9	0.0	0.0–0.0
Mersey	8.2	7.5–9.0	8.1	7.1–9.3	Ragusa	0.0	0.0–0.0	–	
Oxford	8.4	7.5–9.3	8.2	7.0–9.5	Romagna	0.0	0.0–0.0	0.0	0.0–0.0
Thames	7.3	6.8–7.9	7.6	6.9–8.5	Turin	5.8	1.0–27.5	14.4	4.0–42.0
Wessex	7.3	6.6–8.1	7.3	6.3–8.5	Varese	0.0	0.0–0.0	19.0	3.4–64.1
West Midlands	6.3	5.9–6.9	5.8	5.1–6.6	Poland				
Yorkshire	6.0	5.4–6.6	6.3	5.5–7.2	Cracow	12.8	2.3–50.1	22.4	4.1–69.9
France					Warsaw	16.5	3.0–62.0	0.0	0.0–0.0
Amiens	12.5	10.3–15.1	19.1	11.7–29.9	Spain				
Calvados	12.8	10.6–15.5	27.5	18.3–39.3	Basque Country	14.9	4.2–42.4	28.3	8.1–66.9
Doubs	13.4	10.8–16.4	14.4	8.4–23.6	Mallorca	0.0	0.0–0.0	0.0	0.0–0.0

Five-year relative survival (%), with 95% confidence interval (95% CI), by cancer registry and sex for countries with multiple local cancer registries (Contd)

Site / Registry area	Males R_{5y}	95% CI	Females R_{5y}	95% CI
Navarra	0.0	0.0–0.0	33.7	12.1–67.7
Tarragona	0.0	0.0–0.0	38.0	7.0–90.4
Bone				
England				
East Anglia	39.7	22.9–61.4	55.1	29.3–82.5
Mersey	50.5	31.2–71.8	32.8	16.6–56.5
Oxford	46.3	31.3–63.1	54.0	34.5–74.0
Thames	55.5	45.2–65.9	59.2	48.9–69.3
Wessex	44.5	31.9–58.8	52.0	37.5–67.2
West Midlands	53.3	40.0–67.0	55.2	41.3–69.3
Yorkshire	61.2	45.4–76.4	62.9	45.2–79.5
France				
Amiens	29.0	5.3–81.2	44.5	13.1–85.6
Calvados	86.5	57.3–98.9	56.6	27.2–82.6
Doubs	76.8	41.9–95.1	100.0	100.0–100.0
Italy				
Florence	41.8	26.9–59.5	43.4	22.8–67.5
Genoa	0.0	0.0–0.0	49.2	18.2–86.0
Latina	55.2	16.6–93.8	18.6	3.4–62.9
Modena	54.6	10.3–98.9	54.9	10.4–99.5
Parma	0.0	0.0–0.0	–	
Ragusa	0.0	0.0–0.0	0.0	0.0–0.0
Romagna	51.9	22.0–85.6	67.0	20.9–94.3
Turin	34.9	14.4–65.3	64.6	33.6–89.5
Varese	65.2	37.4–89.3	85.4	64.6–99.2
Poland				
Cracow	34.7	14.3–64.9	21.0	3.8–71.1
Warsaw	30.2	12.3–59.8	43.3	20.1–70.7
Spain				
Basque Country	43.8	21.7–70.3	75.1	49.4–92.3
Mallorca	100.0	100.0–100.0	100.0	100.0–100.0
Navarra	53.7	20.1–87.2	56.1	28.8–80.9
Tarragona	43.0	18.1–73.8	66.0	36.2–91.3
Soft tissues				
England				
East Anglia	52.8	41.7–64.5	58.3	46.6–70.2
Mersey	49.3	37.5–62.1	50.7	39.8–62.2
Oxford	59.6	49.2–70.0	60.2	49.2–71.0
Thames	59.6	52.2–66.9	60.0	52.1–67.9
Wessex	56.2	47.6–64.9	50.6	42.1–59.6
West Midlands	53.0	45.6–60.5	58.6	50.9–66.3
Yorkshire	53.4	44.9–62.1	45.2	37.1–53.9
France				
Amiens	56.7	33.8–80.5	49.8	23.1–81.3
Calvados	43.6	26.1–64.3	56.9	35.6–78.8
Doubs	–		72.8	37.6–96.8
Italy				
Florence	57.8	44.2–71.4	64.6	49.6–78.2
Genoa	44.4	25.1–67.9	45.7	26.8–67.1
Latina	66.5	41.1–86.8	68.3	45.8–86.5
Modena	29.8	13.3–56.5	23.2	4.2–72.5
Parma	60.9	36.5–85.4	68.8	41.0–92.0
Ragusa	43.9	12.6–98.4	68.0	30.6–92.2
Romagna	60.3	37.1–83.6	76.0	44.5–98.3
Turin	70.7	50.2–88.1	47.1	28.6–67.4
Varese	68.2	47.4–86.6	54.2	35.3–73.4
Poland				
Cracow	30.6	14.7–54.5	47.7	27.1–71.4
Warsaw	38.7	21.4–60.8	49.7	30.1–71.1
Spain				
Basque Country	62.0	46.0–77.6	53.1	37.6–68.9
Mallorca	73.7	32.3–108.6	73.1	41.4–93.1
Navarra	73.2	48.3–93.7	37.7	17.3–64.7
Tarragona	81.7	62.5–96.5	53.7	33.2–76.1
Melanoma of skin				
England				
East Anglia	71.4	64.9–77.6	81.4	77.1–85.4
Mersey	71.9	64.2–79.2	84.2	79.0–88.8
Oxford	77.5	71.8–82.7	86.3	82.8–89.5
Thames	66.5	62.4–70.5	81.8	79.2–84.3
Wessex	71.5	66.7–76.0	82.7	79.5–85.6
West Midlands	73.2	68.6–77.5	85.1	82.1–87.8
Yorkshire	65.1	59.4–70.7	86.0	82.5–89.2
France				
Amiens	69.6	50.2–86.7	77.2	62.1–89.2
Calvados	69.7	55.7–82.3	80.6	71.0–88.6
Doubs	72.7	56.0–86.5	88.0	76.8–96.1
Italy				
Florence	58.5	50.6–66.3	81.8	75.3–87.4
Genoa	57.0	43.5–70.4	76.0	63.7–86.1
Latina	59.0	36.4–80.7	77.1	52.4–93.4
Modena	49.6	32.9–67.8	68.0	50.8–83.3
Parma	53.4	33.1–75.3	61.0	45.2–75.8
Ragusa	69.2	49.7–85.4	70.4	49.0–87.8
Romagna	52.7	35.7–70.3	79.6	65.7–90.2
Turin	55.3	43.0–67.5	82.6	71.7–91.6
Varese	55.0	44.3–65.7	82.4	73.0–90.2
Poland				
Cracow	43.8	31.3–58.0	67.7	56.6–77.6
Warsaw	41.6	28.1–57.4	53.9	42.2–65.7
Spain				
Basque Country	62.8	48.3–76.9	85.7	77.8–92.2
Mallorca	86.3	60.0–102.9	91.6	73.0–102.7
Navarra	59.4	42.8–75.6	86.7	74.5–95.3
Tarragona	70.7	54.4–85.1	78.8	63.6–90.8

Five-year relative survival (%), with 95% confidence interval (95% CI), by cancer registry and sex for countries with multiple local cancer registries (Contd)

Site / Registry area	Males R_{5y}	95% CI	Females R_{5y}	95% CI
Breast				
England				
East Anglia	47.5	30.6–67.8	67.2	65.6–68.7
Mersey	60.4	38.2–84.8	67.6	66.1–69.0
Oxford	75.9	58.8–90.8	68.8	67.4–70.2
Thames	71.2	59.9–82.3	68.4	67.5–69.3
Wessex	63.2	47.3–79.8	67.3	66.0–68.5
West Midlands	72.0	58.4–85.0	65.4	64.4–66.4
Yorkshire	76.8	60.7–91.6	66.6	65.4–67.8
France				
Amiens	47.1	19.0–85.5	74.7	71.4–77.8
Calvados	76.0	46.1–98.6	79.0	76.3–81.6
Côte d'Or	–		81.0	77.9–83.9
Doubs	100.0	100.0–100.0	85.9	81.6–89.8
Isere	–		84.7	82.3–87.0
Italy				
Florence	73.5	52.3–92.2	77.1	75.3–78.8
Genoa	53.5	20.1–86.9	75.3	72.5–78.1
Latina	63.3	24.3–93.0	74.0	68.7–78.8
Modena	100.0	100.0–100.0	75.8	71.8–79.6
Parma	54.7	10.3–99.1	79.6	75.9–83.1
Ragusa	55.1	16.2–106.0	64.2	59.1–69.0
Romagna	59.6	25.7–93.6	85.7	82.2–88.8
Turin	40.2	18.2–71.5	76.5	74.0–78.9
Varese	68.3	29.0–112.8	78.5	76.4–80.6
Poland				
Cracow	62.3	23.0–108.9	57.0	53.6–60.4
Warsaw	68.3	32.8–99.7	63.5	59.9–66.9
Spain				
Basque Country	84.7	49.5–116.0	69.7	67.1–72.3
Girona	–		73.0	68.9–77.0
Granada	–		63.9	59.0–68.7
Mallorca	100.0	100.0–100.0	80.1	74.9–84.8
Navarra	60.5	22.7–98.3	71.5	68.0–74.9
Tarragona	88.6	50.2–112.9	68.6	65.0–72.1
Switzerland				
Basel	–		78.3	74.9–81.6
Geneva	100.0	100.0–100.0	80.9	77.7–84.0
Cervix uteri				
England				
East Anglia	–		64.7	60.9–68.4
Mersey	–		63.4	60.4–66.3
Oxford	–		69.8	66.3–73.2
Thames	–		61.1	58.8–63.3
Wessex	–		64.9	62.0–67.8
West Midlands	–		66.4	64.3–68.6
Yorkshire	–		67.9	65.5–70.2
France				
Amiens	–		62.8	55.7–69.6
Calvados	–		66.6	59.8–73.1
Côte d'Or	–		65.1	56.0–73.6
Doubs	–		60.4	50.4–70.1
Italy				
Florence	–		58.4	52.3–64.4
Genoa	–		65.1	56.8–73.0
Latina	–		68.4	56.7–78.6
Modena	–		70.7	57.1–82.2
Parma	–		61.3	49.2–72.9
Ragusa	–		53.6	43.1–64.2
Romagna	–		68.1	57.9–77.2
Turin	–		52.3	45.1–59.7
Varese	–		68.3	60.8–75.3
Poland				
Cracow	–		52.2	47.4–57.0
Warsaw	–		53.2	47.6–58.9
Spain				
Basque Country	–		62.3	54.9–69.3
Girona	–		57.6	46.5–68.4
Mallorca	–		63.5	53.3–72.8
Navarra	–		62.9	50.8–73.9
Tarragona	–		63.7	54.8–72.2
Switzerland				
Basel	–		58.7	46.5–70.3
Geneva	–		72.1	61.6–81.4
Corpus uteri				
England				
East Anglia	–		71.1	67.3–74.8
Mersey	–		69.7	65.8–73.5
Oxford	–		75.1	71.7–78.5
Thames	–		73.9	71.6–76.1
Wessex	–		75.2	72.1–78.3
West Midlands	–		73.2	70.6–75.7
Yorkshire	–		73.8	70.5–77.0
France				
Amiens	–		77.6	69.7–84.7
Calvados	–		73.0	65.8–79.6
Côte d'Or	–		72.9	64.4–80.7
Doubs	–		78.1	64.9–89.2
Italy				
Florence	–		74.6	70.6–78.4
Genoa	–		78.0	70.6–84.6
Latina	–		78.7	67.4–87.8
Modena	–		79.9	70.6–87.7
Parma	–		69.8	61.0–77.8

Five-year relative survival (%), with 95% confidence interval (95% CI), by cancer registry and sex for countries with multiple local cancer registries (Contd)

Site / Registry area	Males R_{5y}	95% CI	Females R_{5y}	95% CI
Ragusa	–		74.8	66.0–82.4
Romagna	–		66.1	57.1–74.5
Turin	–		73.8	67.7–79.4
Varese	–		75.9	70.9–80.6
Poland				
Cracow	–		70.2	64.0–76.1
Warsaw	–		73.4	67.1–79.2
Spain				
Basque Country	–		79.2	74.0–83.9
Girona	–		68.4	59.5–76.7
Mallorca	–		76.2	65.4–85.4
Navarra	–		77.6	70.5–83.7
Tarragona	–		75.1	68.2–81.2
Switzerland				
Basel	–		79.2	71.7–85.8
Geneva	–		73.6	66.0–80.6
Ovary				
England				
East Anglia	–		29.6	26.6–32.8
Mersey	–		31.7	28.6–34.9
Oxford	–		37.1	34.1–40.2
Thames	–		31.2	29.4–33.1
Wessex	–		26.7	24.3–29.3
West Midlands	–		32.2	30.2–34.3
Yorkshire	–		30.0	27.5–32.6
France				
Amiens	–		40.5	33.1–48.6
Calvados	–		39.5	32.5–47.1
Côte d'Or	–		33.3	25.4–42.4
Doubs	–		38.4	27.5–51.0
Italy				
Florence	–		36.7	32.1–41.7
Genoa	–		35.8	29.1–43.2
Latina	–		35.0	22.7–50.1
Modena	–		34.9	26.6–44.5
Parma	–		34.6	26.4–44.0
Ragusa	–		23.7	15.1–35.4
Romagna	–		30.5	22.3–40.3
Turin	–		25.8	20.3–32.4
Varese	–		35.7	30.1–41.8
Poland				
Cracow	–		32.0	26.8–37.9
Warsaw	–		27.5	22.3–33.5
Spain				
Basque Country	–		51.7	45.1–58.4
Girona	–		29.7	21.7–39.3
Mallorca	–		63.6	49.2–76.7
Navarra	–		38.2	30.4–46.7
Tarragona	–		43.5	34.9–52.8

Site / Registry area	Males R_{5y}	95% CI	Females R_{5y}	95% CI
Switzerland				
Basel	–		38.5	30.9–46.9
Geneva	–		43.0	35.3–51.3
Vagina and vulva				
England				
East Anglia	–		59.5	50.5–68.7
Mersey	–		52.0	43.8–60.8
Oxford	–		55.0	46.6–63.8
Thames	–		53.2	47.7–58.8
Wessex	–		56.5	49.6–63.7
West Midlands	–		60.4	54.6–66.3
Yorkshire	–		49.9	43.6–56.6
France				
Amiens	–		44.5	29.0–63.0
Calvados	–		44.8	28.8–64.3
Côte d'Or	–		29.0	8.4–71.1
Doubs	–		61.6	33.4–91.5
Italy				
Florence	–		52.5	42.2–63.5
Genoa	–		41.5	26.5–60.2
Latina	–		29.2	13.1–54.7
Modena	–		61.9	41.5–82.7
Parma	–		55.5	34.3–78.9
Ragusa	–		31.9	13.0–62.1
Romagna	–		58.4	38.8–79.3
Turin	–		40.2	25.3–58.8
Varese	–		50.0	35.0–67.2
Poland				
Cracow	–		25.5	14.7–41.4
Warsaw	–		58.6	43.1–74.5
Spain				
Basque Country	–		58.6	47.5–69.8
Girona	–		42.0	21.8–69.0
Mallorca	–		67.3	45.3–88.9
Navarra	–		41.9	26.9–60.3
Tarragona	–		51.6	35.1–70.1
Prostate				
England				
East Anglia	44.4	42.0–47.0	–	
Mersey	46.9	44.2–49.8	–	
Oxford	48.3	45.8–51.0	–	
Thames	45.6	44.0–47.3	–	
Wessex	42.4	40.3–44.4	–	
West Midlands	43.7	41.9–45.5	–	
Yorkshire	44.0	41.9–46.2	–	
France				
Amiens	59.9	54.6–65.3	–	
Calvados	58.5	53.8–63.4	–	
Doubs	79.3	70.4–87.8	–	

Five-year relative survival (%), with 95% confidence interval (95% CI), by cancer registry and sex for countries with multiple local cancer registries (Contd)

Site Registry area	Males R_{5y}	95% CI	Females R_{5y}	95% CI	Site Registry area	Males R_{5y}	95% CI	Females R_{5y}	95% CI
Italy					**Spain**				
Florence	45.4	41.9–49.1	–		Basque Country	92.2	81.1–98.1	–	
Genoa	48.3	42.1–55.0	–		Mallorca	100.0	100.0–100.0	–	
Latina	35.1	25.4–47.0	–		Navarra	93.9	72.9–101.5	–	
Modena	63.1	55.4–71.0	–		Tarragona	86.7	67.5–96.7	–	
Parma	40.1	32.4–48.8	–		**Switzerland**				
Ragusa	28.1	20.6–37.5	–		Basel	95.8	88.5–99.2	–	
Romagna	49.0	41.6–56.9	–		Geneva	96.2	88.2–99.7	–	
Turin	55.0	49.0–61.3	–						
Varese	55.9	51.0–60.9	–		***Penis***				
Poland					**England**				
Cracow	36.7	28.8–45.9	–		East Anglia	70.6	55.1–85.3	–	
Warsaw	37.5	29.8–46.4	–		Mersey	75.5	62.7–87.6	–	
Spain					Oxford	75.5	62.8–87.2	–	
Basque Country	52.9	47.0–59.2	–		Thames	60.6	51.2–70.2	–	
Mallorca	61.3	51.8–71.3	–		Wessex	69.3	57.1–81.2	–	
Navarra	63.6	57.8–69.4	–		West Midlands	76.6	67.5–85.2	–	
Tarragona	40.4	34.4–47.0	–		Yorkshire	69.4	57.9–80.8	–	
Switzerland					**France**				
Basel	80.0	74.1–85.8	–		Amiens	100.0	100.0–100.0	–	
Geneva	62.0	55.8–68.3	–		Calvados	55.8	29.3–86.7	–	
					Doubs	92.7	50.7–106.5	–	
Testis					**Italy**				
England					Florence	69.9	50.5–88.5	–	
East Anglia	91.9	87.6–95.1	–		Genoa	72.7	43.3–97.1	–	
Mersey	89.8	85.5–93.2	–		Latina	100.0	100.0–100.0	–	
Oxford	88.3	84.2–91.6	–		Modena	68.4	20.5–116.2	–	
Thames	92.7	90.5–94.5	–		Parma	100.0	100.0–100.0	–	
Wessex	91.2	87.6–94.0	–		Ragusa	100.0	100.0–100.0	–	
West Midlands	88.4	84.7–91.4	–		Romagna	56.7	26.6–89.9	–	
Yorkshire	87.8	83.8–91.0	–		Turin	72.7	46.5–96.1	–	
France					Varese	76.7	52.8–95.4	–	
Amiens	82.4	69.4–91.1	–		**Poland**				
Calvados	87.7	76.0–94.7	–		Cracow	71.2	34.2–104.0	–	
Doubs	94.3	79.4–99.2	–		Warsaw	51.3	21.6–88.2	–	
Italy					**Spain**				
Florence	88.6	80.4–94.4	–		Basque Country	81.5	63.1–96.9	–	
Genoa	89.3	73.9–96.7	–		Mallorca	79.1	39.6–111.9	–	
Latina	75.1	44.9–93.2	–		Navarra	82.5	54.8–101.3	–	
Modena	97.9	77.9–102.4	–		Tarragona	65.2	37.0–91.1	–	
Parma	88.7	63.5–98.5	–						
Ragusa	83.3	51.1–98.3	–		***Bladder***				
Romagna	98.0	82.7–101.3	–		**England**				
Turin	86.9	73.3–95.0	–		East Anglia	64.2	60.6–67.7	58.1	52.5–63.8
Varese	94.6	87.2–98.6	–		Mersey	67.2	64.0–70.3	62.9	58.5–67.3
Poland					Oxford	69.1	66.1–72.1	60.2	55.3–65.1
Cracow	85.7	72.7–93.7	–		Thames	66.5	64.6–68.5	60.1	57.1–63.1
Warsaw	76.1	64.6–85.2	–		Wessex	72.8	70.3–75.3	59.8	55.8–63.7

Five-year relative survival (%), with 95% confidence interval (95% CI), by cancer registry and sex for countries with multiple local cancer registries (Contd)

Site Registry area	Males R_{5y}	95% CI	Females R_{5y}	95% CI	Site Registry area	Males R_{5y}	95% CI	Females R_{5y}	95% CI
West Midlands	66.0	63.8–68.2	58.5	55.0–61.9	Poland				
Yorkshire	63.2	60.7–65.8	55.6	51.8–59.3	Cracow	27.1	20.4–35.2	33.7	24.6–44.5
France					Warsaw	42.6	35.0–51.0	39.5	31.1–48.9
Amiens	53.2	45.1–61.8	50.5	35.1–67.8	Spain				
Calvados	66.6	59.3–73.9	53.9	40.9–67.8	Basque Country	54.7	47.5–62.0	57.4	47.3–67.4
Doubs	73.1	61.7–83.7	66.5	44.4–87.9	Mallorca	66.8	49.4–83.5	25.6	10.3–52.6
Italy					Navarra	49.4	38.9–60.6	50.0	37.5–63.1
Florence	70.4	67.4–73.3	67.8	61.8–73.7	Tarragona	43.6	31.6–57.2	59.7	41.7–77.4
Genoa	64.0	58.6–69.4	63.6	53.1–73.9	Switzerland				
Latina	63.6	54.2–73.1	52.8	32.1–74.7	Basel	53.3	42.0–65.1	42.5	31.1–55.3
Modena	74.4	67.7–80.7	69.0	54.6–82.5	Geneva	57.3	46.0–68.9	46.6	34.6–59.9
Parma	62.9	55.1–70.6	62.0	46.2–77.2					
Ragusa	39.8	31.1–49.6	52.7	27.7–82.0	***Choroid(melanoma)***				
Romagna	76.3	69.9–82.3	64.6	48.4–80.5	England				
Turin	70.7	66.1–75.3	59.2	50.2–68.3	East Anglia	80.1	49.0–101.0	77.6	39.0–99.7
Varese	68.4	63.3–73.5	61.5	51.3–71.8	Mersey	47.9	25.0–75.6	44.9	16.4–83.1
Poland					Oxford	100.0	100.0–100.0	58.2	32.9–82.1
Cracow	29.0	22.3–37.0	25.9	13.6–44.9	Thames	89.2	74.9–99.0	79.4	63.6–91.5
Warsaw	45.5	37.6–54.2	45.4	33.2–59.1	Wessex	88.6	65.7–102.2	89.9	64.8–105.5
Spain					West Midlands	76.4	60.0–90.2	64.5	46.5–81.1
Basque Country	72.9	68.8–76.9	71.8	61.6–81.3	Yorkshire	82.3	62.2–98.5	62.6	45.8–78.3
Mallorca	72.9	64.3–81.2	75.8	52.8–96.7	France				
Navarra	71.6	65.9–77.2	67.3	52.4–81.6	Amiens	81.0	42.2–112.4	100.0	100.0–100.0
Tarragona	69.1	63.4–74,7	68.1	55.6–80.1	Calvados	78.4	39.4–100.8	100.0	100.0–100.0
					Doubs	0.0	0.0–0.0	69.1	21.5–97.3
Kidney					Italy				
England					Florence	85.4	46.6–105.8	38.5	11.2–80.9
East Anglia	40.9	35.6–46.5	28.3	21.9–36.0	Genoa	–		0.0	0.0–0.0
Mersey	45.3	40.0–50.9	33.6	27.5–40.6	Latina	60.4	11.4–109.5	100.0	100.0–100.0
Oxford	40.7	35.8–45.9	38.4	32.5–44.8	Modena	0.0	0.0–0.0	57.1	10.8–103.4
Thames	40.2	36.8–43.7	36.7	32.5–41.1	Parma	71.0	22.1–100.0	100.0	100.0–100.0
Wessex	41.4	37.2–45.8	40.0	34.5–45.8	Ragusa	0.0	0.0–0.0	–	
West Midlands	37.7	34.2–41.3	38.0	33.7–42.6	Romagna	0.0	0.0–0.0	44.6	13.1–85.9
Yorkshire	39.7	35.5–44.1	36.9	32.0–42.1	Turin	41.6	7.7–99.0	80.5	46.8–97.0
France					Varese	97.4	30.3–137.1	47.1	13.8–90.5
Amiens	49.6	39.9–59.8	56.4	41.6–71.3	Poland				
Calvados	60.4	50.9–69.8	50.6	39.0–62.7	Cracow	100.0	100.0–100.0	–	
Doubs	68.9	52.4–84.4	74.8	57.4–89.7	Warsaw	100.0	100.0–100.0	100.0	100.0–100.0
Italy					Spain				
Florence	55.6	50.3–61.0	59.2	52.0–66.3	Basque Country	–		93.4	61.8–101.9
Genoa	53.7	44.3–63.6	48.7	37.4–60.7	Mallorca	–		100.0	100.0–100.0
Latina	46.0	29.6–64.6	65.5	42.6–86.1	Navarra	75.8	23.6–106.7	37.5	6.9–89.1
Modena	57.4	46.0–69.0	65.4	51.6–78.6					
Parma	46.4	35.7–58.1	38.7	25.2–54.9	***Brain***				
Ragusa	52.7	36.1–69.8	38.9	19.1–64.8	England				
Romagna	59.0	49.4–68.7	57.6	43.5–71.7	East Anglia	10.7	7.7–14.7	12.6	8.9–17.6
Turin	48.0	39.7–56.7	42.8	32.9–53.9	Mersey	11.2	8.1–15.3	17.6	13.3–22.8
Varese	53.2	46.3–60.4	58.8	49.8–67.8	Oxford	19.7	16.0–24.0	21.8	17.7–26.7

Five-year relative survival (%), with 95% confidence interval (95% CI), by cancer registry and sex for countries with multiple local cancer registries (Contd)

Site Registry area	Males R_{5y}	95% CI	Females R_{5y}	95% CI
Thames	18.3	15.8–21.1	20.6	17.6–24.0
Wessex	14.1	11.2–17.5	15.4	12.0–19.5
West Midlands	16.3	13.6–19.4	16.2	13.1–20.0
Yorkshire	16.1	13.0–19.8	15.2	11.8–19.4
France				
Amiens	21.9	12.6–35.5	19.0	9.5–34.9
Calvados	18.8	10.5–31.5	18.7	9.4–34.1
Doubs	25.9	13.7–43.8	28.3	13.9–49.7
Italy				
Florence	14.6	10.5–20.0	18.2	13.0–25.0
Genoa	20.0	12.0–31.6	9.7	4.5–19.8
Latina	34.1	19.5–53.1	36.3	20.8–55.7
Modena	16.5	7.2–33.8	17.3	7.6–35.2
Parma	16.7	7.3–34.5	0.0	0.0–0.0
Ragusa	15.8	7.4–30.9	15.5	6.2–34.1
Romagna	23.3	13.8–36.8	14.8	7.3–27.6
Turin	15.1	9.4–23.6	14.6	8.1–25.3
Varese	14.6	9.2–22.6	22.1	14.9–31.6
Poland				
Cracow	8.0	3.5–17.5	11.7	5.1–24.9
Warsaw	22.5	12.7–37.2	16.5	10.0–25.9
Spain				
Basque Country	14.6	9.9–21.0	16.5	10.9–24.2
Mallorca	12.9	5.6–27.2	16.4	7.2–33.3
Navarra	18.9	12.1–28.4	13.9	7.5–24.5
Tarragona	16.9	9.5–28.5	18.6	10.3–31.4
Switzerland				
Basel	11.9	5.5–23.8	14.2	6.7–28.0
Geneva	29.1	18.8–42.3	20.0	9.8–37.0

Thyroid gland
Site Registry area	Males R_{5y}	95% CI	Females R_{5y}	95% CI
England				
East Anglia	65.0	48.6–80.7	80.5	70.8–88.5
Mersey	68.2	51.7–83.5	75.6	64.2–85.6
Oxford	69.4	55.0–82.1	79.6	71.9–86.1
Thames	59.5	50.0–68.8	73.1	67.1–78.8
Wessex	62.2	48.6–75.5	77.8	70.0–84.7
West Midlands	62.1	52.0–72.0	70.1	63.5–76.4
Yorkshire	66.7	53.1–79.5	77.8	70.4–84.4
France				
Amiens	65.4	38.9–87.3	80.0	65.1–91.3
Calvados	76.6	53.7–92.4	88.9	78.4–95.9
Doubs	78.8	52.4–95.0	84.5	54.0–100.5
Italy				
Florence	77.9	65.6–87.9	84.1	77.3–89.6
Genoa	59.1	37.7–81.0	64.4	52.2–75.7
Latina	70.4	21.9–99.1	85.0	60.9–96.8
Modena	89.4	59.2–102.2	92.6	79.4–99.3
Parma	60.9	37.0–82.7	88.8	76.5–96.3

Site Registry area	Males R_{5y}	95% CI	Females R_{5y}	95% CI
Ragusa	84.4	51.7–99.5	58.4	35.5–79.3
Romagna	80.2	55.8–96.0	93.5	83.9–98.8
Turin	89.0	69.9–98.7	78.8	67.5–87.7
Varese	56.8	42.5–70.7	88.1	80.7–93.6
Poland				
Cracow	38.0	15.9–70.7	61.9	47.0–76.2
Warsaw	67.2	29.5–99.0	69.2	54.5–81.9
Spain				
Basque Country	76.4	54.0–93.5	76.5	65.3–85.6
Mallorca	60.6	11.5–109.7	95.4	75.8–102.3
Navarra	79.3	58.5–93.6	92.6	85.3–97.2
Tarragona	72.0	46.0–92.0	86.3	72.7–95.3

Non-Hodgkin's lymphomas
Site Registry area	Males R_{5y}	95% CI	Females R_{5y}	95% CI
England				
East Anglia	46.9	42.6–51.5	44.8	40.1–49.7
Mersey	45.1	40.3–50.1	51.0	46.3–55.8
Oxford	47.9	43.5–52.4	48.3	43.5–53.4
Thames	47.1	44.3–49.9	47.5	44.7–50.4
Wessex	48.9	45.3–52.5	49.5	45.9–53.3
West Midlands	42.9	39.6–46.3	42.7	39.2–46.2
Yorkshire	45.8	42.1–49.7	42.2	38.4–46.2
France				
Amiens	52.2	41.6–63.4	48.9	38.5–60.1
Calvados	50.7	41.2–60.7	49.8	40.5–59.6
Côte d'Or	54.9	44.9–65.2	52.3	41.6–63.4
Doubs	65.4	51.2–79.2	72.6	57.6–85.6
Italy				
Florence	40.8	35.0–47.1	47.4	41.2–53.9
Genoa	41.2	32.2–51.3	51.3	42.0–61.0
Latina	51.5	36.9–67.1	57.7	41.7–73.0
Modena	46.9	37.4–57.2	49.7	39.3–60.7
Parma	51.9	38.6–66.1	43.3	31.6–56.3
Ragusa	49.6	34.4–66.1	40.5	24.1–61.0
Romagna	54.1	44.2–64.2	51.5	41.8–61.4
Turin	34.4	26.7–43.3	44.3	35.3–53.9
Varese	55.6	48.9–62.4	50.6	44.0–57.5
Poland				
Cracow	29.7	20.2–41.8	25.5	15.7–39.2
Warsaw	40.8	30.8–52.2	38.2	27.3–50.9
Spain				
Basque Country	57.4	49.6–65.2	50.1	41.6–58.8
Mallorca	52.6	38.8–67.2	45.1	30.4–61.7
Navarra	55.4	44.7–66.3	49.5	38.2–61.5
Tarragona	51.3	39.0–64.3	45.1	32.9–58.7
Switzerland				
Basel	47.4	37.0–58.7	51.0	40.1–62.6
Geneva	50.9	40.9–61.4	47.6	37.5–58.5

Five-year relative survival (%), with 95% confidence interval (95% CI), by cancer registry and sex for countries with multiple local cancer registries (Contd)

Site Registry area	Males R_{5y}	95% CI	Females R_{5y}	95% CI	Site Registry area	Males R_{5y}	95% CI	Females R_{5y}	95% CI
Hodgkin's disease					Côte d'Or	30.3	16.5–51.1	35.5	21.0–55.3
England					Doubs	62.5	39.9–85.8	61.3	41.6–80.7
East Anglia	75.4	67.0–82.6	72.0	63.0–80.0	Italy				
Mersey	71.6	63.3–78.9	74.1	63.9–82.8	Florence	27.3	20.5–35.7	30.7	23.2–39.5
Oxford	73.7	66.2–80.3	76.4	68.1–83.5	Genoa	36.9	25.4–51.2	33.7	21.7–49.1
Thames	77.7	73.1–81.8	78.4	73.1–83.0	Latina	37.4	16.9–67.6	39.5	16.4–72.2
Wessex	76.2	69.4–82.1	83.3	75.9–89.2	Modena	51.1	34.6–69.6	43.1	27.3–61.6
West Midlands	68.2	62.5–73.6	72.5	65.7–78.5	Parma	40.7	24.0–62.5	32.3	18.9–50.7
Yorkshire	71.2	64.7–77.2	77.7	70.4–83.9	Ragusa	16.5	7.2–34.2	32.4	17.2–54.3
France					Romagna	31.2	18.6–48.7	32.5	18.0–52.5
Amiens	60.2	42.3–77.2	90.1	70.0–99.1	Turin	28.2	15.9–45.9	22.9	13.2–37.4
Calvados	86.8	72.5–95.7	89.7	72.8–98.1	Varese	25.2	15.8–38.3	27.4	18.5–38.8
Côte d'Or	63.0	43.3–81.4	74.8	50.5–90.5	Poland				
Doubs	67.4	38.6–88.7	95.1	75.2–99.6	Cracow	10.4	3.6–27.3	10.8	3.8–27.5
Italy					Warsaw	22.4	10.6–42.8	9.2	3.2–24.4
Florence	62.3	51.8–72.3	74.1	64.2–82.4	Spain				
Genoa	70.4	54.2–83.8	76.4	58.6–89.2	Basque Country	45.5	32.4–60.5	28.2	18.1–41.6
Latina	74.5	51.3–91.9	82.9	59.4–94.4	Mallorca	61.4	37.6–85.0	44.3	25.0–67.7
Modena	93.8	69.8–102.8	69.8	40.9–90.3	Navarra	41.0	25.9–59.3	30.1	16.6–49.0
Parma	63.0	44.6–79.6	29.2	13.1–54.7	Tarragona	20.0	11.0–34.3	34.8	21.4–52.2
Ragusa	94.2	62.3–102.7	76.1	47.4–92.4	Switzerland				
Romagna	84.9	62.0–97.6	66.9	45.1–84.3	Basel	26.6	11.3–53.4	28.6	14.4–50.4
Turin	66.7	51.4–80.5	64.4	49.3–77.5	Geneva	38.3	23.3–57.6	33.3	19.1–52.9
Varese	68.6	56.6–79.1	78.9	66.9–88.2					
Poland					**Acute lymphatic leukaemia**				
Cracow	63.3	48.3–76.8	70.0	53.9–83.3	England				
Warsaw	56.6	39.4–73.5	82.9	64.4–93.4	East Anglia	5.3	0.9–25.5	12.3	3.4–36.2
Spain					Mersey	39.4	22.8–60.2	33.3	17.8–54.5
Basque Country	67.2	54.9–78.3	61.9	47.6–75.2	Oxford	37.4	22.2–55.9	40.7	24.3–60.5
Mallorca	98.3	62.5–108.4	89.6	64.2–99.5	Thames	30.0	20.5–42.0	30.1	18.4–45.7
Navarra	71.9	56.0–84.8	75.9	55.3–90.4	Wessex	19.1	11.5–30.3	42.2	26.4–60.7
Tarragona	71.3	53.1–85.9	52.4	28.8–76.2	West Midlands	25.9	17.7–36.5	9.9	4.3–21.4
Switzerland					Yorkshire	18.2	9.5–32.3	37.5	22.2–56.3
Basel	77.7	56.7–92.5	88.3	67.2–99.3	France				
Geneva	70.8	51.2–87.7	64.3	41.7–83.2	Amiens	55.1	20.7–89.6	–	
					Calvados	22.0	6.2–57.7	52.8	19.5–92.3
Multiple myeloma					Doubs	25.2	4.6–70.4	51.2	19.2–83.2
England					Italy				
East Anglia	17.2	12.6–23.3	20.1	15.0–26.4	Florence	21.1	8.5–44.3	6.8	1.2–31.0
Mersey	16.9	11.9–23.4	16.7	11.8–23.2	Genoa	19.2	3.5–69.0	27.6	9.8–58.8
Oxford	18.6	14.0–24.4	23.2	18.0–29.6	Latina	13.3	2.4–52.0	100.0	100.0–100.0
Thames	25.6	21.9–29.8	22.1	18.6–26.2	Modena	100.0	100.0–100.0	0.0	0.0–0.0
Wessex	19.1	15.1–23.8	23.3	19.2–28.2	Parma	0.0	0.0–0.0	0.0	0.0–0.0
West Midlands	18.6	15.1–22.6	18.3	14.9–22.4	Ragusa	15.4	2.8–58.1	34.9	10.1–73.2
Yorkshire	23.8	19.6–28.8	24.1	19.7–29.3	Romagna	0.0	0.0–0.0	33.2	9.5–74.4
France					Turin	30.1	10.8–62.4	0.0	0.0–0.0
Amiens	36.8	20.6–58.8	22.3	11.6–39.2	Varese	36.6	16.8–62.8	17.1	4.8–47.7
Calvados	23.8	11.9–43.1	25.3	15.0–39.7					

Five-year relative survival (%), with 95% confidence interval (95% CI), by cancer registry and sex for countries with multiple local cancer registries (Contd)

Site Registry area	Males R_{5y}	95% CI	Females R_{5y}	95% CI
Poland				
Cracow	9.7	1.7–41.3	0.0	0.0–0.0
Warsaw	16.9	3.0–60.6	23.5	4.3–73.5
Spain				
Basque Country	30.1	14.3–54.1	27.2	11.1–52.9
Mallorca	41.4	7.6–98.5	100.0	100.0–100.0
Navarra	0.0	0.0–0.0	52.5	15.8–89.3
Tarragona	30.1	10.8–62.5	19.3	3.5–65.2
Switzerland				
Basel	15.2	2.7–54.6	30.0	5.5–84.0
Geneva	0.0	0.0–0.0	17.0	3.1–61.2
Chronic lymphatic leukaemia				
England				
East Anglia	50.1	41.4–59.4	48.3	36.9–61.1
Mersey	55.4	44.1–67.7	45.1	33.4–58.6
Oxford	26.5	18.5–36.8	30.5	20.7–43.3
Thames	59.2	52.9–65.6	61.4	54.4–68.6
Wessex	51.3	43.6–59.6	62.5	54.2–71.1
West Midlands	50.4	44.3–56.8	52.7	45.1–60.8
Yorkshire	59.4	52.7–66.4	62.4	54.6–70.3
France				
Amiens	69.5	54.4–84.0	81.2	65.0–94.6
Calvados	81.3	63.3–95.9	72.2	46.5–94.0
Côte d'Or	82.9	66.4–97.7	88.6	72.0–101.0
Doubs	89.9	69.5–103.7	94.6	67.2–110.0
Italy				
Florence	39.9	29.3–52.4	51.9	39.1–65.6
Genoa	39.2	23.6–59.4	64.5	45.8–83.0
Latina	52.7	30.2–77.1	75.4	44.2–97.4
Modena	69.4	47.6–90.3	87.6	64.3–101.7
Parma	65.8	40.2–92.2	72.9	39.5–104.0
Ragusa	26.5	7.5–69.5	77.9	34.1–114.7
Romagna	64.6	46.5–82.2	51.7	30.4–75.9
Turin	44.1	22.8–71.4	37.0	16.6–68.6
Varese	67.8	52.4–82.4	73.1	56.3–88.8
Poland				
Cracow	24.6	10.8–49.3	14.2	4.0–41.9
Warsaw	52.0	30.2–78.2	42.1	17.4–76.9
Spain				
Basque Country	84.6	68.8–98.5	76.2	56.5–93.5
Mallorca	62.4	34.7–91.5	66.2	28.5–103.9
Navarra	71.9	52.4–90.3	64.5	44.6–82.7
Tarragona	58.7	42.3–75.6	82.0	57.9–99.5
Switzerland				
Basel	82.6	64.1–98.4	71.6	48.0–91.5
Geneva	53.3	34.5–74.9	80.5	53.2–103.9

Site Registry area	Males R_{5y}	95% CI	Females R_{5y}	95% CI
Acute myeloid leukaemia				
England				
East Anglia	6.8	3.5–13.0	8.8	4.7–15.9
Mersey	7.1	3.6–13.5	9.1	5.0–16.1
Oxford	10.5	6.0–18.1	11.6	7.1–18.4
Thames	8.8	5.9–13.0	14.4	10.5–19.4
Wessex	12.5	8.4–18.2	13.4	9.0–19.6
West Midlands	12.1	8.5–16.9	6.6	4.1–10.3
Yorkshire	15.0	10.3–21.6	10.7	6.9–16.4
France				
Amiens	16.7	6.7–37.1	4.2	0.7–20.6
Calvados	37.3	13.5–72.2	28.8	10.2–62.7
Côte d'Or	11.4	4.5–26.8	18.9	9.4–34.7
Doubs	–		23.4	11.1–43.7
Italy				
Florence	8.8	4.1–18.1	11.5	5.0–24.4
Genoa	15.0	6.0–33.5	20.1	8.9–40.1
Latina	18.7	6.5–44.5	19.4	6.8–44.4
Modena	0.0	0.0–0.0	0.0	0.0–0.0
Parma	10.1	2.8–31.5	5.5	1.0–26.2
Ragusa	8.6	1.5–38.0	9.2	1.6–39.1
Romagna	5.6	1.0–26.4	7.8	1.4–34.9
Turin	8.3	2.9–22.0	4.8	0.8–23.3
Varese	4.4	1.2–14.9	8.8	3.5–20.9
Poland				
Cracow	0.0	0.0–0.0	5.9	1.1–27.7
Warsaw	0.0	0.0–0.0	0.0	0.0–0.0
Spain				
Basque Country	13.5	5.9–28.4	16.5	5.8–39.2
Mallorca	28.1	10.0–59.7	13.8	3.9–39.8
Navarra	14.7	4.1–41.8	21.5	7.5–50.0
Tarragona	21.5	8.7–45.6	0.0	0.0–0.0
Switzerland				
Basel	23.6	9.5–49.6	6.0	1.1–28.7
Geneva	13.3	3.7–39.4	11.2	3.1–34.2
Chronic myeloid leukaemia				
England				
East Anglia	15.2	8.1–27.0	29.7	17.1–47.6
Mersey	27.5	17.0–42.3	18.6	9.6–33.6
Oxford	19.8	12.3–30.8	17.4	9.6–29.8
Thames	25.0	17.5–34.6	26.5	19.3–35.5
Wessex	22.2	15.6–30.8	38.5	28.9–49.6
West Midlands	23.4	17.0–31.4	22.7	15.9–31.6
Yorkshire	24.3	16.9–34.1	22.9	15.2–33.4
France				
Amiens	39.2	20.1–64.8	23.2	6.8–57.1
Calvados	34.6	16.3–61.0	40.3	18.7–67.0
Côte d'Or	31.7	19.7–48.2	57.3	39.1–76.6
Doubs	60.5	27.1–92.0	43.7	9.1–94.1

Five-year relative survival (%), with 95% confidence interval (95% CI), by cancer registry and sex for countries with multiple local cancer registries (Contd)

Site / Registry area	Males R_{5y}	95% CI	Females R_{5y}	95% CI
Italy				
Florence	23.8	14.4–37.1	21.8	10.9–39.3
Genoa	14.7	5.1–37.1	25.7	9.0–58.9
Latina	15.9	2.9–57.1	43.9	16.2–76.8
Modena	9.0	1.6–38.8	27.8	7.9–70.9
Parma	26.1	7.4–66.4	35.1	12.6–70.7
Ragusa	20.6	5.8–55.4	45.0	16.4–83.2
Romagna	40.4	19.7–68.1	33.9	14.0–63.5
Turin	14.2	4.0–41.9	13.2	3.7–39.1
Varese	36.8	23.5–53.5	39.1	23.2–59.1
Poland				
Cracow	11.3	2.0–45.8	10.2	1.8–42.4
Warsaw	0.0	0.0–0.0	8.1	1.4–36.1
Spain				
Basque Country	41.8	23.2–64.9	23.7	6.7–58.5
Mallorca	–		36.5	10.6–76.7
Navarra	33.0	14.8–60.4	26.0	7.4–61.3
Tarragona	38.0	21.1–60.2	52.6	24.9–80.4
Switzerland				
Basel	30.7	10.9–65.4	10.8	1.9–44.8
Geneva	29.7	14.2–54.5	43.1	19.6–75.3

Leukaemia

Site / Registry area	Males R_{5y}	95% CI	Females R_{5y}	95% CI
England				
East Anglia	25.1	20.8–30.1	22.6	18.0–28.2
Mersey	27.4	22.7–32.8	23.6	19.0–29.0
Oxford	19.1	15.3–23.6	18.5	14.7–23.1
Thames	33.3	30.1–36.8	34.6	31.1–38.2
Wessex	27.3	23.8–31.1	36.9	32.7–41.4
West Midlands	28.8	25.8–32.0	23.5	20.4–26.9
Yorkshire	35.7	31.9–39.8	34.5	30.4–39.0
France				
Amiens	47.2	37.6–57.6	46.8	36.3–58.1
Calvados	49.9	38.7–61.9	41.5	29.9–54.9
Côte d'Or	43.8	35.3–53.2	55.7	46.3–65.3
Doubs	58.8	45.8–71.8	53.4	37.8–69.9
Italy				
Florence	22.2	17.6–27.6	25.6	20.0–32.4
Genoa	21.1	14.0–30.8	37.8	28.3–48.9
Latina	30.0	18.9–44.6	44.0	29.4–60.1
Modena	34.7	23.2–49.2	54.0	37.8–70.9
Parma	26.6	17.6–38.8	22.1	12.7–36.0
Ragusa	15.0	7.4–28.5	30.6	17.9–47.9
Romagna	38.6	28.2–50.6	32.1	21.4–45.5
Turin	17.1	10.9–25.9	11.6	6.0–21.6
Varese	34.8	27.8–42.8	35.5	27.9–44.1

Leukaemia (continued)

Site / Registry area	Males R_{5y}	95% CI	Females R_{5y}	95% CI
Poland				
Cracow	11.5	5.9–21.4	6.6	2.5–16.4
Warsaw	18.4	10.5–30.7	13.7	7.1–25.1
Spain				
Basque Country	41.4	33.7–49.9	37.9	28.2–49.2
Mallorca	41.5	26.1–60.5	32.5	18.5–51.5
Navarra	45.6	34.8–57.5	41.4	29.8–54.5
Tarragona	38.6	29.5–49.0	39.9	27.8–54.0
Switzerland				
Basel	54.7	43.7–66.3	34.6	24.0–47.5
Geneva	32.1	22.2–44.7	37.4	25.5–52.0

Malignant neoplasms

Site / Registry area	Males R_{5y}	95% CI	Females R_{5y}	95% CI
England				
East Anglia	31.8	31.0–32.6	46.3	45.4–47.1
Mersey	30.3	29.6–31.1	44.2	43.4–45.0
Oxford	33.0	32.3–33.8	46.9	46.2–47.7
Thames	32.0	31.5–32.5	45.8	45.3–46.3
Wessex	33.3	32.7–34.0	46.1	45.5–46.8
West Midlands	28.1	27.6–28.6	42.8	42.2–43.3
Yorkshire	27.9	27.3–28.5	42.3	41.7–42.9
France				
Amiens	34.1	32.6–35.7	53.6	51.7–55.6
Calvados	37.5	36.0–39.0	60.8	59.0–62.6
Doubs	42.4	40.0–44.7	65.0	62.3–67.7
Italy				
Florence	35.9	35.0–36.8	52.2	51.2–53.3
Genoa	30.6	29.2–32.1	49.0	47.4–50.7
Latina	36.0	33.3–38.7	54.7	51.7–57.7
Modena	38.5	36.6–40.6	51.8	49.6–54.1
Parma	30.8	28.9–32.7	50.2	48.0–52.4
Ragusa	25.5	23.3–27.9	44.5	41.8–47.2
Romagna	37.1	35.2–39.0	54.8	52.7–56.9
Turin	33.9	32.5–35.3	48.8	47.3–50.3
Varese	34.2	33.0–35.4	54.8	53.4–56.1
Poland				
Cracow	18.7	17.3–20.1	38.8	37.2–40.4
Warsaw	23.5	22.0–25.1	37.8	36.2–39.4
Spain				
Basque Country	40.1	39.0–41.3	52.7	51.2–54.1
Navarra	42.6	40.9–44.3	53.3	51.3–55.3
Tarragona	36.2	34.5–37.9	51.4	49.4–53.4
Switzerland				
Basel	44.8	42.7–47.0	57.3	55.1–59.4
Geneva	40.9	38.9–42.9	57.1	55.1–59.1

Chapter 3

General mortality and the survival of cancer patients in Europe

A. Micheli, G. De Angelis, A. Giorgi Rossi and R. Capocaccia

Introduction

Over the past two decades, numerous studies have indicated an overall secular decline in European mortality, which however is not of the same extent in all populations, while in a few populations mortality is actually increasing. Life expectancy reflects the level of economic and social development in a country. The rapid increase in affluence that occurred in many countries after the Second World War is considered to be the principal determinant of the general reduction in European mortality. However, economic, political and social crises can interrupt or change the general trend, so that differences in life expectancy persist.

Observed survival is used to describe the prognosis of cancer patients. However, patients can die of causes unrelated to their cancer. Comparison of observed survival of cancer patients in different populations may therefore be confounded by differing levels of general mortality. For this reason, *relative survival* is usually calculated, as described in Chapter 2. Relative survival is an artificial measure, since it assumes that the cancer in question is the only possible cause of death; nevertheless the relative survival of cancer patients across populations has been shown to correlate with social and economic variables, and so may be used as an indicator of social development (Micheli *et al.*, 1997; see also Chapter 5).

Comparisons of survival of cancer patients usually make use of both observed and relative survival data; this was so in the EUROCARE-1 study (Berrino *et al.*, 1995), and is also the case in the present EUROCARE-2 study. The parameter that relates observed survival to relative survival is the *expected survival*.

This chapter provides information on the general risk of dying in the populations covered by the cancer registries participating in EUROCARE-2, including a brief description of geographical differences in life expectancy and their time trends in each country. The mortality data used by EUROCARE-2 for calculating expected survival at the local level are also presented, and the manipulations performed on them to correct for incompleteness are described.

Methods

The general mortality data from the *Health For All* CD-ROM of the World Health Organization (1998) were the basic starting point. These data are presented as time trends for the participating countries in Figure 1. This diagram shows combined male and female life expectancy at birth for each country participating in EUROCARE-2, from 1978 to 1994.

The registries participating in EUROCARE-2 provided data on their incident cases diagnosed between 1985 and 1989. Registries were asked to include all cases with a minimum follow-up of five years. They also provided life tables for the population in the area they covered, by calendar year, by sex and by age (0 to 99 years) for the years 1985 to 1994, the entire study period including both incidence and follow-up periods. These data were used for calculating relative survival. The registries that participated in EUROCARE-1 had previously provided life tables for 1978 to 1990 and were asked to update this information to 1994; any additional information pertaining to the 1978–90 period was also accepted and used to improve the EUROCARE database.

Unfortunately, complete life tables were not available from all registries. In particular, mortality data on the oldest segment of the population were often missing; in some cases the data were available only for five-year periods, whereas EUROCARE-2 required the data for each year. In other cases, data for particular years were missing (usually the most recent years). In all these cases, the missing data had to be reconstructed. Table 1 gives details of the mortality data provided by each of the cancer registries, noting the years for which data had to be estimated (reconstructed), either by EUROCARE-1 or by the present EUROCARE-2.

The methods used to reconstruct the life tables were as follows.

(a) *Missing mortality data on the oldest section of the population.* When registries did not have mortality data on the oldest age groups, the rates were estimated simply as equal to that of the oldest age available; this figure was assumed constant for each year of age up to 99 years.

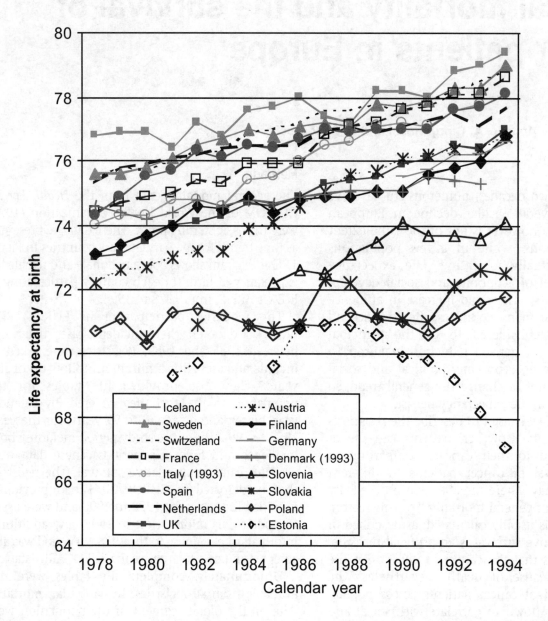

Figure 1. Life expectancy at birth in selected European countries, 1978–1994 (World Health Organization, 1998)

(b) *Age intervals*. When five-year age-specific mortality rates were provided, the required one-year mortality rates were reconstructed from the five-year rates by assuming that the risk of mortality was constant over the five-year period in question.

(c) *Calendar year*. Many registries did not provide data for the whole period covered by EUROCARE-2. When information for the most recent years (after 1990) was missing, the death rate for the unknown years was assumed to be the same as that for the last known year. On some occasions, mortality was provided as constant over a series of years; in such cases no reconstruction was performed. In some cases

information on mortality was completely missing for a number of years; mortality rates were then estimated by a linear interpolation method, independent of age. For example, if data were available only for years 1988 and 1993 (with data missing for the five years in between), the 1989 mortality would be estimated as the sum of the death probability in 1988 multiplied by 4/5, plus the death probability in 1993 multiplied by 1/5. Similarly, the 1990 death rate would be estimated as the death probability in 1988 multiplied by 3/5 plus the death probability in 1993 multiplied by 2/5, and so on. However, in a few cases when data for only one or two

Table 1. Available and estimated (reconstructed) general mortality by registry

Registry	Country	Mortality data provided by the cancer registry for EUROCARE-2			Data reconstructed from EUROCARE-1	Data reconstructed by EUROCARE-2
		Age interval	Up to age of	Period	Period	Period
Basel	CH	5 yrs [a]	105	1991..1993	1978..1990	1994
Basque Country	E	1 yr	100	1980–81, 1985–86, 1990–91		1978, 1979, 1982..1984, 1987..1989, 1992..1994
Calvados	F	1 yr	99	1980..1992		1978, 1979, 1993, 1994
Côte d'Or	F	5 yrs	90	1981–83, 1989–91	1984..1988	1992–94
Cracow [c]	PL	1 yr	100	1976–81, 1981–85, 1986–90		1991–94
Denmark	DK	1 yr	99	1977..1993		1994
Doubs	F	1 yr	99	1978..1993		1994
East Anglia	ENG	5 yrs	85	1990..1992	1978..1989	1993,1994
Eindhoven [d]	NL	1 yr	99	1971–75, 1976–80, 1981–85, 1985–90		1991, 1992, 1993, 1994
Estonia	EST	1 yr	110	1978..1993		1994
Finland	FIN	1 yr	99	1955..1995		
Florence	I	1 yr	99	1978..1994		
Geneva	CH	5 yrs	85[e]	1981..1993	1978..1980	1994
Genoa	I	1 yr	99	1978..1994		
Girona (women only)	E	5 yrs	94[e]	1983..1990	1983, 1984	1978..1983, 1991..1994
Granada	E	1 yr	89	1985..1994	1978..1984	
Iceland	ICE	1 yr	99	1955..1994		
Isère	F	5 yrs	95	1981–83, 1986..1994		1978..1980, 1984,1985
Latina	I	1 yr	99	1978..1994		
Mainz	D	1 yr	90	1982..1984		1978..1980,
childhood		5 yrs	90	1981		1985..1994
Mallorca	E	5 yrs [a]	90[e]	1985–87, 1988–90	1988..1990	1978..1984, 1991..1994
Mersey	ENG	5 yrs	99	1985–87, 1988–90	1978..1984	1991..1994
Modena	I	1 yr	99	1978..1994		
Navarra	E	1 yr	99	1985..1994		1978..1984
Oxford	ENG	5 yrs [a]	85	1981..1994		1978..1980
Parma	I	1 yr	99	1978..1994		
Piedmont	I	1 yr	99	1978..1994		
Ragusa	I	1 yr	99	1978..1994		
Romagna	I	1 yr	99	1978..1994		
Rotterdam [d]	NL	5 yrs	99	1990, 1993		1991, 1992, 1994
Saarland	D	1 yr	99	1978..1984, 1988, 1992	1985..1887	1989..1991, 1993, 1994
Scotland	SCO	1 yr (1978–90)	89	1978..1994		
		5 yrs (1991–94)	100			
Slovakia	SK	1 yr	103	1982, 1984, 1986, 1988, 1990..1993		1978..1981, 1983, 1985, 1987, 1989, 1994
Slovenia	SLO	1 yr	99	1981, 1986, 1991		1978..1980, 1982..1985, 1987..1990, 1992..1994
Somme	F	5 yrs	90	1982–90	1984..1988	1978..1981, 1991..1994
Sweden, South	S	1 yr	110	1976–79, 1980–84, 1985–89, 1990–94		
Tarragona	E	5 yrs	94[e]	1985–92	1978..1984	1993, 1994
Thames, South	ENG	5 yrs	85	1990..1992	1978..1989	1993, 1994
Turin	I	1 yr	99	1978..1994		
Tyrol	A	5 yrs [b]	95	1961..1995		
Varese	I	1 yr	99	1978..1994		
Warsaw [c]	PL	1 yr	100	1990–91		1992..1994
Wessex	ENG	10 yrs [a]	85[e]	1978..1990, 1990–92		1993, 1994
West Midlands	ENG	10 yrs [a]	85[e]	1978..1991		1992..1994
Yorkshire	ENG	5 yrs	85	1978..1990, 1990–92		1993, 1994

[a] Age intervals for the first classes were: 0, 1–4; after that five-year intervals.
[b] The general mortality for 0 age-class was also supplied.
[c] National life tables were used for 1976–90 for Cracow and 1990–91 for Warsaw.
[d] National life tables were used for 1971–90 data from Eindhoven and for 1993 data from Rotterdam.
[e] Information on mortality for all ages combined was also provided, facilitating estimates of mortality rates among the oldest, for whom specific mortality data was not available.
Note: Period: A dash linking two years means that the entry is the mean of all years included in the interval. Dots between years mean that all individual years were available.

years were missing, the unknown death rates were assumed to be the same as that for the previous known year.

Because of the unusual structure of the data provided by the English registries, a special strategy had to be adopted. For the registries that participated in the EUROCARE-1 study (all but Oxford), the reconstructed results for the period 1978–90 were used in the EUROCARE-2 study. From EUROCARE-1, a national life table with one-year age classes until 90 years of age for the calendar year 1981 was also available. For all the registries, data were available only in the age range 0–84 years (never in one-year age intervals, but at least in five years). In the age span 85–89 years, one-year mortality rates were extracted from the available data on 85+ years of age from each registry. For the age span 91–99 years, the national life-table was extended up to 99 years by an exponential regression model, then adopted for the whole time span under consideration. For Oxford this procedure was also used for the age span 85–89 years. For the whole set of English registries, results for 1992 were also applied to 1993 and 1994.

For the Polish (Cracow and Warsaw) and Dutch (Eindhoven and Rotterdam) registries, national life tables were reconstructed and applied at the local level.

By means of such expedients, complete life tables specific for age (from 0 to 99 years), sex and calendar year (from 1978 to 1994) were constructed. Relative survival rates in the present volume were calculated by using these mortality tables for each calendar year from 1978 to 1994.

Trends of life expectancy in Europe

Life expectancy at birth has changed markedly in many European countries over the last two decades, as is illustrated in Figure 1 for the EUROCARE-2 countries from 1978 to 1994. In Sweden, Switzerland and Iceland, life expectancy increased from 76–77 years in 1978 to 79 years in 1994. For France, Italy and Spain, life expectancy increased steeply and uniformly from about 74 years in 1978 to about 78 years in 1994 (1993 in the case of Italy); by 1994, life expectancy was almost 78 years in The Netherlands also. In Finland and the UK, where survival in the 1970s was lower than in other countries of northern Europe, life expectancy rose from about 73 years in 1978 to about 77 years in 1994. By 1994, life expectancy in Austria and Germany was also about

77 years, while Denmark, at about 75 years (1993), had the lowest among the northern European countries.

Life expectancy in Denmark increased less over the period than in many other countries. In contrast, life expectancy in Austria showed the greatest increase, rising by more than four years over 17 years. In all countries of the European Union, life expectancy at birth increased over the period, and the rate of increase was greater in countries with initially low figures, so that differences tended to reduce. In the countries of eastern Europe, on the other hand, life expectancy was lower than in the European Union, and except for Slovenia, did not increase over the period considered, while that in Estonia has been declining since 1988. In 1994, life expectancy was 67 years in Estonia, about 72 years in Poland and Slovakia, and 74 years in Slovenia. Considering all the EUROCARE-2 countries, the range of life expectancy increased over the study period, from extremes of 70.7 in Poland and 76.8 in Iceland in 1978 (data for Estonia, Germany, Slovakia and Slovenia not available) to 67.1 in Estonia to 79.4 in Iceland in 1994 (data for Denmark and Italy up to 1993).

General risk of mortality in the areas covered by the participating registries

Table 2 shows the cumulative general mortality for males and females (per 1000) for the years 1987 and 1991, by registry and age, as calculated from the EUROCARE-2 mortality database (reconstructed where necessary as described above). Note that in this table the cumulative general mortality risk is reported, giving the probability, at the beginning of the age span considered, of dying before the end of that span.

Both absolute mortality and between-registry variation in mortality risk were greater for males than for females. Estonia and Slovakia had the highest risks of cumulative mortality for both sexes and almost all age classes, with risks in 1991 often greater than in 1987. The mortality risks for Poland (the national life-table was used for Warsaw and Cracow due to markedly incomplete data from the individual registries; see Table 1) were very similar to those for Estonia and Slovakia, in both magnitude and time trend. The registries of southern Europe reported the lowest risks of mortality: this was true for most of Spain and for central and southern Italy (Tarragona, Latina and Ragusa, the last reporting a large mortality reduction for both sexes, but especially for females, between 1987 and 1991), whereas for registries in the northern part of

Table 2. Cumulative general mortality risk per 1000 for various age-classes by registry area in 1987 and 1991: mortality data used in EUROCARE-2

(a) Males

Registry	1987							1991						
	0–1	0–14	15–44	45–54	55–64	65–74	0–74	0–1	0–14	15–44	45–54	55–64	65–74	0–74
Basel	8	10	43	51	108	239	344	10	13	39	44	114	232	339
Basque Country	10	17	46	51	124	264	372	10	14	58	49	114	252	362
Calvados	7	12	51	78	144	271	395	7	12	53	69	140	257	382
Côte d'Or	8	14	51	67	124	249	369	8	11	50	59	121	224	348
Cracow	16	20	60	92	192	334	458	17	22	73	106	210	353	480
Denmark	9	13	46	58	145	287	397	9	13	43	55	138	286	392
Doubs	8	15	47	62	127	252	369	8	12	54	57	124	246	364
East Anglia	10	14	29	48	129	273	372	9	13	25	39	114	249	343
Eindhoven	11	14	31	45	126	296	386	8	11	31	43	109	268	357
Estonia	17	27	80	99	193	346	472	15	24	108	121	224	346	492
Finland	7	10	59	68	154	301	416	5	8	54	60	132	279	389
Florence	9	12	31	41	114	246	344	6	9	31	37	100	232	324
Geneva	8	14	40	45	116	249	353	8	13	37	43	110	239	341
Genoa	9	12	38	51	132	275	379	8	11	49	46	118	259	364
Girona	NE	NE	NE	NE	NE	NE	NE	NE	NE	NE	NE	NE	NE	NE
Granada	14	18	42	48	117	252	359	10	14	51	49	109	244	352
Iceland	6	9	37	43	101	234	331	6	9	27	35	89	209	299
Isère	9	13	54	67	139	261	385	8	12	56	60	128	242	366
Latina	11	15	35	45	118	249	353	8	12	41	41	111	254	352
Mainz	10	14	40	56	132	277	383	9	12	36	52	121	258	362
Mallorca	11	17	46	63	140	266	385	6	11	57	55	126	244	365
Mersey	12	17	32	54	146	304	404	12	16	31	53	141	295	395
Modena	10	14	35	47	126	261	365	7	10	39	39	110	234	336
Navarra	11	16	39	44	102	237	339	7	11	40	36	93	220	317
Oxford	11	15	29	37	119	270	362	9	11	28	38	102	261	346
Parma	10	14	38	48	132	264	371	6	10	40	41	120	240	346
Piedmont	9	12	31	41	114	246	344	6	9	31	37	100	232	324
Ragusa	10	14	32	35	103	236	331	8	11	31	36	93	225	316
Romagna	10	13	35	42	113	234	338	7	10	44	36	101	222	324
Rotterdam	11	14	31	45	126	296	386	8	11	31	43	109	268	357
Saarland	10	13	45	57	144	301	405	7	10	44	62	139	297	402
Scotland	10	14	42	64	166	328	432	9	13	40	58	148	315	415
Slovakia	16	21	65	104	205	343	471	14	20	69	107	213	344	475
Slovenia	12	17	67	86	177	319	444	10	14	61	77	176	309	433
Somme	12	17	62	89	155	268	407	10	15	63	76	157	260	399
Sweden, South	7	10	36	44	110	251	349	6	9	33	39	102	236	330
Tarragona	11	15	36	41	99	223	324	8	13	48	39	101	210	320
Thames, South	11	15	29	49	132	278	377	7	11	32	41	138	251	360
Tyrol	13	18	42	47	107	216	329	8	13	35	37	94	212	310
Turin	10	13	36	48	133	269	374	8	11	42	44	119	257	359
Varese	9	13	33	48	141	280	383	8	11	46	42	127	269	372
Warsaw	16	20	60	92	192	334	458	17	22	73	106	210	353	480
Wessex	10	14	29	48	130	275	374	9	12	27	42	115	254	349
West Midlands	12	16	31	54	143	298	398	12	16	26	48	133	287	383
Yorkshire	12	16	32	54	145	301	402	12	16	30	48	138	286	386

Table 2. Cumulative general mortality risk per 1000 for various age-classes by registry area in 1987 and 1991: mortality data used in EUROCARE-2

(b) Females

Registry	1987							1991						
	0–1	0–14	15–44	45–54	55–64	65–74	0–74	0–1	0–14	15–44	45–54	55–64	65–74	0–74
Basel	7	10	22	25	48	133	206	8	10	22	23	55	125	204
Basque Country	9	15	19	22	50	135	208	7	11	23	19	42	121	189
Calvados	5	9	21	27	54	132	209	9	13	20	25	51	125	201
Côte d'Or	6	9	20	23	50	124	196	8	10	20	24	47	108	182
Cracow	13	16	23	39	94	217	311	13	17	27	41	97	225	321
Denmark	7	10	24	41	92	182	283	7	10	22	38	93	185	283
Doubs	8	12	19	25	51	141	213	6	9	26	25	52	130	207
East Anglia	8	11	18	31	76	172	258	6	9	15	28	63	147	224
Eindhoven	8	13	20	28	70	155	241	5[a]	8	18	26	62	144	222
Estonia	15	20	28	36	87	222	313	11	16	32	45	101	223	326
Finland	5	8	21	28	63	172	246	4	7	20	26	55	153	224
Florence	7	10	15	21	54	137	205	4	7	15	19	48	125	189
Geneva	6	10	19	24	54	138	211	6	9	18	23	52	130	201
Genoa	6	8	19	27	59	155	230	7	8	20	25	54	140	213
Girona	7	11	24	31	55	161	239	5	10	23	23	56	158	231
Granada	10	14	16	24	54	152	224	6	9	17	23	50	138	207
Iceland	6	9	15	28	65	154	231	4	5	14	30	54	148	217
Isère	6	9	22	28	56	137	216	5	8	21	25	52	124	199
Latina	8	11	15	23	56	144	216	8	10	15	20	54	142	210
Mainz	8	11	20	28	65	161	241	7	10	18	25	59	147	221
Mallorca	9	13	20	26	59	153	231	6	8	22	23	54	136	209
Mersey	10	14	21	36	90	198	291	9	13	20	34	85	189	280
Modena	8	11	18	25	57	136	213	6	8	19	22	54	128	201
Navarra	11	14	16	19	47	120	190	8	11	16	18	38	105	167
Oxford	7	10	16	28	76	174	255	6	8	16	26	68	166	242
Parma	5	8	18	26	58	137	213	6	8	19	25	53	132	205
Piedmont	7	10	15	21	54	137	205	4	7	15	19	48	125	189
Ragusa	8	11	17	26	61	166	240	9	11	14	23	51	149	216
Romagna	7	10	19	23	53	133	205	7	9	18	20	48	112	182
Rotterdam	8	13	20	28	70	155	241	5[a]	8	18	26	62	144	222
Saarland	9	12	25	27	71	183	264	7	9	24	29	69	172	255
Scotland	7	10	21	38	102	220	314	5	9	22	35	95	212	302
Slovakia	11	14	24	40	95	225	317	12	16	25	41	95	224	318
Slovenia	9	12	25	38	81	201	290	6	9	22	35	76	191	275
Somme	12	17	25	36	56	137	228	9	11	26	29	61	139	225
Sweden, South	5	8	19	26	59	147	221	5	7	17	25	57	139	213
Tarragona	11	14	18	19	46	112	184	6	8	20	25	45	125	194
Thames, South	8	12	18	31	77	173	259	7	9	17	26	62	145	223
Turin	8	10	18	25	61	153	229	7	9	18	22	54	144	214
Tyrol	8	12	19	21	43	128	195	8	10	18	24	46	124	193
Varese	7	10	17	24	58	149	222	6	7	18	22	52	132	201
Warsaw	13	16	23	39	94	217	311	13	17	27	41	97	225	321
Wessex	8	11	18	31	75	171	255	7	11	17	27	61	150	227
West Midlands	9	13	20	34	85	190	280	10	13	19	31	77	172	258
Yorkshire	10	13	21	35	87	193	284	9	14	18	27	77	176	261

The minimum and maximum values for each age-class are in bold type. Minimum and maximum values were chosen before eliminating decimal digits.

NE, not estimated (Girona sent data on females only).

[a] For the Netherlands, 1992 data are presented. Data for 1991 are anomalous and could give erroneous comparisons.

southern Europe (Basque Country, Varese and Turin, but not Piedmont), mortality was above the European mean.

With regard to childhood mortality, the registries in the southernmost regions of Europe were no longer characterized by the much higher rates reported in EUROCARE-1 (Micheli & Capocaccia, 1995). In the present study, high rates are seen in the eastern European countries and England. In 1987 cumulative mortality in the first year of life ranged from 6 per 1000 males in Iceland to 17 per 1000 males in Estonia, and from 5 per 1000 females in Calvados, Finland, Parma and Sweden to 15 per 1000 females in Estonia. In 1991, the ranges for males were from 5 per 1000 in Finland to 17 per 1000 in Poland (12 per 1000 in most of the registries of England), and for females from 4 per 1000 in Finland, Florence, Iceland and Piedmont to 13 per 1000 in Poland (10 per 1000 in West Midlands).

In 1987, the ratio of the highest (Estonia) to the lowest (Tarragona) cumulative death rate for the 0–74-year age span was 1.46 for men and 1.72 for women (Slovakia versus Tarragona). In 1991 the corresponding ratios were 1.64 and 1.95, the figures coming from Estonia and Iceland for men, and from Estonia and Navarra for women. Only four registries (Estonia, Slovakia and the two Polish registries) for males and six registries (Denmark, Estonia, Slovakia, Tarragona and the two Polish registries) for females reported no reduction in mortality between 1987 and 1991. In most registry areas, there was a slight reduction in mortality for males and greater reduction for females over the study period; these reductions were more marked in the South Thames and East Anglia cancer registries.

Basic data for estimating relative survival

The observed rate of survival of cancer patients is the percentage surviving a certain number of years after diagnosis, irrespective of the actual cause of death. The expected survival rate is the survival of the general population of the same age and sex as the cancer patients. Table 3 shows the expected five-year survival rates, by selected ages, of the general population in each of the participating countries in 1987. These figures were arrived at by pooling, on a country basis, the life-table data provided by each cancer registry, reconstructed where necessary. For this purpose, the life-table data were weighted by the population number covered by each registry and the figure obtained was attributed to the country. These pooled estimates of expected survival were used to estimate relative cancer survival rates at both the

national level and the European level. The ratio of the age- and sex-specific observed survival to the five-year expected survival for a given tumour, multiplied by 100, gives, approximately, the relative five-year survival rate used in this volume.

The difference between the observed and relative survival depends, for a given group of cancer patients, on the risk of dying from other causes. In all registries, the differences between the observed and relative survival are zero or very small for the youngest patients (15–44 years) and increase with age. For countries where the risk of dying is high, the difference between the observed and the relative survival in a specific age group is also high. Furthermore, because males have a higher risk of mortality from all causes combined than females, differences between observed and relative survival were greater for males than for females. The risk of dying from cancer reduces during the follow-up of cancer patients. At the same time, due to population ageing, the risk of dying from causes other than the specific cancer increases. These two opposing effects result in a widening of the difference between observed and relative survival during the years of follow-up. However, it must be remembered that selection occurs during follow-up because of the heterogeneity of the patient death risk. As an example, the proportion of patients of young age at diagnosis increases during follow-up, at least for those tumours for which young age is a favourable prognostic factor (Hakulinen, 1982).

Conclusions

The study of survival of cancer patients requires comprehensive information on general mortality. Life expectancy has changed in Europe over the last two decades. In general, in western European countries, life expectancy increased steeply, and more so in countries that initially had low life expectancy than in those with higher initial values; therefore in recent years, inter-country differences in life expectancy have narrowed. The picture in eastern European countries differs starkly, so that across the whole set of EUROCARE-2 countries, the range of life expectancy has widened considerably over recent years.

Comparison of mortality at the level of the individual cancer registries suggests that the areas at low mortality risk are located in the northernmost and southernmost extremes of Europe (Sweden and Iceland, and Spain and Italy), but also in Austria, the Netherlands and some areas of England. The secular decline in mortality in western Europe is tending to

Table 3. Expected five-year survival rates at various ages by country and sex in 1987, estimated by pooling life expectancies from registries by country (as percentage)

Country	Sex	30 yrs	40 yrs	50 yrs	60 yrs	70 yrs	80 yrs
Austria	M	99.46	98.76	96.99	93.24	84.22	60.03
	F	99.79	99.24	98.91	97.21	90.23	71.04
Denmark	M	99.20	98.58	96.12	90.03	77.96	54.45
	F	99.63	99.04	97.38	94.15	87.42	67.85
England	M	99.58	99.00	96.68	90.66	77.49	53.60
	F	99.72	99.28	97.93	94.74	86.96	66.13
Estonia	M	98.77	97.05	93.65	86.86	71.57	46.64
	F	99.59	98.98	97.65	94.35	83.17	57.20
Finland	M	99.00	98.01	95.70	89.38	76.33	52.14
	F	99.69	99.30	98.35	95.85	87.44	63.56
France	M	99.17	98.20	95.31	91.02	80.07	55.78
	F	99.66	99.29	98.28	96.70	90.50	69.46
Germany	M	99.19	98.43	96.39	90.08	75.96	50.57
	F	99.57	99.23	98.56	95.46	86.76	65.22
Iceland	M	99.54	99.00	97.19	93.27	82.33	59.08
	F	99.77	99.61	98.39	95.69	88.83	70.20
Italy	M	99.51	99.05	97.12	91.79	81.00	55.93
	F	99.79	99.43	98.62	96.41	90.05	68.32
Netherlands	M	99.64	98.83	97.15	90.73	76.74	52.37
	F	99.61	99.42	98.23	95.41	89.47	65.95
Poland	M	99.04	97.68	93.91	86.37	72.96	52.77
	F	99.63	99.09	97.60	93.70	83.85	59.05
Scotland	M	99.41	98.48	95.69	88.07	73.44	49.15
	F	99.71	99.21	97.50	93.14	84.03	64.41
Slovakia	M	99.02	97.36	93.21	85.49	72.81	47.48
	F	99.58	99.13	97.53	93.62	83.28	58.36
Slovenia	M	98.99	97.71	94.44	87.95	74.51	48.79
	F	99.65	99.05	97.65	94.68	84.78	59.20
Spain	M	98.89	98.38	96.65	92.28	82.20	58.26
	F	99.70	99.40	98.61	96.71	90.11	65.94
Sweden	M	99.40	98.91	97.17	92.59	80.83	55.40
	F	99.71	99.36	98.42	96.23	89.66	68.79
Switzerland	M	99.30	99.03	96.95	92.76	82.00	58.42
	F	99.64	99.30	98.54	96.75	90.09	70.54

result in similar mortality levels everywhere, and with this reduced variability, areas of lower than average mortality may emerge anywhere. In contrast, the high-risk areas are all located in eastern Europe. In some eastern areas, the risk of dying increased over the last few years of the study period, so that the gap between eastern and western areas widened markedly.

Changes in the risk of dying modify differences between the observed and relative survival of cancer patients. When the risk of mortality from causes other than cancer is high, the difference between the observed and relative survival is marked. Thus the difference between observed and relative survival is greater for males than females, for older patients than younger patients, and for patients in the later years of follow-up compared with those in the early years.

We can conclude that the dramatic secular differentiation of death risk in Europe which has been shown to occur over the last two decades fully justifies the effort made in the EUROCARE project to consider in great detail the effects of general mortality on the survival of cancer patients.

References

Berrino, F., Sant, M., Verdecchia, A, Capocaccia, R., Hakulinen, T. & Esteve, J., eds (1995) *Survival of Cancer Patients in Europe. The EUROCARE Study* (IARC Scientific Publications No. 132), Lyon, IARC

Hakulinen, T. (1982) Cancer survival corrected for heterogeneity in patient withdrawal. *Biometrics*, **39**, 933–942

Micheli, A. & Capocaccia, R. (1995) General mortality and its effect on survival estimates. In: Berrino, F., Sant, M., Verdecchia, A., Capocaccia, R., Hakulinen, T. & Esteve, J., eds, *Survival of Cancer Patients in Europe. The EUROCARE Study* (IARC Scientific Publications No. 132), Lyon, IARC

Micheli, A., Gatta, G. & Verdecchia, A. (1997) Studying survival of cancer patients in different populations: its potential and role. In: Verdecchia, A., Micheli, A. & Gatta, G., eds, Survival of Cancer Patients in Italy. The Itacare Study. *Tumori*, **83**, 3–8

Chapter 4

Results

In this chapter, the detailed results of the EUROCARE-2 study are presented, mainly in tabular form, as described in Chapter 2, with survival figures presented for each cancer site at single country level and at the European level.

LIP (ICD-9 140)

AUSTRIA

AREA	NUMBER OF CASES			PERIOD	MEAN AGE		
	Males	Females	All		Males	Females	All
Tirol	2	0	2	1988-1989	51.0	-	51.0

OBSERVED AND RELATIVE SURVIVAL (%) BY AGE (number of cases in parentheses)

	AGE CLASS										ALL	
	15-44		45-54		55-64		65-74		75-99			
	obs	rel	obs	rel	obs	rel	obs	rel	obs	rel	obs	rel
Males	(0)		(1)		(1)		(0)		(0)		(2)	
1 year	-	-	100	100	100	100	-	-	-	-	100	100
3 years	-	-	100	100	100	100	-	-	-	-	100	100
5 years	-	-	100	100	100	100	-	-	-	-	100	100
Females	(0)		(0)		(0)		(0)		(0)		(0)	
1 year	-	-	-	-	-	-	-	-	-	-	-	-
3 years	-	-	-	-	-	-	-	-	-	-	-	-
5 years	-	-	-	-	-	-	-	-	-	-	-	-
Overall	(0)		(1)		(1)		(0)		(0)		(2)	
1 year	-	-	100	100	100	100	-	-	-	-	100	100
3 years	-	-	100	100	100	100	-	-	-	-	100	100
5 years	-	-	100	100	100	100	-	-	-	-	100	100

DENMARK

AREA	NUMBER OF CASES			PERIOD	MEAN AGE		
	Males	Females	All		Males	Females	All
Denmark	549	79	628	1985-1989	68.1	69.6	68.3

OBSERVED AND RELATIVE SURVIVAL (%) BY AGE (number of cases in parentheses)

	AGE CLASS										ALL	
	15-44		45-54		55-64		65-74		75-99			
	obs	rel	obs	rel	obs	rel	obs	rel	obs	rel	obs	rel
Males	(22)		(63)		(117)		(159)		(188)		(549)	
1 year	100	100	98	99	97	99	96	100	84	94	92	98
3 years	100	100	98	100	91	97	82	94	64	92	80	95
5 years	100	100	98	100	79	89	69	89	49	96	69	93
Females	(5)		(8)		(8)		(24)		(34)		(79)	
1 year	100	100	100	100	100	100	100	100	82	89	92	96
3 years	100	100	88	89	100	100	92	99	68	87	82	94
5 years	100	100	88	90	100	100	88	100	53	84	75	95
Overall	(27)		(71)		(125)		(183)		(222)		(628)	
1 year	100	100	99	99	98	99	96	100	83	93	92	97
3 years	100	100	97	99	92	97	83	94	64	92	81	95
5 years	100	100	97	100	81	90	72	91	50	93	70	93

LIP (ICD-9 140)

ENGLAND

AREA	NUMBER OF CASES			PERIOD	MEAN AGE			5-YR RELATIVE SURVIVAL (%)	
	Males	Females	All		Males	Females	All	Males	Females
East Anglia	133	28	161	1985-1989	69.7	72.0	70.1		
Mersey	9	5	14	1985-1989	66.4	66.2	66.4		
Oxford	112	33	145	1985-1989	67.4	74.1	68.9		
South Thames	80	29	109	1985-1989	66.3	74.2	68.4		
Wessex	61	21	82	1985-1989	70.5	75.3	71.8		
West Midlands	48	14	62	1985-1989	64.3	68.2	65.2		
Yorkshire	68	24	92	1985-1989	68.9	70.0	69.2		
English Registries	511	154	665		68.1	72.5	69.1		

OBSERVED AND RELATIVE SURVIVAL (%) BY AGE (number of cases in parentheses)

	AGE CLASS										ALL	
	15-44		45-54		55-64		65-74		75-99			
	obs	rel	obs	rel	obs	rel	obs	rel	obs	rel	obs	rel
Males	(21)		(46)		(101)		(174)		(169)		(511)	
1 year	100	100	91	92	99	100	94	98	85	95	92	97
3 years	100	100	85	86	92	97	84	95	64	91	80	94
5 years	95	96	83	85	89	98	70	88	50	92	69	92
Females	(5)		(6)		(21)		(48)		(74)		(154)	
1 year	100	100	100	100	95	96	89	91	89	98	91	96
3 years	100	100	100	100	95	98	77	82	74	100	80	94
5 years	100	100	100	100	95	100	70	79	62	100	72	95
Overall	(26)		(52)		(122)		(222)		(243)		(665)	
1 year	100	100	92	93	98	100	93	97	86	96	92	97
3 years	100	100	87	88	93	97	82	92	67	94	80	94
5 years	96	97	85	87	90	98	70	86	53	97	70	92

ESTONIA

AREA	NUMBER OF CASES			PERIOD	MEAN AGE		
	Males	Females	All		Males	Females	All
Estonia	98	25	123	1985-1989	63.3	73.5	65.4

OBSERVED AND RELATIVE SURVIVAL (%) BY AGE (number of cases in parentheses)

	AGE CLASS										ALL	
	15-44		45-54		55-64		65-74		75-99			
	obs	rel	obs	rel	obs	rel	obs	rel	obs	rel	obs	rel
Males	(6)		(22)		(22)		(26)		(22)		(98)	
1 year	83	84	91	92	100	100	88	93	77	90	89	94
3 years	67	68	73	76	82	89	73	86	45	73	68	81
5 years	67	69	68	74	77	91	54	73	32	73	58	77
Females	(0)		(1)		(3)		(7)		(14)		(25)	
1 year	-	-	100	100	100	100	86	87	86	96	88	94
3 years	-	-	100	100	100	100	86	91	57	81	72	89
5 years	-	-	100	100	100	100	86	97	50	93	68	97
Overall	(6)		(23)		(25)		(33)		(36)		(123)	
1 year	83	84	91	92	100	100	88	92	81	92	89	94
3 years	67	68	74	77	84	91	76	87	50	76	69	82
5 years	67	69	70	75	80	93	61	79	39	82	60	81

LIP (ICD-9 140)

FINLAND

AREA	NUMBER OF CASES			PERIOD	MEAN AGE		
	Males	Females	All		Males	Females	All
Finland	552	151	703	1985-1989	67.1	72.9	68.3

OBSERVED AND RELATIVE SURVIVAL (%) BY AGE (number of cases in parentheses)

	AGE CLASS										ALL	
	15-44		45-54		55-64		65-74		75-99			
	obs	rel	obs	rel	obs	rel	obs	rel	obs	rel	obs	rel
Males	(12)		(41)		(174)		(190)		(135)		(552)	
1 year	100	100	98	98	97	98	95	100	88	100	94	99
3 years	100	100	98	100	89	94	84	97	67	99	83	97
5 years	100	100	88	92	76	85	75	96	54	100	72	93
Females	(5)		(1)		(21)		(52)		(72)		(151)	
1 year	100	100	100	100	100	100	92	94	92	100	93	98
3 years	100	100	100	100	100	100	88	95	75	99	84	98
5 years	100	100	100	100	95	100	71	81	51	85	66	87
Overall	(17)		(42)		(195)		(242)		(207)		(703)	
1 year	100	100	98	98	97	99	95	98	89	100	94	99
3 years	100	100	98	100	90	95	85	96	70	99	83	97
5 years	100	100	88	92	78	86	74	92	53	98	71	92

FRANCE

AREA	NUMBER OF CASES			PERIOD	MEAN AGE			5-YR RELATIVE SURVIVAL (%)	
	Males	Females	All		Males	Females	All	Males	Females
Somme	22	5	27	1985-1989	67.2	79.6	69.6		
Calvados	47	11	58	1985-1989	68.2	80.8	70.6		
Doubs	7	0	7	1985-1989	64.6	-	64.6		
French Registries	76	16	92		67.6	80.6	69.9		

OBSERVED AND RELATIVE SURVIVAL (%) BY AGE (number of cases in parentheses)

	AGE CLASS										ALL	
	15-44		45-54		55-64		65-74		75-99			
	obs	rel	obs	rel	obs	rel	obs	rel	obs	rel	obs	rel
Males	(3)		(9)		(16)		(19)		(29)		(76)	
1 year	100	100	89	90	100	100	84	87	86	95	89	94
3 years	100	100	78	80	75	79	68	77	68	92	72	84
5 years	100	100	67	71	62	68	63	77	60	100	64	83
Females	(0)		(0)		(1)		(1)		(14)		(16)	
1 year	-	-	-	-	100	100	0	0	71	79	69	75
3 years	-	-	-	-	100	100	0	0	57	78	56	74
5 years	-	-	-	-	100	100	0	0	36	65	38	62
Overall	(3)		(9)		(17)		(20)		(43)		(92)	
1 year	100	100	89	90	100	100	80	83	81	89	86	91
3 years	100	100	78	80	76	81	65	72	64	87	69	82
5 years	100	100	67	71	64	70	60	73	52	90	59	80

LIP   (ICD-9 140)

GERMANY

AREA	NUMBER OF CASES			PERIOD	MEAN AGE		
	Males	Females	All		Males	Females	All
Saarland	48	5	53	1985-1989	69.4	55.8	68.1

OBSERVED AND RELATIVE SURVIVAL (%) BY AGE (number of cases in parentheses)

	AGE CLASS									ALL	
	15-44		45-54		55-64		65-74		75-99			
	obs	rel	obs	rel	obs	rel	obs	rel	obs	rel	obs	rel
Males	(0)		(4)		(13)		(15)		(16)		(48)	
1 year	-	-	100	100	100	100	100	100	94	100	98	100
3 years	-	-	75	77	92	98	93	100	63	90	81	97
5 years	-	-	75	79	84	94	79	100	49	96	70	96
Females	(1)		(1)		(1)		(2)		(0)		(5)	
1 year	100	100	100	100	100	100	100	100	-	-	100	100
3 years	100	100	100	100	100	100	100	100	-	-	100	100
5 years	-	-	100	100	-	-	100	100	-	-	100	100
Overall	(1)		(5)		(14)		(17)		(16)		(53)	
1 year	100	100	100	100	100	100	100	100	94	100	98	100
3 years	100	100	80	82	93	99	94	100	63	90	83	98
5 years	-	-	80	83	85	95	80	100	49	96	72	97

ICELAND

AREA	NUMBER OF CASES			PERIOD	MEAN AGE		
	Males	Females	All		Males	Females	All
Iceland	21	2	23	1985-1989	74.1	67.0	73.6

OBSERVED AND RELATIVE SURVIVAL (%) BY AGE (number of cases in parentheses)

	AGE CLASS									ALL	
	15-44		45-54		55-64		65-74		75-99			
	obs	rel	obs	rel	obs	rel	obs	rel	obs	rel	obs	rel
Males	(0)		(0)		(2)		(10)		(9)		(21)	
1 year	-	-	-	-	100	100	90	93	100	100	95	100
3 years	-	-	-	-	100	100	80	89	67	94	76	92
5 years	-	-	-	-	100	100	70	84	56	100	67	93
Females	(0)		(0)		(1)		(0)		(1)		(2)	
1 year	-	-	-	-	100	100	-	-	100	100	100	100
3 years	-	-	-	-	100	100	-	-	100	100	100	100
5 years	-	-	-	-	100	100	-	-	100	100	100	100
Overall	(0)		(0)		(3)		(10)		(10)		(23)	
1 year	-	-	-	-	100	100	90	93	100	100	96	100
3 years	-	-	-	-	100	100	80	89	70	96	78	94
5 years	-	-	-	-	100	100	70	84	60	100	70	95

LIP (ICD-9 140)

ITALY

AREA	NUMBER OF CASES			PERIOD	MEAN AGE			5-YR RELATIVE SURVIVAL (%)	
	Males	Females	All		Males	Females	All	Males	Females
Florence	47	11	58	1985-1989	64.7	74.4	66.6		
Genoa	9	1	10	1986-1988	65.1	60.0	64.7		
Latina	19	3	22	1985-1987	63.2	59.0	62.7		
Modena	3	0	3	1988-1989	72.7	-	72.7		
Parma	5	0	5	1985-1987	62.6	-	62.6		
Ragusa	51	4	55	1985-1989	67.8	74.0	68.3		
Romagna	4	0	4	1986-1988	59.3	-	59.3		
Turin	42	15	57	1985-1987	63.4	66.3	64.1		
Varese	26	2	28	1985-1989	65.8	78.0	66.7		
Italian Registries	206	36	242		65.2	69.6	65.9		

OBSERVED AND RELATIVE SURVIVAL (%) BY AGE (number of cases in parentheses)

	AGE CLASS										ALL	
	15-44		45-54		55-64		65-74		75-99			
	obs	rel	obs	rel	obs	rel	obs	rel	obs	rel	obs	rel
Males	(10)		(25)		(68)		(51)		(52)		(206)	
1 year	90	90	96	97	97	98	90	93	85	95	92	96
3 years	90	90	88	89	88	92	76	85	56	78	77	87
5 years	90	91	84	87	84	91	65	79	40	73	68	84
Females	(1)		(3)		(8)		(10)		(14)		(36)	
1 year	100	100	100	100	100	100	90	92	77	85	89	92
3 years	100	100	100	100	100	100	90	96	62	82	83	94
5 years	100	100	100	100	100	100	80	90	46	76	74	91
Overall	(11)		(28)		(76)		(61)		(66)		(242)	
1 year	91	91	96	97	97	99	90	93	83	93	91	95
3 years	91	91	89	91	89	93	79	87	57	79	78	88
5 years	91	92	86	88	86	92	67	81	42	74	69	85

NETHERLANDS

AREA	NUMBER OF CASES			PERIOD	MEAN AGE		
	Males	Females	All		Males	Females	All
Eindhoven	44	5	49	1985-1989	67.0	60.0	66.3

OBSERVED AND RELATIVE SURVIVAL (%) BY AGE (number of cases in parentheses)

	AGE CLASS										ALL	
	15-44		45-54		55-64		65-74		75-99			
	obs	rel	obs	rel	obs	rel	obs	rel	obs	rel	obs	rel
Males	(2)		(6)		(10)		(14)		(12)		(44)	
1 year	100	100	83	84	100	100	93	97	83	93	91	95
3 years	100	100	67	68	80	85	71	83	56	81	70	82
5 years	100	100	67	69	70	78	50	65	56	100	61	79
Females	(1)		(1)		(1)		(1)		(1)		(5)	
1 year	100	100	100	100	100	100	0	0	100	100	80	82
3 years	100	100	100	100	100	100	0	0	100	100	80	85
5 years	100	100	100	100	100	100	0	0	0	0	60	67
Overall	(3)		(7)		(11)		(15)		(13)		(49)	
1 year	100	100	86	86	100	100	87	90	85	95	90	94
3 years	100	100	71	72	82	86	67	77	60	86	71	82
5 years	100	100	71	73	73	80	47	60	51	97	61	77

LIP (ICD-9 140)

POLAND

AREA	NUMBER OF CASES			PERIOD	MEAN AGE			5-YR RELATIVE SURVIVAL (%)	
	Males	Females	All		Males	Females	All	Males	Females
Cracow	29	3	32	1985-1989	69.1	68.7	69.1		
Warsaw	25	2	27	1988-1989	64.4	65.5	64.6		
Polish Registries	54	5	59		67.0	67.8	67.1		

OBSERVED AND RELATIVE SURVIVAL (%) BY AGE (number of cases in parentheses)

	AGE CLASS										ALL	
	15-44		45-54		55-64		65-74		75-99			
	obs	rel	obs	rel	obs	rel	obs	rel	obs	rel	obs	rel
Males	(1)		(6)		(18)		(15)		(14)		(54)	
1 year	100	100	83	84	89	91	86	91	92	100	88	94
3 years	100	100	83	86	78	86	72	85	59	90	73	87
5 years	100	100	83	89	67	79	57	79	8	18	53	72
Females	(0)		(0)		(2)		(2)		(1)		(5)	
1 year	-	-	-	-	100	100	100	100	100	100	100	100
3 years	-	-	-	-	100	100	100	100	-	-	100	100
5 years	-	-	-	-	100	100	100	100	-	-	100	100
Overall	(1)		(6)		(20)		(17)		(15)		(59)	
1 year	100	100	83	84	90	92	88	92	93	100	89	94
3 years	100	100	83	86	79	87	75	89	59	90	74	88
5 years	100	100	83	89	69	81	63	85	8	18	56	75

SCOTLAND

AREA	NUMBER OF CASES			PERIOD	MEAN AGE		
	Males	Females	All		Males	Females	All
Scotland	253	66	319	1985-1989	68.4	69.5	68.7

OBSERVED AND RELATIVE SURVIVAL (%) BY AGE (number of cases in parentheses)

	AGE CLASS										ALL	
	15-44		45-54		55-64		65-74		75-99			
	obs	rel	obs	rel	obs	rel	obs	rel	obs	rel	obs	rel
Males	(9)		(23)		(49)		(96)		(76)		(253)	
1 year	100	100	100	100	88	90	94	98	93	100	93	99
3 years	100	100	91	94	78	83	79	93	68	100	77	94
5 years	100	100	91	96	67	76	72	95	53	100	68	94
Females	(4)		(8)		(5)		(20)		(29)		(66)	
1 year	100	100	100	100	100	100	95	98	86	94	92	97
3 years	100	100	100	100	80	84	95	100	66	88	82	95
5 years	100	100	88	90	80	87	90	100	41	70	68	89
Overall	(13)		(31)		(54)		(116)		(105)		(319)	
1 year	100	100	100	100	89	91	94	98	91	100	93	99
3 years	100	100	94	96	78	83	82	95	68	99	78	94
5 years	100	100	90	94	68	77	75	98	50	97	68	93

LIP (ICD-9 140)

SLOVAKIA

AREA	NUMBER OF CASES			PERIOD	MEAN AGE		
	Males	Females	All		Males	Females	All
Slovakia	664	147	811	1985-1989	65.2	71.1	66.3

OBSERVED AND RELATIVE SURVIVAL (%) BY AGE (number of cases in parentheses)

	AGE CLASS										ALL	
	15-44		45-54		55-64		65-74		75-99			
	obs	rel	obs	rel	obs	rel	obs	rel	obs	rel	obs	rel
Males	(32)		(94)		(191)		(175)		(172)		(664)	
1 year	97	97	97	98	95	98	95	100	81	93	92	97
3 years	91	92	88	92	86	94	83	99	63	98	80	96
5 years	87	89	83	89	78	91	78	100	54	100	73	99
Females	(2)		(10)		(28)		(42)		(65)		(147)	
1 year	100	100	100	100	100	100	93	96	89	100	93	99
3 years	100	100	100	100	96	100	86	95	75	100	84	100
5 years	100	100	100	100	96	100	73	88	59	100	73	100
Overall	(34)		(104)		(219)		(217)		(237)		(811)	
1 year	97	97	97	98	96	98	94	99	83	95	92	98
3 years	91	92	89	93	87	95	84	99	67	100	81	97
5 years	88	90	84	90	80	93	77	100	55	100	73	99

SLOVENIA

AREA	NUMBER OF CASES			PERIOD	MEAN AGE		
	Males	Females	All		Males	Females	All
Slovenia	120	36	156	1985-1989	63.7	70.9	65.4

OBSERVED AND RELATIVE SURVIVAL (%) BY AGE (number of cases in parentheses)

	AGE CLASS										ALL	
	15-44		45-54		55-64		65-74		75-99			
	obs	rel	obs	rel	obs	rel	obs	rel	obs	rel	obs	rel
Males	(7)		(22)		(39)		(23)		(29)		(120)	
1 year	100	100	95	96	92	94	96	100	79	90	91	95
3 years	71	72	86	89	74	80	78	92	45	68	70	81
5 years	71	73	86	92	74	84	65	87	38	81	66	85
Females	(0)		(4)		(11)		(6)		(15)		(36)	
1 year	-	-	100	100	91	92	100	100	87	100	92	99
3 years	-	-	100	100	91	94	100	100	40	68	72	90
5 years	-	-	100	100	91	96	100	100	20	53	64	92
Overall	(7)		(26)		(50)		(29)		(44)		(156)	
1 year	100	100	96	97	92	94	97	100	82	94	91	96
3 years	71	72	88	91	78	83	83	96	43	68	71	83
5 years	71	73	88	94	78	87	72	94	32	73	65	86

LIP   (ICD-9 140)

SPAIN

AREA	NUMBER OF CASES			PERIOD	MEAN AGE			5-YR RELATIVE SURVIVAL (%)	
	Males	Females	All		Males	Females	All	Males	Females
Basque Country	164	11	175	1986-1988	62.3	70.0	62.8		
Mallorca	47	9	56	1988-1989	62.4	71.1	63.9		
Navarra	137	5	142	1985-1989	65.6	81.0	66.2		
Tarragona	102	14	116	1985-1989	65.8	72.3	66.6		
Spanish Registries	450	39	489		64.1	72.6	64.8		

OBSERVED AND RELATIVE SURVIVAL (%) BY AGE (number of cases in parentheses)

	AGE CLASS										ALL	
	15-44		45-54		55-64		65-74		75-99			
	obs	rel	obs	rel	obs	rel	obs	rel	obs	rel	obs	rel
Males	(31)		(66)		(131)		(121)		(101)		(450)	
1 year	100	100	100	100	98	100	97	100	91	100	97	100
3 years	100	100	94	96	92	96	89	99	76	100	89	99
5 years	100	100	92	95	90	96	81	97	62	100	82	99
Females	(1)		(2)		(7)		(9)		(20)		(39)	
1 year	100	100	100	100	100	100	100	100	100	100	100	100
3 years	100	100	100	100	100	100	89	93	80	100	87	100
5 years	100	100	100	100	100	100	76	84	80	100	84	100
Overall	(32)		(68)		(138)		(130)		(121)		(489)	
1 year	100	100	100	100	99	100	97	100	93	100	97	100
3 years	100	100	94	96	93	96	89	98	77	100	89	99
5 years	100	100	93	96	90	97	80	96	65	100	82	99

SWEDEN

AREA	NUMBER OF CASES			PERIOD	MEAN AGE		
	Males	Females	All		Males	Females	All
South Sweden	133	46	179	1985-1989	69.4	70.8	69.8

OBSERVED AND RELATIVE SURVIVAL (%) BY AGE (number of cases in parentheses)

	AGE CLASS										ALL	
	15-44		45-54		55-64		65-74		75-99			
	obs	rel	obs	rel	obs	rel	obs	rel	obs	rel	obs	rel
Males	(3)		(11)		(24)		(48)		(47)		(133)	
1 year	100	100	100	100	96	97	98	100	91	100	95	100
3 years	100	100	91	92	92	96	94	100	66	93	83	98
5 years	100	100	91	94	92	99	90	100	34	62	71	93
Females	(2)		(4)		(7)		(13)		(20)		(46)	
1 year	100	100	100	100	100	100	100	100	90	100	96	100
3 years	100	100	100	100	86	87	92	98	75	100	85	99
5 years	100	100	100	100	86	89	92	100	55	98	76	98
Overall	(5)		(15)		(31)		(61)		(67)		(179)	
1 year	100	100	100	100	97	98	98	100	91	100	96	100
3 years	100	100	93	95	90	94	93	100	69	96	84	98
5 years	100	100	93	96	90	97	90	100	40	73	72	95

LIP

(ICD-9 140)

SWITZERLAND

AREA	NUMBER OF CASES			PERIOD	MEAN AGE		
	Males	Females	All		Males	Females	All
Geneva	19	4	23	1985-1989	59.0	61.0	59.4

OBSERVED AND RELATIVE SURVIVAL (%) BY AGE (number of cases in parentheses)

	AGE CLASS										ALL	
	15-44		45-54		55-64		65-74		75-99			
	obs	rel	obs	rel	obs	rel	obs	rel	obs	rel	obs	rel
Males	(3)		(5)		(3)		(5)		(3)		(19)	
1 year	100	100	100	100	100	100	100	100	67	73	95	97
3 years	67	67	80	81	50	52	100	100	67	88	78	84
5 years	67	68	80	83	50	54	100	100	33	55	72	83
Females	(0)		(2)		(0)		(1)		(1)		(4)	
1 year	-	-	100	100	-	-	100	100	100	100	100	100
3 years	-	-	100	100	-	-	100	100	0	0	75	78
5 years	-	-	100	100	-	-	100	100	0	0	75	80
Overall	(3)		(7)		(3)		(6)		(4)		(23)	
1 year	100	100	100	100	100	100	100	100	75	81	96	98
3 years	67	67	86	87	50	52	100	100	50	63	77	83
5 years	67	68	86	88	50	54	100	100	25	38	73	82

LIP (ICD-9 140)

EUROPE, 1985-89

Weighted analyses

COUNTRY	% COVERAGE WITH C.R.s	YEARLY NO. OF CASES (Mean No. of cases recorded) Males	Females	All
AUSTRIA	8	2	0	2
DENMARK	100	110	16	126
ENGLAND	50	102	31	133
ESTONIA	100	20	5	25
FINLAND	100	110	30	140
FRANCE	3	16	3	19
GERMANY	2	10	1	11
ICELAND	100	4	0	4
ITALY	10	55	10	65
NETHERLANDS	6	9	1	10
POLAND	6	18	2	20
SCOTLAND	100	51	13	64
SLOVAKIA	100	133	29	162
SLOVENIA	100	24	7	31
SPAIN	10	126	12	138
SWEDEN	17	27	9	36
SWITZERLAND	6	4	1	5

RELATIVE SURVIVAL (%) (Age-standardized)

□ 1 year ■ 5 years

OBSERVED AND RELATIVE SURVIVAL (%) BY AGE

	AGE CLASS										ALL	
	15-44 obs	rel	45-54 obs	rel	55-64 obs	rel	65-74 obs	rel	75-99 obs	rel	obs	rel
Males												
1 year	98	98	96	96	98	99	94	97	88	97	94	98
3 years	97	97	86	88	87	92	83	92	66	92	81	93
5 years	97	97	83	87	81	89	73	89	50	87	71	91
Females												
1 year	100	100	100	100	99	100	78	79	87	93	90	94
3 years	100	100	100	100	98	98	73	77	68	89	81	93
5 years	100	100	99	99	97	99	67	73	52	81	72	90
Overall												
1 year	99	99	96	97	98	99	92	94	88	97	93	97
3 years	98	98	88	90	88	93	82	90	67	92	81	93
5 years	97	97	85	88	83	90	72	87	50	86	71	91

AGE STANDARDIZED RELATIVE SURVIVAL(%)

COUNTRY	MALES 1-year (95% C.I.)	5-years (95% C.I.)	FEMALES 1-year (95% C.I.)	5-years (95% C.I.)
AUSTRIA	-	-	-	-
DENMARK	97.7 (95.4 - 99.9)	92.5 (87.1 - 98.1)	96.6 (92.3 -101.0)	93.9 (84.5 -104.3)
ENGLAND	96.9 (94.5 - 99.4)	91.9 (86.6 - 97.6)	95.9 (91.8 -100.3)	93.7 (86.3 -101.8)
ESTONIA	93.3 (85.9 -101.3)	77.0 (61.8 - 95.9)	-	-
FINLAND	99.2 (96.9 -101.5)	94.2 (88.4 -100.4)	98.3 (95.3 -101.5)	89.6 (82.3 - 97.6)
FRANCE	93.4 (86.5 -100.8)	82.4 (69.0 - 98.4)	-	-
GERMANY	-	-	-	-
ICELAND	-	-	-	-
ITALY	95.2 (90.7 - 99.8)	81.2 (72.3 - 91.1)	92.8 (83.6 -103.0)	89.3 (74.5 -107.1)
NETHERLANDS	95.3 (86.6 -104.9)	81.0 (61.7 -106.4)	70.1 (69.8 - 70.4)	38.7 (38.3 - 39.2)
POLAND	93.4 (84.8 -103.0)	61.7 (47.2 - 80.5)	-	-
SCOTLAND	97.1 (93.8 -100.5)	92.5 (83.9 -102.0)	97.6 (92.5 -103.0)	86.4 (73.3 -101.8)
SLOVAKIA	96.8 (94.3 - 99.4)	96.3 (90.4 -102.6)	98.8 (95.2 -102.4)	96.4 (87.5 -106.2)
SLOVENIA	95.2 (89.1 -101.7)	84.2 (70.7 -100.4)	-	-
SPAIN	99.9 (97.7 -102.1)	97.7 (91.5 -104.2)	100.0 (100.0 -100.0)	95.1 (82.8 -109.3)
SWEDEN	99.3 (95.8 -103.0)	87.3 (78.7 - 96.8)	99.9 (95.4 -104.5)	96.5 (83.0 -112.2)
SWITZERLAND	91.4 (74.9 -111.7)	71.7 (45.1 -114.0)	-	-
EUROPE, 1985-89	97.3 (95.7 - 98.9)	88.6 (84.6 - 92.9)	91.4 (89.1 - 93.7)	85.7 (80.5 - 91.2)

TONGUE (ICD-9 141)

AUSTRIA

AREA	NUMBER OF CASES			PERIOD	MEAN AGE		
	Males	Females	All		Males	Females	All
Tirol	12	1	13	1988-1989	55.7	55.0	55.7

OBSERVED AND RELATIVE SURVIVAL (%) BY AGE (number of cases in parentheses)

	AGE CLASS										ALL	
	15-44		45-54		55-64		65-74		75-99			
	obs	rel	obs	rel	obs	rel	obs	rel	obs	rel	obs	rel
Males	(2)		(4)		(3)		(2)		(1)		(12)	
1 year	50	50	75	75	67	67	100	100	100	100	75	76
3 years	0	0	50	51	67	69	50	54	100	100	50	52
5 years	0	0	50	51	67	71	0	0	100	100	42	45
Females	(0)		(0)		(1)		(0)		(0)		(1)	
1 year	-	-	-	-	100	100	-	-	-	-	100	100
3 years	-	-	-	-	100	100	-	-	-	-	100	100
5 years	-	-	-	-	100	100	-	-	-	-	100	100
Overall	(2)		(4)		(4)		(2)		(1)		(13)	
1 year	50	50	75	75	75	76	100	100	100	100	77	78
3 years	0	0	50	51	75	77	50	54	100	100	54	56
5 years	0	0	50	51	75	79	0	0	100	100	46	49

DENMARK

AREA	NUMBER OF CASES			PERIOD	MEAN AGE		
	Males	Females	All		Males	Females	All
Denmark	196	127	323	1985-1989	61.8	66.9	63.8

OBSERVED AND RELATIVE SURVIVAL (%) BY AGE (number of cases in parentheses)

	AGE CLASS										ALL	
	15-44		45-54		55-64		65-74		75-99			
	obs	rel	obs	rel	obs	rel	obs	rel	obs	rel	obs	rel
Males	(16)		(40)		(58)		(54)		(28)		(196)	
1 year	88	88	70	70	53	54	57	60	36	40	58	60
3 years	44	44	48	49	34	36	33	38	11	16	34	38
5 years	44	44	45	47	24	27	22	28	7	14	27	33
Females	(8)		(13)		(36)		(27)		(43)		(127)	
1 year	75	75	62	62	75	76	63	64	67	74	69	71
3 years	50	50	31	31	53	55	44	48	47	62	46	52
5 years	50	50	23	24	50	53	37	42	33	55	39	47
Overall	(24)		(53)		(94)		(81)		(71)		(323)	
1 year	83	84	68	68	62	63	59	61	55	61	62	64
3 years	46	46	43	44	41	44	37	41	32	45	39	44
5 years	46	46	40	41	34	37	27	33	23	40	32	38

TONGUE (ICD-9 141)

ENGLAND

AREA	NUMBER OF CASES			PERIOD	MEAN AGE			5-YR RELATIVE SURVIVAL (%)	
	Males	Females	All		Males	Females	All	Males	Females
East Anglia	52	52	104	1985-1989	64.7	68.4	66.6		
Mersey	117	66	183	1985-1989	62.3	69.2	64.8		
Oxford	85	57	142	1985-1989	63.0	66.7	64.5		
South Thames	173	128	301	1985-1989	64.3	68.8	66.2		
Wessex	96	84	180	1985-1989	65.4	68.4	66.8		
West Midlands	188	111	299	1985-1989	60.8	66.9	63.1		
Yorkshire	123	73	196	1985-1989	64.4	64.5	64.5		
English Registries	834	571	1405		63.3	67.6	65.1		

OBSERVED AND RELATIVE SURVIVAL (%) BY AGE (number of cases in parentheses)

	AGE CLASS										ALL	
	15-44		45-54		55-64		65-74		75-99			
	obs	rel	obs	rel	obs	rel	obs	rel	obs	rel	obs	rel
Males	(79)		(127)		(218)		(239)		(171)		(834)	
1 year	73	74	73	74	64	65	65	68	48	54	63	66
3 years	53	53	49	50	42	44	35	40	21	30	38	43
5 years	47	47	46	47	33	36	29	36	17	32	32	39
Females	(51)		(51)		(92)		(172)		(205)		(571)	
1 year	86	86	86	87	75	76	71	72	59	64	70	73
3 years	65	65	63	63	49	50	47	51	32	42	45	51
5 years	61	61	55	56	43	46	44	50	24	39	39	48
Overall	(130)		(178)		(310)		(411)		(376)		(1405)	
1 year	78	79	77	77	67	68	68	70	54	59	66	69
3 years	58	58	53	54	44	46	40	44	27	37	41	46
5 years	52	53	48	50	36	39	35	42	21	36	35	43

ESTONIA

AREA	NUMBER OF CASES			PERIOD	MEAN AGE		
	Males	Females	All		Males	Females	All
Estonia	71	14	85	1985-1989	57.2	65.4	58.5

OBSERVED AND RELATIVE SURVIVAL (%) BY AGE (number of cases in parentheses)

	AGE CLASS										ALL	
	15-44		45-54		55-64		65-74		75-99			
	obs	rel	obs	rel	obs	rel	obs	rel	obs	rel	obs	rel
Males	(5)		(29)		(25)		(6)		(6)		(71)	
1 year	80	80	69	70	68	70	33	35	50	58	65	67
3 years	60	61	31	32	24	26	17	20	17	27	28	31
5 years	60	62	24	26	8	9	17	23	0	0	18	22
Females	(3)		(1)		(2)		(3)		(5)		(14)	
1 year	33	33	0	0	0	0	33	34	0	0	14	15
3 years	0	0	0	0	0	0	0	0	0	0	0	0
5 years	0	0	0	0	0	0	0	0	0	0	0	0
Overall	(8)		(30)		(27)		(9)		(11)		(85)	
1 year	63	63	67	68	63	65	33	35	27	31	56	58
3 years	38	38	30	31	22	24	11	13	9	14	24	26
5 years	38	39	23	25	7	9	11	15	0	0	15	18

TONGUE (ICD-9 141)

FINLAND

AREA	NUMBER OF CASES			PERIOD	MEAN AGE		
	Males	Females	All		Males	Females	All
Finland	137	99	236	1985-1989	59.1	70.5	63.9

OBSERVED AND RELATIVE SURVIVAL (%) BY AGE (number of cases in parentheses)

	AGE CLASS										ALL	
	15-44		45-54		55-64		65-74		75-99			
	obs	rel	obs	rel	obs	rel	obs	rel	obs	rel	obs	rel
Males	(16)		(33)		(43)		(28)		(17)		(137)	
1 year	88	88	76	76	74	76	71	75	71	78	75	77
3 years	63	63	48	50	40	42	46	54	29	41	45	49
5 years	63	63	24	25	33	36	36	46	18	32	33	38
Females	(4)		(6)		(17)		(32)		(40)		(99)	
1 year	75	75	100	100	88	89	84	86	50	55	72	75
3 years	75	75	83	84	71	72	72	78	28	38	55	63
5 years	75	75	67	68	59	61	53	61	20	35	42	55
Overall	(20)		(39)		(60)		(60)		(57)		(236)	
1 year	85	85	79	80	78	80	78	81	56	62	74	77
3 years	65	65	54	55	48	51	60	67	28	39	49	55
5 years	65	66	31	32	40	44	45	55	19	34	37	45

FRANCE

AREA	NUMBER OF CASES			PERIOD	MEAN AGE			5-YR RELATIVE SURVIVAL (%)	
	Males	Females	All		Males	Females	All	Males	Females
Somme	120	14	134	1985-1989	57.4	63.6	58.1		
Calvados	128	17	145	1985-1989	57.7	61.2	58.1		
Doubs	85	13	98	1985-1989	58.0	62.8	58.6		
French Registries	333	44	377		57.7	62.5	58.2		

OBSERVED AND RELATIVE SURVIVAL (%) BY AGE (number of cases in parentheses)

	AGE CLASS										ALL	
	15-44		45-54		55-64		65-74		75-99			
	obs	rel	obs	rel	obs	rel	obs	rel	obs	rel	obs	rel
Males	(37)		(98)		(108)		(65)		(25)		(333)	
1 year	72	72	70	71	62	63	67	69	35	39	65	66
3 years	45	45	37	38	37	39	42	47	25	34	38	40
5 years	38	39	30	31	28	31	28	35	19	31	29	33
Females	(2)		(7)		(20)		(9)		(6)		(44)	
1 year	100	100	57	57	80	80	76	78	60	66	74	75
3 years	-	-	14	14	69	70	64	67	40	55	54	57
5 years	-	-	14	15	69	71	64	71	40	71	54	60
Overall	(39)		(105)		(128)		(74)		(31)		(377)	
1 year	73	73	70	70	65	66	68	70	40	44	66	67
3 years	45	46	36	37	42	44	44	49	28	37	40	42
5 years	38	39	29	30	35	38	32	40	23	39	32	36

TONGUE (ICD-9 141)

GERMANY

AREA	NUMBER OF CASES			PERIOD	MEAN AGE		
	Males	Females	All		Males	Females	All
Saarland	153	27	180	1985-1989	56.5	63.1	57.5

OBSERVED AND RELATIVE SURVIVAL (%) BY AGE (number of cases in parentheses)

	AGE CLASS										ALL	
	15-44		45-54		55-64		65-74		75-99			
	obs	rel	obs	rel	obs	rel	obs	rel	obs	rel	obs	rel
Males	(28)		(44)		(41)		(25)		(15)		(153)	
1 year	79	79	70	71	68	69	72	75	40	45	69	70
3 years	57	58	48	49	54	57	32	37	33	48	47	51
5 years	57	58	39	41	38	42	27	35	33	66	40	45
Females	(1)		(8)		(7)		(3)		(8)		(27)	
1 year	0	0	88	88	71	72	100	100	88	95	81	84
3 years	0	0	63	63	57	59	0	0	63	82	52	57
5 years	0	0	63	64	57	60	0	0	49	79	48	56
Overall	(29)		(52)		(48)		(28)		(23)		(180)	
1 year	76	76	73	73	69	70	75	78	57	63	71	72
3 years	55	56	50	51	54	57	29	33	43	61	48	52
5 years	55	56	43	45	41	45	24	30	38	69	41	47

ICELAND

AREA	NUMBER OF CASES			PERIOD	MEAN AGE		
	Males	Females	All		Males	Females	All
Iceland	4	2	6	1985-1989	60.8	68.5	63.5

OBSERVED AND RELATIVE SURVIVAL (%) BY AGE (number of cases in parentheses)

	AGE CLASS										ALL	
	15-44		45-54		55-64		65-74		75-99			
	obs	rel	obs	rel	obs	rel	obs	rel	obs	rel	obs	rel
Males	(0)		(2)		(0)		(2)		(0)		(4)	
1 year	-	-	100	100	-	-	50	52	-	-	75	77
3 years	-	-	0	0	-	-	50	57	-	-	25	27
5 years	-	-	0	0	-	-	0	0	-	-	0	0
Females	(0)		(0)		(0)		(2)		(0)		(2)	
1 year	-	-	-	-	-	-	50	51	-	-	50	51
3 years	-	-	-	-	-	-	0	0	-	-	0	0
5 years	-	-	-	-	-	-	0	0	-	-	0	0
Overall	(0)		(2)		(0)		(4)		(0)		(6)	
1 year	-	-	100	100	-	-	50	52	-	-	67	68
3 years	-	-	0	0	-	-	25	28	-	-	17	18
5 years	-	-	0	0	-	-	0	0	-	-	0	0

TONGUE

(ICD-9 141)

ITALY

AREA	NUMBER OF CASES			PERIOD	MEAN AGE		
	Males	Females	All		Males	Females	All
Florence	67	27	94	1985-1989	61.2	65.9	62.5
Genoa	36	17	53	1986-1988	64.4	66.2	65.0
Latina	13	2	15	1985-1987	59.2	53.0	58.4
Modena	12	3	15	1988-1989	62.9	70.7	64.5
Parma	23	7	30	1985-1987	59.5	65.9	61.0
Ragusa	11	3	14	1985-1989	65.1	59.7	64.0
Romagna	14	3	17	1986-1988	56.9	57.0	57.0
Turin	47	22	69	1985-1987	61.7	61.5	61.6
Varese	74	18	92	1985-1989	61.2	68.4	62.6
Italian Registries	297	102	399		61.5	65.0	62.4

5-YR RELATIVE SURVIVAL (%)

OBSERVED AND RELATIVE SURVIVAL (%) BY AGE (number of cases in parentheses)

	AGE CLASS										ALL	
	15-44		45-54		55-64		65-74		75-99			
	obs	rel	obs	rel	obs	rel	obs	rel	obs	rel	obs	rel
Males	(19)		(59)		(105)		(73)		(41)		(297)	
1 year	79	79	62	62	72	73	74	77	51	56	68	70
3 years	47	48	43	44	37	39	37	42	22	30	37	40
5 years	42	43	36	37	33	36	34	42	17	29	32	38
Females	(9)		(13)		(24)		(25)		(31)		(102)	
1 year	89	89	92	93	63	63	79	81	71	76	75	77
3 years	67	67	77	78	38	38	58	62	42	53	52	58
5 years	67	67	62	62	38	39	50	56	29	44	44	50
Overall	(28)		(72)		(129)		(98)		(72)		(399)	
1 year	82	82	68	68	71	71	75	78	60	65	70	72
3 years	54	54	49	50	37	39	42	47	31	40	41	44
5 years	50	50	41	42	34	37	38	46	22	36	35	41

NETHERLANDS

AREA	NUMBER OF CASES			PERIOD	MEAN AGE		
	Males	Females	All		Males	Females	All
Eindhoven	24	22	46	1985-1989	64.5	59.9	62.3

OBSERVED AND RELATIVE SURVIVAL (%) BY AGE (number of cases in parentheses)

	AGE CLASS										ALL	
	15-44		45-54		55-64		65-74		75-99			
	obs	rel	obs	rel	obs	rel	obs	rel	obs	rel	obs	rel
Males	(4)		(3)		(2)		(9)		(6)		(24)	
1 year	100	100	0	0	100	100	56	58	67	77	63	66
3 years	100	100	0	0	100	100	22	26	50	79	46	54
5 years	100	100	0	0	100	100	22	29	0	0	33	44
Females	(4)		(3)		(6)		(4)		(5)		(22)	
1 year	100	100	100	100	83	84	75	77	20	22	73	75
3 years	75	75	67	67	50	51	75	79	0	0	50	54
5 years	75	75	67	68	33	34	75	84	0	0	45	52
Overall	(8)		(6)		(8)		(13)		(11)		(46)	
1 year	100	100	50	50	88	88	62	64	45	51	67	70
3 years	88	88	33	34	63	64	38	43	27	40	48	54
5 years	88	88	33	34	50	52	38	48	0	0	39	48

TONGUE   (ICD-9 141)

POLAND

| AREA | NUMBER OF CASES | | | PERIOD | MEAN AGE | | | 5-YR RELATIVE SURVIVAL (%) | |
	Males	Females	All		Males	Females	All	Males	Females
Cracow	34	6	40	1985-1989	55.9	58.7	56.3		
Warsaw	34	14	48	1988-1989	58.7	61.1	59.4		
Polish Registries	68	20	88		57.3	60.5	58.0		

OBSERVED AND RELATIVE SURVIVAL (%) BY AGE (number of cases in parentheses)

| | AGE CLASS | | | | | | | | | | ALL | |
| | 15-44 | | 45-54 | | 55-64 | | 65-74 | | 75-99 | | | |
	obs	rel	obs	rel	obs	rel	obs	rel	obs	rel	obs	rel
Males	(5)		(20)		(28)		(13)		(2)		(68)	
1 year	60	60	30	30	43	44	31	32	50	56	38	39
3 years	40	41	5	5	18	19	31	36	0	0	18	19
5 years	40	41	5	5	14	17	15	20	0	0	13	15
Females	(2)		(5)		(7)		(2)		(4)		(20)	
1 year	100	100	40	40	69	70	100	100	50	58	66	68
3 years	100	100	0	0	69	72	50	54	0	0	40	43
5 years	100	100	0	0	69	74	50	57	0	0	40	45
Overall	(7)		(25)		(35)		(15)		(6)		(88)	
1 year	71	72	32	32	47	48	40	42	53	61	44	45
3 years	57	58	4	4	25	27	33	39	0	0	22	24
5 years	57	58	4	4	22	26	20	26	0	0	18	21

SCOTLAND

| AREA | NUMBER OF CASES | | | PERIOD | MEAN AGE | | |
	Males	Females	All		Males	Females	All
Scotland	250	156	406	1985-1989	62.4	69.1	65.0

OBSERVED AND RELATIVE SURVIVAL (%) BY AGE (number of cases in parentheses)

| | AGE CLASS | | | | | | | | | | ALL | |
| | 15-44 | | 45-54 | | 55-64 | | 65-74 | | 75-99 | | | |
	obs	rel	obs	rel	obs	rel	obs	rel	obs	rel	obs	rel
Males	(20)		(45)		(73)		(70)		(42)		(250)	
1 year	70	70	71	72	67	69	60	63	55	62	64	67
3 years	50	50	47	48	40	43	41	48	26	39	40	45
5 years	40	41	36	37	30	34	29	38	14	29	29	36
Females	(8)		(12)		(36)		(40)		(60)		(156)	
1 year	100	100	92	92	67	67	65	67	40	44	60	63
3 years	88	88	75	76	39	40	43	47	22	30	38	45
5 years	63	63	58	60	33	36	40	47	15	27	31	41
Overall	(28)		(57)		(109)		(110)		(102)		(406)	
1 year	79	79	75	76	67	68	62	64	46	52	62	65
3 years	61	61	53	54	39	42	42	48	24	34	39	45
5 years	46	47	40	42	31	35	33	41	15	28	30	38

TONGUE   (ICD-9 141)

SLOVAKIA

AREA	NUMBER OF CASES			PERIOD	MEAN AGE		
	Males	Females	All		Males	Females	All
Slovakia	563	40	603	1985-1989	54.7	60.7	55.1

OBSERVED AND RELATIVE SURVIVAL (%) BY AGE (number of cases in parentheses)

	AGE CLASS										ALL	
	15-44		45-54		55-64		65-74		75-99			
	obs	rel	obs	rel	obs	rel	obs	rel	obs	rel	obs	rel
Males	(108)		(182)		(168)		(75)		(30)		(563)	
1 year	43	43	54	55	53	54	36	38	37	42	48	50
3 years	12	12	23	24	18	19	16	19	20	31	18	20
5 years	6	6	18	19	13	15	15	20	16	34	14	16
Females	(10)		(4)		(6)		(9)		(11)		(40)	
1 year	100	100	50	50	83	84	67	69	55	59	73	75
3 years	50	50	25	25	67	69	44	49	18	24	40	44
5 years	50	50	0	0	67	70	-	-	18	30	37	44
Overall	(118)		(186)		(174)		(84)		(41)		(603)	
1 year	47	48	54	55	54	55	39	41	41	47	50	51
3 years	15	15	23	24	20	21	19	22	20	29	20	21
5 years	10	10	17	19	15	18	18	24	17	32	15	18

SLOVENIA

AREA	NUMBER OF CASES			PERIOD	MEAN AGE		
	Males	Females	All		Males	Females	All
Slovenia	187	24	211	1985-1989	56.4	64.2	57.3

OBSERVED AND RELATIVE SURVIVAL (%) BY AGE (number of cases in parentheses)

	AGE CLASS										ALL	
	15-44		45-54		55-64		65-74		75-99			
	obs	rel	obs	rel	obs	rel	obs	rel	obs	rel	obs	rel
Males	(19)		(60)		(73)		(25)		(10)		(187)	
1 year	47	48	60	61	49	50	56	59	50	55	53	55
3 years	21	21	32	33	22	23	16	19	30	41	25	26
5 years	16	16	18	19	16	18	8	10	30	53	16	19
Females	(1)		(4)		(8)		(6)		(5)		(24)	
1 year	100	100	100	100	63	63	100	100	60	68	79	82
3 years	100	100	100	100	38	38	67	73	0	0	50	56
5 years	100	100	100	100	25	26	33	40	0	0	38	45
Overall	(20)		(64)		(81)		(31)		(15)		(211)	
1 year	50	50	63	63	51	52	65	67	53	59	56	58
3 years	25	25	36	37	23	25	26	30	20	28	27	30
5 years	20	20	23	25	17	19	13	16	20	37	19	21

TONGUE   (ICD-9 141)

SPAIN

AREA	NUMBER OF CASES			PERIOD	MEAN AGE			5-YR RELATIVE SURVIVAL (%)	
	Males	Females	All		Males	Females	All	Males	Females
Basque Country	173	25	198	1986-1988	58.8	63.2	59.4		
Mallorca	21	4	25	1988-1989	58.2	66.5	59.6		
Navarra	26	10	36	1985-1989	56.5	64.4	58.8		
Tarragona	33	6	39	1985-1989	60.0	64.7	60.7		
Spanish Registries	253	45	298		58.7	64.0	59.5		

OBSERVED AND RELATIVE SURVIVAL (%) BY AGE (number of cases in parentheses)

	AGE CLASS										ALL	
	15-44		45-54		55-64		65-74		75-99			
	obs	rel	obs	rel	obs	rel	obs	rel	obs	rel	obs	rel
Males	(35)		(44)		(95)		(54)		(25)		(253)	
1 year	74	74	75	75	58	59	61	63	32	35	61	63
3 years	49	49	48	49	36	37	41	45	16	21	39	41
5 years	46	46	37	38	31	33	31	37	16	26	33	37
Females	(4)		(8)		(10)		(9)		(14)		(45)	
1 year	100	100	75	75	100	100	89	90	36	39	73	75
3 years	75	75	63	63	70	71	89	93	21	28	58	63
5 years	75	75	63	63	70	72	89	97	14	22	55	64
Overall	(39)		(52)		(105)		(63)		(39)		(298)	
1 year	77	77	75	75	62	63	65	67	33	36	63	64
3 years	51	52	50	51	39	41	48	52	18	23	42	45
5 years	49	49	41	43	34	37	40	47	15	24	36	41

SWEDEN

AREA	NUMBER OF CASES			PERIOD	MEAN AGE		
	Males	Females	All		Males	Females	All
South Sweden	56	33	89	1985-1989	62.4	67.9	64.5

OBSERVED AND RELATIVE SURVIVAL (%) BY AGE (number of cases in parentheses)

	AGE CLASS										ALL	
	15-44		45-54		55-64		65-74		75-99			
	obs	rel	obs	rel	obs	rel	obs	rel	obs	rel	obs	rel
Males	(7)		(10)		(9)		(20)		(10)		(56)	
1 year	100	100	80	80	89	90	90	93	60	66	84	87
3 years	43	43	50	51	78	81	60	67	50	68	57	63
5 years	43	43	30	31	56	60	55	68	20	35	43	51
Females	(5)		(4)		(5)		(4)		(15)		(33)	
1 year	80	80	100	100	80	80	75	76	60	68	73	77
3 years	80	80	75	76	60	61	25	27	27	39	45	54
5 years	80	81	75	76	60	62	25	28	13	26	39	52
Overall	(12)		(14)		(14)		(24)		(25)		(89)	
1 year	92	92	86	86	86	87	88	90	60	67	80	83
3 years	58	59	57	58	71	74	54	60	36	51	53	60
5 years	58	59	43	44	57	60	50	61	16	30	42	51

TONGUE   (ICD-9 141)

SWITZERLAND

AREA	NUMBER OF CASES			PERIOD	MEAN AGE			5-YR RELATIVE SURVIVAL (%)	
	Males	Females	All		Males	Females	All	Males	Females
Basel	26	8	34	1985-1988	59.2	64.1	60.4		
Geneva	52	16	68	1985-1989	57.5	69.2	60.3		
Swiss Registries	78	24	102		58.1	67.6	60.3		

OBSERVED AND RELATIVE SURVIVAL (%) BY AGE (number of cases in parentheses)

	AGE CLASS										ALL	
	15-44		45-54		55-64		65-74		75-99			
	obs	rel	obs	rel	obs	rel	obs	rel	obs	rel	obs	rel
Males	(15)		(11)		(29)		(17)		(6)		(78)	
1 year	100	100	91	91	69	70	47	49	33	36	71	72
3 years	80	80	64	65	52	54	41	46	17	22	54	57
5 years	73	74	64	66	41	44	24	29	17	27	44	50
Females	(1)		(4)		(4)		(7)		(8)		(24)	
1 year	100	100	100	100	75	75	43	44	63	68	66	69
3 years	100	100	33	34	50	51	29	30	25	32	35	39
5 years	100	100	0	0	50	52	29	32	13	20	27	32
Overall	(16)		(15)		(33)		(24)		(14)		(102)	
1 year	100	100	93	94	70	71	46	47	50	54	70	71
3 years	81	82	57	58	52	54	38	41	21	28	50	53
5 years	74	75	50	52	42	45	25	30	14	23	40	46

TONGUE (ICD-9 141)

EUROPE, 1985-89
Weighted analyses

COUNTRY	% COVERAGE WITH C.R.s	YEARLY NO. OF CASES (Mean No. of cases recorded)		
		Males	Females	All
AUSTRIA	8	6	1	7
DENMARK	100	39	25	64
ENGLAND	50	167	114	281
ESTONIA	100	14	3	17
FINLAND	100	27	20	47
FRANCE	3	67	9	76
GERMANY	2	31	5	36
ICELAND	100	1	0	1
ITALY	10	81	28	109
NETHERLANDS	6	5	4	9
POLAND	6	24	8	32
SCOTLAND	100	50	31	81
SLOVAKIA	100	113	8	121
SLOVENIA	100	37	5	42
SPAIN	10	81	14	95
SWEDEN	17	11	7	18
SWITZERLAND	11	17	5	22

RELATIVE SURVIVAL (%) (Age-standardized) — Males / Females

□ 1 year ■ 5 years

OBSERVED AND RELATIVE SURVIVAL (%) BY AGE

	AGE CLASS										ALL	
	15-44		45-54		55-64		65-74		75-99			
	obs	rel	obs	rel	obs	rel	obs	rel	obs	rel	obs	rel
Males												
1 year	75	75	67	68	64	65	66	68	41	45	64	66
3 years	49	50	41	42	42	44	37	42	25	35	39	43
5 years	46	46	33	35	33	36	28	35	21	38	32	37
Females												
1 year	76	76	79	79	75	76	82	83	62	68	74	76
3 years	57	57	51	51	56	57	47	50	36	47	50	54
5 years	56	56	46	46	54	57	45	50	28	46	46	53
Overall												
1 year	75	75	70	70	66	67	69	71	45	50	66	68
3 years	51	51	43	44	44	46	39	43	27	37	41	45
5 years	47	48	36	37	37	40	31	37	23	39	35	40

AGE STANDARDIZED RELATIVE SURVIVAL(%)

COUNTRY	MALES		FEMALES	
	1-year (95% C.I.)	5-years (95% C.I.)	1-year (95% C.I.)	5-years (95% C.I.)
AUSTRIA	80.7 (63.9 -101.8)	48.3 (32.8 - 71.2)	-	-
DENMARK	59.8 (53.3 - 67.2)	30.7 (24.2 - 38.8)	69.9 (61.5 - 79.4)	44.8 (35.8 - 56.0)
ENGLAND	66.2 (63.0 - 69.7)	38.9 (35.2 - 42.9)	76.0 (72.2 - 80.0)	49.2 (44.4 - 54.5)
ESTONIA	60.8 (47.9 - 77.3)	20.0 (11.0 - 36.2)	11.6 (3.5 - 38.9)	0.0 (0.0 - 0.0)
FINLAND	77.5 (70.0 - 85.7)	38.5 (29.7 - 49.9)	82.8 (75.5 - 90.8)	59.2 (47.8 - 73.3)
FRANCE	62.6 (56.8 - 68.9)	32.9 (26.3 - 41.2)	74.7 (61.9 - 90.2)	-
GERMANY	67.6 (59.7 - 76.5)	46.1 (35.7 - 59.6)	78.0 (67.4 - 90.3)	43.7 (30.0 - 63.8)
ICELAND	-	-	-	-
ITALY	69.5 (64.1 - 75.3)	37.2 (31.2 - 44.3)	78.1 (70.3 - 86.8)	51.3 (41.6 - 63.3)
NETHERLANDS	66.4 (56.1 - 78.6)	45.5 (38.0 - 54.6)	75.7 (62.2 - 92.1)	50.5 (34.4 - 74.1)
POLAND	42.5 (28.2 - 64.2)	14.9 (8.1 - 27.3)	72.1 (54.9 - 94.8)	44.9 (27.9 - 72.1)
SCOTLAND	66.9 (60.9 - 73.4)	35.2 (28.8 - 43.1)	71.4 (64.9 - 78.6)	44.5 (35.8 - 55.2)
SLOVAKIA	47.1 (42.1 - 52.7)	19.6 (14.3 - 26.8)	71.0 (56.8 - 88.8)	-
SLOVENIA	54.8 (46.4 - 64.8)	22.6 (14.3 - 35.9)	83.7 (71.7 - 97.7)	47.0 (35.2 - 62.9)
SPAIN	60.3 (54.3 - 66.9)	35.0 (28.3 - 43.4)	81.6 (72.9 - 91.2)	67.2 (54.9 - 82.4)
SWEDEN	85.5 (75.9 - 96.4)	49.6 (36.1 - 68.0)	80.9 (66.9 - 98.0)	52.3 (35.7 - 76.6)
SWITZERLAND	66.3 (56.0 - 78.4)	44.9 (33.2 - 60.6)	74.1 (59.5 - 92.2)	36.4 (22.2 - 59.5)
EUROPE, 1985-89	63.8 (60.7 - 67.1)	36.8 (32.8 - 41.3)	76.6 (72.5 - 80.8)	50.9 (45.1 - 57.6)

SALIVARY GLANDS   (ICD-9 142)

AUSTRIA

AREA	NUMBER OF CASES			PERIOD	MEAN AGE		
	Males	Females	All		Males	Females	All
Tirol	4	3	7	1988-1989	59.5	57.7	58.9

OBSERVED AND RELATIVE SURVIVAL (%) BY AGE (number of cases in parentheses)

	AGE CLASS										ALL	
	15-44		45-54		55-64		65-74		75-99			
	obs	rel	obs	rel	obs	rel	obs	rel	obs	rel	obs	rel
Males	(1)		(0)		(1)		(0)		(2)		(4)	
1 year	100	100	-	-	100	100	-	-	50	53	75	78
3 years	100	100	-	-	0	0	-	-	50	61	50	56
5 years	100	100	-	-	0	0	-	-	0	0	25	30
Females	(1)		(0)		(1)		(0)		(1)		(3)	
1 year	100	100	-	-	100	100	-	-	0	0	67	68
3 years	100	100	-	-	100	100	-	-	0	0	67	72
5 years	100	100	-	-	100	100	-	-	0	0	67	77
Overall	(2)		(0)		(2)		(0)		(3)		(7)	
1 year	100	100	-	-	100	100	-	-	33	36	71	74
3 years	100	100	-	-	50	51	-	-	33	41	57	63
5 years	100	100	-	-	50	52	-	-	0	0	43	51

DENMARK

AREA	NUMBER OF CASES			PERIOD	MEAN AGE		
	Males	Females	All		Males	Females	All
Denmark	124	105	229	1985-1989	63.9	62.2	63.1

OBSERVED AND RELATIVE SURVIVAL (%) BY AGE (number of cases in parentheses)

	AGE CLASS										ALL	
	15-44		45-54		55-64		65-74		75-99			
	obs	rel	obs	rel	obs	rel	obs	rel	obs	rel	obs	rel
Males	(12)		(19)		(28)		(30)		(35)		(124)	
1 year	100	100	100	100	71	73	73	76	60	67	76	79
3 years	100	100	79	81	43	45	53	61	31	45	53	61
5 years	83	84	63	66	43	47	30	38	26	49	42	53
Females	(20)		(11)		(21)		(24)		(29)		(105)	
1 year	100	100	91	91	76	77	83	85	69	74	82	84
3 years	90	90	73	74	71	74	71	77	52	66	70	76
5 years	90	91	73	75	71	76	63	72	48	76	67	78
Overall	(32)		(30)		(49)		(54)		(64)		(229)	
1 year	100	100	97	97	73	75	78	80	64	70	79	82
3 years	94	94	77	78	55	58	61	68	41	55	61	68
5 years	88	88	67	69	55	60	44	54	36	62	53	65

SALIVARY GLANDS (ICD-9 142)

ENGLAND

AREA	NUMBER OF CASES			PERIOD	MEAN AGE			5-YR RELATIVE SURVIVAL (%)	
	Males	Females	All		Males	Females	All	Males	Females
East Anglia	30	28	58	1985-1989	70.3	62.6	66.6		
Mersey	30	38	68	1985-1989	64.8	63.7	64.2		
Oxford	45	37	82	1985-1989	63.9	59.9	62.1		
South Thames	100	105	205	1985-1989	62.1	69.3	65.8		
Wessex	59	49	108	1985-1989	67.8	64.8	66.4		
West Midlands	75	70	145	1985-1989	61.7	63.9	62.8		
Yorkshire	54	44	98	1985-1989	63.5	68.8	65.9		
English Registries	393	371	764		64.1	65.6	64.8		

OBSERVED AND RELATIVE SURVIVAL (%) BY AGE (number of cases in parentheses)

	AGE CLASS										ALL	
	15-44		45-54		55-64		65-74		75-99			
	obs	rel	obs	rel	obs	rel	obs	rel	obs	rel	obs	rel
Males	(48)		(58)		(67)		(109)		(111)		(393)	
1 year	92	92	86	87	84	85	75	78	52	59	74	78
3 years	83	84	62	63	63	66	46	52	26	39	50	58
5 years	83	84	57	59	55	60	36	46	19	37	43	55
Females	(50)		(35)		(67)		(94)		(125)		(371)	
1 year	96	96	91	91	81	81	80	81	58	64	76	79
3 years	86	86	76	77	69	71	63	67	41	56	61	69
5 years	86	86	70	72	64	67	53	60	30	52	53	65
Overall	(98)		(93)		(134)		(203)		(236)		(764)	
1 year	94	94	88	88	82	83	77	80	56	62	75	78
3 years	85	85	67	68	66	68	54	60	34	48	55	63
5 years	85	85	62	64	60	64	44	53	25	46	48	60

ESTONIA

AREA	NUMBER OF CASES			PERIOD	MEAN AGE		
	Males	Females	All		Males	Females	All
Estonia	21	31	52	1985-1989	58.5	63.0	61.2

OBSERVED AND RELATIVE SURVIVAL (%) BY AGE (number of cases in parentheses)

	AGE CLASS										ALL	
	15-44		45-54		55-64		65-74		75-99			
	obs	rel	obs	rel	obs	rel	obs	rel	obs	rel	obs	rel
Males	(5)		(3)		(4)		(5)		(4)		(21)	
1 year	60	60	67	68	100	100	60	63	0	0	57	60
3 years	60	61	33	35	25	28	0	0	0	0	24	27
5 years	60	61	33	36	25	30	0	0	0	0	24	30
Females	(6)		(4)		(4)		(10)		(7)		(31)	
1 year	83	83	75	75	50	50	70	73	29	32	61	64
3 years	67	67	75	76	50	52	40	45	29	42	48	55
5 years	67	67	75	77	50	53	30	38	0	0	39	48
Overall	(11)		(7)		(8)		(15)		(11)		(52)	
1 year	73	73	71	72	75	77	67	70	18	21	60	62
3 years	64	64	57	59	38	40	27	31	18	27	38	44
5 years	64	65	57	60	38	42	20	26	0	0	33	41

SALIVARY GLANDS (ICD-9 142)

FINLAND

AREA	NUMBER OF CASES			PERIOD	MEAN AGE		
	Males	Females	All		Males	Females	All
Finland	78	99	177	1985-1989	56.4	59.2	58.0

OBSERVED AND RELATIVE SURVIVAL (%) BY AGE (number of cases in parentheses)

	AGE CLASS										ALL	
	15-44		45-54		55-64		65-74		75-99			
	obs	rel	obs	rel	obs	rel	obs	rel	obs	rel	obs	rel
Males	(21)		(11)		(15)		(22)		(9)		(78)	
1 year	100	100	100	100	73	75	64	67	44	49	78	80
3 years	86	86	73	75	60	64	36	42	22	30	58	63
5 years	76	77	64	66	47	52	32	41	11	19	49	57
Females	(22)		(15)		(15)		(24)		(23)		(99)	
1 year	100	100	87	87	100	100	79	81	65	71	85	87
3 years	95	96	87	87	93	95	63	66	35	45	72	77
5 years	91	91	80	81	87	90	54	60	30	48	66	75
Overall	(43)		(26)		(30)		(46)		(32)		(177)	
1 year	100	100	92	93	87	88	72	74	59	65	82	84
3 years	91	91	81	82	77	80	50	55	31	41	66	71
5 years	84	84	73	75	67	72	43	52	25	40	58	67

FRANCE

AREA	NUMBER OF CASES			PERIOD	MEAN AGE			5-YR RELATIVE SURVIVAL (%)	
	Males	Females	All		Males	Females	All	Males	Females
Somme	7	4	11	1985-1989	66.4	54.8	62.3		
Calvados	14	6	20	1985-1989	55.9	58.5	56.8		
Doubs	8	9	17	1985-1989	61.0	60.3	60.7		
French Registries	29	19	48		60.0	58.7	59.5		

OBSERVED AND RELATIVE SURVIVAL (%) BY AGE (number of cases in parentheses)

	AGE CLASS										ALL	
	15-44		45-54		55-64		65-74		75-99			
	obs	rel	obs	rel	obs	rel	obs	rel	obs	rel	obs	rel
Males	(6)		(1)		(6)		(10)		(6)		(29)	
1 year	100	100	100	100	67	68	70	73	100	100	83	86
3 years	100	100	100	100	17	18	60	68	67	87	62	69
5 years	100	100	100	100	17	18	60	75	50	82	57	69
Females	(4)		(4)		(4)		(3)		(4)		(19)	
1 year	100	100	67	67	100	100	100	100	50	59	81	85
3 years	100	100	67	67	100	100	50	53	50	83	74	83
5 years	100	100	67	68	75	78	50	55	0	0	59	71
Overall	(10)		(5)		(10)		(13)		(10)		(48)	
1 year	100	100	75	75	80	81	76	79	80	90	82	86
3 years	100	100	75	76	50	52	57	64	60	85	66	74
5 years	100	100	75	77	40	43	57	70	36	67	58	70

SALIVARY GLANDS (ICD-9 142)

GERMANY

AREA	NUMBER OF CASES			PERIOD	MEAN AGE		
	Males	Females	All		Males	Females	All
Saarland	30	20	50	1985-1989	59.8	67.8	63.1

OBSERVED AND RELATIVE SURVIVAL (%) BY AGE (number of cases in parentheses)

	AGE CLASS										ALL	
	15-44		45-54		55-64		65-74		75-99			
	obs	rel	obs	rel	obs	rel	obs	rel	obs	rel	obs	rel
Males	(3)		(7)		(9)		(6)		(5)		(30)	
1 year	100	100	86	86	67	68	67	70	60	68	73	76
3 years	100	100	71	73	44	47	33	38	40	59	53	59
5 years	100	100	56	58	30	33	33	43	40	84	45	54
Females	(1)		(4)		(3)		(3)		(9)		(20)	
1 year	100	100	100	100	100	100	100	100	44	49	75	79
3 years	100	100	100	100	100	100	100	100	33	44	70	80
5 years	100	100	100	100	100	100	100	100	22	37	65	83
Overall	(4)		(11)		(12)		(9)		(14)		(50)	
1 year	100	100	91	91	75	76	78	81	50	55	74	77
3 years	100	100	82	83	58	61	56	63	36	49	60	68
5 years	100	100	71	73	49	53	56	70	29	52	53	66

ICELAND

AREA	NUMBER OF CASES			PERIOD	MEAN AGE		
	Males	Females	All		Males	Females	All
Iceland	2	0	2	1985-1989	62.0	-	62.0

OBSERVED AND RELATIVE SURVIVAL (%) BY AGE (number of cases in parentheses)

	AGE CLASS										ALL	
	15-44		45-54		55-64		65-74		75-99			
	obs	rel	obs	rel	obs	rel	obs	rel	obs	rel	obs	rel
Males	(0)		(0)		(1)		(1)		(0)		(2)	
1 year	-	-	-	-	100	100	100	100	-	-	100	100
3 years	-	-	-	-	0	0	100	100	-	-	50	52
5 years	-	-	-	-	0	0	100	100	-	-	50	54
Females	(0)		(0)		(0)		(0)		(0)		(0)	
1 year	-	-	-	-	-	-	-	-	-	-	-	-
3 years	-	-	-	-	-	-	-	-	-	-	-	-
5 years	-	-	-	-	-	-	-	-	-	-	-	-
Overall	(0)		(0)		(1)		(1)		(0)		(2)	
1 year	-	-	-	-	100	100	100	100	-	-	100	100
3 years	-	-	-	-	0	0	100	100	-	-	50	52
5 years	-	-	-	-	0	0	100	100	-	-	50	54

SALIVARY GLANDS (ICD-9 142)

ITALY

AREA	NUMBER OF CASES			PERIOD	MEAN AGE			5-YR RELATIVE SURVIVAL (%)	
	Males	Females	All		Males	Females	All	Males	Females
Florence	22	22	44	1985-1989	58.6	59.3	59.0		
Genoa	8	10	18	1986-1988	59.1	66.6	63.3		
Latina	11	5	16	1985-1987	56.1	59.8	57.3		
Modena	7	2	9	1988-1989	64.7	70.0	66.0		
Parma	8	3	11	1985-1987	68.8	75.3	70.6		
Ragusa	8	4	12	1985-1989	72.9	67.5	71.2		
Romagna	7	10	17	1986-1988	67.7	51.9	58.5		
Turin	14	11	25	1985-1987	56.1	68.2	61.5		
Varese	18	16	34	1985-1989	57.8	63.3	60.4		
Italian Registries	103	83	186		60.9	62.6	61.7		

OBSERVED AND RELATIVE SURVIVAL (%) BY AGE (number of cases in parentheses)

	AGE CLASS										ALL	
	15-44		45-54		55-64		65-74		75-99			
	obs	rel	obs	rel	obs	rel	obs	rel	obs	rel	obs	rel
Males	(13)		(14)		(32)		(27)		(17)		(103)	
1 year	100	100	86	86	84	86	67	69	53	59	77	79
3 years	92	93	50	51	63	66	44	50	18	24	52	58
5 years	92	93	50	51	53	58	33	41	18	32	47	55
Females	(11)		(13)		(17)		(22)		(20)		(83)	
1 year	91	91	100	100	94	95	95	97	58	62	86	88
3 years	91	91	62	62	82	84	75	80	42	52	69	74
5 years	91	91	54	55	82	86	65	72	42	61	65	73
Overall	(24)		(27)		(49)		(49)		(37)		(186)	
1 year	96	96	93	93	88	89	79	81	56	61	81	83
3 years	92	92	56	56	69	72	58	63	31	40	60	65
5 years	92	92	52	53	63	68	47	55	31	49	55	63

NETHERLANDS

AREA	NUMBER OF CASES			PERIOD	MEAN AGE		
	Males	Females	All		Males	Females	All
Eindhoven	16	11	27	1985-1989	59.3	66.4	62.2

OBSERVED AND RELATIVE SURVIVAL (%) BY AGE (number of cases in parentheses)

	AGE CLASS										ALL	
	15-44		45-54		55-64		65-74		75-99			
	obs	rel	obs	rel	obs	rel	obs	rel	obs	rel	obs	rel
Males	(4)		(1)		(6)		(3)		(2)		(16)	
1 year	75	75	100	100	100	100	100	100	50	55	88	90
3 years	50	50	100	100	83	88	100	100	50	69	75	81
5 years	50	51	0	0	67	73	33	42	50	90	50	58
Females	(1)		(0)		(3)		(4)		(3)		(11)	
1 year	100	100	-	-	100	100	100	100	100	100	100	100
3 years	0	0	-	-	100	100	75	80	67	89	73	80
5 years	0	0	-	-	67	69	75	83	67	100	64	75
Overall	(5)		(1)		(9)		(7)		(5)		(27)	
1 year	80	80	100	100	100	100	100	100	80	88	93	95
3 years	40	40	100	100	89	93	86	93	60	81	74	81
5 years	40	40	0	0	67	72	57	67	60	100	56	65

SALIVARY GLANDS (ICD-9 142)

POLAND

AREA	NUMBER OF CASES			PERIOD	MEAN AGE			5-YR RELATIVE SURVIVAL (%)	
	Males	Females	All		Males	Females	All	Males	Females
Cracow	13	15	28	1985-1989	54.5	61.5	58.3		
Warsaw	4	3	7	1988-1989	57.0	48.0	53.3		
Polish Registries	17	18	35		55.2	59.4	57.4		

OBSERVED AND RELATIVE SURVIVAL (%) BY AGE (number of cases in parentheses)

	15-44		45-54		55-64		65-74		75-99		ALL	
	obs	rel	obs	rel	obs	rel	obs	rel	obs	rel	obs	rel
Males	(3)		(4)		(8)		(1)		(1)		(17)	
1 year	100	100	0	0	63	64	0	0	0	0	47	48
3 years	67	67	0	0	25	27	0	0	0	0	24	25
5 years	67	68	0	0	25	30	0	0	0	0	24	27
Females	(4)		(4)		(3)		(5)		(2)		(18)	
1 year	75	75	100	100	67	68	13	14	0	0	55	56
3 years	75	75	75	76	33	35	-	-	0	0	43	46
5 years	75	76	75	77	33	37	-	-	0	0	43	49
Overall	(7)		(8)		(11)		(6)		(3)		(35)	
1 year	86	86	50	50	64	65	10	10	0	0	51	52
3 years	71	72	38	38	27	30	-	-	0	0	33	36
5 years	71	73	38	39	27	32	-	-	0	0	33	38

SCOTLAND

AREA	NUMBER OF CASES			PERIOD	MEAN AGE		
	Males	Females	All		Males	Females	All
Scotland	137	122	259	1985-1989	62.6	57.5	60.2

OBSERVED AND RELATIVE SURVIVAL (%) BY AGE (number of cases in parentheses)

	15-44		45-54		55-64		65-74		75-99		ALL	
	obs	rel	obs	rel	obs	rel	obs	rel	obs	rel	obs	rel
Males	(23)		(15)		(29)		(36)		(34)		(137)	
1 year	91	92	80	81	83	84	72	76	53	60	74	77
3 years	91	92	73	75	59	62	47	56	35	53	57	66
5 years	87	88	67	69	52	58	28	37	24	48	46	59
Females	(38)		(16)		(19)		(15)		(34)		(122)	
1 year	100	100	100	100	100	100	93	96	62	68	89	91
3 years	100	100	94	95	100	100	87	95	47	64	83	91
5 years	95	95	94	96	84	90	73	86	32	56	73	86
Overall	(61)		(31)		(48)		(51)		(68)		(259)	
1 year	97	97	90	91	90	91	78	82	57	64	81	84
3 years	97	97	84	85	75	79	59	68	41	59	69	78
5 years	92	93	81	83	65	71	41	53	28	52	59	72

SALIVARY GLANDS (ICD-9 142)

SLOVAKIA

AREA	NUMBER OF CASES			PERIOD	MEAN AGE		
	Males	Females	All		Males	Females	All
Slovakia	94	59	153	1985-1989	62.6	67.0	64.3

OBSERVED AND RELATIVE SURVIVAL (%) BY AGE (number of cases in parentheses)

	AGE CLASS										ALL	
	15-44		45-54		55-64		65-74		75-99			
	obs	rel	obs	rel	obs	rel	obs	rel	obs	rel	obs	rel
Males	(7)		(15)		(33)		(22)		(17)		(94)	
1 year	57	57	40	41	61	62	50	53	59	67	54	57
3 years	43	43	27	28	24	26	32	38	41	62	31	36
5 years	43	44	27	29	19	23	25	35	29	59	25	33
Females	(4)		(7)		(14)		(10)		(24)		(59)	
1 year	100	100	100	100	93	94	90	93	29	32	68	71
3 years	75	75	86	87	50	52	60	67	29	40	49	57
5 years	75	75	86	88	36	38	60	73	17	30	40	52
Overall	(11)		(22)		(47)		(32)		(41)		(153)	
1 year	73	73	59	60	70	72	63	66	41	46	59	62
3 years	55	55	45	47	32	34	41	48	34	49	38	44
5 years	55	56	45	48	24	28	36	49	21	39	31	40

SLOVENIA

AREA	NUMBER OF CASES			PERIOD	MEAN AGE		
	Males	Females	All		Males	Females	All
Slovenia	14	14	28	1985-1989	62.9	67.4	65.2

OBSERVED AND RELATIVE SURVIVAL (%) BY AGE (number of cases in parentheses)

	AGE CLASS										ALL	
	15-44		45-54		55-64		65-74		75-99			
	obs	rel	obs	rel	obs	rel	obs	rel	obs	rel	obs	rel
Males	(0)		(2)		(8)		(2)		(2)		(14)	
1 year	-	-	100	100	75	77	50	53	100	100	79	81
3 years	-	-	100	100	50	54	50	59	50	69	57	64
5 years	-	-	100	100	38	43	0	0	0	0	36	44
Females	(1)		(2)		(2)		(5)		(4)		(14)	
1 year	100	100	50	50	100	100	80	83	50	58	71	75
3 years	100	100	50	51	100	100	60	67	0	0	50	58
5 years	100	100	50	51	100	100	40	49	0	0	43	55
Overall	(1)		(4)		(10)		(7)		(6)		(28)	
1 year	100	100	75	76	80	82	71	74	67	76	75	78
3 years	100	100	75	77	60	64	57	64	17	25	54	61
5 years	100	100	75	78	50	56	29	36	0	0	39	49

SALIVARY GLANDS (ICD-9 142)

SPAIN

AREA	NUMBER OF CASES			PERIOD	MEAN AGE			5-YR RELATIVE SURVIVAL (%)	
	Males	Females	All		Males	Females	All	Males	Females
Basque Country	20	19	39	1986-1988	62.3	67.5	64.9		
Mallorca	1	2	3	1988-1989	52.0	63.0	59.7		
Navarra	10	4	14	1985-1989	67.7	55.3	64.2		
Tarragona	9	9	18	1985-1989	60.2	56.4	58.4		
Spanish Registries	40	34	74		63.0	63.0	63.0		

OBSERVED AND RELATIVE SURVIVAL (%) BY AGE (number of cases in parentheses)

	AGE CLASS										ALL	
	15-44		45-54		55-64		65-74		75-99			
	obs	rel	obs	rel	obs	rel	obs	rel	obs	rel	obs	rel
Males	(4)		(7)		(8)		(11)		(10)		(40)	
1 year	100	100	86	86	88	89	91	94	60	66	83	85
3 years	75	76	43	44	50	52	64	71	20	27	48	53
5 years	75	76	43	44	38	40	54	65	20	34	42	51
Females	(6)		(4)		(5)		(7)		(12)		(34)	
1 year	100	100	100	100	80	80	100	100	83	89	91	94
3 years	67	67	100	100	60	61	86	90	42	52	65	71
5 years	67	67	100	100	60	62	57	63	42	63	58	67
Overall	(10)		(11)		(13)		(18)		(22)		(74)	
1 year	100	100	91	91	85	85	94	97	73	79	86	89
3 years	70	70	64	65	54	55	72	79	32	41	55	61
5 years	70	71	64	65	46	49	55	64	32	51	50	59

SWEDEN

AREA	NUMBER OF CASES			PERIOD	MEAN AGE		
	Males	Females	All		Males	Females	All
South Sweden	39	45	84	1985-1989	65.0	62.9	63.9

OBSERVED AND RELATIVE SURVIVAL (%) BY AGE (number of cases in parentheses)

	AGE CLASS										ALL	
	15-44		45-54		55-64		65-74		75-99			
	obs	rel	obs	rel	obs	rel	obs	rel	obs	rel	obs	rel
Males	(4)		(2)		(10)		(14)		(9)		(39)	
1 year	100	100	100	100	100	100	86	89	56	62	85	88
3 years	100	100	100	100	90	94	71	80	22	31	69	79
5 years	100	100	100	100	90	97	64	79	11	21	64	80
Females	(8)		(6)		(6)		(10)		(15)		(45)	
1 year	100	100	100	100	83	84	90	91	93	100	93	96
3 years	100	100	83	84	67	68	80	84	60	76	76	83
5 years	100	100	83	85	67	70	70	77	47	71	69	80
Overall	(12)		(8)		(16)		(24)		(24)		(84)	
1 year	100	100	100	100	94	95	88	90	79	86	89	92
3 years	100	100	88	88	81	84	75	82	46	60	73	81
5 years	100	100	88	89	81	87	67	78	33	55	67	80

SALIVARY GLANDS (ICD-9 142)

SWITZERLAND

AREA	NUMBER OF CASES			PERIOD	MEAN AGE		
	Males	Females	All		Males	Females	All
Geneva	9	6	15	1985-1989	66.1	70.7	68.0

OBSERVED AND RELATIVE SURVIVAL (%) BY AGE (number of cases in parentheses)

	AGE CLASS										ALL	
	15-44		45-54		55-64		65-74		75-99			
	obs	rel	obs	rel	obs	rel	obs	rel	obs	rel	obs	rel
Males	(0)		(2)		(1)		(5)		(1)		(9)	
1 year	-	-	100	100	0	0	80	83	0	0	67	69
3 years	-	-	100	100	0	0	60	67	0	0	56	62
5 years	-	-	50	52	0	0	60	73	0	0	44	54
Females	(0)		(0)		(2)		(2)		(2)		(6)	
1 year	-	-	-	-	100	100	100	100	50	61	83	89
3 years	-	-	-	-	50	51	100	100	0	0	50	60
5 years	-	-	-	-	50	51	100	100	0	0	50	64
Overall	(0)		(2)		(3)		(7)		(3)		(15)	
1 year	-	-	100	100	67	67	86	88	33	40	73	77
3 years	-	-	100	100	33	34	71	78	0	0	53	61
5 years	-	-	50	52	33	35	71	84	0	0	47	58

SALIVARY GLANDS (ICD-9 142)

EUROPE, 1985-89

Weighted analyses

COUNTRY	% COVERAGE WITH C.R.s	YEARLY NO. OF CASES (Mean No. of cases recorded)			RELATIVE SURVIVAL (%) (Age-standardized)
		Males	Females	All	
AUSTRIA	8	2	2	4	
DENMARK	100	25	21	46	
ENGLAND	50	79	74	153	
ESTONIA	100	4	6	10	
FINLAND	100	16	20	36	
FRANCE	3	6	4	10	
GERMANY	2	6	4	10	
ICELAND	100	1	0	1	
ITALY	10	29	22	51	
NETHERLANDS	6	3	2	5	
POLAND	6	7	6	13	
SCOTLAND	100	27	24	51	
SLOVAKIA	100	19	12	31	
SLOVENIA	100	3	3	6	
SPAIN	10	12	10	22	
SWEDEN	17	8	9	17	
SWITZERLAND	6	2	1	3	

□ 1 year   ■ 5 years

OBSERVED AND RELATIVE SURVIVAL (%) BY AGE

	AGE CLASS										ALL	
	15-44		45-54		55-64		65-74		75-99			
	obs	rel	obs	rel	obs	rel	obs	rel	obs	rel	obs	rel
Males												
1 year	97	97	83	83	75	76	67	70	57	62	75	77
3 years	89	89	65	66	46	49	46	51	32	45	52	59
5 years	89	89	55	56	38	42	38	47	27	51	45	55
Females												
1 year	96	96	94	94	90	91	88	88	54	59	80	83
3 years	87	88	80	81	80	81	77	80	38	51	66	74
5 years	87	87	78	78	75	77	69	75	27	42	60	72
Overall												
1 year	97	97	87	88	82	83	76	78	55	60	77	80
3 years	88	89	72	72	61	63	59	64	35	47	59	65
5 years	88	88	65	66	54	57	52	59	27	47	52	62

AGE STANDARDIZED RELATIVE SURVIVAL(%)

COUNTRY	MALES		FEMALES	
	1-year (95% C.I.)	5-years (95% C.I.)	1-year (95% C.I.)	5-years (95% C.I.)
AUSTRIA	-	-	-	-
DENMARK	79.7 (72.9 - 87.3)	53.3 (43.6 - 65.3)	83.7 (76.5 - 91.5)	77.0 (66.7 - 88.9)
ENGLAND	77.8 (73.6 - 82.2)	53.9 (48.3 - 60.2)	80.5 (76.5 - 84.7)	65.1 (59.5 - 71.2)
ESTONIA	54.2 (41.3 - 71.2)	20.2 (9.8 - 41.6)	59.4 (44.2 - 79.9)	40.6 (27.3 - 60.4)
FINLAND	73.0 (62.1 - 85.7)	46.2 (34.6 - 61.8)	85.8 (78.8 - 93.4)	70.8 (60.8 - 82.5)
FRANCE	86.6 (76.4 - 98.0)	72.3 (54.2 - 96.6)	84.7 (69.6 -103.2)	53.7 (35.6 - 81.1)
GERMANY	75.6 (59.8 - 95.6)	62.3 (39.6 - 98.0)	86.4 (77.5 - 96.4)	83.4 (72.2 - 96.3)
ICELAND	-	-	-	-
ITALY	76.6 (68.1 - 86.2)	51.3 (40.8 - 64.4)	86.8 (79.6 - 94.7)	72.8 (61.9 - 85.7)
NETHERLANDS	84.5 (65.6 -108.7)	56.9 (28.9 -112.0)	-	-
POLAND	28.4 (22.1 - 36.5)	16.4 (8.4 - 32.2)	41.8 (28.9 - 60.4)	-
SCOTLAND	76.5 (69.2 - 84.5)	56.3 (46.5 - 68.1)	90.5 (85.0 - 96.5)	81.7 (71.9 - 93.0)
SLOVAKIA	57.6 (47.1 - 70.4)	39.3 (26.5 - 58.2)	79.1 (71.8 - 87.1)	56.7 (43.7 - 73.5)
SLOVENIA	-	-	78.0 (60.6 -100.3)	54.5 (40.7 - 73.0)
SPAIN	85.3 (74.6 - 97.6)	50.8 (35.5 - 72.5)	93.1 (84.1 -103.0)	68.0 (51.9 - 89.1)
SWEDEN	87.2 (77.1 - 98.5)	73.3 (61.1 - 87.9)	94.6 (86.4 -103.5)	78.5 (64.2 - 95.8)
SWITZERLAND	-	-	-	-
EUROPE, 1985-89	74.9 (69.6 - 80.6)	54.7 (46.4 - 64.5)	82.8 (79.0 - 86.7)	68.8 (63.2 - 75.0)

103

ORAL CAVITY (ICD-9 143-145)

AUSTRIA

AREA	NUMBER OF CASES			PERIOD	MEAN AGE		
	Males	Females	All		Males	Females	All
Tirol	28	14	42	1988-1989	60.7	60.1	60.5

OBSERVED AND RELATIVE SURVIVAL (%) BY AGE (number of cases in parentheses)

	15-44		45-54		55-64		65-74		75-99		ALL	
	obs	rel	obs	rel	obs	rel	obs	rel	obs	rel	obs	rel
Males	(4)		(5)		(10)		(4)		(5)		(28)	
1 year	100	100	80	80	90	91	100	100	60	67	86	88
3 years	50	50	60	61	60	62	50	55	20	29	50	55
5 years	50	51	60	61	50	53	50	60	20	39	46	54
Females	(1)		(4)		(3)		(4)		(2)		(14)	
1 year	100	100	100	100	100	100	100	100	100	100	100	100
3 years	0	0	100	100	67	68	50	52	50	56	64	66
5 years	0	0	75	76	67	68	50	53	50	62	57	60
Overall	(5)		(9)		(13)		(8)		(7)		(42)	
1 year	100	100	89	89	92	93	100	100	71	78	90	93
3 years	40	40	78	79	62	64	50	53	29	38	55	59
5 years	40	40	67	68	54	57	50	56	29	48	50	56

DENMARK

AREA	NUMBER OF CASES			PERIOD	MEAN AGE		
	Males	Females	All		Males	Females	All
Denmark	399	283	682	1985-1989	62.4	67.0	64.3

OBSERVED AND RELATIVE SURVIVAL (%) BY AGE (number of cases in parentheses)

	15-44		45-54		55-64		65-74		75-99		ALL	
	obs	rel	obs	rel	obs	rel	obs	rel	obs	rel	obs	rel
Males	(32)		(74)		(114)		(111)		(68)		(399)	
1 year	84	85	81	82	77	79	74	77	63	71	75	78
3 years	66	66	54	55	45	47	39	44	35	51	45	50
5 years	50	51	45	46	32	36	28	35	24	45	33	40
Females	(20)		(29)		(65)		(75)		(94)		(283)	
1 year	85	85	83	83	78	79	73	75	55	60	70	73
3 years	85	85	72	73	57	59	56	60	31	41	52	58
5 years	80	81	69	71	42	44	48	55	21	35	42	51
Overall	(52)		(103)		(179)		(186)		(162)		(682)	
1 year	85	85	82	82	78	79	74	76	59	65	73	76
3 years	73	74	59	60	49	52	46	51	33	45	48	53
5 years	62	62	51	53	36	39	36	44	22	39	37	45

ORAL CAVITY (ICD-9 143-145)

ENGLAND

AREA	NUMBER OF CASES			PERIOD	MEAN AGE			5-YR RELATIVE SURVIVAL (%)	
	Males	Females	All		Males	Females	All	Males	Females
East Anglia	79	60	139	1985-1989	63.2	69.8	66.1		
Mersey	180	79	259	1985-1989	63.2	65.4	63.9		
Oxford	93	64	157	1985-1989	62.9	65.9	64.1		
South Thames	220	174	394	1985-1989	64.3	70.3	66.9		
Wessex	96	90	186	1985-1989	65.1	69.7	67.3		
West Midlands	245	155	400	1985-1989	62.1	64.8	63.2		
Yorkshire	198	122	320	1985-1989	63.5	68.8	65.5		
English Registries	1111	744	1855		63.4	67.9	65.2		

OBSERVED AND RELATIVE SURVIVAL (%) BY AGE (number of cases in parentheses)

	AGE CLASS										ALL	
	15-44		45-54		55-64		65-74		75-99			
	obs	rel	obs	rel	obs	rel	obs	rel	obs	rel	obs	rel
Males	(75)		(186)		(299)		(336)		(215)		(1111)	
1 year	77	77	78	79	75	77	70	73	56	62	71	73
3 years	56	56	50	51	53	56	45	51	35	49	47	52
5 years	53	54	41	43	45	50	33	41	19	36	36	44
Females	(52)		(62)		(160)		(207)		(263)		(744)	
1 year	88	89	84	84	76	77	75	77	56	62	70	73
3 years	75	75	74	75	59	61	58	63	35	47	53	60
5 years	75	75	69	71	51	53	51	57	26	42	45	55
Overall	(127)		(248)		(459)		(543)		(478)		(1855)	
1 year	82	82	80	80	76	77	72	74	56	62	70	73
3 years	64	64	56	57	55	58	50	55	35	48	49	55
5 years	62	63	48	50	47	51	40	48	23	40	40	49

ESTONIA

AREA	NUMBER OF CASES			PERIOD	MEAN AGE		
	Males	Females	All		Males	Females	All
Estonia	132	21	153	1985-1989	55.2	62.5	56.2

OBSERVED AND RELATIVE SURVIVAL (%) BY AGE (number of cases in parentheses)

	AGE CLASS										ALL	
	15-44		45-54		55-64		65-74		75-99			
	obs	rel	obs	rel	obs	rel	obs	rel	obs	rel	obs	rel
Males	(19)		(46)		(46)		(19)		(2)		(132)	
1 year	58	58	72	73	50	51	26	28	50	56	55	57
3 years	16	16	33	34	22	24	16	19	0	0	23	25
5 years	16	16	26	28	20	23	11	14	0	0	20	23
Females	(1)		(3)		(9)		(4)		(4)		(21)	
1 year	0	0	0	0	56	56	50	52	50	54	43	44
3 years	0	0	0	0	33	34	25	28	25	32	24	26
5 years	0	0	0	0	22	24	25	30	0	0	14	16
Overall	(20)		(49)		(55)		(23)		(6)		(153)	
1 year	55	55	67	68	51	52	30	32	50	55	54	55
3 years	15	15	31	32	24	26	17	20	17	22	24	25
5 years	15	16	24	27	20	23	13	17	0	0	19	22

ORAL CAVITY   (ICD-9 143-145)

FINLAND

AREA	NUMBER OF CASES			PERIOD	MEAN AGE		
	Males	Females	All		Males	Females	All
Finland	133	128	261	1985-1989	60.0	66.0	62.9

OBSERVED AND RELATIVE SURVIVAL (%) BY AGE (number of cases in parentheses)

	AGE CLASS										ALL	
	15-44		45-54		55-64		65-74		75-99			
	obs	rel	obs	rel	obs	rel	obs	rel	obs	rel	obs	rel
Males	(13)		(31)		(39)		(36)		(14)		(133)	
1 year	100	100	81	81	87	89	69	73	57	64	79	81
3 years	77	78	45	46	51	54	47	54	36	52	50	55
5 years	69	70	45	47	36	40	42	54	14	28	41	48
Females	(16)		(17)		(17)		(30)		(48)		(128)	
1 year	94	94	82	83	71	71	63	65	54	59	67	70
3 years	63	63	76	77	65	66	40	43	33	44	48	55
5 years	63	63	76	78	65	68	33	39	25	42	44	54
Overall	(29)		(48)		(56)		(66)		(62)		(261)	
1 year	97	97	81	82	82	83	67	69	55	60	73	76
3 years	69	69	56	57	55	58	44	49	34	46	49	55
5 years	66	66	56	58	45	48	38	46	23	39	42	51

FRANCE

AREA	NUMBER OF CASES			PERIOD	MEAN AGE			5-YR RELATIVE SURVIVAL (%)	
	Males	Females	All		Males	Females	All	Males	Females
Somme	139	25	164	1985-1989	57.8	65.8	59.0		
Calvados	167	18	185	1985-1989	57.2	61.6	57.6		
Doubs	86	18	104	1985-1989	58.9	61.5	59.4		
French Registries	392	61	453		57.8	63.3	58.5		

OBSERVED AND RELATIVE SURVIVAL (%) BY AGE (number of cases in parentheses)

	AGE CLASS										ALL	
	15-44		45-54		55-64		65-74		75-99			
	obs	rel	obs	rel	obs	rel	obs	rel	obs	rel	obs	rel
Males	(37)		(119)		(137)		(72)		(27)		(392)	
1 year	89	89	87	88	78	79	72	75	58	64	79	81
3 years	36	37	66	68	40	42	44	50	34	47	48	51
5 years	33	34	57	60	30	33	31	38	21	38	39	43
Females	(8)		(10)		(12)		(13)		(18)		(61)	
1 year	100	100	68	69	75	75	92	93	58	62	76	78
3 years	63	63	57	58	48	49	84	87	51	65	60	65
5 years	63	63	57	58	48	49	66	72	51	82	56	65
Overall	(45)		(129)		(149)		(85)		(45)		(453)	
1 year	91	91	86	86	78	79	75	78	58	63	79	81
3 years	41	41	66	67	40	42	50	56	41	54	50	53
5 years	39	39	57	60	32	35	37	44	33	55	41	46

ORAL CAVITY (ICD-9 143-145)

GERMANY

AREA	NUMBER OF CASES			PERIOD	MEAN AGE		
	Males	Females	All		Males	Females	All
Saarland	185	33	218	1985-1989	54.8	57.5	55.2

OBSERVED AND RELATIVE SURVIVAL (%) BY AGE (number of cases in parentheses)

	AGE CLASS										ALL	
	15-44		45-54		55-64		65-74		75-99			
	obs	rel	obs	rel	obs	rel	obs	rel	obs	rel	obs	rel
Males	(23)		(72)		(58)		(27)		(5)		(185)	
1 year	91	92	72	73	76	77	81	84	40	44	76	77
3 years	65	66	54	55	55	58	48	54	20	27	54	57
5 years	55	55	44	46	40	44	30	37	0	0	41	45
Females	(6)		(7)		(9)		(6)		(5)		(33)	
1 year	83	83	71	72	67	67	83	85	40	43	70	71
3 years	67	67	57	58	33	34	83	89	20	25	52	54
5 years	50	50	21	22	33	35	83	93	20	31	41	45
Overall	(29)		(79)		(67)		(33)		(10)		(218)	
1 year	90	90	72	73	75	76	82	85	40	43	75	76
3 years	66	66	54	56	52	55	55	61	20	26	54	56
5 years	53	54	42	44	39	43	40	49	10	16	41	45

ICELAND

AREA	NUMBER OF CASES			PERIOD	MEAN AGE		
	Males	Females	All		Males	Females	All
Iceland	8	12	20	1985-1989	64.9	66.8	66.1

OBSERVED AND RELATIVE SURVIVAL (%) BY AGE (number of cases in parentheses)

	AGE CLASS										ALL	
	15-44		45-54		55-64		65-74		75-99			
	obs	rel	obs	rel	obs	rel	obs	rel	obs	rel	obs	rel
Males	(1)		(1)		(1)		(1)		(4)		(8)	
1 year	100	100	100	100	100	100	0	0	100	100	88	94
3 years	100	100	100	100	100	100	0	0	25	38	50	61
5 years	100	100	100	100	100	100	0	0	25	47	50	68
Females	(1)		(1)		(2)		(4)		(4)		(12)	
1 year	100	100	100	100	100	100	100	100	75	83	92	95
3 years	100	100	0	0	50	52	50	53	75	99	58	65
5 years	100	100	0	0	50	53	50	55	75	100	58	70
Overall	(2)		(2)		(3)		(5)		(8)		(20)	
1 year	100	100	100	100	100	100	80	81	88	98	90	95
3 years	100	100	50	50	67	69	40	43	50	70	55	64
5 years	100	100	50	51	67	70	40	45	50	86	55	69

ORAL CAVITY (ICD-9 143-145)

ITALY

AREA	NUMBER OF CASES			PERIOD	MEAN AGE			5-YR RELATIVE SURVIVAL (%)	
	Males	Females	All		Males	Females	All	Males	Females
Florence	97	45	142	1985-1989	62.9	68.9	64.8		
Genoa	48	25	73	1986-1988	62.1	73.8	66.1		
Latina	9	3	12	1985-1987	56.2	68.0	59.3		
Modena	13	7	20	1988-1989	60.9	69.9	64.1		
Parma	27	7	34	1985-1987	63.3	72.3	65.1		
Ragusa	10	4	14	1985-1989	66.8	69.8	67.7		
Romagna	12	5	17	1986-1988	63.8	70.6	65.8		
Turin	70	18	88	1985-1987	60.2	68.1	61.9		
Varese	70	22	92	1985-1989	60.5	62.0	60.9		
Italian Registries	356	136	492		61.8	68.9	63.7		

OBSERVED AND RELATIVE SURVIVAL (%) BY AGE (number of cases in parentheses)

	AGE CLASS										ALL	
	15-44		45-54		55-64		65-74		75-99			
	obs	rel	obs	rel	obs	rel	obs	rel	obs	rel	obs	rel
Males	(17)		(79)		(120)		(94)		(46)		(356)	
1 year	71	71	75	75	79	80	74	77	55	60	73	75
3 years	47	47	48	49	54	57	43	48	27	37	46	50
5 years	47	48	44	46	42	45	31	38	21	34	37	43
Females	(6)		(16)		(31)		(24)		(59)		(136)	
1 year	100	100	88	88	81	81	63	64	51	55	66	69
3 years	50	50	69	69	48	49	46	48	31	40	43	48
5 years	50	50	69	70	45	47	46	51	19	30	37	45
Overall	(23)		(95)		(151)		(118)		(105)		(492)	
1 year	78	78	77	77	79	80	72	74	53	57	71	74
3 years	48	48	52	52	53	55	43	48	29	39	45	50
5 years	48	48	48	50	42	46	34	41	19	32	37	43

NETHERLANDS

AREA	NUMBER OF CASES			PERIOD	MEAN AGE		
	Males	Females	All		Males	Females	All
Eindhoven	36	30	66	1985-1989	58.4	61.1	59.7

OBSERVED AND RELATIVE SURVIVAL (%) BY AGE (number of cases in parentheses)

	AGE CLASS										ALL	
	15-44		45-54		55-64		65-74		75-99			
	obs	rel	obs	rel	obs	rel	obs	rel	obs	rel	obs	rel
Males	(5)		(7)		(13)		(9)		(2)		(36)	
1 year	100	100	100	100	92	94	56	58	50	56	83	85
3 years	60	60	86	87	68	71	22	26	50	68	58	62
5 years	60	61	86	89	68	73	22	29	50	87	58	65
Females	(7)		(2)		(7)		(6)		(8)		(30)	
1 year	86	86	100	100	71	72	83	85	35	38	70	72
3 years	71	72	100	100	43	44	83	89	35	48	59	65
5 years	71	72	100	100	43	44	67	75	17	30	51	60
Overall	(12)		(9)		(20)		(15)		(10)		(66)	
1 year	92	92	100	100	85	86	67	69	38	42	77	79
3 years	66	66	89	90	59	61	47	52	38	52	58	63
5 years	66	67	89	92	59	63	40	49	25	45	55	63

ORAL CAVITY (ICD-9 143-145)

POLAND

AREA	NUMBER OF CASES			PERIOD	MEAN AGE			5-YR RELATIVE SURVIVAL (%)	
	Males	Females	All		Males	Females	All	Males	Females
Cracow	31	10	41	1985-1989	56.4	54.7	56.0		
Warsaw	12	7	19	1988-1989	53.7	65.4	58.1		
Polish Registries	43	17	60		55.7	59.2	56.7		

OBSERVED AND RELATIVE SURVIVAL (%) BY AGE (number of cases in parentheses)

	AGE CLASS										ALL	
	15-44		45-54		55-64		65-74		75-99			
	obs	rel	obs	rel	obs	rel	obs	rel	obs	rel	obs	rel
Males	(3)		(14)		(21)		(4)		(1)		(43)	
1 year	67	67	71	72	62	63	75	79	100	100	67	69
3 years	67	68	43	44	43	46	50	58	0	0	44	47
5 years	67	69	43	46	43	49	25	33	0	0	42	48
Females	(4)		(3)		(5)		(2)		(3)		(17)	
1 year	50	50	100	100	20	20	50	51	33	39	47	49
3 years	50	50	67	68	20	21	0	0	33	51	35	39
5 years	50	51	67	69	20	22	0	0	0	0	29	34
Overall	(7)		(17)		(26)		(6)		(4)		(60)	
1 year	57	57	76	77	54	55	67	69	50	58	62	63
3 years	57	58	47	49	38	41	33	38	25	38	42	45
5 years	57	58	47	50	38	44	17	21	0	0	38	44

SCOTLAND

AREA	NUMBER OF CASES			PERIOD	MEAN AGE		
	Males	Females	All		Males	Females	All
Scotland	405	254	659	1985-1989	62.6	67.4	64.4

OBSERVED AND RELATIVE SURVIVAL (%) BY AGE (number of cases in parentheses)

	AGE CLASS										ALL	
	15-44		45-54		55-64		65-74		75-99			
	obs	rel	obs	rel	obs	rel	obs	rel	obs	rel	obs	rel
Males	(25)		(80)		(115)		(111)		(74)		(405)	
1 year	80	80	80	81	78	80	77	80	55	63	74	77
3 years	56	56	64	65	53	57	45	52	26	37	48	55
5 years	56	57	51	53	34	38	35	46	20	40	37	45
Females	(14)		(28)		(55)		(76)		(81)		(254)	
1 year	71	72	93	93	75	75	79	81	56	61	72	75
3 years	71	72	82	83	53	55	54	59	31	42	50	57
5 years	71	72	68	69	45	49	39	47	26	44	41	52
Overall	(39)		(108)		(170)		(187)		(155)		(659)	
1 year	77	77	83	84	77	78	78	81	55	62	73	76
3 years	62	62	69	70	53	56	49	55	28	40	49	56
5 years	62	62	56	58	38	42	37	46	23	42	38	48

ORAL CAVITY (ICD-9 143-145)

SLOVAKIA

AREA	NUMBER OF CASES			PERIOD	MEAN AGE		
	Males	Females	All		Males	Females	All
Slovakia	627	51	678	1985-1989	54.7	59.8	55.1

OBSERVED AND RELATIVE SURVIVAL (%) BY AGE (number of cases in parentheses)

	AGE CLASS										ALL	
	15-44		45-54		55-64		65-74		75-99			
	obs	rel	obs	rel	obs	rel	obs	rel	obs	rel	obs	rel
Males	(99)		(207)		(225)		(78)		(18)		(627)	
1 year	68	68	63	64	53	55	50	53	39	44	58	59
3 years	41	42	26	27	22	24	28	33	22	32	27	29
5 years	31	32	22	24	18	21	21	29	7	14	21	24
Females	(8)		(8)		(14)		(11)		(10)		(51)	
1 year	100	100	63	63	64	65	82	84	40	44	69	71
3 years	88	88	50	51	50	52	64	70	10	14	51	56
5 years	88	88	50	51	50	53	64	75	10	18	51	60
Overall	(107)		(215)		(239)		(89)		(28)		(678)	
1 year	70	70	63	64	54	55	54	57	39	44	59	60
3 years	45	46	27	28	24	26	33	38	18	25	29	31
5 years	35	36	23	25	20	23	27	36	9	17	24	27

SLOVENIA

AREA	NUMBER OF CASES			PERIOD	MEAN AGE		
	Males	Females	All		Males	Females	All
Slovenia	281	30	311	1985-1989	56.8	57.3	56.8

OBSERVED AND RELATIVE SURVIVAL (%) BY AGE (number of cases in parentheses)

	AGE CLASS										ALL	
	15-44		45-54		55-64		65-74		75-99			
	obs	rel	obs	rel	obs	rel	obs	rel	obs	rel	obs	rel
Males	(20)		(93)		(120)		(38)		(10)		(281)	
1 year	75	75	63	64	57	58	63	66	50	55	61	62
3 years	50	51	41	42	28	29	37	43	40	54	35	38
5 years	45	46	33	35	16	18	26	34	40	70	26	29
Females	(2)		(8)		(13)		(6)		(1)		(30)	
1 year	50	50	75	75	85	85	67	68	0	0	73	74
3 years	50	50	38	38	54	55	50	54	0	0	47	49
5 years	50	50	38	38	38	40	50	58	0	0	40	43
Overall	(22)		(101)		(133)		(44)		(11)		(311)	
1 year	73	73	64	65	59	61	64	66	45	50	62	63
3 years	50	51	41	42	30	32	39	44	36	50	36	39
5 years	45	46	34	35	18	20	30	38	36	64	27	31

ORAL CAVITY   (ICD-9 143-145)

SPAIN

AREA	NUMBER OF CASES			PERIOD	MEAN AGE			5-YR RELATIVE SURVIVAL (%)	
	Males	Females	All		Males	Females	All	Males	Females
Basque Country	185	38	223	1986-1988	58.1	67.0	59.6		
Mallorca	31	6	37	1988-1989	58.0	74.3	60.6		
Navarra	64	6	70	1985-1989	59.3	65.3	59.9		
Tarragona	49	7	56	1985-1989	63.0	55.7	62.1		
Spanish Registries	329	57	386		59.1	66.3	60.1		

OBSERVED AND RELATIVE SURVIVAL (%) BY AGE (number of cases in parentheses)

	AGE CLASS										ALL	
	15-44		45-54		55-64		65-74		75-99			
	obs	rel	obs	rel	obs	rel	obs	rel	obs	rel	obs	rel
Males	(32)		(68)		(126)		(76)		(27)		(329)	
1 year	75	75	82	83	75	76	68	71	44	49	72	74
3 years	47	47	57	58	44	45	43	48	33	45	46	49
5 years	42	43	50	52	33	36	36	42	30	50	38	42
Females	(6)		(6)		(8)		(19)		(18)		(57)	
1 year	83	83	83	84	75	75	84	85	56	61	74	76
3 years	83	84	50	50	50	51	58	61	22	29	47	52
5 years	83	84	50	51	50	51	50	54	-	-	44	52
Overall	(38)		(74)		(134)		(95)		(45)		(386)	
1 year	76	76	82	83	75	76	72	74	49	54	73	74
3 years	53	53	57	58	44	46	46	51	29	39	46	49
5 years	48	49	50	52	34	37	38	45	26	44	39	44

SWEDEN

AREA	NUMBER OF CASES			PERIOD	MEAN AGE		
	Males	Females	All		Males	Females	All
South Sweden	96	61	157	1985-1989	62.9	69.5	65.5

OBSERVED AND RELATIVE SURVIVAL (%) BY AGE (number of cases in parentheses)

	AGE CLASS										ALL	
	15-44		45-54		55-64		65-74		75-99			
	obs	rel	obs	rel	obs	rel	obs	rel	obs	rel	obs	rel
Males	(9)		(12)		(29)		(31)		(15)		(96)	
1 year	89	89	100	100	93	94	65	67	40	46	76	79
3 years	78	78	75	76	76	79	45	50	27	41	58	65
5 years	67	67	67	69	76	82	42	50	13	28	53	63
Females	(3)		(3)		(12)		(17)		(26)		(61)	
1 year	100	100	100	100	100	100	94	96	62	66	82	85
3 years	100	100	100	100	83	85	88	93	46	59	70	79
5 years	100	100	100	100	58	60	76	85	31	48	56	68
Overall	(12)		(15)		(41)		(48)		(41)		(157)	
1 year	92	92	100	100	95	96	75	77	54	59	78	81
3 years	83	84	80	81	78	81	60	66	39	53	63	70
5 years	75	76	73	76	71	75	54	63	24	42	54	65

ORAL CAVITY (ICD-9 143-145)

SWITZERLAND

AREA	NUMBER OF CASES			PERIOD	MEAN AGE			5-YR RELATIVE SURVIVAL (%)	
	Males	Females	All		Males	Females	All	Males	Females
Basel	23	12	35	1985-1988	51.1	66.4	56.4		
Geneva	41	22	63	1985-1989	57.2	63.1	59.3		
Swiss Registries	64	34	98		55.0	64.4	58.3		

OBSERVED AND RELATIVE SURVIVAL (%) BY AGE (number of cases in parentheses)

	AGE CLASS										ALL	
	15-44		45-54		55-64		65-74		75-99			
	obs	rel	obs	rel	obs	rel	obs	rel	obs	rel	obs	rel
Males	(9)		(27)		(15)		(9)		(4)		(64)	
1 year	100	100	78	78	87	88	67	69	75	82	81	82
3 years	56	56	48	49	53	56	44	49	50	66	50	52
5 years	56	56	37	38	47	51	30	36	50	82	42	46
Females	(2)		(8)		(10)		(3)		(11)		(34)	
1 year	100	100	75	75	90	90	67	68	36	40	68	70
3 years	50	50	38	38	80	81	67	70	36	48	53	58
5 years	50	50	38	38	80	82	67	72	18	31	47	56
Overall	(11)		(35)		(25)		(12)		(15)		(98)	
1 year	100	100	77	77	88	89	67	69	47	51	77	78
3 years	55	55	46	46	64	66	50	55	40	53	51	54
5 years	55	55	37	38	60	64	40	47	27	45	44	49

ORAL CAVITY (ICD-9 143-145)

EUROPE, 1985-89

Weighted analyses

COUNTRY	% COVERAGE WITH C.R.s	Males	Females	All
AUSTRIA	8	14	7	21
DENMARK	100	80	57	137
ENGLAND	50	222	149	371
ESTONIA	100	26	4	30
FINLAND	100	27	26	53
FRANCE	3	78	12	90
GERMANY	2	37	7	44
ICELAND	100	2	3	5
ITALY	10	97	37	134
NETHERLANDS	6	7	6	13
POLAND	6	18	9	27
SCOTLAND	100	81	51	132
SLOVAKIA	100	125	10	135
SLOVENIA	100	56	6	62
SPAIN	10	100	18	118
SWEDEN	17	19	12	31
SWITZERLAND	11	14	7	21

YEARLY NO. OF CASES (Mean No. of cases recorded)

RELATIVE SURVIVAL (%) (Age-standardized)

□ 1 year ■ 5 years

OBSERVED AND RELATIVE SURVIVAL (%) BY AGE

	15-44 obs	15-44 rel	45-54 obs	45-54 rel	55-64 obs	55-64 rel	65-74 obs	65-74 rel	75-99 obs	75-99 rel	ALL obs	ALL rel
Males												
1 year	84	85	80	80	77	78	74	77	52	57	76	77
3 years	51	51	57	59	48	51	45	50	28	39	49	52
5 years	46	46	50	52	37	41	31	39	16	29	39	44
Females												
1 year	89	89	82	82	73	74	78	80	51	56	71	73
3 years	63	63	67	67	48	50	63	67	34	44	52	57
5 years	60	61	58	59	45	47	56	63	27	42	45	53
Overall												
1 year	85	86	80	81	76	77	75	77	52	57	75	76
3 years	53	54	59	60	48	50	48	54	30	40	49	53
5 years	49	49	51	53	39	42	37	44	19	32	40	46

AGE STANDARDIZED RELATIVE SURVIVAL(%)

COUNTRY	MALES 1-year (95% C.I.)	MALES 5-years (95% C.I.)	FEMALES 1-year (95% C.I.)	FEMALES 5-years (95% C.I.)
AUSTRIA	87.5 (75.8 -100.9)	53.6 (34.8 - 82.5)	100.0 (100.0 -100.0)	59.2 (37.6 - 93.3)
DENMARK	78.0 (73.7 - 82.5)	40.9 (35.4 - 47.2)	76.1 (71.0 - 81.6)	53.7 (47.5 - 60.8)
ENGLAND	73.6 (70.9 - 76.4)	44.1 (40.8 - 47.7)	76.5 (73.3 - 80.0)	57.8 (53.7 - 62.3)
ESTONIA	51.6 (37.9 - 70.2)	17.3 (11.7 - 25.5)	38.3 (23.9 - 61.4)	14.1 (4.9 - 40.5)
FINLAND	79.9 (72.6 - 88.0)	44.9 (35.7 - 56.6)	71.8 (63.4 - 81.4)	57.7 (48.3 - 68.8)
FRANCE	78.1 (73.0 - 83.5)	40.9 (34.2 - 48.9)	78.0 (67.7 - 89.9)	63.6 (50.2 - 80.6)
GERMANY	73.2 (63.8 - 84.0)	35.8 (29.0 - 44.4)	69.3 (55.0 - 87.2)	46.7 (32.0 - 68.1)
ICELAND	76.3 (76.1 - 76.5)	66.8 (53.7 - 83.0)	96.9 (88.8 -105.8)	55.4 (33.6 - 91.2)
ITALY	74.0 (69.1 - 79.2)	41.8 (36.1 - 48.5)	75.3 (68.2 - 83.1)	49.6 (40.6 - 60.6)
NETHERLANDS	80.1 (65.1 - 98.6)	67.3 (46.0 - 98.5)	75.8 (62.9 - 91.3)	62.7 (47.2 - 83.4)
POLAND	75.7 (63.0 - 91.1)	37.5 (24.0 - 58.7)	49.6 (31.2 - 79.0)	24.6 (12.7 - 47.6)
SCOTLAND	77.0 (72.7 - 81.5)	45.0 (39.5 - 51.2)	77.5 (72.3 - 83.1)	53.8 (47.0 - 61.5)
SLOVAKIA	55.2 (49.6 - 61.4)	23.1 (17.7 - 30.1)	68.4 (56.5 - 82.7)	54.8 (41.7 - 71.9)
SLOVENIA	62.1 (54.4 - 70.7)	37.1 (27.5 - 50.0)	60.7 (48.3 - 76.2)	37.7 (24.3 - 58.3)
SPAIN	71.0 (65.7 - 76.8)	43.8 (37.0 - 51.8)	77.4 (65.9 - 91.0)	-
SWEDEN	79.6 (72.6 - 87.4)	60.7 (50.3 - 73.2)	92.9 (88.5 - 97.5)	75.4 (65.0 - 87.4)
SWITZERLAND	81.3 (69.5 - 95.1)	50.6 (34.4 - 74.4)	73.6 (59.0 - 91.7)	58.9 (42.4 - 82.0)
EUROPE, 1985-89	75.0 (71.8 - 78.3)	40.8 (37.2 - 44.9)	74.9 (70.9 - 79.1)	53.7 (48.7 - 59.1)

OROPHARYNX   (ICD-9 146)

AUSTRIA

AREA	NUMBER OF CASES			PERIOD	MEAN AGE		
	Males	Females	All		Males	Females	All
Tirol	8	4	12	1988-1989	64.3	64.5	64.4

OBSERVED AND RELATIVE SURVIVAL (%) BY AGE (number of cases in parentheses)

	AGE CLASS										ALL	
	15-44		45-54		55-64		65-74		75-99			
	obs	rel	obs	rel	obs	rel	obs	rel	obs	rel	obs	rel
Males	(0)		(2)		(2)		(2)		(2)		(8)	
1 year	-	-	0	0	0	0	50	51	100	100	38	39
3 years	-	-	0	0	0	0	50	54	100	100	38	41
5 years	-	-	0	0	0	0	0	0	50	77	13	15
Females	(1)		(0)		(1)		(0)		(2)		(4)	
1 year	100	100	-	-	100	100	-	-	0	0	50	51
3 years	100	100	-	-	0	0	-	-	0	0	25	27
5 years	0	0	-	-	0	0	-	-	0	0	0	0
Overall	(1)		(2)		(3)		(2)		(4)		(12)	
1 year	100	100	0	0	33	34	50	51	50	53	42	43
3 years	100	100	0	0	0	0	50	54	50	59	33	36
5 years	0	0	0	0	0	0	0	0	25	34	8	10

DENMARK

AREA	NUMBER OF CASES			PERIOD	MEAN AGE		
	Males	Females	All		Males	Females	All
Denmark	255	105	360	1985-1989	60.4	63.0	61.2

OBSERVED AND RELATIVE SURVIVAL (%) BY AGE (number of cases in parentheses)

	AGE CLASS										ALL	
	15-44		45-54		55-64		65-74		75-99			
	obs	rel	obs	rel	obs	rel	obs	rel	obs	rel	obs	rel
Males	(25)		(60)		(71)		(67)		(32)		(255)	
1 year	80	80	78	79	51	52	48	50	56	62	60	62
3 years	56	57	45	46	30	31	28	32	31	43	36	39
5 years	44	45	37	38	25	28	25	32	13	22	28	33
Females	(6)		(23)		(29)		(26)		(21)		(105)	
1 year	50	50	83	83	76	77	77	79	48	51	70	72
3 years	50	50	61	62	62	64	54	58	19	24	50	54
5 years	33	34	48	49	62	66	46	53	14	22	44	50
Overall	(31)		(83)		(100)		(93)		(53)		(360)	
1 year	74	74	80	80	58	59	56	58	53	58	63	65
3 years	55	55	49	50	39	41	35	40	26	35	40	44
5 years	42	43	40	41	36	39	31	38	13	22	33	38

OROPHARYNX (ICD-9 146)

ENGLAND

AREA	NUMBER OF CASES			PERIOD	MEAN AGE			5-YR RELATIVE SURVIVAL (%)	
	Males	Females	All		Males	Females	All	Males	Females
East Anglia	38	21	59	1985-1989	65.5	68.0	66.4		
Mersey	77	25	102	1985-1989	59.7	65.2	61.1		
Oxford	45	22	67	1985-1989	62.5	64.3	63.1		
South Thames	131	58	189	1985-1989	63.2	63.8	63.4		
Wessex	38	24	62	1985-1989	63.7	67.8	65.3		
West Midlands	119	48	167	1985-1989	62.0	67.6	63.6		
Yorkshire	65	24	89	1985-1989	58.8	66.2	60.8		
English Registries	513	222	735		62.0	65.9	63.2		

OBSERVED AND RELATIVE SURVIVAL (%) BY AGE (number of cases in parentheses)

	AGE CLASS										ALL	
	15-44		45-54		55-64		65-74		75-99			
	obs	rel	obs	rel	obs	rel	obs	rel	obs	rel	obs	rel
Males	(42)		(93)		(160)		(147)		(71)		(513)	
1 year	90	91	72	72	61	62	62	64	54	60	65	67
3 years	74	74	41	42	34	36	33	38	31	45	38	42
5 years	62	62	35	37	24	26	24	30	24	45	29	34
Females	(15)		(27)		(48)		(77)		(55)		(222)	
1 year	93	93	81	82	79	80	62	64	40	44	65	67
3 years	80	80	59	60	46	47	38	40	18	24	40	44
5 years	80	81	48	49	35	37	32	37	11	18	33	39
Overall	(57)		(120)		(208)		(224)		(126)		(735)	
1 year	91	91	74	75	65	66	62	64	48	53	65	67
3 years	75	76	45	46	37	38	35	39	25	35	39	43
5 years	66	67	38	40	26	29	27	32	18	32	30	36

ESTONIA

AREA	NUMBER OF CASES			PERIOD	MEAN AGE		
	Males	Females	All		Males	Females	All
Estonia	107	13	120	1985-1989	55.5	59.1	55.9

OBSERVED AND RELATIVE SURVIVAL (%) BY AGE (number of cases in parentheses)

	AGE CLASS										ALL	
	15-44		45-54		55-64		65-74		75-99			
	obs	rel	obs	rel	obs	rel	obs	rel	obs	rel	obs	rel
Males	(12)		(43)		(34)		(14)		(4)		(107)	
1 year	33	34	58	59	32	33	50	52	0	0	44	45
3 years	0	0	19	19	21	22	21	25	0	0	17	18
5 years	0	0	9	10	18	21	21	28	0	0	12	14
Females	(1)		(4)		(6)		(1)		(1)		(13)	
1 year	0	0	100	100	67	67	100	100	0	0	69	70
3 years	0	0	25	25	50	52	0	0	0	0	31	32
5 years	0	0	0	0	33	36	0	0	0	0	15	17
Overall	(13)		(47)		(40)		(15)		(5)		(120)	
1 year	31	31	62	62	38	38	53	56	0	0	47	48
3 years	0	0	19	20	25	27	20	23	0	0	18	20
5 years	0	0	9	9	20	23	20	27	0	0	13	14

OROPHARYNX (ICD-9 146)

FINLAND

AREA	NUMBER OF CASES			PERIOD	MEAN AGE		
	Males	Females	All		Males	Females	All
Finland	58	16	74	1985-1989	61.2	65.6	62.1

OBSERVED AND RELATIVE SURVIVAL (%) BY AGE (number of cases in parentheses)

	AGE CLASS										ALL	
	15-44		45-54		55-64		65-74		75-99			
	obs	rel	obs	rel	obs	rel	obs	rel	obs	rel	obs	rel
Males	(5)		(8)		(29)		(5)		(11)		(58)	
1 year	60	60	75	76	79	81	40	42	55	61	69	71
3 years	40	40	25	26	34	36	20	23	18	26	29	32
5 years	40	41	25	26	24	27	20	26	9	17	22	27
Females	(2)		(0)		(2)		(8)		(4)		(16)	
1 year	100	100	-	-	0	0	50	51	50	54	50	52
3 years	100	100	-	-	0	0	38	40	25	33	38	41
5 years	100	100	-	-	0	0	13	14	25	40	25	29
Overall	(7)		(8)		(31)		(13)		(15)		(74)	
1 year	71	72	75	76	74	75	46	47	53	59	65	67
3 years	57	58	25	26	32	34	31	34	20	28	31	34
5 years	57	58	25	26	23	25	15	18	13	24	23	27

FRANCE

AREA	NUMBER OF CASES			PERIOD	MEAN AGE			5-YR RELATIVE SURVIVAL (%)	
	Males	Females	All		Males	Females	All	Males	Females
Somme	206	15	221	1985-1989	56.8	58.5	57.0		
Calvados	196	17	213	1985-1989	58.9	59.5	58.9		
Doubs	140	8	148	1985-1989	59.3	65.9	59.7		
French Registries	542	40	582		58.2	60.5	58.4		

OBSERVED AND RELATIVE SURVIVAL (%) BY AGE (number of cases in parentheses)

	AGE CLASS										ALL	
	15-44		45-54		55-64		65-74		75-99			
	obs	rel	obs	rel	obs	rel	obs	rel	obs	rel	obs	rel
Males	(50)		(148)		(209)		(84)		(51)		(542)	
1 year	81	81	76	76	73	74	69	71	39	42	70	72
3 years	59	59	37	38	39	41	35	40	15	20	38	40
5 years	51	52	32	33	25	27	25	31	12	20	28	32
Females	(4)		(10)		(11)		(10)		(5)		(40)	
1 year	50	50	70	70	73	73	90	91	26	28	69	70
3 years	50	50	30	30	45	46	80	84	-	-	48	50
5 years	50	50	20	20	45	47	68	75	-	-	42	45
Overall	(54)		(158)		(220)		(94)		(56)		(582)	
1 year	79	79	75	76	73	74	71	73	38	41	70	72
3 years	58	59	36	37	39	41	41	45	15	19	38	41
5 years	51	52	31	32	26	29	30	36	12	20	29	33

OROPHARYNX

(ICD-9 146)

GERMANY

AREA	NUMBER OF CASES			PERIOD	MEAN AGE		
	Males	Females	All		Males	Females	All
Saarland	93	23	116	1985-1989	55.3	64.7	57.2

OBSERVED AND RELATIVE SURVIVAL (%) BY AGE (number of cases in parentheses)

	AGE CLASS										ALL	
	15-44		45-54		55-64		65-74		75-99			
	obs	rel	obs	rel	obs	rel	obs	rel	obs	rel	obs	rel
Males	(18)		(27)		(25)		(16)		(7)		(93)	
1 year	83	84	70	71	76	77	44	45	86	96	71	72
3 years	44	45	48	49	48	51	13	14	29	40	40	42
5 years	35	35	33	34	34	38	-	-	29	54	28	32
Females	(0)		(6)		(4)		(7)		(6)		(23)	
1 year	-	-	67	67	75	76	71	73	50	56	65	68
3 years	-	-	33	34	50	51	57	61	17	23	39	43
5 years	-	-	33	34	50	52	57	64	17	29	39	46
Overall	(18)		(33)		(29)		(23)		(13)		(116)	
1 year	83	84	70	70	76	77	52	54	69	77	70	71
3 years	44	45	45	46	48	51	26	29	23	32	40	43
5 years	35	35	33	34	36	39	21	26	23	42	31	35

ICELAND

AREA	NUMBER OF CASES			PERIOD	MEAN AGE		
	Males	Females	All		Males	Females	All
Iceland	2	1	3	1985-1989	71.0	82.0	75.0

OBSERVED AND RELATIVE SURVIVAL (%) BY AGE (number of cases in parentheses)

	AGE CLASS										ALL	
	15-44		45-54		55-64		65-74		75-99			
	obs	rel	obs	rel	obs	rel	obs	rel	obs	rel	obs	rel
Males	(0)		(0)		(1)		(0)		(1)		(2)	
1 year	-	-	-	-	100	100	-	-	100	100	100	100
3 years	-	-	-	-	0	0	-	-	100	100	50	57
5 years	-	-	-	-	0	0	-	-	100	100	50	64
Females	(0)		(0)		(0)		(0)		(1)		(1)	
1 year	-	-	-	-	-	-	-	-	100	100	100	100
3 years	-	-	-	-	-	-	-	-	100	100	100	100
5 years	-	-	-	-	-	-	-	-	100	100	100	100
Overall	(0)		(0)		(1)		(0)		(2)		(3)	
1 year	-	-	-	-	100	100	-	-	100	100	100	100
3 years	-	-	-	-	0	0	-	-	100	100	67	79
5 years	-	-	-	-	0	0	-	-	100	100	67	92

OROPHARYNX $\qquad$ (ICD-9 146)

ITALY

AREA	NUMBER OF CASES			PERIOD	MEAN AGE			5-YR RELATIVE SURVIVAL (%)	
	Males	Females	All		Males	Females	All	Males	Females
Florence	47	25	72	1985-1989	63.0	65.1	63.7		
Genoa	30	9	39	1986-1988	57.7	61.9	58.7		
Latina	9	1	10	1985-1987	59.0	64.0	59.6		
Modena	11	3	14	1988-1989	66.3	61.0	65.2		
Parma	14	3	17	1985-1987	60.1	66.7	61.4		
Ragusa	3	0	3	1985-1989	53.7	-	53.7		
Romagna	8	1	9	1986-1988	64.3	73.0	65.3		
Turin	54	18	72	1985-1987	63.1	63.7	63.3		
Varese	93	15	108	1985-1989	60.6	63.3	61.0		
Italian Registries	269	75	344		61.4	64.1	62.0		

OBSERVED AND RELATIVE SURVIVAL (%) BY AGE (number of cases in parentheses)

	AGE CLASS										ALL	
	15-44		45-54		55-64		65-74		75-99			
	obs	rel	obs	rel	obs	rel	obs	rel	obs	rel	obs	rel
Males	(14)		(50)		(100)		(78)		(27)		(269)	
1 year	71	72	70	70	64	65	68	70	52	56	65	67
3 years	50	50	36	37	32	34	35	39	33	43	35	38
5 years	50	51	30	31	22	24	23	28	19	29	25	29
Females	(5)		(11)		(20)		(25)		(14)		(75)	
1 year	80	80	73	73	80	81	72	73	57	61	72	73
3 years	20	20	55	55	55	56	52	55	29	35	47	50
5 years	20	20	45	46	45	47	48	54	14	20	39	43
Overall	(19)		(61)		(120)		(103)		(41)		(344)	
1 year	74	74	70	71	66	67	69	71	54	58	67	68
3 years	42	42	39	40	36	38	39	43	32	40	37	40
5 years	42	43	33	34	26	28	29	35	17	26	28	32

NETHERLANDS

AREA	NUMBER OF CASES			PERIOD	MEAN AGE		
	Males	Females	All		Males	Females	All
Eindhoven	20	6	26	1985-1989	58.1	59.2	58.4

OBSERVED AND RELATIVE SURVIVAL (%) BY AGE (number of cases in parentheses)

	AGE CLASS										ALL	
	15-44		45-54		55-64		65-74		75-99			
	obs	rel	obs	rel	obs	rel	obs	rel	obs	rel	obs	rel
Males	(1)		(7)		(6)		(4)		(2)		(20)	
1 year	100	100	85	85	50	51	75	78	50	54	70	71
3 years	0	0	68	69	17	17	50	57	50	67	43	46
5 years	0	0	68	70	17	18	25	31	0	0	32	36
Females	(0)		(2)		(2)		(2)		(0)		(6)	
1 year	-	-	50	50	50	50	100	100	-	-	67	67
3 years	-	-	50	50	50	51	100	100	-	-	67	69
5 years	-	-	0	0	50	51	50	56	-	-	33	35
Overall	(1)		(9)		(8)		(6)		(2)		(26)	
1 year	100	100	76	77	50	51	83	86	50	54	69	70
3 years	0	0	64	65	25	26	67	74	50	67	49	52
5 years	0	0	51	52	25	26	33	40	0	0	32	36

OROPHARYNX   (ICD-9 146)

POLAND

AREA	NUMBER OF CASES			PERIOD	MEAN AGE			5-YR RELATIVE SURVIVAL (%)	
	Males	Females	All		Males	Females	All	Males	Females
Cracow	37	7	44	1985-1989	58.4	46.3	56.5		
Warsaw	43	14	57	1988-1989	58.0	60.4	58.6		
Polish Registries	80	21	101		58.2	55.8	57.7		

OBSERVED AND RELATIVE SURVIVAL (%) BY AGE (number of cases in parentheses)

	AGE CLASS										ALL	
	15-44		45-54		55-64		65-74		75-99			
	obs	rel	obs	rel	obs	rel	obs	rel	obs	rel	obs	rel
Males	(6)		(21)		(32)		(17)		(4)		(80)	
1 year	33	33	29	29	50	51	65	68	75	83	48	49
3 years	33	34	14	15	22	24	20	23	0	0	19	21
5 years	33	34	14	15	19	22	7	9	0	0	15	18
Females	(6)		(4)		(6)		(2)		(3)		(21)	
1 year	67	67	100	100	67	67	50	51	33	36	67	68
3 years	67	67	50	51	50	52	50	54	0	0	48	50
5 years	67	67	50	52	33	36	50	57	0	0	43	47
Overall	(12)		(25)		(38)		(19)		(7)		(101)	
1 year	50	50	40	40	53	54	63	66	57	62	51	53
3 years	50	51	20	21	26	28	23	27	0	0	25	27
5 years	50	51	20	21	21	24	12	15	0	0	21	25

SCOTLAND

AREA	NUMBER OF CASES			PERIOD	MEAN AGE		
	Males	Females	All		Males	Females	All
Scotland	128	50	178	1985-1989	62.4	66.3	63.5

OBSERVED AND RELATIVE SURVIVAL (%) BY AGE (number of cases in parentheses)

	AGE CLASS										ALL	
	15-44		45-54		55-64		65-74		75-99			
	obs	rel	obs	rel	obs	rel	obs	rel	obs	rel	obs	rel
Males	(6)		(30)		(36)		(37)		(19)		(128)	
1 year	67	67	67	67	72	74	57	59	37	42	61	63
3 years	33	34	47	48	42	44	32	38	11	16	35	40
5 years	33	34	43	45	33	37	22	28	0	0	27	34
Females	(0)		(9)		(15)		(13)		(13)		(50)	
1 year	-	-	56	56	53	54	62	64	31	34	50	52
3 years	-	-	44	45	27	28	46	51	0	0	28	31
5 years	-	-	44	46	20	21	31	37	0	0	22	27
Overall	(6)		(39)		(51)		(50)		(32)		(178)	
1 year	67	67	64	65	67	68	58	61	34	39	58	60
3 years	33	34	46	47	37	39	36	41	6	9	33	37
5 years	33	34	44	45	29	32	24	31	0	0	26	32

OROPHARYNX (ICD-9 146)

SLOVAKIA

AREA	NUMBER OF CASES			PERIOD	MEAN AGE		
	Males	Females	All		Males	Females	All
Slovakia	563	47	610	1985-1989	54.8	59.9	55.2

OBSERVED AND RELATIVE SURVIVAL (%) BY AGE (number of cases in parentheses)

	AGE CLASS										ALL	
	15-44		45-54		55-64		65-74		75-99			
	obs	rel	obs	rel	obs	rel	obs	rel	obs	rel	obs	rel
Males	(110)		(184)		(164)		(81)		(24)		(563)	
1 year	53	53	48	48	52	54	43	46	50	57	50	51
3 years	21	21	19	20	23	25	22	26	25	37	21	23
5 years	16	17	15	16	16	18	19	26	25	50	16	19
Females	(7)		(8)		(13)		(8)		(11)		(47)	
1 year	100	100	50	50	69	70	75	77	27	30	62	63
3 years	86	86	25	25	38	40	25	27	18	24	36	40
5 years	86	86	25	26	38	41	25	29	9	15	33	39
Overall	(117)		(192)		(177)		(89)		(35)		(610)	
1 year	56	56	48	48	54	55	46	48	43	48	50	52
3 years	25	25	19	20	24	26	22	26	23	33	22	24
5 years	20	21	16	17	17	20	20	26	19	36	18	20

SLOVENIA

AREA	NUMBER OF CASES			PERIOD	MEAN AGE		
	Males	Females	All		Males	Females	All
Slovenia	337	27	364	1985-1989	56.6	61.4	57.0

OBSERVED AND RELATIVE SURVIVAL (%) BY AGE (number of cases in parentheses)

	AGE CLASS										ALL	
	15-44		45-54		55-64		65-74		75-99			
	obs	rel	obs	rel	obs	rel	obs	rel	obs	rel	obs	rel
Males	(35)		(103)		(129)		(55)		(15)		(337)	
1 year	38	39	51	52	52	53	58	61	33	37	50	52
3 years	21	21	27	28	23	25	20	23	27	37	24	26
5 years	18	18	18	19	14	16	16	21	20	37	16	18
Females	(1)		(5)		(14)		(2)		(5)		(27)	
1 year	100	100	60	60	57	58	50	51	40	43	56	57
3 years	0	0	60	61	36	37	50	53	40	50	41	43
5 years	0	0	60	61	29	30	50	56	20	30	33	37
Overall	(36)		(108)		(143)		(57)		(20)		(364)	
1 year	40	40	51	52	52	53	58	61	35	38	51	52
3 years	20	20	29	30	24	26	21	24	30	41	25	27
5 years	17	18	20	21	15	17	18	23	20	35	17	20

OROPHARYNX (ICD-9 146)

SPAIN

AREA	NUMBER OF CASES			PERIOD	MEAN AGE			5-YR RELATIVE SURVIVAL (%)	
	Males	Females	All		Males	Females	All	Males	Females
Basque Country	136	12	148	1986-1988	56.7	65.5	57.4		
Mallorca	15	3	18	1988-1989	58.0	60.7	58.5		
Navarra	29	3	32	1985-1989	56.4	65.3	57.3		
Tarragona	32	6	38	1985-1989	58.4	68.8	60.1		
Spanish Registries	212	24	236		57.0	65.9	57.9		

(5-YR RELATIVE SURVIVAL chart: Males scale 100 80 60 40 20 0; Females scale 0 20 40 60 80 100; bars labelled Basque, Mallor, Navarr, Tarrag)

OBSERVED AND RELATIVE SURVIVAL (%) BY AGE (number of cases in parentheses)

	AGE CLASS										ALL	
	15-44		45-54		55-64		65-74		75-99			
	obs	rel	obs	rel	obs	rel	obs	rel	obs	rel	obs	rel
Males	(26)		(54)		(84)		(35)		(13)		(212)	
1 year	69	69	65	65	57	58	57	59	31	33	59	60
3 years	27	27	31	32	29	30	31	35	8	10	28	30
5 years	22	23	29	30	20	22	27	32	-	-	23	25
Females	(2)		(4)		(5)		(7)		(6)		(24)	
1 year	50	50	100	100	80	80	86	87	67	73	79	81
3 years	50	50	75	76	60	61	71	76	33	44	58	64
5 years	50	50	75	76	60	62	29	32	33	58	43	50
Overall	(28)		(58)		(89)		(42)		(19)		(236)	
1 year	68	68	67	68	58	59	62	64	42	46	61	62
3 years	29	29	34	35	30	32	38	42	16	21	31	33
5 years	24	25	32	33	22	24	25	29	16	26	25	28

SWEDEN

AREA	NUMBER OF CASES			PERIOD	MEAN AGE		
	Males	Females	All		Males	Females	All
South Sweden	39	14	53	1985-1989	60.6	59.2	60.3

OBSERVED AND RELATIVE SURVIVAL (%) BY AGE (number of cases in parentheses)

	AGE CLASS										ALL	
	15-44		45-54		55-64		65-74		75-99			
	obs	rel	obs	rel	obs	rel	obs	rel	obs	rel	obs	rel
Males	(2)		(10)		(14)		(8)		(5)		(39)	
1 year	100	100	80	80	64	65	75	77	40	45	69	71
3 years	50	50	80	81	29	30	38	41	0	0	41	44
5 years	50	50	80	82	21	23	0	0	0	0	31	35
Females	(0)		(4)		(5)		(5)		(0)		(14)	
1 year	-	-	100	100	80	80	60	61	-	-	79	79
3 years	-	-	75	76	60	61	40	42	-	-	57	59
5 years	-	-	75	76	60	62	0	0	-	-	43	45
Overall	(2)		(14)		(19)		(13)		(5)		(53)	
1 year	100	100	86	86	68	69	69	71	40	45	72	73
3 years	50	50	79	80	37	38	38	42	0	0	45	48
5 years	50	50	79	81	32	34	0	0	0	0	34	38

OROPHARYNX   (ICD-9 146)

SWITZERLAND

AREA	NUMBER OF CASES			PERIOD	MEAN AGE			5-YR RELATIVE SURVIVAL (%)	
	Males	Females	All		Males	Females	All	Males	Females
Basel	22	5	27	1985-1988	60.0	68.0	61.6		
Geneva	52	14	66	1985-1989	60.7	58.4	60.2		
Swiss Registries	74	19	93		60.5	61.1	60.6		

OBSERVED AND RELATIVE SURVIVAL (%) BY AGE (number of cases in parentheses)

	AGE CLASS										ALL	
	15-44		45-54		55-64		65-74		75-99			
	obs	rel	obs	rel	obs	rel	obs	rel	obs	rel	obs	rel
Males	(4)		(20)		(24)		(16)		(10)		(74)	
1 year	50	50	80	80	83	84	63	65	60	66	73	75
3 years	0	0	45	46	71	74	38	42	30	40	47	51
5 years	0	0	40	41	44	47	13	15	30	50	32	36
Females	(3)		(5)		(4)		(2)		(5)		(19)	
1 year	100	100	80	80	67	67	100	100	80	89	84	86
3 years	33	33	60	60	67	68	100	100	40	55	56	61
5 years	33	34	60	61	33	35	100	100	40	70	50	58
Overall	(7)		(25)		(28)		(18)		(15)		(93)	
1 year	71	72	80	80	82	82	67	69	67	73	75	77
3 years	14	14	48	49	70	73	44	49	33	45	49	53
5 years	14	14	44	45	42	46	22	27	33	57	35	41

OROPHARYNX (ICD-9 146)

EUROPE, 1985-89

Weighted analyses

COUNTRY	% COVERAGE WITH C.R.s	YEARLY NO. OF CASES (Mean No. of cases recorded)		
		Males	Females	All
AUSTRIA	8	4	2	6
DENMARK	100	51	21	72
ENGLAND	50	103	44	147
ESTONIA	100	21	3	24
FINLAND	100	12	3	15
FRANCE	3	108	8	116
GERMANY	2	19	5	24
ICELAND	100	0	0	0
ITALY	10	73	20	93
NETHERLANDS	6	4	1	5
POLAND	6	29	8	37
SCOTLAND	100	26	10	36
SLOVAKIA	100	113	9	122
SLOVENIA	100	67	5	72
SPAIN	10	65	7	72
SWEDEN	17	8	3	11
SWITZERLAND	11	16	4	20

RELATIVE SURVIVAL (%) (Age-standardized)

□ 1 year ■ 5 years

OBSERVED AND RELATIVE SURVIVAL (%) BY AGE

	AGE CLASS										ALL	
	15-44		45-54		55-64		65-74		75-99			
	obs	rel	obs	rel	obs	rel	obs	rel	obs	rel	obs	rel
Males												
1 year	75	75	69	70	68	69	62	65	50	55	66	68
3 years	49	49	37	38	37	39	30	34	19	26	35	38
5 years	43	43	31	32	25	28	23	28	16	27	26	30
Females												
1 year	69	69	76	76	74	75	75	76	43	47	69	70
3 years	50	50	45	46	49	51	61	65	19	25	46	49
5 years	46	47	39	40	44	46	53	59	15	24	39	44
Overall												
1 year	74	74	70	71	69	70	64	66	49	54	67	68
3 years	49	49	38	39	39	41	35	38	19	25	37	40
5 years	43	44	32	33	28	30	27	32	16	27	28	32

AGE STANDARDIZED RELATIVE SURVIVAL(%)

COUNTRY	MALES		FEMALES	
	1-year (95% C.I.)	5-years (95% C.I.)	1-year (95% C.I.)	5-years (95% C.I.)
AUSTRIA	-	-	-	-
DENMARK	61.9 (56.2 - 68.2)	32.4 (26.6 - 39.4)	73.1 (64.8 - 82.4)	50.8 (41.4 - 62.4)
ENGLAND	67.9 (63.8 - 72.2)	35.4 (31.0 - 40.4)	74.2 (68.3 - 80.5)	42.3 (35.4 - 50.5)
ESTONIA	39.9 (31.8 - 50.2)	15.3 (9.0 - 26.1)	67.9 (56.6 - 81.6)	11.7 (3.8 - 36.2)
FINLAND	66.8 (53.9 - 82.7)	26.7 (15.3 - 46.4)	-	-
FRANCE	71.0 (67.1 - 75.2)	31.3 (26.9 - 36.5)	68.9 (56.3 - 84.2)	-
GERMANY	71.5 (62.5 - 81.8)	-	-	-
ICELAND	-	-	-	-
ITALY	67.0 (61.3 - 73.3)	30.0 (24.4 - 36.9)	74.8 (65.0 - 86.2)	42.4 (31.7 - 56.7)
NETHERLANDS	70.4 (53.4 - 93.0)	29.6 (16.1 - 54.4)	-	-
POLAND	51.1 (41.0 - 63.6)	16.2 (9.7 - 27.2)	68.3 (50.2 - 92.9)	43.4 (24.4 - 77.4)
SCOTLAND	64.8 (56.6 - 74.1)	32.7 (24.9 - 43.1)	-	-
SLOVAKIA	50.9 (46.3 - 56.0)	22.7 (17.9 - 28.8)	65.2 (52.6 - 80.7)	36.4 (24.3 - 54.4)
SLOVENIA	51.0 (45.5 - 57.2)	20.2 (15.1 - 27.1)	59.5 (41.8 - 84.6)	40.2 (23.2 - 69.9)
SPAIN	58.3 (51.8 - 65.6)	-	82.7 (68.7 - 99.6)	57.3 (39.0 - 84.3)
SWEDEN	72.8 (60.5 - 87.5)	32.8 (22.7 - 47.5)	-	-
SWITZERLAND	73.6 (63.8 - 84.8)	34.3 (24.7 - 47.7)	83.2 (65.4 -105.8)	59.0 (39.8 - 87.6)
EUROPE, 1985-89	67.3 (64.6 - 70.1)	30.3 (27.2 - 33.9)	71.8 (65.6 - 78.6)	44.8 (37.6 - 53.3)

NASOPHARYNX   (ICD-9 147)

AUSTRIA

AREA	NUMBER OF CASES			PERIOD	MEAN AGE		
	Males	Females	All		Males	Females	All
Tirol	4	1	5	1988-1989	56.8	53.0	56.2

OBSERVED AND RELATIVE SURVIVAL (%) BY AGE (number of cases in parentheses)

	AGE CLASS										ALL	
	15-44		45-54		55-64		65-74		75-99			
	obs	rel	obs	rel	obs	rel	obs	rel	obs	rel	obs	rel
Males	(1)		(1)		(0)		(1)		(1)		(4)	
1 year	100	100	100	100	-	-	100	100	100	100	100	100
3 years	100	100	0	0	-	-	100	100	100	100	75	80
5 years	100	100	0	0	-	-	100	100	100	100	75	84
Females	(0)		(1)		(0)		(0)		(0)		(1)	
1 year	-	-	100	100	-	-	-	-	-	-	100	100
3 years	-	-	0	0	-	-	-	-	-	-	0	0
5 years	-	-	0	0	-	-	-	-	-	-	0	0
Overall	(1)		(2)		(0)		(1)		(1)		(5)	
1 year	100	100	100	100	-	-	100	100	100	100	100	100
3 years	100	100	0	0	-	-	100	100	100	100	60	63
5 years	100	100	0	0	-	-	100	100	100	100	60	66

DENMARK

AREA	NUMBER OF CASES			PERIOD	MEAN AGE		
	Males	Females	All		Males	Females	All
Denmark	81	35	116	1985-1989	60.7	57.1	59.6

OBSERVED AND RELATIVE SURVIVAL (%) BY AGE (number of cases in parentheses)

	AGE CLASS										ALL	
	15-44		45-54		55-64		65-74		75-99			
	obs	rel	obs	rel	obs	rel	obs	rel	obs	rel	obs	rel
Males	(7)		(12)		(25)		(28)		(9)		(81)	
1 year	86	86	75	75	68	69	61	63	33	38	64	66
3 years	86	86	58	59	32	34	29	33	0	0	36	40
5 years	71	72	50	52	20	22	18	23	0	0	26	31
Females	(4)		(12)		(10)		(6)		(3)		(35)	
1 year	100	100	75	75	80	81	67	68	33	35	74	75
3 years	50	50	58	59	40	41	17	18	0	0	40	42
5 years	50	50	42	43	30	32	0	0	0	0	29	31
Overall	(11)		(24)		(35)		(34)		(12)		(116)	
1 year	91	91	75	75	71	72	62	64	33	37	67	69
3 years	73	73	58	59	34	36	26	30	0	0	37	40
5 years	64	64	46	47	23	25	15	18	0	0	27	31

NASOPHARYNX (ICD-9 147)

ENGLAND

AREA	NUMBER OF CASES			PERIOD	MEAN AGE			5-YR RELATIVE SURVIVAL (%)	
	Males	Females	All		Males	Females	All	Males	Females
East Anglia	20	10	30	1985-1989	64.6	58.0	62.4		
Mersey	32	22	54	1985-1989	57.6	57.5	57.6		
Oxford	30	18	48	1985-1989	56.4	62.3	58.7		
South Thames	77	27	104	1985-1989	56.4	54.5	55.9		
Wessex	31	24	55	1985-1989	54.4	60.9	57.2		
West Midlands	61	27	88	1985-1989	60.5	58.8	60.0		
Yorkshire	25	19	44	1985-1989	55.4	50.3	53.2		
English Registries	276	147	423		57.8	57.5	57.7		

OBSERVED AND RELATIVE SURVIVAL (%) BY AGE (number of cases in parentheses)

	AGE CLASS										ALL	
	15-44		45-54		55-64		65-74		75-99			
	obs	rel	obs	rel	obs	rel	obs	rel	obs	rel	obs	rel
Males	(53)		(50)		(66)		(72)		(35)		(276)	
1 year	79	79	80	80	70	71	56	58	34	38	65	67
3 years	57	57	52	53	42	45	32	36	17	23	41	45
5 years	45	46	44	46	29	32	17	21	14	24	30	34
Females	(30)		(26)		(34)		(38)		(19)		(147)	
1 year	93	93	69	69	62	62	63	65	42	46	67	69
3 years	67	67	42	43	50	51	34	37	16	21	44	46
5 years	53	54	38	39	34	36	26	30	11	17	34	38
Overall	(83)		(76)		(100)		(110)		(54)		(423)	
1 year	84	84	76	77	67	68	58	60	37	41	66	68
3 years	60	60	49	49	45	47	33	37	17	22	42	45
5 years	48	48	42	43	31	33	20	24	13	22	31	36

ESTONIA

AREA	NUMBER OF CASES			PERIOD	MEAN AGE		
	Males	Females	All		Males	Females	All
Estonia	21	15	36	1985-1989	51.3	61.2	55.4

OBSERVED AND RELATIVE SURVIVAL (%) BY AGE (number of cases in parentheses)

	AGE CLASS										ALL	
	15-44		45-54		55-64		65-74		75-99			
	obs	rel	obs	rel	obs	rel	obs	rel	obs	rel	obs	rel
Males	(5)		(6)		(8)		(1)		(1)		(21)	
1 year	80	80	67	68	75	77	100	100	0	0	71	73
3 years	40	41	33	35	50	54	100	100	0	0	43	46
5 years	20	21	33	36	50	58	0	0	0	0	33	38
Females	(3)		(1)		(5)		(3)		(3)		(15)	
1 year	100	100	100	100	80	81	67	69	67	75	80	83
3 years	100	100	0	0	40	41	33	37	0	0	40	44
5 years	100	100	0	0	20	21	0	0	0	0	27	32
Overall	(8)		(7)		(13)		(4)		(4)		(36)	
1 year	88	88	71	72	77	78	75	78	50	56	75	77
3 years	63	63	29	30	46	49	50	57	0	0	42	45
5 years	50	51	29	31	38	43	0	0	0	0	31	35

NASOPHARYNX   (ICD-9 147)

FINLAND

AREA	NUMBER OF CASES			PERIOD	MEAN AGE		
	Males	Females	All		Males	Females	All
Finland	38	27	65	1985-1989	53.5	62.7	57.4

OBSERVED AND RELATIVE SURVIVAL (%) BY AGE (number of cases in parentheses)

	AGE CLASS										ALL	
	15-44		45-54		55-64		65-74		75-99			
	obs	rel	obs	rel	obs	rel	obs	rel	obs	rel	obs	rel
Males	(11)		(6)		(12)		(7)		(2)		(38)	
1 year	91	91	100	100	67	68	86	90	100	100	84	86
3 years	73	73	67	68	50	53	57	66	50	64	61	64
5 years	36	37	50	52	50	56	43	55	0	0	42	47
Females	(5)		(1)		(5)		(8)		(8)		(27)	
1 year	100	100	100	100	80	81	38	38	38	41	59	61
3 years	100	100	0	0	60	61	13	13	13	17	37	41
5 years	80	80	0	0	60	62	0	0	13	21	30	35
Overall	(16)		(7)		(17)		(15)		(10)		(65)	
1 year	94	94	100	100	71	72	60	62	50	55	74	76
3 years	81	82	57	58	53	56	33	37	20	27	51	55
5 years	50	51	43	44	53	58	20	24	10	17	37	42

FRANCE

AREA	NUMBER OF CASES			PERIOD	MEAN AGE			5-YR RELATIVE SURVIVAL (%)	
	Males	Females	All		Males	Females	All	Males	Females
Somme	10	2	12	1985-1989	59.4	28.0	54.3		
Calvados	9	2	11	1985-1989	49.0	63.0	51.6		
Doubs	9	3	12	1985-1989	59.2	56.3	58.6		
French Registries	28	7	35		56.1	50.6	55.0		

OBSERVED AND RELATIVE SURVIVAL (%) BY AGE (number of cases in parentheses)

	AGE CLASS										ALL	
	15-44		45-54		55-64		65-74		75-99			
	obs	rel	obs	rel	obs	rel	obs	rel	obs	rel	obs	rel
Males	(3)		(8)		(8)		(8)		(1)		(28)	
1 year	100	100	61	61	75	76	87	90	0	0	74	75
3 years	100	100	40	42	25	26	18	20	0	0	32	34
5 years	100	100	40	43	25	27	-	-	0	0	32	36
Females	(3)		(1)		(1)		(0)		(2)		(7)	
1 year	100	100	100	100	100	100	-	-	50	52	86	87
3 years	100	100	0	0	-	-	-	-	-	-	57	59
5 years	100	100	0	0	-	-	-	-	-	-	57	60
Overall	(6)		(9)		(9)		(8)		(3)		(35)	
1 year	100	100	65	66	78	79	87	90	33	35	76	77
3 years	100	100	33	33	26	27	18	20	-	-	37	39
5 years	100	100	33	34	26	28	-	-	-	-	37	40

NASOPHARYNX   (ICD-9 147)

GERMANY

AREA	NUMBER OF CASES			PERIOD	MEAN AGE		
	Males	Females	All		Males	Females	All
Saarland	23	11	34	1985-1989	53.0	56.1	54.0

OBSERVED AND RELATIVE SURVIVAL (%) BY AGE (number of cases in parentheses)

	15-44		45-54		55-64		65-74		75-99		ALL	
	obs	rel	obs	rel	obs	rel	obs	rel	obs	rel	obs	rel
Males	(8)		(7)		(2)		(4)		(2)		(23)	
1 year	63	63	71	72	100	100	100	100	50	56	74	76
3 years	25	25	29	29	0	0	75	87	0	0	30	33
5 years	-	-	0	0	0	0	38	51	0	0	14	16
Females	(2)		(1)		(3)		(4)		(1)		(11)	
1 year	100	100	100	100	100	100	50	51	0	0	73	74
3 years	50	50	0	0	67	68	50	53	0	0	45	47
5 years	50	50	0	0	33	35	25	28	0	0	27	29
Overall	(10)		(8)		(5)		(8)		(3)		(34)	
1 year	70	70	75	76	100	100	75	77	33	37	74	75
3 years	30	30	25	26	40	42	63	69	0	0	35	38
5 years	30	30	0	0	20	21	31	38	0	0	18	20

ICELAND

AREA	NUMBER OF CASES			PERIOD	MEAN AGE		
	Males	Females	All		Males	Females	All
Iceland	4	0	4	1985-1989	53.0	-	53.0

OBSERVED AND RELATIVE SURVIVAL (%) BY AGE (number of cases in parentheses)

	15-44		45-54		55-64		65-74		75-99		ALL	
	obs	rel	obs	rel	obs	rel	obs	rel	obs	rel	obs	rel
Males	(2)		(1)		(0)		(0)		(1)		(4)	
1 year	100	100	100	100	-	-	-	-	0	0	75	76
3 years	100	100	100	100	-	-	-	-	0	0	75	79
5 years	100	100	100	100	-	-	-	-	0	0	75	83
Females	(0)		(0)		(0)		(0)		(0)		(0)	
1 year	-	-	-	-	-	-	-	-	-	-	-	-
3 years	-	-	-	-	-	-	-	-	-	-	-	-
5 years	-	-	-	-	-	-	-	-	-	-	-	-
Overall	(2)		(1)		(0)		(0)		(1)		(4)	
1 year	100	100	100	100	-	-	-	-	0	0	75	76
3 years	100	100	100	100	-	-	-	-	0	0	75	79
5 years	100	100	100	100	-	-	-	-	0	0	75	83

NASOPHARYNX (ICD-9 147)

ITALY

AREA	NUMBER OF CASES			PERIOD	MEAN AGE			5-YR RELATIVE SURVIVAL (%)	
	Males	Females	All		Males	Females	All	Males	Females
Florence	40	13	53	1985-1989	52.7	57.1	53.8		
Genoa	18	10	28	1986-1988	58.2	56.6	57.6		
Latina	3	0	3	1985-1987	36.3	-	36.3		
Modena	5	2	7	1988-1989	53.2	59.0	55.0		
Parma	5	4	9	1985-1987	63.4	51.8	58.3		
Ragusa	8	5	13	1985-1989	58.8	40.0	51.6		
Romagna	13	2	15	1986-1988	58.1	63.5	58.9		
Turin	15	3	18	1985-1987	51.7	34.0	48.8		
Varese	19	10	29	1985-1989	54.4	56.5	55.1		
Italian Registries	126	49	175		54.7	53.8	54.4		

OBSERVED AND RELATIVE SURVIVAL (%) BY AGE (number of cases in parentheses)

	AGE CLASS										ALL	
	15-44		45-54		55-64		65-74		75-99			
	obs	rel	obs	rel	obs	rel	obs	rel	obs	rel	obs	rel
Males	(22)		(31)		(43)		(25)		(5)		(126)	
1 year	91	91	74	75	81	82	64	66	60	65	77	78
3 years	64	64	52	53	49	51	40	44	0	0	48	51
5 years	50	50	45	47	27	29	24	29	0	0	34	37
Females	(15)		(14)		(7)		(7)		(6)		(49)	
1 year	80	80	86	86	71	72	86	87	50	54	78	79
3 years	67	67	50	50	29	29	29	30	17	22	45	47
5 years	67	67	50	51	29	29	29	31	17	27	45	48
Overall	(37)		(45)		(50)		(32)		(11)		(175)	
1 year	86	87	78	78	79	80	69	71	55	59	77	78
3 years	65	65	51	52	46	48	38	41	9	12	47	50
5 years	57	57	47	48	27	29	25	30	9	15	37	40

NETHERLANDS

AREA	NUMBER OF CASES			PERIOD	MEAN AGE		
	Males	Females	All		Males	Females	All
Eindhoven	8	4	12	1985-1989	54.9	41.8	50.6

OBSERVED AND RELATIVE SURVIVAL (%) BY AGE (number of cases in parentheses)

	AGE CLASS										ALL	
	15-44		45-54		55-64		65-74		75-99			
	obs	rel	obs	rel	obs	rel	obs	rel	obs	rel	obs	rel
Males	(3)		(1)		(3)		(0)		(1)		(8)	
1 year	100	100	100	100	67	68	-	-	100	100	88	89
3 years	100	100	100	100	67	72	-	-	100	100	88	93
5 years	100	100	100	100	67	76	-	-	0	0	75	84
Females	(1)		(2)		(1)		(0)		(0)		(4)	
1 year	100	100	0	0	0	0	-	-	-	-	25	25
3 years	100	100	0	0	0	0	-	-	-	-	25	25
5 years	100	100	0	0	0	0	-	-	-	-	25	25
Overall	(4)		(3)		(4)		(0)		(1)		(12)	
1 year	100	100	33	33	50	51	-	-	100	100	67	68
3 years	100	100	33	34	50	53	-	-	100	100	67	70
5 years	100	100	33	34	50	56	-	-	0	0	58	63

NASOPHARYNX (ICD-9 147)

POLAND

AREA	NUMBER OF CASES			PERIOD	MEAN AGE			5-YR RELATIVE SURVIVAL (%)	
	Males	Females	All		Males	Females	All	Males	Females
Cracow	8	5	13	1985-1989	61.0	62.0	61.5		
Warsaw	8	2	10	1988-1989	57.1	41.5	54.1		
Polish Registries	16	7	23		59.2	56.4	58.3		

OBSERVED AND RELATIVE SURVIVAL (%) BY AGE (number of cases in parentheses)

	15-44 obs rel		45-54 obs rel		55-64 obs rel		65-74 obs rel		75-99 obs rel		ALL obs rel	
Males	(3)		(1)		(6)		(3)		(3)		(16)	
1 year	67	67	100	100	67	68	67	70	33	39	63	65
3 years	33	34	100	100	33	36	0	0	0	0	25	29
5 years	33	34	100	100	33	39	0	0	0	0	25	32
Females	(2)		(1)		(2)		(2)		(0)		(7)	
1 year	50	50	100	100	0	0	50	51	-	-	40	40
3 years	50	50	-	-	0	0	0	0	-	-	20	21
5 years	0	0	-	-	0	0	0	0	-	-	0	0
Overall	(5)		(2)		(8)		(5)		(3)		(23)	
1 year	60	60	100	100	50	51	60	62	33	39	56	58
3 years	40	40	100	100	25	27	0	0	0	0	23	26
5 years	13	14	100	100	25	29	0	0	0	0	18	22

SCOTLAND

AREA	NUMBER OF CASES			PERIOD	MEAN AGE		
	Males	Females	All		Males	Females	All
Scotland	70	22	92	1985-1989	56.2	58.0	56.7

OBSERVED AND RELATIVE SURVIVAL (%) BY AGE (number of cases in parentheses)

	15-44 obs rel		45-54 obs rel		55-64 obs rel		65-74 obs rel		75-99 obs rel		ALL obs rel	
Males	(12)		(17)		(18)		(18)		(5)		(70)	
1 year	92	92	88	89	72	74	61	64	0	0	71	73
3 years	58	59	53	54	17	18	33	39	0	0	36	39
5 years	33	34	41	43	11	12	28	36	0	0	26	30
Females	(6)		(1)		(5)		(4)		(6)		(22)	
1 year	67	67	0	0	20	20	50	51	33	35	41	42
3 years	50	50	0	0	0	0	25	27	17	20	23	24
5 years	50	50	0	0	0	0	25	29	0	0	18	21
Overall	(18)		(18)		(23)		(22)		(11)		(92)	
1 year	83	83	83	84	61	62	59	62	18	20	64	66
3 years	56	56	50	51	13	14	32	36	9	12	33	35
5 years	39	39	39	40	9	10	27	35	0	0	24	27

NASOPHARYNX (ICD-9 147)

SLOVAKIA

AREA	NUMBER OF CASES			PERIOD	MEAN AGE		
	Males	Females	All		Males	Females	All
Slovakia	87	27	114	1985-1989	54.0	52.0	53.6

OBSERVED AND RELATIVE SURVIVAL (%) BY AGE (number of cases in parentheses)

	AGE CLASS										ALL	
	15-44		45-54		55-64		65-74		75-99			
	obs	rel	obs	rel	obs	rel	obs	rel	obs	rel	obs	rel
Males	(21)		(23)		(23)		(11)		(9)		(87)	
1 year	76	76	65	66	57	58	55	58	33	38	61	63
3 years	57	58	48	50	26	28	18	22	22	34	38	42
5 years	36	37	37	40	26	30	18	25	22	47	30	36
Females	(11)		(4)		(5)		(2)		(5)		(27)	
1 year	91	91	75	75	60	61	0	0	40	43	67	68
3 years	82	82	50	51	20	21	0	0	20	26	48	51
5 years	60	60	50	52	20	21	0	0	-	-	39	44
Overall	(32)		(27)		(28)		(13)		(14)		(114)	
1 year	81	81	67	67	57	58	46	48	36	40	62	64
3 years	66	66	48	50	25	27	15	18	21	31	40	44
5 years	45	46	39	42	25	29	15	20	21	41	33	38

SLOVENIA

AREA	NUMBER OF CASES			PERIOD	MEAN AGE		
	Males	Females	All		Males	Females	All
Slovenia	19	22	41	1985-1989	52.4	56.4	54.6

OBSERVED AND RELATIVE SURVIVAL (%) BY AGE (number of cases in parentheses)

	AGE CLASS										ALL	
	15-44		45-54		55-64		65-74		75-99			
	obs	rel	obs	rel	obs	rel	obs	rel	obs	rel	obs	rel
Males	(5)		(4)		(6)		(4)		(0)		(19)	
1 year	100	100	75	76	67	68	50	52	-	-	74	75
3 years	80	81	75	77	50	53	0	0	-	-	53	56
5 years	80	81	75	79	50	56	0	0	-	-	53	59
Females	(5)		(4)		(6)		(3)		(4)		(22)	
1 year	100	100	100	100	100	100	33	34	25	27	77	79
3 years	100	100	75	76	83	85	0	0	0	0	59	63
5 years	100	100	75	77	17	17	0	0	0	0	41	46
Overall	(10)		(8)		(12)		(7)		(4)		(41)	
1 year	100	100	88	88	83	84	43	45	25	27	76	77
3 years	90	91	75	77	67	70	0	0	0	0	56	60
5 years	90	91	75	78	33	36	0	0	0	0	46	52

NASOPHARYNX (ICD-9 147)

SPAIN

AREA	NUMBER OF CASES			PERIOD	MEAN AGE			5-YR RELATIVE SURVIVAL (%)	
	Males	Females	All		Males	Females	All	Males	Females
Basque Country	43	18	61	1986-1988	52.4	51.8	52.3		
Mallorca	9	3	12	1988-1989	58.0	59.0	58.3		
Navarra	14	3	17	1985-1989	49.6	65.3	52.5		
Tarragona	17	2	19	1985-1989	48.4	62.5	49.9		
Spanish Registries	83	26	109		51.8	55.2	52.6		

OBSERVED AND RELATIVE SURVIVAL (%) BY AGE (number of cases in parentheses)

	AGE CLASS										ALL	
	15-44		45-54		55-64		65-74		75-99			
	obs	rel	obs	rel	obs	rel	obs	rel	obs	rel	obs	rel
Males	(24)		(19)		(24)		(11)		(5)		(83)	
1 year	83	83	84	85	75	76	55	56	40	43	75	76
3 years	46	46	42	43	29	30	45	49	0	0	37	39
5 years	37	37	32	33	19	21	35	41	0	0	28	30
Females	(7)		(7)		(4)		(4)		(4)		(26)	
1 year	86	86	100	100	100	100	50	51	0	0	73	74
3 years	57	57	71	72	75	76	25	26	0	0	50	53
5 years	29	29	71	72	-	-	25	28	0	0	39	43
Overall	(31)		(26)		(28)		(15)		(9)		(109)	
1 year	84	84	88	89	79	79	53	55	22	24	74	75
3 years	48	49	50	51	36	37	40	43	0	0	40	42
5 years	35	35	42	43	24	25	33	38	0	0	31	33

SWEDEN

AREA	NUMBER OF CASES			PERIOD	MEAN AGE		
	Males	Females	All		Males	Females	All
South Sweden	21	11	32	1985-1989	59.9	57.5	59.1

OBSERVED AND RELATIVE SURVIVAL (%) BY AGE (number of cases in parentheses)

	AGE CLASS										ALL	
	15-44		45-54		55-64		65-74		75-99			
	obs	rel	obs	rel	obs	rel	obs	rel	obs	rel	obs	rel
Males	(3)		(3)		(6)		(8)		(1)		(21)	
1 year	100	100	100	100	67	68	50	52	0	0	67	68
3 years	100	100	100	100	67	69	38	42	0	0	62	66
5 years	100	100	100	100	67	72	38	46	0	0	62	70
Females	(4)		(1)		(3)		(0)		(3)		(11)	
1 year	50	50	100	100	100	100	-	-	33	36	64	65
3 years	25	25	100	100	100	100	-	-	33	44	55	59
5 years	25	25	100	100	100	100	-	-	0	0	45	51
Overall	(7)		(4)		(9)		(8)		(4)		(32)	
1 year	71	72	100	100	78	79	50	52	25	27	66	67
3 years	57	57	100	100	78	80	38	42	25	33	59	64
5 years	57	58	100	100	78	83	38	46	0	0	56	63

NASOPHARYNX   (ICD-9 147)

SWITZERLAND

AREA	NUMBER OF CASES			PERIOD	MEAN AGE		
	Males	Females	All		Males	Females	All
Geneva	6	2	8	1985-1989	51.3	46.0	50.1

OBSERVED AND RELATIVE SURVIVAL (%) BY AGE (number of cases in parentheses)

	AGE CLASS										ALL	
	15-44		45-54		55-64		65-74		75-99			
	obs	rel	obs	rel	obs	rel	obs	rel	obs	rel	obs	rel
Males	(2)		(2)		(1)		(1)		(0)		(6)	
1 year	100	100	50	50	100	100	0	0	-	-	67	68
3 years	100	100	-	-	100	100	0	0	-	-	67	70
5 years	100	100	-	-	100	100	0	0	-	-	67	72
Females	(1)		(0)		(1)		(0)		(0)		(2)	
1 year	100	100	-	-	0	0	-	-	-	-	50	50
3 years	100	100	-	-	0	0	-	-	-	-	50	50
5 years	-	-	-	-	0	0	-	-	-	-	-	-
Overall	(3)		(2)		(2)		(1)		(0)		(8)	
1 year	100	100	50	50	50	50	0	0	-	-	63	63
3 years	100	100	-	-	50	52	0	0	-	-	63	65
5 years	100	100	-	-	50	53	0	0	-	-	63	67

NASOPHARYNX (ICD-9 147)

EUROPE, 1985-89

Weighted analyses

COUNTRY	% COVERAGE WITH C.R.s	YEARLY NO. OF CASES (Mean No. of cases recorded)			RELATIVE SURVIVAL (%) (Age-standardized)
		Males	Females	All	
AUSTRIA	8	2	1	3	A
DENMARK	100	16	7	23	DK
ENGLAND	50	55	29	84	ENG
ESTONIA	100	4	3	7	EST
FINLAND	100	8	5	13	FIN
FRANCE	3	6	1	7	F
GERMANY	2	5	2	7	D
ICELAND	100	2	0	2	IS
ITALY	10	34	13	47	I
NETHERLANDS	6	2	1	3	NL
POLAND	6	10	3	13	PL
SCOTLAND	100	14	4	18	SCO
SLOVAKIA	100	17	5	22	SK
SLOVENIA	100	4	4	8	SLO
SPAIN	10	25	9	34	E
SWEDEN	17	4	2	6	S
SWITZERLAND	6	1	0	1	CH
					EUR

□ 1 year ■ 5 years

OBSERVED AND RELATIVE SURVIVAL (%) BY AGE

	AGE CLASS										ALL	
	15-44		45-54		55-64		65-74		75-99			
	obs	rel	obs	rel	obs	rel	obs	rel	obs	rel	obs	rel
Males												
1 year	83	83	78	78	79	80	71	73	41	45	73	75
3 years	57	57	50	51	32	33	40	45	6	6	40	42
5 years	56	57	41	42	24	26	27	33	3	4	30	34
Females												
1 year	87	87	90	90	76	76	61	62	26	28	70	71
3 years	64	64	34	34	47	48	31	32	8	11	44	46
5 years	52	53	33	34	28	29	22	25	6	10	34	37
Overall												
1 year	84	84	81	82	78	79	68	70	37	41	72	74
3 years	59	59	46	46	36	37	37	41	6	8	41	43
5 years	55	56	39	39	25	27	26	31	4	6	31	35

AGE STANDARDIZED RELATIVE SURVIVAL(%)

COUNTRY	MALES		FEMALES	
	1-year (95% C.I.)	5-years (95% C.I.)	1-year (95% C.I.)	5-years (95% C.I.)
AUSTRIA	-	-	-	-
DENMARK	69.3 (59.5 - 80.6)	36.5 (26.9 - 49.4)	76.1 (64.0 - 90.5)	27.8 (16.6 - 46.7)
ENGLAND	68.2 (63.0 - 73.9)	34.5 (28.9 - 41.1)	69.1 (62.2 - 76.8)	37.1 (29.8 - 46.2)
ESTONIA	72.3 (60.0 - 87.0)	26.8 (15.1 - 47.6)	85.6 (70.8 -103.5)	27.0 (18.8 - 38.7)
FINLAND	87.6 (78.3 - 98.0)	44.6 (30.7 - 64.8)	75.3 (63.9 - 88.8)	35.7 (23.8 - 53.5)
FRANCE	72.7 (61.7 - 85.7)	-	-	-
GERMANY	81.5 (69.4 - 95.7)	-	78.5 (68.6 - 89.9)	25.7 (10.5 - 63.0)
ICELAND	-	-	-	-
ITALY	77.1 (69.2 - 86.0)	34.0 (26.7 - 43.2)	77.8 (66.0 - 91.7)	41.9 (29.3 - 59.9)
NETHERLANDS	-	-	-	-
POLAND	71.6 (53.7 - 95.3)	37.6 (24.4 - 57.9)	-	-
SCOTLAND	70.5 (62.3 - 79.8)	26.9 (18.2 - 39.6)	34.3 (21.0 - 56.1)	16.9 (7.6 - 37.6)
SLOVAKIA	61.3 (51.3 - 73.2)	34.2 (23.4 - 50.0)	55.3 (41.8 - 73.3)	-
SLOVENIA	-	-	77.9 (66.2 - 91.8)	41.5 (31.2 - 55.3)
SPAIN	71.5 (61.7 - 82.8)	28.9 (20.1 - 41.5)	75.5 (64.4 - 88.5)	-
SWEDEN	70.3 (58.8 - 84.0)	70.1 (57.7 - 85.3)	-	-
SWITZERLAND	-	-	-	-
EUROPE, 1985-89	75.0 (70.4 - 79.9)	34.9 (29.2 - 41.8)	72.7 (67.1 - 78.8)	32.1 (23.5 - 43.9)

HYPOPHARYNX   (ICD-9 148)

AUSTRIA

AREA	NUMBER OF CASES			PERIOD	MEAN AGE		
	Males	Females	All		Males	Females	All
Tirol	7	4	11	1988-1989	54.0	59.5	56.1

OBSERVED AND RELATIVE SURVIVAL (%) BY AGE (number of cases in parentheses)

	AGE CLASS										ALL	
	15-44		45-54		55-64		65-74		75-99			
	obs	rel	obs	rel	obs	rel	obs	rel	obs	rel	obs	rel
Males	(0)		(4)		(3)		(0)		(0)		(7)	
1 year	-	-	75	75	67	67	-	-	-	-	71	72
3 years	-	-	50	51	33	35	-	-	-	-	43	44
5 years	-	-	25	26	33	36	-	-	-	-	29	30
Females	(2)		(0)		(0)		(1)		(1)		(4)	
1 year	100	100	-	-	-	-	100	100	100	100	100	100
3 years	100	100	-	-	-	-	0	0	100	100	75	80
5 years	50	50	-	-	-	-	0	0	100	100	50	56
Overall	(2)		(4)		(3)		(1)		(1)		(11)	
1 year	100	100	75	75	67	67	100	100	100	100	82	83
3 years	100	100	50	51	33	35	0	0	100	100	55	57
5 years	50	50	25	26	33	36	0	0	100	100	36	39

DENMARK

AREA	NUMBER OF CASES			PERIOD	MEAN AGE		
	Males	Females	All		Males	Females	All
Denmark	130	43	173	1985-1989	62.7	65.3	63.4

OBSERVED AND RELATIVE SURVIVAL (%) BY AGE (number of cases in parentheses)

	AGE CLASS										ALL	
	15-44		45-54		55-64		65-74		75-99			
	obs	rel	obs	rel	obs	rel	obs	rel	obs	rel	obs	rel
Males	(7)		(29)		(34)		(38)		(22)		(130)	
1 year	71	72	45	45	50	51	47	49	45	50	48	50
3 years	43	43	14	14	12	12	21	24	5	6	15	17
5 years	14	15	10	11	12	13	16	20	0	0	11	13
Females	(0)		(9)		(13)		(10)		(11)		(43)	
1 year	-	-	22	22	69	70	60	61	36	39	49	50
3 years	-	-	11	11	38	40	20	22	9	12	21	23
5 years	-	-	0	0	31	33	0	0	0	0	9	11
Overall	(7)		(38)		(47)		(48)		(33)		(173)	
1 year	71	72	39	40	55	56	50	52	42	46	49	50
3 years	43	43	13	13	19	20	21	23	6	8	17	19
5 years	14	15	8	8	17	19	13	16	0	0	10	12

HYPOPHARYNX (ICD-9 148)

ENGLAND

AREA	NUMBER OF CASES			PERIOD	MEAN AGE			5-YR RELATIVE SURVIVAL (%)	
	Males	Females	All		Males	Females	All	Males	Females
East Anglia	47	35	82	1985-1989	68.9	71.1	69.9		
Mersey	92	50	142	1985-1989	64.1	68.1	65.5		
Oxford	34	27	61	1985-1989	69.5	70.0	69.8		
South Thames	114	82	196	1985-1989	64.6	69.5	66.6		
Wessex	51	31	82	1985-1989	66.2	73.3	68.9		
West Midlands	123	64	187	1985-1989	64.6	66.6	65.3		
Yorkshire	81	51	132	1985-1989	66.1	68.2	66.9		
English Registries	542	340	882		65.6	69.1	67.0		

OBSERVED AND RELATIVE SURVIVAL (%) BY AGE (number of cases in parentheses)

	AGE CLASS										ALL	
	15-44		45-54		55-64		65-74		75-99			
	obs	rel	obs	rel	obs	rel	obs	rel	obs	rel	obs	rel
Males	(13)		(66)		(170)		(178)		(115)		(542)	
1 year	62	62	65	66	51	52	52	54	37	41	50	53
3 years	38	39	32	32	26	28	26	30	16	22	25	29
5 years	23	23	27	28	22	24	18	23	10	19	19	24
Females	(11)		(24)		(71)		(122)		(112)		(340)	
1 year	45	46	83	84	56	57	44	45	32	35	46	47
3 years	9	9	25	25	32	33	22	24	16	21	22	25
5 years	0	0	25	26	27	28	19	21	10	16	17	21
Overall	(24)		(90)		(241)		(300)		(227)		(882)	
1 year	54	54	70	70	53	53	49	51	34	38	49	51
3 years	25	25	30	31	28	30	25	27	16	22	24	27
5 years	13	13	27	28	23	25	18	22	10	17	18	23

ESTONIA

AREA	NUMBER OF CASES			PERIOD	MEAN AGE		
	Males	Females	All		Males	Females	All
Estonia	59	2	61	1985-1989	57.6	64.0	57.8

OBSERVED AND RELATIVE SURVIVAL (%) BY AGE (number of cases in parentheses)

	AGE CLASS										ALL	
	15-44		45-54		55-64		65-74		75-99			
	obs	rel	obs	rel	obs	rel	obs	rel	obs	rel	obs	rel
Males	(2)		(21)		(23)		(9)		(4)		(59)	
1 year	0	0	62	63	48	49	56	58	0	0	49	51
3 years	0	0	27	28	17	19	33	39	0	0	21	24
5 years	0	0	21	23	17	20	11	15	0	0	16	19
Females	(0)		(0)		(1)		(1)		(0)		(2)	
1 year	-	-	-	-	100	100	0	0	-	-	50	51
3 years	-	-	-	-	100	100	0	0	-	-	50	53
5 years	-	-	-	-	100	100	0	0	-	-	50	55
Overall	(2)		(21)		(24)		(10)		(4)		(61)	
1 year	0	0	62	63	50	51	50	52	0	0	49	51
3 years	0	0	27	28	21	23	30	35	0	0	22	25
5 years	0	0	21	23	21	24	10	13	0	0	17	20

HYPOPHARYNX (ICD-9 148)

FINLAND

AREA	NUMBER OF CASES			PERIOD	MEAN AGE		
	Males	Females	All		Males	Females	All
Finland	64	29	93	1985-1989	64.2	67.0	65.1

OBSERVED AND RELATIVE SURVIVAL (%) BY AGE (number of cases in parentheses)

	AGE CLASS										ALL	
	15-44		45-54		55-64		65-74		75-99			
	obs	rel	obs	rel	obs	rel	obs	rel	obs	rel	obs	rel
Males	(4)		(5)		(23)		(21)		(11)		(64)	
1 year	25	25	80	81	52	53	43	45	36	41	47	49
3 years	25	25	60	62	13	14	14	16	18	26	19	21
5 years	25	26	40	42	4	5	10	12	0	0	9	12
Females	(1)		(3)		(8)		(10)		(7)		(29)	
1 year	100	100	100	100	38	38	80	82	57	62	66	67
3 years	100	100	67	67	38	38	50	53	14	18	41	45
5 years	100	100	33	34	38	39	40	45	0	0	31	36
Overall	(5)		(8)		(31)		(31)		(18)		(93)	
1 year	40	40	88	88	48	49	55	57	44	49	53	55
3 years	40	40	63	64	19	20	26	29	17	23	26	29
5 years	40	41	38	39	13	14	19	24	0	0	16	20

FRANCE

AREA	NUMBER OF CASES			PERIOD	MEAN AGE			5-YR RELATIVE SURVIVAL (%)	
	Males	Females	All		Males	Females	All	Males	Females
Somme	141	6	147	1985-1989	57.7	52.5	57.5		
Calvados	241	4	245	1985-1989	58.4	59.0	58.4		
Doubs	121	3	124	1985-1989	60.3	65.3	60.4		
French Registries	503	13	516		58.6	57.7	58.6		

OBSERVED AND RELATIVE SURVIVAL (%) BY AGE (number of cases in parentheses)

	AGE CLASS										ALL	
	15-44		45-54		55-64		65-74		75-99			
	obs	rel	obs	rel	obs	rel	obs	rel	obs	rel	obs	rel
Males	(46)		(121)		(210)		(88)		(38)		(503)	
1 year	76	76	68	68	71	72	54	56	49	54	66	67
3 years	49	50	36	38	33	35	24	27	20	27	33	35
5 years	32	33	24	25	22	24	20	24	10	17	22	25
Females	(3)		(2)		(4)		(3)		(1)		(13)	
1 year	100	100	50	50	71	72	100	100	0	0	76	77
3 years	67	67	50	51	0	0	60	63	0	0	38	40
5 years	67	67	50	51	0	0	60	66	0	0	38	41
Overall	(49)		(123)		(214)		(91)		(39)		(516)	
1 year	77	78	67	68	71	72	56	58	47	52	66	68
3 years	50	50	37	38	33	34	25	28	20	26	33	35
5 years	35	35	24	26	22	24	21	25	10	17	23	26

HYPOPHARYNX (ICD-9 148)

GERMANY

AREA	NUMBER OF CASES			PERIOD	MEAN AGE		
	Males	Females	All		Males	Females	All
Saarland	83	10	93	1985-1989	54.8	58.4	55.2

OBSERVED AND RELATIVE SURVIVAL (%) BY AGE (number of cases in parentheses)

	AGE CLASS										ALL	
	15-44		45-54		55-64		65-74		75-99			
	obs	rel	obs	rel	obs	rel	obs	rel	obs	rel	obs	rel
Males	(11)		(33)		(28)		(10)		(1)		(83)	
1 year	64	64	61	61	61	62	60	63	100	100	61	62
3 years	27	28	27	28	32	34	40	46	0	0	30	32
5 years	27	28	20	21	32	36	10	13	0	0	23	25
Females	(2)		(1)		(5)		(1)		(1)		(10)	
1 year	50	50	0	0	100	100	100	100	100	100	80	81
3 years	50	50	0	0	20	21	0	0	100	100	30	31
5 years	50	51	0	0	-	-	0	0	100	100	30	32
Overall	(13)		(34)		(33)		(11)		(2)		(93)	
1 year	62	62	59	59	67	68	64	66	100	100	63	64
3 years	31	31	26	27	30	32	36	42	50	61	30	32
5 years	31	31	19	20	30	33	9	12	50	72	24	26

ICELAND

AREA	NUMBER OF CASES			PERIOD	MEAN AGE		
	Males	Females	All		Males	Females	All
Iceland	1	0	1	1985-1989	82.0	-	82.0

OBSERVED AND RELATIVE SURVIVAL (%) BY AGE (number of cases in parentheses)

	AGE CLASS										ALL	
	15-44		45-54		55-64		65-74		75-99			
	obs	rel	obs	rel	obs	rel	obs	rel	obs	rel	obs	rel
Males	(0)		(0)		(0)		(0)		(1)		(1)	
1 year	-	-	-	-	-	-	-	-	0	0	0	0
3 years	-	-	-	-	-	-	-	-	0	0	0	0
5 years	-	-	-	-	-	-	-	-	0	0	0	0
Females	(0)		(0)		(0)		(0)		(0)		(0)	
1 year	-	-	-	-	-	-	-	-	-	-	-	-
3 years	-	-	-	-	-	-	-	-	-	-	-	-
5 years	-	-	-	-	-	-	-	-	-	-	-	-
Overall	(0)		(0)		(0)		(0)		(1)		(1)	
1 year	-	-	-	-	-	-	-	-	0	0	0	0
3 years	-	-	-	-	-	-	-	-	0	0	0	0
5 years	-	-	-	-	-	-	-	-	0	0	0	0

HYPOPHARYNX   (ICD-9 148)

ITALY

AREA	NUMBER OF CASES			PERIOD	MEAN AGE			5-YR RELATIVE SURVIVAL (%)	
	Males	Females	All		Males	Females	All	Males	Females
Florence	44	7	51	1985-1989	59.3	67.3	60.4		
Genoa	21	6	27	1986-1988	58.6	61.7	59.3		
Latina	1	0	1	1985-1987	51.0	-	51.0		
Modena	14	2	16	1988-1989	56.9	52.5	56.4		
Parma	19	0	19	1985-1987	71.1	-	71.1		
Ragusa	2	0	2	1985-1989	65.0	-	65.0		
Romagna	4	2	6	1986-1988	59.5	57.0	58.8		
Turin	16	1	17	1985-1987	63.5	51.0	62.8		
Varese	54	6	60	1985-1989	60.2	65.7	60.8		
Italian Registries	175	24	199		61.0	63.0	61.3		

OBSERVED AND RELATIVE SURVIVAL (%) BY AGE (number of cases in parentheses)

	AGE CLASS										ALL	
	15-44		45-54		55-64		65-74		75-99			
	obs	rel	obs	rel	obs	rel	obs	rel	obs	rel	obs	rel
Males	(6)		(42)		(62)		(43)		(22)		(175)	
1 year	67	67	60	60	65	65	63	65	59	65	62	64
3 years	33	34	36	36	21	22	33	36	9	12	26	28
5 years	33	34	26	27	19	21	28	34	5	8	22	25
Females	(2)		(6)		(6)		(4)		(6)		(24)	
1 year	100	100	50	50	67	67	25	25	17	18	46	47
3 years	0	0	33	34	17	17	0	0	17	22	17	18
5 years	0	0	33	34	17	17	0	0	0	0	13	14
Overall	(8)		(48)		(68)		(47)		(28)		(199)	
1 year	75	75	58	59	65	66	60	61	50	55	60	62
3 years	25	25	35	36	21	21	30	33	11	14	25	27
5 years	25	25	27	28	19	21	26	31	4	6	21	24

NETHERLANDS

AREA	NUMBER OF CASES			PERIOD	MEAN AGE		
	Males	Females	All		Males	Females	All
Eindhoven	15	4	19	1985-1989	65.9	62.3	65.2

OBSERVED AND RELATIVE SURVIVAL (%) BY AGE (number of cases in parentheses)

	AGE CLASS										ALL	
	15-44		45-54		55-64		65-74		75-99			
	obs	rel	obs	rel	obs	rel	obs	rel	obs	rel	obs	rel
Males	(0)		(0)		(7)		(4)		(4)		(15)	
1 year	-	-	-	-	71	72	75	78	50	55	67	70
3 years	-	-	-	-	29	30	75	85	50	66	47	53
5 years	-	-	-	-	14	15	0	0	25	41	13	16
Females	(1)		(0)		(1)		(1)		(1)		(4)	
1 year	100	100	-	-	0	0	0	0	100	100	50	52
3 years	0	0	-	-	0	0	0	0	0	0	0	0
5 years	0	0	-	-	0	0	0	0	0	0	0	0
Overall	(1)		(0)		(8)		(5)		(5)		(19)	
1 year	100	100	-	-	63	63	60	62	60	66	63	66
3 years	0	0	-	-	25	26	60	67	40	55	37	42
5 years	0	0	-	-	13	13	0	0	20	34	11	13

HYPOPHARYNX (ICD-9 148)

POLAND

AREA	NUMBER OF CASES			PERIOD	MEAN AGE			5-YR RELATIVE SURVIVAL (%)	
	Males	Females	All		Males	Females	All	Males	Females
Cracow	5	3	8	1985-1989	57.2	60.7	58.6		
Warsaw	8	0	8	1988-1989	64.4	-	64.4		
Polish Registries	13	3	16		61.8	61.0	61.6		

100 80 60 40 20 0   0 20 40 60 80 100

Cracow
Warsaw

OBSERVED AND RELATIVE SURVIVAL (%) BY AGE (number of cases in parentheses)

	AGE CLASS										ALL	
	15-44		45-54		55-64		65-74		75-99			
	obs	rel	obs	rel	obs	rel	obs	rel	obs	rel	obs	rel
Males	(1)		(1)		(7)		(3)		(1)		(13)	
1 year	0	0	0	0	29	29	67	71	0	0	31	32
3 years	0	0	0	0	29	31	0	0	0	0	15	17
5 years	0	0	0	0	29	34	0	0	0	0	15	19
Females	(0)		(1)		(1)		(1)		(0)		(3)	
1 year	-	-	100	100	0	0	0	0	-	-	33	34
3 years	-	-	100	100	0	0	0	0	-	-	33	35
5 years	-	-	0	0	0	0	0	0	-	-	0	0
Overall	(1)		(2)		(8)		(4)		(1)		(16)	
1 year	0	0	50	51	25	26	50	52	0	0	31	32
3 years	0	0	50	52	25	27	0	0	0	0	19	21
5 years	0	0	0	0	25	29	0	0	0	0	13	15

SCOTLAND

AREA	NUMBER OF CASES			PERIOD	MEAN AGE		
	Males	Females	All		Males	Females	All
Scotland	134	65	199	1985-1989	64.9	66.0	65.3

OBSERVED AND RELATIVE SURVIVAL (%) BY AGE (number of cases in parentheses)

	AGE CLASS										ALL	
	15-44		45-54		55-64		65-74		75-99			
	obs	rel	obs	rel	obs	rel	obs	rel	obs	rel	obs	rel
Males	(4)		(22)		(37)		(42)		(29)		(134)	
1 year	75	75	59	60	49	50	52	55	31	36	49	51
3 years	25	25	23	23	19	20	21	25	7	11	18	21
5 years	25	25	14	14	14	15	12	16	0	0	10	13
Females	(3)		(0)		(29)		(20)		(13)		(65)	
1 year	100	100	-	-	62	63	55	57	38	42	57	59
3 years	67	67	-	-	31	32	30	33	8	10	28	30
5 years	67	67	-	-	17	18	15	18	8	13	17	20
Overall	(7)		(22)		(66)		(62)		(42)		(199)	
1 year	86	86	59	60	55	55	53	55	33	38	51	54
3 years	43	43	23	23	24	25	24	28	7	10	21	24
5 years	43	43	14	14	15	17	13	16	2	5	13	16

HYPOPHARYNX   (ICD-9 148)

SLOVAKIA

AREA	NUMBER OF CASES			PERIOD	MEAN AGE		
	Males	Females	All		Males	Females	All
Slovakia	423	14	437	1985-1989	55.0	61.2	55.2

OBSERVED AND RELATIVE SURVIVAL (%) BY AGE (number of cases in parentheses)

	AGE CLASS										ALL	
	15-44		45-54		55-64		65-74		75-99			
	obs	rel	obs	rel	obs	rel	obs	rel	obs	rel	obs	rel
Males	(72)		(137)		(142)		(54)		(18)		(423)	
1 year	38	38	47	47	45	46	37	39	28	32	43	44
3 years	6	6	15	16	18	19	13	15	6	8	14	15
5 years	4	4	13	14	14	16	13	17	-	-	12	13
Females	(1)		(4)		(4)		(2)		(3)		(14)	
1 year	100	100	75	75	75	76	100	100	33	37	71	73
3 years	100	100	50	51	75	79	0	0	0	0	43	47
5 years	100	100	50	51	75	82	0	0	0	0	43	50
Overall	(73)		(141)		(146)		(56)		(21)		(437)	
1 year	38	39	48	48	46	47	39	41	29	32	43	45
3 years	7	7	16	17	19	21	13	15	5	7	15	16
5 years	5	5	15	16	16	18	13	17	-	-	13	14

SLOVENIA

AREA	NUMBER OF CASES			PERIOD	MEAN AGE		
	Males	Females	All		Males	Females	All
Slovenia	191	13	204	1985-1989	57.3	60.4	57.5

OBSERVED AND RELATIVE SURVIVAL (%) BY AGE (number of cases in parentheses)

	AGE CLASS										ALL	
	15-44		45-54		55-64		65-74		75-99			
	obs	rel	obs	rel	obs	rel	obs	rel	obs	rel	obs	rel
Males	(8)		(69)		(73)		(34)		(7)		(191)	
1 year	50	50	49	50	49	50	50	52	29	32	49	50
3 years	25	25	17	18	18	19	21	24	0	0	18	19
5 years	0	0	6	7	10	11	6	8	0	0	7	8
Females	(2)		(2)		(3)		(4)		(2)		(13)	
1 year	0	0	100	100	33	34	75	76	0	0	46	47
3 years	0	0	50	51	0	0	25	27	0	0	15	16
5 years	0	0	50	51	0	0	0	0	0	0	8	9
Overall	(10)		(71)		(76)		(38)		(9)		(204)	
1 year	40	40	51	51	49	50	53	55	22	24	49	50
3 years	20	20	18	18	17	18	21	24	0	0	18	19
5 years	0	0	7	8	9	10	5	7	0	0	7	8

HYPOPHARYNX (ICD-9 148)

SPAIN

AREA	NUMBER OF CASES			PERIOD	MEAN AGE			5-YR RELATIVE SURVIVAL (%)	
	Males	Females	All		Males	Females	All	Males	Females
Basque Country	134	3	137	1986-1988	57.3	52.7	57.2		
Mallorca	21	0	21	1988-1989	53.6	-	53.6		
Navarra	19	1	20	1985-1989	57.6	48.0	57.2		
Tarragona	22	0	22	1985-1989	56.0	-	56.0		
Spanish Registries	196	4	200		56.8	52.0	56.7		

OBSERVED AND RELATIVE SURVIVAL (%) BY AGE (number of cases in parentheses)

	AGE CLASS										ALL	
	15-44		45-54		55-64		65-74		75-99			
	obs	rel	obs	rel	obs	rel	obs	rel	obs	rel	obs	rel
Males	(22)		(65)		(68)		(31)		(10)		(196)	
1 year	64	64	55	56	65	66	65	67	80	86	62	63
3 years	23	23	22	22	31	32	19	22	30	37	25	26
5 years	23	23	20	21	27	29	19	23	0	0	22	24
Females	(0)		(3)		(1)		(0)		(0)		(4)	
1 year	-	-	67	67	0	0	-	-	-	-	50	50
3 years	-	-	67	67	0	0	-	-	-	-	50	50
5 years	-	-	67	67	0	0	-	-	-	-	50	51
Overall	(22)		(68)		(69)		(31)		(10)		(200)	
1 year	64	64	56	56	64	65	65	67	80	86	62	63
3 years	23	23	24	24	30	32	19	22	30	37	26	27
5 years	23	23	22	23	27	29	19	23	0	0	23	25

SWEDEN

AREA	NUMBER OF CASES			PERIOD	MEAN AGE		
	Males	Females	All		Males	Females	All
South Sweden	51	8	59	1985-1989	64.7	63.6	64.6

OBSERVED AND RELATIVE SURVIVAL (%) BY AGE (number of cases in parentheses)

	AGE CLASS										ALL	
	15-44		45-54		55-64		65-74		75-99			
	obs	rel	obs	rel	obs	rel	obs	rel	obs	rel	obs	rel
Males	(1)		(8)		(16)		(16)		(10)		(51)	
1 year	100	100	50	50	56	57	63	65	30	33	53	55
3 years	100	100	38	38	38	39	38	42	0	0	31	35
5 years	100	100	38	39	31	34	25	30	0	0	25	31
Females	(1)		(2)		(1)		(2)		(2)		(8)	
1 year	0	0	50	50	100	100	100	100	0	0	50	52
3 years	0	0	50	50	100	100	50	53	0	0	38	42
5 years	0	0	50	51	100	100	50	56	0	0	38	45
Overall	(2)		(10)		(17)		(18)		(12)		(59)	
1 year	50	50	50	50	59	60	67	69	25	28	53	54
3 years	50	50	40	41	41	43	39	43	0	0	32	36
5 years	50	51	40	41	35	38	28	33	0	0	27	33

HYPOPHARYNX (ICD-9 148)

SWITZERLAND

AREA	NUMBER OF CASES			PERIOD	MEAN AGE			5-YR RELATIVE SURVIVAL (%)	
	Males	Females	All		Males	Females	All	Males	Females
Basel	23	0	23	1985-1988	61.1	-	61.1		
Geneva	45	6	51	1985-1989	59.8	67.2	60.7		
Swiss Registries	68	6	74		60.3	67.3	60.8		

OBSERVED AND RELATIVE SURVIVAL (%) BY AGE (number of cases in parentheses)

	AGE CLASS										ALL	
	15-44		45-54		55-64		65-74		75-99			
	obs	rel	obs	rel	obs	rel	obs	rel	obs	rel	obs	rel
Males	(2)		(14)		(34)		(12)		(6)		(68)	
1 year	100	100	50	50	71	72	58	60	17	18	60	62
3 years	50	50	21	22	32	34	17	19	17	21	26	28
5 years	50	51	21	22	24	25	0	0	17	27	19	21
Females	(0)		(0)		(3)		(1)		(2)		(6)	
1 year	-	-	-	-	67	67	100	100	0	0	50	52
3 years					33	34	100	100	0	0	33	37
5 years	-	-	-	-	33	34	100	100	0	0	33	40
Overall	(2)		(14)		(37)		(13)		(8)		(74)	
1 year	100	100	50	50	70	71	62	64	13	14	59	61
3 years	50	50	21	22	32	34	23	26	13	16	27	29
5 years	50	51	21	22	24	26	8	9	13	20	20	23

HYPOPHARYNX (ICD-9 148)

EUROPE, 1985-89
Weighted analyses

COUNTRY	% COVERAGE WITH C.R.s	YEARLY NO. OF CASES (Mean No. of cases recorded)		
		Males	Females	All
AUSTRIA	8	4	2	6
DENMARK	100	26	9	35
ENGLAND	50	108	68	176
ESTONIA	100	12	0	12
FINLAND	100	13	6	19
FRANCE	3	101	3	104
GERMANY	2	17	2	19
ICELAND	100	1	0	1
ITALY	10	48	7	55
NETHERLANDS	6	3	1	4
POLAND	6	10	1	11
SCOTLAND	100	27	13	40
SLOVAKIA	100	85	3	88
SLOVENIA	100	38	3	41
SPAIN	10	63	1	64
SWEDEN	17	10	2	12
SWITZERLAND	11	15	1	16

RELATIVE SURVIVAL (%) (Age-standardized)

Males / Females

☐ 1 year ■ 5 years

OBSERVED AND RELATIVE SURVIVAL (%) BY AGE

	AGE CLASS										ALL	
	15-44		45-54		55-64		65-74		75-99			
	obs	rel	obs	rel	obs	rel	obs	rel	obs	rel	obs	rel
Males												
1 year	69	70	62	62	65	66	57	59	58	62	62	64
3 years	40	40	32	32	31	33	26	30	16	21	30	32
5 years	30	30	22	23	24	26	17	22	7	12	22	24
Females												
1 year	70	70	50	50	67	67	68	68	45	46	62	63
3 years	36	36	29	29	21	21	21	22	36	38	30	32
5 years	31	31	25	26	18	19	19	21	32	33	25	28
Overall												
1 year	69	70	61	61	66	67	58	60	57	60	62	64
3 years	39	40	31	32	30	32	26	29	18	23	30	32
5 years	30	30	23	24	24	26	17	21	9	13	22	25

AGE STANDARDIZED RELATIVE SURVIVAL(%)

COUNTRY	MALES		FEMALES	
	1-year (95% C.I.)	5-years (95% C.I.)	1-year (95% C.I.)	5-years (95% C.I.)
AUSTRIA	-	-	-	-
DENMARK	50.6 (42.4 - 60.4)	12.5 (7.6 - 20.5)	-	-
ENGLAND	54.6 (50.1 - 59.4)	23.9 (20.0 - 28.6)	55.9 (50.2 - 62.3)	22.2 (17.1 - 28.7)
ESTONIA	43.7 (33.5 - 57.0)	15.3 (8.0 - 29.1)	-	-
FINLAND	53.3 (41.9 - 67.7)	15.2 (7.3 - 31.8)	69.3 (56.6 - 84.9)	38.2 (23.6 - 62.0)
FRANCE	65.1 (60.6 - 69.9)	24.1 (19.6 - 29.7)	65.6 (47.0 - 91.6)	31.2 (15.3 - 63.6)
GERMANY	67.4 (57.6 - 78.9)	21.5 (13.8 - 33.3)	75.0 (70.3 - 80.1)	-
ICELAND	-	-	-	-
ITALY	64.1 (57.0 - 72.1)	24.3 (18.3 - 32.3)	48.9 (33.2 - 72.2)	13.0 (4.7 - 35.9)
NETHERLANDS	-	-	-	-
POLAND	26.6 (13.7 - 51.7)	11.3 (3.5 - 36.4)	-	-
SCOTLAND	52.8 (44.5 - 62.6)	13.6 (8.3 - 22.4)	-	-
SLOVAKIA	42.0 (36.6 - 48.2)	-	77.7 (60.8 - 99.3)	45.6 (30.1 - 69.1)
SLOVENIA	48.0 (40.1 - 57.3)	6.8 (3.9 - 11.8)	50.8 (33.8 - 76.5)	11.0 (2.8 - 44.1)
SPAIN	66.4 (59.4 - 74.3)	21.4 (16.1 - 28.5)	-	-
SWEDEN	56.9 (45.1 - 72.0)	33.8 (23.2 - 49.1)	68.0 (54.6 - 84.7)	57.7 (38.2 - 86.9)
SWITZERLAND	58.7 (48.5 - 71.1)	20.6 (12.1 - 35.1)	-	-
EUROPE, 1985-89	63.4 (60.3 - 66.7)	22.7 (19.3 - 26.8)	61.0 (55.2 - 67.4)	23.7 (16.7 - 33.8)

HEAD & NECK   (ICD-9 141,143-148)

AUSTRIA

AREA	NUMBER OF CASES			PERIOD	MEAN AGE		
	Males	Females	All		Males	Females	All
Tirol	59	24	83	1988-1989	59.2	60.4	59.5

OBSERVED AND RELATIVE SURVIVAL (%) BY AGE (number of cases in parentheses)

	AGE CLASS										ALL	
	15-44		45-54		55-64		65-74		75-99			
	obs	rel	obs	rel	obs	rel	obs	rel	obs	rel	obs	rel
Males	(7)		(16)		(18)		(9)		(9)		(59)	
1 year	86	86	69	69	72	73	89	91	78	85	76	78
3 years	43	43	44	44	50	52	56	60	56	74	49	53
5 years	43	43	38	38	44	48	33	39	44	75	41	46
Females	(4)		(5)		(5)		(5)		(5)		(24)	
1 year	100	100	100	100	100	100	100	100	60	62	92	93
3 years	75	75	80	81	60	61	40	42	40	46	58	61
5 years	25	25	60	61	60	62	40	43	40	51	46	49
Overall	(11)		(21)		(23)		(14)		(14)		(83)	
1 year	91	91	76	76	78	79	93	95	71	77	81	82
3 years	55	55	52	53	52	54	50	53	50	63	52	55
5 years	36	37	43	44	48	51	36	40	43	65	42	47

DENMARK

AREA	NUMBER OF CASES			PERIOD	MEAN AGE		
	Males	Females	All		Males	Females	All
Denmark	1061	593	1654	1985-1989	61.7	65.5	63.1

OBSERVED AND RELATIVE SURVIVAL (%) BY AGE (number of cases in parentheses)

	AGE CLASS										ALL	
	15-44		45-54		55-64		65-74		75-99			
	obs	rel	obs	rel	obs	rel	obs	rel	obs	rel	obs	rel
Males	(87)		(215)		(302)		(298)		(159)		(1061)	
1 year	83	83	73	73	63	64	60	63	53	59	64	66
3 years	59	59	45	46	34	36	32	37	24	34	36	40
5 years	46	47	38	40	26	29	24	30	14	26	28	33
Females	(38)		(86)		(153)		(144)		(172)		(593)	
1 year	79	79	72	72	76	77	71	72	56	61	69	71
3 years	68	69	55	55	54	56	49	53	31	41	47	52
5 years	63	64	45	47	46	49	40	46	22	35	38	46
Overall	(125)		(301)		(455)		(442)		(331)		(1654)	
1 year	82	82	73	73	67	68	64	66	54	60	66	68
3 years	62	62	48	49	41	43	38	42	28	38	40	45
5 years	51	52	40	42	33	36	29	36	18	31	31	38

HEAD & NECK   (ICD-9 141,143-148)

ENGLAND

AREA	NUMBER OF CASES			PERIOD	MEAN AGE			5-YR RELATIVE SURVIVAL (%)	
	Males	Females	All		Males	Females	All	Males	Females
East Anglia	236	178	414	1985-1989	65.2	68.8	66.7		
Mersey	498	242	740	1985-1989	62.3	66.3	63.6		
Oxford	287	188	475	1985-1989	63.0	66.2	64.3		
South Thames	715	469	1184	1985-1989	63.3	68.0	65.2		
Wessex	312	253	565	1985-1989	64.1	68.7	66.2		
West Midlands	736	405	1141	1985-1989	62.1	65.6	63.3		
Yorkshire	492	289	781	1985-1989	63.2	66.2	64.3		
English Registries	3276	2024	5300		63.0	67.1	64.6		

OBSERVED AND RELATIVE SURVIVAL (%) BY AGE (number of cases in parentheses)

	AGE CLASS										ALL	
	15-44		45-54		55-64		65-74		75-99			
	obs	rel	obs	rel	obs	rel	obs	rel	obs	rel	obs	rel
Males	(262)		(522)		(913)		(972)		(607)		(3276)	
1 year	78	78	74	75	65	66	63	66	48	54	64	66
3 years	57	58	46	47	41	44	36	41	26	37	39	44
5 years	50	50	40	41	33	36	26	33	17	32	31	37
Females	(159)		(190)		(405)		(616)		(654)		(2024)	
1 year	86	86	82	82	72	72	65	67	51	56	65	68
3 years	66	66	58	59	50	51	44	47	29	38	43	49
5 years	62	62	53	54	42	44	39	44	21	34	37	44
Overall	(421)		(712)		(1318)		(1588)		(1261)		(5300)	
1 year	81	81	77	77	67	68	64	66	50	55	64	67
3 years	61	61	49	50	44	46	39	44	28	38	41	46
5 years	54	55	43	45	36	39	31	38	19	33	33	40

ESTONIA

AREA	NUMBER OF CASES			PERIOD	MEAN AGE		
	Males	Females	All		Males	Females	All
Estonia	390	65	455	1985-1989	55.8	62.2	56.7

OBSERVED AND RELATIVE SURVIVAL (%) BY AGE (number of cases in parentheses)

	AGE CLASS										ALL	
	15-44		45-54		55-64		65-74		75-99			
	obs	rel	obs	rel	obs	rel	obs	rel	obs	rel	obs	rel
Males	(43)		(145)		(136)		(49)		(17)		(390)	
1 year	53	54	66	66	50	51	41	43	24	27	54	55
3 years	19	19	27	29	23	25	22	26	6	9	23	25
5 years	16	17	20	22	18	22	14	19	0	0	18	20
Females	(8)		(9)		(23)		(12)		(13)		(65)	
1 year	50	50	56	56	61	61	50	52	31	34	51	52
3 years	38	38	11	11	39	41	17	18	8	10	25	27
5 years	38	38	0	0	26	28	8	10	0	0	15	18
Overall	(51)		(154)		(159)		(61)		(30)		(455)	
1 year	53	53	65	66	52	53	43	45	27	30	53	55
3 years	22	22	26	28	25	27	21	25	7	10	23	26
5 years	20	20	19	21	19	23	13	17	0	0	17	20

HEAD & NECK   (ICD-9 141,143-148)

FINLAND

AREA	NUMBER OF CASES			PERIOD	MEAN AGE		
	Males	Females	All		Males	Females	All
Finland	430	299	729	1985-1989	59.9	67.3	62.9

OBSERVED AND RELATIVE SURVIVAL (%) BY AGE (number of cases in parentheses)

	AGE CLASS										ALL	
	15-44		45-54		55-64		65-74		75-99			
	obs	rel	obs	rel	obs	rel	obs	rel	obs	rel	obs	rel
Males	(49)		(83)		(146)		(97)		(55)		(430)	
1 year	84	84	80	80	75	76	64	67	58	65	72	74
3 years	63	64	47	48	38	41	39	45	27	39	42	46
5 years	53	54	35	36	29	32	32	41	11	20	31	37
Females	(28)		(27)		(49)		(88)		(107)		(299)	
1 year	93	93	89	89	69	70	69	71	51	56	67	70
3 years	75	75	74	75	59	61	50	54	28	38	48	55
5 years	71	72	67	68	55	58	36	42	21	35	40	49
Overall	(77)		(110)		(195)		(185)		(162)		(729)	
1 year	87	87	82	82	73	74	66	69	54	59	70	72
3 years	68	68	54	55	44	46	44	49	28	38	44	49
5 years	60	60	43	44	35	39	34	41	17	30	35	42

FRANCE

AREA	NUMBER OF CASES			PERIOD	MEAN AGE			5-YR RELATIVE SURVIVAL (%)	
	Males	Females	All		Males	Females	All	Males	Females
Somme	616	62	678	1985-1989	57.4	61.1	57.7		
Calvados	741	58	799	1985-1989	58.0	60.8	58.2		
Doubs	441	45	486	1985-1989	59.2	62.6	59.6		
French Registries	1798	165	1963		58.1	61.4	58.4		

OBSERVED AND RELATIVE SURVIVAL (%) BY AGE (number of cases in parentheses)

	AGE CLASS										ALL	
	15-44		45-54		55-64		65-74		75-99			
	obs	rel	obs	rel	obs	rel	obs	rel	obs	rel	obs	rel
Males	(173)		(494)		(672)		(317)		(142)		(1798)	
1 year	80	80	75	76	71	73	65	68	44	49	70	72
3 years	49	49	44	45	37	39	35	40	22	30	39	41
5 years	40	41	36	37	26	28	26	31	14	24	29	33
Females	(20)		(30)		(48)		(35)		(32)		(165)	
1 year	90	90	66	66	77	77	88	90	50	54	74	76
3 years	64	64	35	35	53	54	76	80	42	54	54	57
5 years	64	65	31	31	53	55	66	72	42	68	51	57
Overall	(193)		(524)		(720)		(352)		(174)		(1963)	
1 year	81	81	75	75	72	73	68	70	45	50	70	72
3 years	50	51	43	45	38	40	39	44	26	34	40	43
5 years	43	44	35	37	28	30	30	36	19	33	31	35

HEAD & NECK   (ICD-9 141,143-148)

GERMANY

AREA	NUMBER OF CASES			PERIOD	MEAN AGE		
	Males	Females	All		Males	Females	All
Saarland	537	104	641	1985-1989	55.3	60.5	56.2

OBSERVED AND RELATIVE SURVIVAL (%) BY AGE (number of cases in parentheses)

	15-44		45-54		55-64		65-74		75-99		ALL	
	obs	rel	obs	rel	obs	rel	obs	rel	obs	rel	obs	rel
Males	(88)		(183)		(154)		(82)		(30)		(537)	
1 year	80	80	69	70	71	73	70	72	53	60	71	72
3 years	50	50	46	47	49	51	37	42	27	38	45	48
5 years	45	46	35	37	36	40	21	27	22	42	34	38
Females	(11)		(23)		(28)		(21)		(21)		(104)	
1 year	73	73	74	74	79	79	76	78	62	67	73	75
3 years	55	55	48	48	43	44	52	56	38	49	46	49
5 years	45	46	38	39	38	40	48	53	33	53	40	45
Overall	(99)		(206)		(182)		(103)		(51)		(641)	
1 year	79	79	70	70	73	74	71	73	57	63	71	73
3 years	51	51	46	47	48	50	40	45	31	43	45	48
5 years	45	46	36	37	37	40	27	34	27	47	35	39

ICELAND

AREA	NUMBER OF CASES			PERIOD	MEAN AGE		
	Males	Females	All		Males	Females	All
Iceland	19	15	34	1985-1989	63.3	68.1	65.4

OBSERVED AND RELATIVE SURVIVAL (%) BY AGE (number of cases in parentheses)

	15-44		45-54		55-64		65-74		75-99		ALL	
	obs	rel	obs	rel	obs	rel	obs	rel	obs	rel	obs	rel
Males	(3)		(4)		(2)		(3)		(7)		(19)	
1 year	100	100	100	100	100	100	33	35	71	80	79	83
3 years	100	100	50	51	50	52	33	38	29	40	47	55
5 years	100	100	50	51	50	54	0	0	29	50	42	53
Females	(1)		(1)		(2)		(6)		(5)		(15)	
1 year	100	100	100	100	100	100	83	85	80	88	87	90
3 years	100	100	0	0	50	52	33	35	80	100	53	60
5 years	100	100	0	0	50	53	33	37	80	100	53	64
Overall	(4)		(5)		(4)		(9)		(12)		(34)	
1 year	100	100	100	100	100	100	67	68	75	83	82	86
3 years	100	100	40	40	50	52	33	36	50	69	50	57
5 years	100	100	40	41	50	53	22	26	50	84	47	58

HEAD & NECK   (ICD-9 141,143-148)

ITALY

AREA	NUMBER OF CASES			PERIOD	MEAN AGE		
	Males	Females	All		Males	Females	All
Florence	295	117	412	1985-1989	60.6	66.0	62.1
Genoa	153	67	220	1986-1988	60.9	66.7	62.6
Latina	35	6	41	1985-1987	56.3	62.7	57.2
Modena	55	17	72	1988-1989	60.8	65.4	61.9
Parma	88	21	109	1985-1987	63.5	65.6	63.9
Ragusa	34	12	46	1985-1989	63.2	55.0	61.1
Romagna	51	13	64	1986-1988	60.3	64.8	61.2
Turin	202	62	264	1985-1987	61.0	62.6	61.4
Varese	310	71	381	1985-1989	60.3	63.5	60.9
Italian Registries	1223	386	1609		60.8	64.7	61.7

5-YR RELATIVE SURVIVAL (%)

Males   Females

100 80 60 40 20 0   0 20 40 60 80 100

Floren
Genoa
Latina
Modena
Parma
Ragusa
Romagn
Turin
Varese

OBSERVED AND RELATIVE SURVIVAL (%) BY AGE (number of cases in parentheses)

	AGE CLASS										ALL	
	15-44		45-54		55-64		65-74		75-99			
	obs	rel	obs	rel	obs	rel	obs	rel	obs	rel	obs	rel
Males	(78)		(261)		(430)		(313)		(141)		(1223)	
1 year	78	78	68	69	72	73	70	73	54	59	69	71
3 years	51	52	43	44	40	41	38	42	23	31	39	42
5 years	46	47	37	38	30	33	29	35	16	26	31	35
Females	(37)		(60)		(88)		(85)		(116)		(386)	
1 year	86	87	82	82	74	74	70	72	55	60	70	72
3 years	54	54	60	60	43	44	48	50	32	41	44	49
5 years	54	54	55	56	40	41	44	49	20	31	38	45
Overall	(115)		(321)		(518)		(398)		(257)		(1609)	
1 year	81	81	71	71	72	73	70	73	55	59	69	71
3 years	52	52	46	47	40	42	40	44	27	35	40	43
5 years	49	49	40	41	32	35	32	38	18	28	33	37

NETHERLANDS

AREA	NUMBER OF CASES			PERIOD	MEAN AGE		
	Males	Females	All		Males	Females	All
Eindhoven	103	66	169	1985-1989	60.6	59.5	60.2

OBSERVED AND RELATIVE SURVIVAL (%) BY AGE (number of cases in parentheses)

	AGE CLASS										ALL	
	15-44		45-54		55-64		65-74		75-99			
	obs	rel	obs	rel	obs	rel	obs	rel	obs	rel	obs	rel
Males	(13)		(18)		(31)		(26)		(15)		(103)	
1 year	100	100	77	78	77	79	62	64	60	67	74	76
3 years	77	77	65	66	51	53	35	40	53	76	53	58
5 years	77	78	65	67	48	52	19	25	13	25	42	49
Females	(13)		(9)		(17)		(13)		(14)		(66)	
1 year	92	92	67	67	65	65	77	78	34	37	66	68
3 years	69	69	56	56	41	42	77	82	17	23	51	55
5 years	69	70	44	45	35	36	62	69	9	15	43	48
Overall	(26)		(27)		(48)		(39)		(29)		(169)	
1 year	96	96	74	74	73	74	67	69	48	53	71	73
3 years	73	73	62	63	47	49	49	55	37	51	52	57
5 years	73	74	58	60	43	46	33	41	11	20	42	49

HEAD & NECK   (ICD-9 141,143-148)

POLAND

AREA	NUMBER OF CASES			PERIOD	MEAN AGE			5-YR RELATIVE SURVIVAL (%)	
	Males	Females	All		Males	Females	All	Males	Females
Cracow	115	31	146	1985-1989	57.3	55.5	56.9		
Warsaw	105	37	142	1988-1989	58.2	60.6	58.8		
Polish Registries	220	68	288		57.7	58.3	57.8		

OBSERVED AND RELATIVE SURVIVAL (%) BY AGE (number of cases in parentheses)

	AGE CLASS										ALL	
	15-44		45-54		55-64		65-74		75-99			
	obs	rel	obs	rel	obs	rel	obs	rel	obs	rel	obs	rel
Males	(18)		(57)		(94)		(40)		(11)		(220)	
1 year	50	50	40	41	50	51	55	58	55	61	49	50
3 years	39	39	19	20	27	29	24	28	0	0	24	26
5 years	39	40	19	21	24	28	11	14	0	0	21	24
Females	(14)		(14)		(21)		(9)		(10)		(68)	
1 year	64	64	78	78	45	46	56	57	39	44	57	58
3 years	64	65	39	40	40	42	22	24	13	18	39	42
5 years	57	58	31	32	34	37	22	26	0	0	33	37
Overall	(32)		(71)		(115)		(49)		(21)		(288)	
1 year	56	56	48	48	49	50	55	58	48	55	51	52
3 years	50	51	23	24	29	31	23	27	5	8	27	30
5 years	47	48	22	23	26	30	13	17	0	0	23	27

SCOTLAND

AREA	NUMBER OF CASES			PERIOD	MEAN AGE		
	Males	Females	All		Males	Females	All
Scotland	987	547	1534	1985-1989	62.4	67.2	64.1

OBSERVED AND RELATIVE SURVIVAL (%) BY AGE (number of cases in parentheses)

	AGE CLASS										ALL	
	15-44		45-54		55-64		65-74		75-99			
	obs	rel	obs	rel	obs	rel	obs	rel	obs	rel	obs	rel
Males	(67)		(194)		(279)		(278)		(169)		(987)	
1 year	78	78	74	75	70	72	65	68	47	54	66	69
3 years	51	51	52	53	41	44	38	44	20	30	39	45
5 years	43	44	41	43	29	32	28	36	12	25	29	36
Females	(31)		(50)		(140)		(153)		(173)		(547)	
1 year	81	81	84	84	66	66	70	72	46	51	63	66
3 years	71	71	72	73	40	42	46	51	23	31	41	47
5 years	65	65	60	61	32	34	35	42	18	31	33	41
Overall	(98)		(244)		(419)		(431)		(342)		(1534)	
1 year	79	79	76	77	69	70	67	70	47	52	65	68
3 years	57	58	56	57	41	43	41	47	22	31	40	45
5 years	50	51	45	47	30	33	30	38	15	28	30	38

HEAD & NECK   (ICD-9 141,143-148)

SLOVAKIA

AREA	NUMBER OF CASES			PERIOD	MEAN AGE		
	Males	Females	All		Males	Females	All
Slovakia	2263	179	2442	1985-1989	54.8	59.0	55.1

OBSERVED AND RELATIVE SURVIVAL (%) BY AGE (number of cases in parentheses)

	AGE CLASS										ALL	
	15-44		45-54		55-64		65-74		75-99			
	obs	rel	obs	rel	obs	rel	obs	rel	obs	rel	obs	rel
Males	(410)		(733)		(722)		(299)		(99)		(2263)	
1 year	52	52	54	55	52	53	42	45	38	44	51	52
3 years	23	23	22	23	21	22	20	24	19	29	21	23
5 years	16	17	18	19	16	18	18	24	15	30	17	19
Females	(37)		(28)		(42)		(32)		(40)		(179)	
1 year	97	97	61	61	69	70	72	74	40	44	68	69
3 years	76	76	39	40	48	49	41	44	15	20	44	48
5 years	69	70	36	36	48	51	41	48	11	19	41	48
Overall	(447)		(761)		(764)		(331)		(139)		(2442)	
1 year	56	56	54	55	52	54	45	48	39	44	52	53
3 years	27	27	23	24	22	24	22	26	18	26	23	25
5 years	21	21	19	20	18	20	20	26	14	27	19	21

SLOVENIA

AREA	NUMBER OF CASES			PERIOD	MEAN AGE		
	Males	Females	All		Males	Females	All
Slovenia	1015	116	1131	1985-1989	56.7	59.9	57.0

OBSERVED AND RELATIVE SURVIVAL (%) BY AGE (number of cases in parentheses)

	AGE CLASS										ALL	
	15-44		45-54		55-64		65-74		75-99			
	obs	rel	obs	rel	obs	rel	obs	rel	obs	rel	obs	rel
Males	(87)		(329)		(401)		(156)		(42)		(1015)	
1 year	54	54	56	57	53	54	57	60	40	45	54	55
3 years	31	32	30	31	24	25	23	27	26	36	27	28
5 years	26	26	21	22	15	16	15	19	24	43	18	20
Females	(11)		(23)		(44)		(21)		(17)		(116)	
1 year	73	73	83	83	70	71	71	73	35	38	68	70
3 years	64	64	61	62	45	47	43	46	12	16	45	48
5 years	64	64	61	62	27	29	29	33	6	10	34	39
Overall	(98)		(352)		(445)		(177)		(59)		(1131)	
1 year	56	56	58	58	54	55	59	61	39	43	55	57
3 years	35	36	32	33	26	27	25	29	22	30	28	30
5 years	30	31	23	25	16	18	16	21	19	33	20	22

HEAD & NECK (ICD-9 141,143-148)

SPAIN

AREA	NUMBER OF CASES			PERIOD	MEAN AGE			5-YR RELATIVE SURVIVAL (%)	
	Males	Females	All		Males	Females	All	Males	Females
Basque Country	671	96	767	1986-1988	57.5	62.6	58.1		
Mallorca	97	16	113	1988-1989	57.1	67.1	58.6		
Navarra	152	23	175	1985-1989	57.2	64.3	58.2		
Tarragona	153	21	174	1985-1989	58.8	62.8	59.3		
Spanish Registries	1073	156	1229		57.6	63.3	58.3		

OBSERVED AND RELATIVE SURVIVAL (%) BY AGE (number of cases in parentheses)

	AGE CLASS										ALL	
	15-44		45-54		55-64		65-74		75-99			
	obs	rel	obs	rel	obs	rel	obs	rel	obs	rel	obs	rel
Males	(139)		(250)		(397)		(207)		(80)		(1073)	
1 year	73	74	70	71	65	66	63	65	43	46	65	67
3 years	40	40	40	40	36	37	37	41	21	28	36	38
5 years	35	36	34	35	28	30	31	36	17	28	30	33
Females	(19)		(28)		(28)		(39)		(42)		(156)	
1 year	84	84	86	86	86	86	82	83	45	49	74	76
3 years	68	69	64	65	61	62	64	67	21	28	53	57
5 years	56	56	64	65	61	62	51	56	17	27	47	54
Overall	(158)		(278)		(425)		(246)		(122)		(1229)	
1 year	75	75	72	72	67	67	66	68	43	47	66	68
3 years	43	43	42	43	37	39	41	45	21	28	38	41
5 years	38	38	37	38	30	32	34	40	17	28	32	36

SWEDEN

AREA	NUMBER OF CASES			PERIOD	MEAN AGE		
	Males	Females	All		Males	Females	All
South Sweden	263	127	390	1985-1989	62.6	66.6	63.9

OBSERVED AND RELATIVE SURVIVAL (%) BY AGE (number of cases in parentheses)

	AGE CLASS										ALL	
	15-44		45-54		55-64		65-74		75-99			
	obs	rel	obs	rel	obs	rel	obs	rel	obs	rel	obs	rel
Males	(22)		(43)		(74)		(83)		(41)		(263)	
1 year	95	96	81	82	77	78	70	72	41	46	71	74
3 years	68	69	65	66	58	61	46	51	22	31	51	56
5 years	64	64	58	60	53	57	37	45	10	18	43	51
Females	(13)		(14)		(26)		(28)		(46)		(127)	
1 year	69	69	93	93	92	93	86	87	57	62	76	78
3 years	62	62	79	79	77	78	68	72	37	49	59	66
5 years	62	62	79	80	65	68	54	60	22	37	48	58
Overall	(35)		(57)		(100)		(111)		(87)		(390)	
1 year	86	86	84	85	81	82	74	76	49	55	73	75
3 years	66	66	68	69	63	65	51	56	30	41	53	59
5 years	63	63	63	65	56	60	41	49	16	29	45	53

HEAD & NECK   (ICD-9 141,143-148)

SWITZERLAND

AREA	NUMBER OF CASES			PERIOD	MEAN AGE			5-YR RELATIVE SURVIVAL (%)	
	Males	Females	All		Males	Females	All	Males	Females
Basel	94	25	119	1985-1988	57.9	66.1	59.6		
Geneva	196	60	256	1985-1989	58.6	63.5	59.8		
Swiss Registries	290	85	375		58.4	64.3	59.8		

OBSERVED AND RELATIVE SURVIVAL (%) BY AGE (number of cases in parentheses)

	AGE CLASS										ALL	
	15-44		45-54		55-64		65-74		75-99			
	obs	rel	obs	rel	obs	rel	obs	rel	obs	rel	obs	rel
Males	(32)		(74)		(103)		(55)		(26)		(290)	
1 year	94	94	74	75	76	77	56	58	46	50	71	72
3 years	62	63	44	45	50	53	35	39	27	35	45	48
5 years	59	60	39	40	37	40	15	19	27	44	35	39
Females	(7)		(17)		(22)		(13)		(26)		(85)	
1 year	100	100	82	82	76	77	62	62	50	55	69	71
3 years	57	57	44	45	62	63	54	57	31	44	47	52
5 years	57	57	38	38	57	59	54	59	19	32	41	48
Overall	(39)		(91)		(125)		(68)		(52)		(375)	
1 year	95	95	76	76	76	77	57	59	48	52	71	72
3 years	61	62	44	45	52	54	38	42	29	38	46	49
5 years	59	59	39	40	41	44	23	27	23	38	36	41

HEAD & NECK   (ICD-9 141,143-148)

EUROPE, 1985-89

Weighted analyses

COUNTRY	% COVERAGE WITH C.R.s	YEARLY NO. OF CASES (Mean No. of cases recorded) Males	Females	All
AUSTRIA	8	30	12	42
DENMARK	100	212	119	331
ENGLAND	50	655	405	1060
ESTONIA	100	78	13	91
FINLAND	100	86	60	146
FRANCE	3	360	33	393
GERMANY	2	107	21	128
ICELAND	100	4	3	7
ITALY	10	332	105	437
NETHERLANDS	6	21	13	34
POLAND	6	76	25	101
SCOTLAND	100	197	109	306
SLOVAKIA	100	453	36	489
SLOVENIA	100	203	23	226
SPAIN	10	333	49	382
SWEDEN	17	53	25	78
SWITZERLAND	11	63	18	81

RELATIVE SURVIVAL (%) (Age-standardized)

□ 1 year   ■ 5 years

OBSERVED AND RELATIVE SURVIVAL (%) BY AGE

	15-44 obs	15-44 rel	45-54 obs	45-54 rel	55-64 obs	55-64 rel	65-74 obs	65-74 rel	75-99 obs	75-99 rel	ALL obs	ALL rel
Males												
1 year	78	78	71	71	69	70	66	68	48	53	68	70
3 years	48	49	43	44	40	42	36	40	23	32	39	42
5 years	42	43	35	37	30	33	25	31	17	29	30	34
Females												
1 year	83	83	77	78	75	75	75	76	52	57	70	72
3 years	62	62	52	53	49	50	54	57	32	41	48	52
5 years	56	57	46	47	45	47	48	53	25	40	41	48
Overall												
1 year	79	79	72	72	70	71	67	70	49	54	69	70
3 years	51	51	45	45	41	43	39	43	25	33	41	44
5 years	45	45	37	39	32	35	29	34	18	31	32	37

AGE STANDARDIZED RELATIVE SURVIVAL(%)

COUNTRY	MALES 1-year (95% C.I.)	MALES 5-years (95% C.I.)	FEMALES 1-year (95% C.I.)	FEMALES 5-years (95% C.I.)
AUSTRIA	79.6 (69.5 - 91.0)	47.4 (34.3 - 65.5)	94.1 (87.3 -101.4)	51.9 (34.2 - 78.7)
DENMARK	66.8 (63.9 - 69.8)	32.7 (29.6 - 36.1)	72.7 (69.0 - 76.6)	47.0 (42.7 - 51.8)
ENGLAND	67.3 (65.6 - 69.0)	37.4 (35.5 - 39.4)	72.0 (69.9 - 74.2)	46.2 (43.7 - 48.9)
ESTONIA	49.0 (43.3 - 55.3)	17.3 (13.5 - 22.1)	52.5 (41.3 - 66.8)	14.6 (8.4 - 25.2)
FINLAND	73.8 (69.5 - 78.4)	35.3 (30.5 - 40.8)	74.4 (69.1 - 80.1)	53.9 (47.4 - 61.3)
FRANCE	69.1 (66.8 - 71.6)	31.6 (28.8 - 34.6)	75.4 (69.0 - 82.4)	56.9 (48.7 - 66.6)
GERMANY	70.6 (66.0 - 75.6)	37.3 (31.6 - 44.2)	75.2 (67.1 - 84.3)	45.4 (35.7 - 57.7)
ICELAND	81.8 (68.9 - 97.1)	44.9 (25.0 - 80.8)	94.6 (85.8 -104.3)	50.2 (30.2 - 83.5)
ITALY	70.4 (67.8 - 73.2)	34.9 (32.0 - 38.1)	74.2 (69.8 - 78.9)	45.8 (40.5 - 51.6)
NETHERLANDS	75.4 (67.2 - 84.7)	47.2 (37.8 - 58.9)	67.0 (56.1 - 79.9)	45.7 (34.3 - 60.7)
POLAND	52.0 (44.6 - 60.6)	20.2 (15.5 - 26.4)	56.8 (45.3 - 71.3)	29.7 (20.0 - 44.1)
SCOTLAND	69.3 (66.4 - 72.4)	35.4 (32.1 - 39.1)	70.5 (66.5 - 74.8)	44.4 (39.7 - 49.6)
SLOVAKIA	49.9 (47.3 - 52.6)	21.5 (18.7 - 24.7)	67.6 (60.6 - 75.3)	44.0 (36.4 - 53.2)
SLOVENIA	54.3 (50.6 - 58.3)	23.3 (19.3 - 28.1)	69.1 (61.2 - 78.0)	37.5 (29.5 - 47.6)
SPAIN	64.5 (61.5 - 67.8)	32.8 (29.5 - 36.6)	79.4 (73.4 - 86.0)	55.4 (47.2 - 65.1)
SWEDEN	74.3 (69.2 - 79.8)	49.5 (43.3 - 56.6)	84.4 (78.3 - 90.9)	62.9 (54.0 - 73.3)
SWITZERLAND	69.7 (64.2 - 75.6)	37.8 (31.7 - 45.2)	73.5 (64.4 - 83.9)	50.4 (39.6 - 64.0)
EUROPE, 1985-89	68.2 (66.7 - 69.7)	33.6 (31.7 - 35.5)	73.9 (71.4 - 76.5)	48.2 (45.0 - 51.5)

OESOPHAGUS (ICD-9 150)

AUSTRIA

AREA	NUMBER OF CASES			PERIOD	MEAN AGE		
	Males	Females	All		Males	Females	All
Tirol	28	4	32	1988-1989	63.5	62.3	63.4

OBSERVED AND RELATIVE SURVIVAL (%) BY AGE (number of cases in parentheses)

	15-44		45-54		55-64		65-74		75-99		ALL	
	obs	rel	obs	rel	obs	rel	obs	rel	obs	rel	obs	rel
Males	(2)		(6)		(5)		(9)		(6)		(28)	
1 year	50	50	17	17	20	20	33	34	50	54	32	33
3 years	50	50	0	0	0	0	22	24	33	44	18	20
5 years	50	51	0	0	0	0	11	13	33	55	14	17
Females	(0)		(1)		(1)		(1)		(1)		(4)	
1 year	-	-	0	0	100	100	0	0	0	0	25	25
3 years	-	-	0	0	0	0	0	0	0	0	0	0
5 years	-	-	0	0	0	0	0	0	0	0	0	0
Overall	(2)		(7)		(6)		(10)		(7)		(32)	
1 year	50	50	14	14	33	34	30	31	43	46	31	32
3 years	50	50	0	0	0	0	20	22	29	36	16	17
5 years	50	51	0	0	0	0	10	12	29	44	13	14

DENMARK

AREA	NUMBER OF CASES			PERIOD	MEAN AGE		
	Males	Females	All		Males	Females	All
Denmark	777	352	1129	1985-1989	67.4	72.0	68.8

OBSERVED AND RELATIVE SURVIVAL (%) BY AGE (number of cases in parentheses)

	15-44		45-54		55-64		65-74		75-99		ALL	
	obs	rel	obs	rel	obs	rel	obs	rel	obs	rel	obs	rel
Males	(24)		(82)		(186)		(264)		(221)		(777)	
1 year	25	25	28	28	20	21	19	20	15	17	19	20
3 years	4	4	7	7	3	3	5	6	4	5	4	5
5 years	4	4	5	5	2	2	2	2	0	1	2	2
Females	(3)		(23)		(68)		(100)		(158)		(352)	
1 year	0	0	48	48	37	37	32	33	19	21	28	29
3 years	0	0	13	13	12	12	14	15	4	6	9	11
5 years	0	0	9	9	7	8	12	14	4	7	7	9
Overall	(27)		(105)		(254)		(364)		(379)		(1129)	
1 year	22	22	32	33	25	25	23	23	17	18	22	23
3 years	4	4	9	9	5	5	8	9	4	6	6	7
5 years	4	4	6	6	3	3	5	6	2	3	3	5

OESOPHAGUS (ICD-9 150)

ENGLAND

AREA	NUMBER OF CASES			PERIOD	MEAN AGE			5-YR RELATIVE SURVIVAL (%)	
	Males	Females	All		Males	Females	All	Males	Females
East Anglia	549	344	893	1985-1989	69.3	74.7	71.4		
Mersey	652	532	1184	1985-1989	67.5	72.7	69.8		
Oxford	450	366	816	1985-1989	69.4	73.5	71.2		
South Thames	1339	1011	2350	1985-1989	68.8	73.8	70.9		
Wessex	892	570	1462	1985-1989	68.6	73.6	70.6		
West Midlands	1318	922	2240	1985-1989	67.5	72.3	69.5		
Yorkshire	808	589	1397	1985-1989	67.9	73.1	70.1		
English Registries	6008	4334	10342		68.3	73.3	70.4		

5-YR RELATIVE SURVIVAL (%) chart scale: 100 80 60 40 20 0 (Males) | 0 20 40 60 80 100 (Females); bars labelled E.Angl, Mersey, Oxford, S.Tham, Wessex, W.Midl, Yorksh

OBSERVED AND RELATIVE SURVIVAL (%) BY AGE (number of cases in parentheses)

	15-44 obs rel		45-54 obs rel		55-64 obs rel		65-74 obs rel		75-99 obs rel		ALL obs rel	
Males	(126)		(509)		(1429)		(2136)		(1808)		(6008)	
1 year	40	40	33	33	29	29	23	24	17	19	24	25
3 years	17	18	12	12	11	11	7	8	4	6	8	9
5 years	14	14	11	11	8	8	5	6	3	6	6	8
Females	(58)		(182)		(669)		(1210)		(2215)		(4334)	
1 year	48	48	37	37	38	38	30	31	17	18	25	26
3 years	22	23	20	20	17	17	13	14	6	7	10	12
5 years	17	17	17	17	14	15	11	12	4	7	8	11
Overall	(184)		(691)		(2098)		(3346)		(4023)		(10342)	
1 year	42	42	34	34	32	32	25	26	17	19	24	25
3 years	19	19	14	14	13	13	9	10	5	7	9	10
5 years	15	15	12	13	10	10	7	9	4	7	7	9

ESTONIA

AREA	NUMBER OF CASES			PERIOD	MEAN AGE		
	Males	Females	All		Males	Females	All
Estonia	206	37	243	1985-1989	62.4	69.6	63.5

OBSERVED AND RELATIVE SURVIVAL (%) BY AGE (number of cases in parentheses)

	15-44 obs rel		45-54 obs rel		55-64 obs rel		65-74 obs rel		75-99 obs rel		ALL obs rel	
Males	(4)		(53)		(73)		(37)		(39)		(206)	
1 year	25	25	15	15	27	28	18	19	21	24	21	22
3 years	25	26	4	4	4	4	3	4	8	12	5	6
5 years	-	-	4	4	3	3	0	0	3	5	3	4
Females	(2)		(4)		(6)		(7)		(18)		(37)	
1 year	0	0	50	50	50	51	14	15	39	43	35	37
3 years	0	0	0	0	0	0	0	0	6	8	3	3
5 years	0	0	0	0	0	0	0	0	0	0	0	0
Overall	(6)		(57)		(79)		(44)		(57)		(243)	
1 year	17	17	18	18	29	30	17	18	26	30	23	25
3 years	17	17	4	4	4	4	2	3	7	10	5	5
5 years	-	-	4	4	3	3	0	0	2	4	2	3

OESOPHAGUS (ICD-9 150)

FINLAND

AREA	NUMBER OF CASES			PERIOD	MEAN AGE		
	Males	Females	All		Males	Females	All
Finland	445	474	919	1985-1989	68.8	73.7	71.4

OBSERVED AND RELATIVE SURVIVAL (%) BY AGE (number of cases in parentheses)

	AGE CLASS										ALL	
	15-44		45-54		55-64		65-74		75-99			
	obs	rel	obs	rel	obs	rel	obs	rel	obs	rel	obs	rel
Males	(10)		(44)		(97)		(141)		(153)		(445)	
1 year	20	20	25	25	28	28	30	32	18	21	25	27
3 years	20	20	7	7	8	9	11	13	3	5	8	9
5 years	20	20	2	2	6	7	8	10	2	4	5	7
Females	(6)		(14)		(57)		(148)		(249)		(474)	
1 year	50	50	29	29	51	51	45	46	28	30	36	38
3 years	17	17	7	7	19	20	16	17	5	7	11	12
5 years	0	0	7	7	11	11	13	15	2	4	7	9
Overall	(16)		(58)		(154)		(289)		(402)		(919)	
1 year	31	31	26	26	36	37	38	39	24	27	31	33
3 years	19	19	7	7	12	13	14	15	4	6	9	11
5 years	13	13	3	4	8	8	10	13	2	4	6	8

FRANCE

AREA	NUMBER OF CASES			PERIOD	MEAN AGE			5-YR RELATIVE SURVIVAL (%)	
	Males	Females	All		Males	Females	All	Males	Females
Somme	345	31	376	1985-1989	61.1	70.9	61.9		
Calvados	436	35	471	1985-1989	62.7	67.7	63.1		
Côte d'Or	176	16	192	1985-1989	62.3	68.8	62.9		
Doubs	180	20	200	1985-1989	63.1	68.5	63.6		
French Registries	1137	102	1239		62.2	69.0	62.8		

OBSERVED AND RELATIVE SURVIVAL (%) BY AGE (number of cases in parentheses)

	AGE CLASS										ALL	
	15-44		45-54		55-64		65-74		75-99			
	obs	rel	obs	rel	obs	rel	obs	rel	obs	rel	obs	rel
Males	(55)		(221)		(432)		(247)		(182)		(1137)	
1 year	58	58	40	40	43	44	31	32	29	32	38	39
3 years	22	22	12	12	12	12	8	9	7	10	11	12
5 years	14	14	9	10	8	9	3	4	4	7	7	8
Females	(2)		(16)		(19)		(25)		(40)		(102)	
1 year	50	50	61	61	26	26	46	47	42	45	43	44
3 years	50	50	27	27	16	16	10	11	15	20	17	19
5 years	50	50	20	21	-	-	5	6	12	19	12	14
Overall	(57)		(237)		(451)		(272)		(222)		(1239)	
1 year	57	57	41	41	42	43	32	33	31	34	38	40
3 years	23	24	13	13	12	13	8	9	9	12	11	12
5 years	15	16	10	10	8	9	3	4	6	10	7	9

OESOPHAGUS (ICD-9 150)

GERMANY

AREA	NUMBER OF CASES			PERIOD	MEAN AGE		
	Males	Females	All		Males	Females	All
Saarland	196	47	243	1985-1989	60.0	70.1	62.0

OBSERVED AND RELATIVE SURVIVAL (%) BY AGE (number of cases in parentheses)

	AGE CLASS										ALL	
	15-44		45-54		55-64		65-74		75-99			
	obs	rel	obs	rel	obs	rel	obs	rel	obs	rel	obs	rel
Males	(12)		(53)		(74)		(32)		(25)		(196)	
1 year	42	42	40	40	35	36	34	36	20	22	35	36
3 years	17	17	8	8	5	6	16	18	0	0	8	8
5 years	17	17	4	4	3	3	16	21	0	0	5	6
Females	(0)		(4)		(14)		(11)		(18)		(47)	
1 year	-	-	50	50	43	43	36	37	17	18	32	33
3 years	-	-	25	25	14	15	18	20	0	0	11	12
5 years	-	-	-	-	14	15	18	21	0	0	11	14
Overall	(12)		(57)		(88)		(43)		(43)		(243)	
1 year	42	42	40	41	36	37	35	36	19	21	34	35
3 years	17	17	9	9	7	7	16	19	0	0	8	9
5 years	17	17	5	5	5	5	16	21	0	0	6	8

ICELAND

AREA	NUMBER OF CASES			PERIOD	MEAN AGE		
	Males	Females	All		Males	Females	All
Iceland	31	16	47	1985-1989	68.5	78.6	72.0

OBSERVED AND RELATIVE SURVIVAL (%) BY AGE (number of cases in parentheses)

	AGE CLASS										ALL	
	15-44		45-54		55-64		65-74		75-99			
	obs	rel	obs	rel	obs	rel	obs	rel	obs	rel	obs	rel
Males	(0)		(3)		(8)		(12)		(8)		(31)	
1 year	-	-	33	33	38	38	58	60	50	56	48	51
3 years	-	-	33	34	13	13	50	55	0	0	26	30
5 years	-	-	33	34	13	13	42	50	0	0	23	28
Females	(0)		(0)		(0)		(6)		(10)		(16)	
1 year	-	-	-	-	-	-	33	34	20	23	25	27
3 years	-	-	-	-	-	-	33	36	10	14	19	24
5 years	-	-	-	-	-	-	33	38	0	0	13	18
Overall	(0)		(3)		(8)		(18)		(18)		(47)	
1 year	-	-	33	33	38	38	50	51	33	38	40	43
3 years	-	-	33	34	13	13	44	49	6	8	23	28
5 years	-	-	33	34	13	13	39	46	0	0	19	25

OESOPHAGUS (ICD-9 150)

ITALY

AREA	NUMBER OF CASES			PERIOD	MEAN AGE		
	Males	Females	All		Males	Females	All
Florence	161	60	221	1985-1989	66.8	72.7	68.4
Genoa	65	24	89	1986-1988	66.5	71.1	67.7
Latina	17	3	20	1985-1987	65.1	70.3	65.9
Modena	20	11	31	1988-1989	64.0	76.3	68.4
Parma	40	8	48	1985-1987	64.2	70.0	65.1
Ragusa	15	3	18	1985-1989	71.6	67.7	71.0
Romagna	22	9	31	1986-1988	66.1	67.7	66.6
Turin	86	31	117	1985-1987	63.1	68.4	64.5
Varese	188	27	215	1985-1989	63.3	72.5	64.4
Italian Registries	614	176	790		65.0	71.5	66.4

5-YR RELATIVE SURVIVAL (%)

Males — Females

Floren, Genoa, Latina, Modena, Parma, Ragusa, Romagn, Turin, Varese

OBSERVED AND RELATIVE SURVIVAL (%) BY AGE (number of cases in parentheses)

	15-44		45-54		55-64		65-74		75-99		ALL	
	obs	rel	obs	rel	obs	rel	obs	rel	obs	rel	obs	rel
Males	(17)		(84)		(207)		(171)		(135)		(614)	
1 year	41	41	37	37	30	31	23	24	20	23	27	28
3 years	24	24	15	16	10	11	4	4	5	6	8	9
5 years	18	18	13	14	6	6	3	4	3	5	6	7
Females	(2)		(14)		(34)		(41)		(85)		(176)	
1 year	50	50	50	50	21	21	37	37	23	24	28	29
3 years	50	50	30	30	12	12	15	15	6	8	12	14
5 years	50	50	29	29	12	12	10	11	6	9	10	13
Overall	(19)		(98)		(241)		(212)		(220)		(790)	
1 year	42	42	39	39	29	29	26	27	21	23	28	29
3 years	26	26	18	19	10	11	6	6	5	7	9	10
5 years	21	21	15	16	7	7	4	5	4	7	7	8

NETHERLANDS

AREA	NUMBER OF CASES			PERIOD	MEAN AGE		
	Males	Females	All		Males	Females	All
Eindhoven	75	30	105	1985-1989	64.1	65.8	64.6

OBSERVED AND RELATIVE SURVIVAL (%) BY AGE (number of cases in parentheses)

	15-44		45-54		55-64		65-74		75-99		ALL	
	obs	rel	obs	rel	obs	rel	obs	rel	obs	rel	obs	rel
Males	(2)		(12)		(23)		(28)		(10)		(75)	
1 year	50	50	50	50	30	31	29	30	40	45	35	36
3 years	50	50	8	8	4	5	14	17	0	0	9	10
5 years	50	50	8	9	4	5	11	14	0	0	8	10
Females	(1)		(6)		(5)		(8)		(10)		(30)	
1 year	100	100	67	67	40	40	38	38	30	32	43	44
3 years	100	100	17	17	20	20	25	26	0	0	17	18
5 years	100	100	17	17	20	21	25	28	0	0	17	19
Overall	(3)		(18)		(28)		(36)		(20)		(105)	
1 year	67	67	56	56	32	33	31	32	35	38	37	38
3 years	67	67	11	11	7	7	17	19	0	0	11	13
5 years	67	67	11	11	7	8	14	17	0	0	10	12

OESOPHAGUS (ICD-9 150)

POLAND

AREA	NUMBER OF CASES			PERIOD	MEAN AGE			5-YR RELATIVE SURVIVAL (%)	
	Males	Females	All		Males	Females	All	Males	Females
Cracow	74	21	95	1985-1989	62.8	65.8	63.4		
Warsaw	91	33	124	1988-1989	63.5	72.1	65.8		
Polish Registries	165	54	219		63.2	69.7	64.8		

OBSERVED AND RELATIVE SURVIVAL (%) BY AGE (number of cases in parentheses)

	AGE CLASS										ALL	
	15-44		45-54		55-64		65-74		75-99			
	obs	rel	obs	rel	obs	rel	obs	rel	obs	rel	obs	rel
Males	(6)		(33)		(59)		(33)		(34)		(165)	
1 year	33	33	18	18	20	21	18	19	15	17	19	20
3 years	17	17	3	3	3	4	3	4	6	9	4	5
5 years	17	17	0	0	2	2	3	4	3	6	2	3
Females	(0)		(6)		(10)		(18)		(20)		(54)	
1 year	-	-	0	0	20	20	0	0	30	33	15	15
3 years	-	-	0	0	10	10	0	0	5	7	4	4
5 years	-	-	0	0	10	11	0	0	5	8	4	5
Overall	(6)		(39)		(69)		(51)		(54)		(219)	
1 year	33	33	15	16	20	21	12	12	20	23	18	19
3 years	17	17	3	3	4	5	2	2	6	8	4	5
5 years	17	17	0	0	3	3	2	3	4	7	3	3

SCOTLAND

AREA	NUMBER OF CASES			PERIOD	MEAN AGE		
	Males	Females	All		Males	Females	All
Scotland	1457	1193	2650	1985-1989	67.4	73.0	69.9

OBSERVED AND RELATIVE SURVIVAL (%) BY AGE (number of cases in parentheses)

	AGE CLASS										ALL	
	15-44		45-54		55-64		65-74		75-99			
	obs	rel	obs	rel	obs	rel	obs	rel	obs	rel	obs	rel
Males	(41)		(136)		(370)		(511)		(399)		(1457)	
1 year	34	34	29	30	27	27	27	28	12	13	23	25
3 years	15	15	12	12	9	9	7	8	4	5	7	8
5 years	12	12	5	5	6	7	4	5	2	4	4	6
Females	(10)		(51)		(200)		(341)		(591)		(1193)	
1 year	60	60	41	41	35	35	29	30	15	16	24	25
3 years	30	30	20	20	14	15	12	14	4	6	9	11
5 years	30	30	14	14	12	12	9	11	3	5	7	9
Overall	(51)		(187)		(570)		(852)		(990)		(2650)	
1 year	39	39	33	33	30	30	28	29	14	15	23	25
3 years	18	18	14	14	11	11	9	10	4	6	8	9
5 years	16	16	7	8	8	9	6	8	3	5	5	7

OESOPHAGUS (ICD-9 150)

SLOVAKIA

AREA	NUMBER OF CASES			PERIOD	MEAN AGE		
	Males	Females	All		Males	Females	All
Slovakia	755	81	836	1985-1989	59.5	68.2	60.4

OBSERVED AND RELATIVE SURVIVAL (%) BY AGE (number of cases in parentheses)

	AGE CLASS										ALL	
	15-44		45-54		55-64		65-74		75-99			
	obs	rel	obs	rel	obs	rel	obs	rel	obs	rel	obs	rel
Males	(62)		(206)		(251)		(139)		(97)		(755)	
1 year	19	19	21	21	16	16	18	19	11	13	17	18
3 years	6	7	7	7	7	7	7	9	4	6	6	7
5 years	6	7	6	7	6	7	5	7	4	8	6	7
Females	(2)		(8)		(25)		(16)		(30)		(81)	
1 year	0	0	25	25	32	32	13	13	17	19	21	22
3 years	0	0	25	25	24	25	6	7	13	19	16	19
5 years	0	0	13	13	16	17	6	8	13	24	12	15
Overall	(64)		(214)		(276)		(155)		(127)		(836)	
1 year	19	19	21	21	17	17	17	18	13	14	18	18
3 years	6	6	7	8	8	9	7	8	6	9	7	8
5 years	6	6	6	7	7	8	5	7	6	12	6	8

SLOVENIA

AREA	NUMBER OF CASES			PERIOD	MEAN AGE		
	Males	Females	All		Males	Females	All
Slovenia	354	49	403	1985-1989	61.1	69.9	62.1

OBSERVED AND RELATIVE SURVIVAL (%) BY AGE (number of cases in parentheses)

	AGE CLASS										ALL	
	15-44		45-54		55-64		65-74		75-99			
	obs	rel	obs	rel	obs	rel	obs	rel	obs	rel	obs	rel
Males	(16)		(86)		(132)		(69)		(51)		(354)	
1 year	25	25	23	23	25	26	17	18	14	16	22	22
3 years	13	13	3	4	5	6	3	3	6	9	5	5
5 years	0	0	3	4	5	5	1	2	2	4	3	4
Females	(0)		(7)		(11)		(9)		(22)		(49)	
1 year	-	-	29	29	18	18	22	23	5	5	14	15
3 years	-	-	14	14	0	0	11	12	0	0	4	5
5 years	-	-	0	0	0	0	0	0	0	0	0	0
Overall	(16)		(93)		(143)		(78)		(73)		(403)	
1 year	25	25	24	24	25	25	18	19	11	13	21	22
3 years	13	13	4	4	5	5	4	4	4	6	5	5
5 years	0	0	3	3	4	5	1	2	1	3	3	3

OESOPHAGUS (ICD-9 150)

SPAIN

AREA	NUMBER OF CASES			PERIOD	MEAN AGE			5-YR RELATIVE SURVIVAL (%)	
	Males	Females	All		Males	Females	All	Males	Females
Basque Country	355	33	388	1986-1988	60.3	71.2	61.2		
Mallorca	39	5	44	1988-1989	59.8	77.4	61.8		
Navarra	108	16	124	1985-1989	61.5	67.7	62.3		
Tarragona	87	3	90	1985-1989	62.0	73.7	62.4		
Spanish Registries	589	57	646		60.7	71.0	61.6		

OBSERVED AND RELATIVE SURVIVAL (%) BY AGE (number of cases in parentheses)

	AGE CLASS										ALL	
	15-44		45-54		55-64		65-74		75-99			
	obs	rel	obs	rel	obs	rel	obs	rel	obs	rel	obs	rel
Males	(46)		(134)		(194)		(147)		(68)		(589)	
1 year	33	33	34	35	35	35	28	29	25	28	32	33
3 years	13	13	7	8	12	12	10	11	9	12	10	11
5 years	13	13	4	4	9	10	6	7	5	9	7	8
Females	(3)		(6)		(8)		(11)		(29)		(57)	
1 year	33	33	50	50	75	75	45	46	28	30	40	42
3 years	33	33	33	34	50	51	0	0	14	18	19	22
5 years	33	33	17	17	38	38	0	0	-	-	13	17
Overall	(49)		(140)		(202)		(158)		(97)		(646)	
1 year	33	33	35	35	37	37	29	30	26	28	33	33
3 years	14	14	9	9	13	14	9	11	10	14	11	12
5 years	14	14	4	5	10	11	5	7	6	10	8	9

SWEDEN

AREA	NUMBER OF CASES			PERIOD	MEAN AGE		
	Males	Females	All		Males	Females	All
South Sweden	220	79	299	1985-1989	68.9	73.4	70.1

OBSERVED AND RELATIVE SURVIVAL (%) BY AGE (number of cases in parentheses)

	AGE CLASS										ALL	
	15-44		45-54		55-64		65-74		75-99			
	obs	rel	obs	rel	obs	rel	obs	rel	obs	rel	obs	rel
Males	(0)		(14)		(53)		(92)		(61)		(220)	
1 year	-	-	50	50	34	34	34	35	25	27	32	34
3 years	-	-	36	36	11	12	13	15	10	14	13	15
5 years	-	-	36	37	9	10	9	11	3	6	9	12
Females	(0)		(4)		(7)		(29)		(39)		(79)	
1 year	-	-	50	50	100	100	45	46	26	28	41	42
3 years	-	-	50	50	86	88	21	22	8	10	22	25
5 years	-	-	50	51	57	59	17	19	5	8	16	21
Overall	(0)		(18)		(60)		(121)		(100)		(299)	
1 year	-	-	50	50	42	42	36	37	25	27	34	36
3 years	-	-	39	39	20	21	15	16	9	12	15	18
5 years	-	-	39	40	15	16	11	13	4	7	11	14

OESOPHAGUS (ICD-9 150)

SWITZERLAND

AREA	NUMBER OF CASES			PERIOD	MEAN AGE			5-YR RELATIVE SURVIVAL (%)	
	Males	Females	All		Males	Females	All	Males	Females
Basel	47	19	66	1985-1988	66.0	73.2	68.1		
Geneva	80	22	102	1985-1989	63.3	68.6	64.5		
Swiss Registries	127	41	168		64.3	70.8	65.9		

100 80 60 40 20 0   0 20 40 60 80 100

Basel
Geneva

OBSERVED AND RELATIVE SURVIVAL (%) BY AGE (number of cases in parentheses)

	AGE CLASS										ALL	
	15-44		45-54		55-64		65-74		75-99			
	obs	rel	obs	rel	obs	rel	obs	rel	obs	rel	obs	rel
Males	(4)		(22)		(42)		(34)		(25)		(127)	
1 year	50	50	32	32	45	46	38	40	12	13	35	36
3 years	25	25	18	18	26	27	18	20	4	6	18	20
5 years	25	25	14	14	19	21	12	14	0	0	13	15
Females	(2)		(3)		(8)		(10)		(18)		(41)	
1 year	50	50	67	67	63	63	60	61	22	24	44	46
3 years	50	50	33	34	13	13	10	11	11	14	15	17
5 years	50	50	0	0	13	13	10	11	6	9	10	12
Overall	(6)		(25)		(50)		(44)		(43)		(168)	
1 year	50	50	36	36	48	49	43	45	16	18	37	38
3 years	33	34	20	20	24	25	16	18	7	10	17	19
5 years	33	34	12	12	18	19	11	14	2	4	12	15

OESOPHAGUS   (ICD-9 150)

EUROPE, 1985-89

Weighted analyses

COUNTRY	% COVERAGE WITH C.R.s	YEARLY NO. OF CASES (Mean No. of cases recorded)			RELATIVE SURVIVAL (%) (Age-standardized)
		Males	Females	All	
AUSTRIA	8	14	2	16	
DENMARK	100	155	70	225	
ENGLAND	50	1202	867	2069	
ESTONIA	100	41	7	48	
FINLAND	100	89	95	184	
FRANCE	4	227	20	247	
GERMANY	2	39	9	48	
ICELAND	100	6	3	9	
ITALY	10	160	49	209	
NETHERLANDS	6	15	6	21	
POLAND	6	60	21	81	
SCOTLAND	100	291	239	530	
SLOVAKIA	100	151	16	167	
SLOVENIA	100	71	10	81	
SPAIN	10	177	17	194	
SWEDEN	17	44	16	60	
SWITZERLAND	11	28	9	37	

□ 1 year ■ 5 years

OBSERVED AND RELATIVE SURVIVAL (%) BY AGE

	AGE CLASS										ALL	
	15-44		45-54		55-64		65-74		75-99			
	obs	rel	obs	rel	obs	rel	obs	rel	obs	rel	obs	rel
Males												
1 year	45	45	36	36	35	36	28	29	23	26	32	33
3 years	20	20	11	11	10	10	9	10	6	8	9	10
5 years	16	16	8	8	7	7	6	7	3	6	6	8
Females												
1 year	49	49	42	42	38	38	33	33	22	24	29	31
3 years	34	34	22	23	18	18	12	13	6	8	11	13
5 years	31	31	17	17	15	16	10	11	5	7	9	12
Overall												
1 year	46	46	37	37	36	36	29	30	23	25	31	32
3 years	23	23	13	13	11	12	10	11	6	8	10	11
5 years	19	19	10	10	9	9	7	8	4	7	7	9

AGE STANDARDIZED RELATIVE SURVIVAL(%)

COUNTRY	MALES		FEMALES	
	1-year (95% C.I.)	5-years (95% C.I.)	1-year (95% C.I.)	5-years (95% C.I.)
AUSTRIA	36.4 (21.2 - 62.5)	23.7 (9.3 - 60.5)	-	-
DENMARK	19.9 (17.2 - 23.1)	2.1 (1.2 - 3.5)	30.5 (25.9 - 35.9)	9.1 (6.3 - 13.3)
ENGLAND	24.8 (23.7 - 26.0)	7.4 (6.7 - 8.2)	29.2 (27.8 - 30.8)	11.5 (10.4 - 12.8)
ESTONIA	22.5 (16.5 - 30.6)	-	35.9 (23.1 - 55.8)	0.0 (0.0 - 0.0)
FINLAND	26.3 (22.4 - 30.9)	6.7 (4.5 - 10.0)	40.4 (35.5 - 45.9)	9.1 (6.4 - 12.9)
FRANCE	36.1 (32.9 - 39.6)	7.2 (5.2 - 9.9)	43.0 (34.0 - 54.4)	-
GERMANY	31.9 (24.5 - 41.6)	7.8 (4.0 - 15.1)	-	-
ICELAND	-	-	-	-
ITALY	26.9 (23.4 - 31.0)	6.2 (4.3 - 9.0)	30.7 (24.3 - 38.7)	13.4 (8.8 - 20.5)
NETHERLANDS	37.7 (26.2 - 54.5)	7.4 (3.5 - 15.6)	41.0 (26.4 - 63.7)	17.5 (8.1 - 37.9)
POLAND	19.0 (13.2 - 27.2)	4.1 (1.3 - 12.6)	-	-
SCOTLAND	23.3 (21.2 - 25.6)	5.3 (4.1 - 6.9)	28.6 (25.8 - 31.6)	10.1 (8.2 - 12.5)
SLOVAKIA	16.4 (13.3 - 20.1)	7.3 (4.7 - 11.3)	20.3 (13.1 - 31.4)	15.7 (8.5 - 29.0)
SLOVENIA	20.0 (15.5 - 25.8)	3.5 (1.5 - 8.4)	-	-
SPAIN	30.7 (26.2 - 35.9)	8.3 (5.2 - 13.3)	47.7 (35.8 - 63.4)	-
SWEDEN	-	-	-	-
SWITZERLAND	31.7 (24.5 - 41.1)	11.2 (7.0 - 18.0)	49.2 (36.2 - 67.0)	10.7 (4.1 - 28.1)
EUROPE, 1985-89	30.7 (28.9 - 32.6)	7.4 (6.1 - 8.9)	32.6 (30.2 - 35.3)	12.2 (10.3 - 14.4)

STOMACH (ICD-9 151)

AUSTRIA

AREA	NUMBER OF CASES			PERIOD	MEAN AGE		
	Males	Females	All		Males	Females	All
Tirol	174	188	362	1988-1989	69.0	71.9	70.5

OBSERVED AND RELATIVE SURVIVAL (%) BY AGE (number of cases in parentheses)

	AGE CLASS										ALL	
	15-44		45-54		55-64		65-74		75-99			
	obs	rel	obs	rel	obs	rel	obs	rel	obs	rel	obs	rel
Males	(7)		(9)		(44)		(49)		(65)		(174)	
1 year	71	72	44	45	50	51	37	38	40	44	43	45
3 years	43	43	33	34	32	33	20	22	18	25	24	28
5 years	43	43	33	34	32	34	12	14	12	20	20	25
Females	(9)		(11)		(20)		(50)		(98)		(188)	
1 year	44	44	73	73	65	65	62	63	42	45	52	54
3 years	44	45	55	55	40	41	40	42	22	28	32	36
5 years	44	45	45	46	25	26	32	35	17	25	25	31
Overall	(16)		(20)		(64)		(99)		(163)		(362)	
1 year	56	56	60	60	55	55	49	51	41	44	48	50
3 years	44	44	45	45	34	36	30	32	21	26	28	32
5 years	44	44	40	41	30	31	22	25	15	24	22	28

DENMARK

AREA	NUMBER OF CASES			PERIOD	MEAN AGE		
	Males	Females	All		Males	Females	All
Denmark	2110	1435	3545	1985-1989	69.4	72.5	70.6

OBSERVED AND RELATIVE SURVIVAL (%) BY AGE (number of cases in parentheses)

	AGE CLASS										ALL	
	15-44		45-54		55-64		65-74		75-99			
	obs	rel	obs	rel	obs	rel	obs	rel	obs	rel	obs	rel
Males	(69)		(172)		(398)		(703)		(768)		(2110)	
1 year	41	41	43	43	35	36	33	35	20	22	30	32
3 years	19	19	21	21	17	18	16	18	8	11	14	16
5 years	12	12	17	18	12	13	12	15	5	9	9	13
Females	(51)		(88)		(183)		(374)		(739)		(1435)	
1 year	31	31	41	41	37	38	37	38	19	21	28	29
3 years	14	14	20	21	22	23	22	24	8	11	15	17
5 years	8	8	18	19	18	19	17	20	5	9	11	15
Overall	(120)		(260)		(581)		(1077)		(1507)		(3545)	
1 year	37	37	42	43	36	36	35	36	19	21	29	31
3 years	17	17	21	21	18	19	18	20	8	11	14	17
5 years	10	10	18	18	14	15	13	17	5	9	10	14

STOMACH (ICD-9 151)

ENGLAND

AREA	NUMBER OF CASES			PERIOD	MEAN AGE			5-YR RELATIVE SURVIVAL (%)	
	Males	Females	All		Males	Females	All	Males	Females
East Anglia	1162	617	1779	1985-1989	71.0	75.2	72.4		
Mersey	1573	1081	2654	1985-1989	68.9	74.0	71.0		
Oxford	1379	783	2162	1985-1989	69.5	74.0	71.1		
South Thames	2854	1710	4564	1985-1989	70.1	74.4	71.7		
Wessex	1686	889	2575	1985-1989	70.5	74.9	72.0		
West Midlands	3695	2149	5844	1985-1989	69.0	73.8	70.8		
Yorkshire	2257	1457	3714	1985-1989	68.4	74.5	70.8		
English Registries	14606	8686	23292		69.5	74.3	71.3		

OBSERVED AND RELATIVE SURVIVAL (%) BY AGE (number of cases in parentheses)

	AGE CLASS										ALL	
	15-44		45-54		55-64		65-74		75-99			
	obs	rel	obs	rel	obs	rel	obs	rel	obs	rel	obs	rel
Males	(297)		(941)		(3011)		(5251)		(5106)		(14606)	
1 year	39	39	40	40	34	34	26	27	18	20	26	27
3 years	23	23	21	21	17	18	11	13	7	10	12	14
5 years	21	21	16	17	13	14	8	10	5	9	9	12
Females	(159)		(292)		(1042)		(2306)		(4887)		(8686)	
1 year	43	43	49	49	38	38	31	32	19	20	26	27
3 years	26	26	26	27	18	19	15	16	7	9	11	14
5 years	23	23	21	22	15	16	12	13	5	8	9	12
Overall	(456)		(1233)		(4053)		(7557)		(9993)		(23292)	
1 year	40	40	42	42	35	35	27	28	18	20	26	27
3 years	24	24	22	22	17	18	12	14	7	10	12	14
5 years	22	22	17	18	14	15	9	11	5	8	9	12

ESTONIA

AREA	NUMBER OF CASES			PERIOD	MEAN AGE		
	Males	Females	All		Males	Females	All
Estonia	1372	1167	2539	1985-1989	62.1	66.4	64.1

OBSERVED AND RELATIVE SURVIVAL (%) BY AGE (number of cases in parentheses)

	AGE CLASS										ALL	
	15-44		45-54		55-64		65-74		75-99			
	obs	rel	obs	rel	obs	rel	obs	rel	obs	rel	obs	rel
Males	(97)		(250)		(439)		(336)		(250)		(1372)	
1 year	45	46	48	49	35	36	31	33	22	25	35	37
3 years	25	25	30	31	19	21	16	19	9	13	19	22
5 years	23	23	24	26	16	19	11	15	6	11	15	19
Females	(78)		(135)		(267)		(322)		(365)		(1167)	
1 year	44	44	59	59	43	44	32	33	22	24	35	37
3 years	21	21	31	32	28	29	15	16	9	12	18	21
5 years	17	17	28	29	23	25	11	13	7	12	15	19
Overall	(175)		(385)		(706)		(658)		(615)		(2539)	
1 year	45	45	52	52	38	39	32	33	22	24	35	37
3 years	23	23	30	31	22	24	16	18	9	12	19	21
5 years	20	20	26	27	19	21	11	14	6	12	15	19

STOMACH (ICD-9 151)

FINLAND

AREA	NUMBER OF CASES			PERIOD	MEAN AGE		
	Males	Females	All		Males	Females	All
Finland	2553	2257	4810	1985-1989	67.7	70.9	69.2

OBSERVED AND RELATIVE SURVIVAL (%) BY AGE (number of cases in parentheses)

	AGE CLASS										ALL	
	15-44		45-54		55-64		65-74		75-99			
	obs	rel	obs	rel	obs	rel	obs	rel	obs	rel	obs	rel
Males	(106)		(230)		(608)		(798)		(811)		(2553)	
1 year	49	49	51	51	48	49	38	40	26	29	38	40
3 years	36	36	29	30	28	30	19	22	11	16	20	24
5 years	31	32	21	22	23	26	15	20	8	14	16	21
Females	(115)		(149)		(324)		(614)		(1055)		(2257)	
1 year	50	50	57	57	55	55	38	39	27	30	37	39
3 years	27	27	37	37	33	34	23	24	12	17	21	24
5 years	23	23	31	31	29	30	17	20	8	13	16	20
Overall	(221)		(379)		(932)		(1412)		(1866)		(4810)	
1 year	50	50	53	54	50	51	38	40	27	30	38	40
3 years	31	31	32	33	30	31	21	23	12	16	20	24
5 years	27	27	25	26	25	27	16	20	8	14	16	21

FRANCE

AREA	NUMBER OF CASES			PERIOD	MEAN AGE			5-YR RELATIVE SURVIVAL (%)	
	Males	Females	All		Males	Females	All	Males	Females
Somme	242	155	397	1985-1989	70.4	74.0	71.8		
Calvados	270	161	431	1985-1989	69.2	73.3	70.7		
Côte d'Or	212	137	349	1985-1989	69.2	74.4	71.2		
Doubs	189	113	302	1985-1989	66.8	73.7	69.4		
French Registries	913	566	1479		69.0	73.8	70.9		

OBSERVED AND RELATIVE SURVIVAL (%) BY AGE (number of cases in parentheses)

	AGE CLASS										ALL	
	15-44		45-54		55-64		65-74		75-99			
	obs	rel	obs	rel	obs	rel	obs	rel	obs	rel	obs	rel
Males	(25)		(78)		(200)		(287)		(323)		(913)	
1 year	63	63	59	59	48	49	48	50	29	33	43	45
3 years	41	41	36	36	32	33	26	29	13	18	24	28
5 years	36	36	31	33	27	29	20	25	9	17	19	25
Females	(21)		(26)		(68)		(123)		(328)		(566)	
1 year	54	54	69	69	59	59	55	56	41	45	48	51
3 years	43	43	48	49	34	34	29	31	19	26	25	30
5 years	38	38	35	36	31	32	25	28	12	20	19	26
Overall	(46)		(104)		(268)		(410)		(651)		(1479)	
1 year	59	59	61	62	51	52	50	52	35	39	45	47
3 years	42	42	39	39	32	34	27	30	16	22	24	29
5 years	37	37	32	33	28	30	21	26	10	19	19	25

STOMACH   (ICD-9 151)

GERMANY

AREA	NUMBER OF CASES			PERIOD	MEAN AGE		
	Males	Females	All		Males	Females	All
Saarland	686	621	1307	1985-1989	67.0	71.4	69.1

OBSERVED AND RELATIVE SURVIVAL (%) BY AGE (number of cases in parentheses)

	AGE CLASS										ALL	
	15-44		45-54		55-64		65-74		75-99			
	obs	rel	obs	rel	obs	rel	obs	rel	obs	rel	obs	rel
Males	(27)		(83)		(170)		(183)		(223)		(686)	
1 year	67	67	51	51	51	52	41	43	30	33	42	44
3 years	48	49	34	34	29	31	27	31	13	19	25	29
5 years	48	49	27	28	22	25	21	27	9	19	19	26
Females	(22)		(47)		(78)		(176)		(298)		(621)	
1 year	82	82	68	68	49	49	40	41	31	34	40	42
3 years	68	68	51	52	36	37	26	28	17	22	26	31
5 years	50	51	42	43	32	33	22	26	11	19	21	27
Overall	(49)		(130)		(248)		(359)		(521)		(1307)	
1 year	73	74	57	57	50	51	41	42	30	33	41	43
3 years	57	58	40	41	31	33	26	30	15	21	25	30
5 years	49	49	33	34	25	27	21	26	10	19	20	27

ICELAND

AREA	NUMBER OF CASES			PERIOD	MEAN AGE		
	Males	Females	All		Males	Females	All
Iceland	166	84	250	1985-1989	68.5	72.6	69.9

OBSERVED AND RELATIVE SURVIVAL (%) BY AGE (number of cases in parentheses)

	AGE CLASS										ALL	
	15-44		45-54		55-64		65-74		75-99			
	obs	rel	obs	rel	obs	rel	obs	rel	obs	rel	obs	rel
Males	(8)		(13)		(34)		(55)		(56)		(166)	
1 year	88	88	62	62	53	54	38	39	23	26	40	42
3 years	50	50	15	16	26	27	22	24	18	25	22	26
5 years	38	38	8	8	24	25	20	24	7	12	16	21
Females	(2)		(6)		(12)		(21)		(43)		(84)	
1 year	100	100	50	50	67	67	52	53	37	41	48	50
3 years	100	100	17	17	58	60	43	46	21	28	33	39
5 years	100	100	17	17	50	52	29	32	12	19	24	31
Overall	(10)		(19)		(46)		(76)		(99)		(250)	
1 year	90	90	58	58	57	57	42	43	29	32	43	45
3 years	60	60	16	16	35	36	28	30	19	26	26	30
5 years	50	50	11	11	30	32	22	26	9	16	19	24

STOMACH (ICD-9 151)

ITALY

AREA	NUMBER OF CASES			PERIOD	MEAN AGE			5-YR RELATIVE SURVIVAL (%)	
	Males	Females	All		Males	Females	All	Males	Females
Florence	1941	1342	3283	1985-1989	69.4	73.2	70.9		
Genoa	377	294	671	1986-1988	69.3	72.7	70.8		
Latina	138	87	225	1985-1987	66.1	66.2	66.2		
Modena	270	189	459	1988-1989	68.5	71.9	69.9		
Parma	422	282	704	1985-1987	69.5	73.0	70.9		
Ragusa	178	108	286	1985-1989	71.3	71.7	71.5		
Romagna	480	343	823	1986-1988	70.0	72.7	71.1		
Turin	438	297	735	1985-1987	66.4	70.2	67.9		
Varese	753	579	1332	1985-1989	67.6	72.2	69.6		
Italian Registries	4997	3521	8518		68.8	72.4	70.3		

OBSERVED AND RELATIVE SURVIVAL (%) BY AGE (number of cases in parentheses)

	AGE CLASS										ALL	
	15-44		45-54		55-64		65-74		75-99			
	obs	rel	obs	rel	obs	rel	obs	rel	obs	rel	obs	rel
Males	(142)		(398)		(1117)		(1610)		(1730)		(4997)	
1 year	68	68	57	57	47	48	38	40	31	34	40	42
3 years	53	53	40	40	28	29	20	23	12	17	22	25
5 years	49	50	35	36	22	24	16	19	8	13	17	22
Females	(104)		(195)		(506)		(907)		(1809)		(3521)	
1 year	57	57	64	64	59	60	48	49	35	38	44	46
3 years	38	38	45	45	38	38	32	33	18	22	26	30
5 years	33	33	39	40	33	34	27	29	13	20	21	27
Overall	(246)		(593)		(1623)		(2517)		(3539)		(8518)	
1 year	63	63	59	59	51	51	42	43	33	36	42	44
3 years	46	46	41	42	31	32	24	27	15	20	23	27
5 years	42	42	36	37	25	27	20	23	10	17	19	24

NETHERLANDS

AREA	NUMBER OF CASES			PERIOD	MEAN AGE			5-YR RELATIVE SURVIVAL (%)	
	Males	Females	All		Males	Females	All	Males	Females
Eindhoven	467	310	777	1985-1989	66.9	71.7	68.8		
Rotterdam	165	84	249	1987-1989	70.3	75.0	71.9		
Dutch Registries	632	394	1026		67.8	72.4	69.5		

OBSERVED AND RELATIVE SURVIVAL (%) BY AGE (number of cases in parentheses)

	AGE CLASS										ALL	
	15-44		45-54		55-64		65-74		75-99			
	obs	rel	obs	rel	obs	rel	obs	rel	obs	rel	obs	rel
Males	(24)		(66)		(132)		(226)		(184)		(632)	
1 year	63	63	45	45	49	50	38	40	29	33	40	42
3 years	37	37	28	28	18	19	19	22	11	17	18	22
5 years	31	32	23	24	17	18	15	20	7	14	15	19
Females	(15)		(17)		(48)		(111)		(203)		(394)	
1 year	73	73	53	53	50	50	40	40	26	29	36	38
3 years	47	47	35	36	33	34	23	25	13	17	21	24
5 years	40	40	29	30	31	32	18	20	9	14	16	21
Overall	(39)		(83)		(180)		(337)		(387)		(1026)	
1 year	67	67	46	47	49	50	39	40	28	31	38	40
3 years	41	41	29	30	22	23	21	23	12	17	19	23
5 years	35	35	24	25	21	22	16	20	8	14	15	20

STOMACH (ICD-9 151)

POLAND

AREA	NUMBER OF CASES			PERIOD	MEAN AGE			5-YR RELATIVE SURVIVAL (%)	
	Males	Females	All		Males	Females	All	Males	Females
Cracow	397	215	612	1985-1989	65.5	69.9	67.1		
Warsaw	354	214	568	1988-1989	66.9	69.0	67.7		
Polish Registries	751	429	1180		66.2	69.4	67.4		

OBSERVED AND RELATIVE SURVIVAL (%) BY AGE (number of cases in parentheses)

	AGE CLASS										ALL	
	15-44		45-54		55-64		65-74		75-99			
	obs	rel	obs	rel	obs	rel	obs	rel	obs	rel	obs	rel
Males	(32)		(78)		(212)		(223)		(206)		(751)	
1 year	41	41	27	27	27	28	23	24	15	17	23	25
3 years	19	19	14	15	13	15	9	11	5	7	10	12
5 years	16	16	12	12	10	12	7	9	2	5	7	10
Females	(28)		(21)		(82)		(110)		(188)		(429)	
1 year	54	54	43	43	32	33	25	26	16	17	25	26
3 years	36	36	19	19	17	18	14	15	5	7	12	14
5 years	29	29	14	15	15	16	9	11	3	4	9	11
Overall	(60)		(99)		(294)		(333)		(394)		(1180)	
1 year	47	47	30	31	29	29	24	25	15	17	24	25
3 years	27	27	15	16	14	16	11	12	5	7	11	13
5 years	22	22	12	13	12	13	7	10	3	5	8	11

SCOTLAND

AREA	NUMBER OF CASES			PERIOD	MEAN AGE		
	Males	Females	All		Males	Females	All
Scotland	3294	2303	5597	1985-1989	68.6	73.0	70.4

OBSERVED AND RELATIVE SURVIVAL (%) BY AGE (number of cases in parentheses)

	AGE CLASS										ALL	
	15-44		45-54		55-64		65-74		75-99			
	obs	rel	obs	rel	obs	rel	obs	rel	obs	rel	obs	rel
Males	(66)		(248)		(773)		(1174)		(1033)		(3294)	
1 year	39	39	35	35	31	32	27	28	18	21	26	28
3 years	18	18	17	17	14	15	12	14	7	10	11	13
5 years	18	18	13	13	10	11	8	11	3	7	7	10
Females	(46)		(93)		(345)		(658)		(1161)		(2303)	
1 year	43	44	47	48	34	35	30	31	16	18	25	26
3 years	26	26	34	35	16	17	14	15	6	9	12	14
5 years	26	26	32	33	14	15	10	12	4	7	9	12
Overall	(112)		(341)		(1118)		(1832)		(2194)		(5597)	
1 year	41	41	38	38	32	33	28	29	17	19	25	27
3 years	21	22	22	22	15	16	13	14	6	9	11	14
5 years	21	22	18	19	11	12	9	11	4	7	8	11

STOMACH   (ICD-9 151)

SLOVAKIA

AREA	NUMBER OF CASES			PERIOD	MEAN AGE		
	Males	Females	All		Males	Females	All
Slovakia	3263	1938	5201	1985-1989	65.6	67.7	66.4

OBSERVED AND RELATIVE SURVIVAL (%) BY AGE (number of cases in parentheses)

	AGE CLASS										ALL	
	15-44		45-54		55-64		65-74		75-99			
	obs	rel	obs	rel	obs	rel	obs	rel	obs	rel	obs	rel
Males	(158)		(383)		(885)		(1011)		(826)		(3263)	
1 year	42	42	44	44	36	37	30	32	21	24	32	33
3 years	25	25	24	25	17	19	16	19	11	17	16	19
5 years	24	25	20	21	14	17	13	18	9	18	14	19
Females	(118)		(163)		(390)		(568)		(699)		(1938)	
1 year	43	43	53	54	41	41	35	36	28	31	36	37
3 years	29	29	31	32	24	25	19	21	14	18	20	23
5 years	22	22	28	29	20	22	15	18	10	18	16	20
Overall	(276)		(546)		(1275)		(1579)		(1525)		(5201)	
1 year	42	43	47	47	37	38	32	34	24	27	33	35
3 years	26	27	26	27	19	21	17	20	12	17	18	21
5 years	23	23	22	23	16	18	14	18	10	18	15	19

SLOVENIA

AREA	NUMBER OF CASES			PERIOD	MEAN AGE		
	Males	Females	All		Males	Females	All
Slovenia	1416	967	2383	1985-1989	64.9	68.1	66.2

OBSERVED AND RELATIVE SURVIVAL (%) BY AGE (number of cases in parentheses)

	AGE CLASS										ALL	
	15-44		45-54		55-64		65-74		75-99			
	obs	rel	obs	rel	obs	rel	obs	rel	obs	rel	obs	rel
Males	(69)		(197)		(411)		(390)		(349)		(1416)	
1 year	51	51	46	47	36	37	28	29	18	20	31	33
3 years	32	32	26	27	17	19	11	13	8	11	15	18
5 years	30	31	18	19	13	15	8	11	4	8	11	14
Females	(64)		(86)		(185)		(245)		(387)		(967)	
1 year	53	53	44	44	42	42	33	34	23	25	33	34
3 years	31	31	25	25	24	25	17	19	11	15	18	20
5 years	25	25	22	23	20	21	14	17	6	11	14	17
Overall	(133)		(283)		(596)		(635)		(736)		(2383)	
1 year	52	52	46	46	38	38	30	31	20	22	32	34
3 years	32	32	26	26	19	20	13	15	9	13	16	19
5 years	28	28	19	20	15	17	11	13	5	10	12	16

STOMACH (ICD-9 151)

SPAIN

AREA	NUMBER OF CASES			PERIOD	MEAN AGE			5-YR RELATIVE SURVIVAL (%)	
	Males	Females	All		Males	Females	All	Males	Females
Basque Country	927	507	1434	1986-1988	64.8	69.7	66.6		
Granada	185	117	302	1985-1989	65.4	66.7	65.9		
Mallorca	83	47	130	1988-1989	68.2	70.0	68.8		
Navarra	458	266	724	1985-1989	66.2	69.2	67.3		
Tarragona	270	155	425	1985-1989	68.3	68.7	68.4		
Spanish Registries	1923	1092	3015		65.8	69.2	67.0		

OBSERVED AND RELATIVE SURVIVAL (%) BY AGE (number of cases in parentheses)

	AGE CLASS										ALL	
	15-44		45-54		55-64		65-74		75-99			
	obs	rel	obs	rel	obs	rel	obs	rel	obs	rel	obs	rel
Males	(106)		(235)		(486)		(585)		(511)		(1923)	
1 year	70	70	55	56	48	48	42	43	29	32	43	45
3 years	54	54	40	40	30	32	24	27	14	19	27	30
5 years	50	51	35	37	26	28	20	24	12	20	23	28
Females	(71)		(80)		(180)		(318)		(443)		(1092)	
1 year	55	55	56	56	51	51	47	48	35	37	44	45
3 years	35	35	35	35	29	29	31	33	20	25	27	30
5 years	32	32	33	34	26	27	28	31	17	25	24	29
Overall	(177)		(315)		(666)		(903)		(954)		(3015)	
1 year	64	64	56	56	48	49	44	45	32	35	43	45
3 years	46	46	38	39	30	31	27	29	17	22	27	30
5 years	43	43	35	36	26	28	23	27	14	23	23	28

SWEDEN

AREA	NUMBER OF CASES			PERIOD	MEAN AGE		
	Males	Females	All		Males	Females	All
South Sweden	823	453	1276	1985-1989	71.6	72.9	72.0

OBSERVED AND RELATIVE SURVIVAL (%) BY AGE (number of cases in parentheses)

	AGE CLASS										ALL	
	15-44		45-54		55-64		65-74		75-99			
	obs	rel	obs	rel	obs	rel	obs	rel	obs	rel	obs	rel
Males	(24)		(39)		(112)		(279)		(369)		(823)	
1 year	67	67	54	54	45	45	37	38	31	35	37	39
3 years	33	34	26	26	28	29	18	20	14	20	18	22
5 years	33	34	23	24	21	22	13	16	8	15	13	18
Females	(16)		(20)		(60)		(104)		(253)		(453)	
1 year	38	38	50	50	45	45	43	44	33	35	38	40
3 years	25	25	20	20	28	29	15	16	16	20	18	21
5 years	25	25	10	10	27	28	11	12	10	15	13	17
Overall	(40)		(59)		(172)		(383)		(622)		(1276)	
1 year	55	55	53	53	45	45	38	40	32	35	37	39
3 years	30	30	24	24	28	29	17	19	15	20	18	22
5 years	30	30	19	19	23	24	12	15	9	15	13	17

STOMACH (ICD-9 151)

SWITZERLAND

AREA	NUMBER OF CASES			PERIOD	MEAN AGE			5-YR RELATIVE SURVIVAL (%)	
	Males	Females	All		Males	Females	All	Males	Females
Basel	177	114	291	1985-1988	67.6	73.0	69.7		
Geneva	161	103	264	1985-1989	67.3	74.6	70.2		
Swiss Registries	338	217	555		67.5	73.7	69.9		

OBSERVED AND RELATIVE SURVIVAL (%) BY AGE (number of cases in parentheses)

	AGE CLASS										ALL	
	15-44		45-54		55-64		65-74		75-99			
	obs	rel	obs	rel	obs	rel	obs	rel	obs	rel	obs	rel
Males	(20)		(40)		(78)		(72)		(128)		(338)	
1 year	84	84	44	45	50	51	47	49	30	33	43	45
3 years	40	41	21	21	32	33	25	28	9	12	20	24
5 years	40	41	21	22	29	31	19	23	7	13	18	23
Females	(7)		(15)		(23)		(45)		(127)		(217)	
1 year	86	86	53	53	61	61	47	48	31	34	41	43
3 years	34	34	33	34	37	38	35	37	18	24	25	30
5 years	17	17	33	34	23	24	26	28	14	23	19	25
Overall	(27)		(55)		(101)		(117)		(255)		(555)	
1 year	84	84	47	47	52	53	47	48	31	34	42	44
3 years	39	39	24	25	33	34	29	31	13	18	22	26
5 years	34	34	24	25	28	30	21	25	10	18	18	24

STOMACH (ICD-9 151)

EUROPE, 1985-89
Weighted analyses

COUNTRY	% COVERAGE WITH C.R.s	YEARLY NO. OF CASES (Mean No. of cases recorded) Males	Females	All
AUSTRIA	8	87	94	181
DENMARK	100	422	287	709
ENGLAND	50	2921	1737	4658
ESTONIA	100	274	233	507
FINLAND	100	511	451	962
FRANCE	4	183	113	296
GERMANY	2	137	124	261
ICELAND	100	33	17	50
ITALY	10	1328	935	2263
NETHERLANDS	20	258	146	404
POLAND	6	256	150	406
SCOTLAND	100	659	461	1120
SLOVAKIA	100	653	388	1041
SLOVENIA	100	283	193	476
SPAIN	11	558	316	874
SWEDEN	17	165	91	256
SWITZERLAND	11	77	49	126

RELATIVE SURVIVAL (%) (Age-standardized)

□ 1 year ■ 5 years

OBSERVED AND RELATIVE SURVIVAL (%) BY AGE

	15-44 obs	15-44 rel	45-54 obs	45-54 rel	55-64 obs	55-64 rel	65-74 obs	65-74 rel	75-99 obs	75-99 rel	ALL obs	ALL rel
Males												
1 year	60	60	50	50	44	45	37	38	27	30	37	39
3 years	41	42	32	32	25	27	20	23	11	16	20	24
5 years	39	39	27	28	21	23	15	19	8	14	16	21
Females												
1 year	60	60	60	61	51	51	43	44	31	33	40	42
3 years	43	43	41	41	32	32	26	28	15	20	23	27
5 years	35	35	34	35	27	29	22	24	11	17	18	24
Overall												
1 year	60	60	54	54	47	47	39	41	29	31	38	40
3 years	42	42	35	36	28	29	23	25	13	18	21	25
5 years	37	38	30	31	23	25	18	21	9	16	17	22

AGE STANDARDIZED RELATIVE SURVIVAL(%)

COUNTRY	MALES 1-year (95% C.I.)	MALES 5-years (95% C.I.)	FEMALES 1-year (95% C.I.)	FEMALES 5-years (95% C.I.)
AUSTRIA	44.2 (37.1 - 52.7)	23.0 (16.8 - 31.6)	56.4 (49.4 - 64.4)	30.6 (23.8 - 39.2)
DENMARK	30.8 (28.8 - 32.9)	12.2 (10.6 - 14.0)	31.2 (28.8 - 33.9)	15.0 (13.0 - 17.3)
ENGLAND	26.9 (26.2 - 27.6)	11.2 (10.6 - 11.8)	30.2 (29.2 - 31.3)	12.7 (11.8 - 13.6)
ESTONIA	32.1 (29.2 - 35.2)	15.2 (12.6 - 18.2)	33.8 (31.2 - 36.8)	16.3 (14.0 - 19.1)
FINLAND	38.6 (36.7 - 40.7)	19.3 (17.5 - 21.3)	40.3 (38.3 - 42.4)	20.2 (18.4 - 22.2)
FRANCE	44.2 (40.9 - 47.6)	23.8 (20.6 - 27.5)	53.2 (48.8 - 57.9)	26.3 (22.2 - 31.2)
GERMANY	42.3 (38.6 - 46.5)	24.5 (20.4 - 29.3)	43.1 (39.3 - 47.3)	26.6 (22.7 - 31.1)
ICELAND	40.1 (33.3 - 48.2)	19.0 (13.2 - 27.3)	52.5 (42.6 - 64.6)	32.1 (22.8 - 45.2)
ITALY	41.1 (39.7 - 42.6)	20.2 (18.9 - 21.5)	48.3 (46.6 - 50.0)	27.4 (25.8 - 29.2)
NETHERLANDS	40.5 (36.6 - 44.8)	18.0 (14.5 - 22.3)	39.7 (34.9 - 45.2)	21.6 (17.3 - 26.9)
POLAND	23.0 (20.0 - 26.4)	8.4 (6.3 - 11.2)	26.0 (22.1 - 30.8)	10.1 (7.3 - 13.9)
SCOTLAND	26.7 (25.2 - 28.3)	9.6 (8.4 - 10.9)	28.2 (26.3 - 30.3)	12.3 (10.9 - 14.0)
SLOVAKIA	31.0 (29.3 - 32.7)	18.4 (16.6 - 20.4)	36.6 (34.4 - 38.9)	19.6 (17.5 - 21.9)
SLOVENIA	29.1 (26.7 - 31.8)	12.0 (10.0 - 14.3)	33.4 (30.5 - 36.7)	16.0 (13.5 - 18.9)
SPAIN	41.8 (39.5 - 44.3)	25.3 (22.8 - 27.9)	45.0 (42.1 - 48.2)	28.3 (25.4 - 31.6)
SWEDEN	40.3 (36.9 - 44.0)	17.9 (15.0 - 21.3)	41.1 (36.5 - 46.3)	16.6 (13.1 - 21.1)
SWITZERLAND	43.8 (38.5 - 49.8)	21.2 (16.5 - 27.2)	46.8 (40.0 - 54.6)	25.4 (19.2 - 33.8)
EUROPE, 1985-89	37.9 (37.0 - 38.9)	19.3 (18.4 - 20.3)	42.9 (41.7 - 44.2)	23.6 (22.4 - 24.8)

SMALL INTESTINE   (ICD-9 152)

AUSTRIA

AREA	NUMBER OF CASES			PERIOD	MEAN AGE		
	Males	Females	All		Males	Females	All
Tirol	6	2	8	1988-1989	63.5	78.0	67.3

OBSERVED AND RELATIVE SURVIVAL (%) BY AGE (number of cases in parentheses)

	15-44		45-54		55-64		65-74		75-99		ALL	
	obs	rel	obs	rel	obs	rel	obs	rel	obs	rel	obs	rel
Males	(0)		(1)		(3)		(0)		(2)		(6)	
1 year	-	-	100	100	67	67	-	-	0	0	50	51
3 years	-	-	100	100	67	69	-	-	0	0	50	54
5 years	-	-	100	100	67	71	-	-	0	0	50	58
Females	(0)		(0)		(0)		(0)		(2)		(2)	
1 year	-	-	-	-	-	-	-	-	100	100	100	100
3 years	-	-	-	-	-	-	-	-	100	100	100	100
5 years	-	-	-	-	-	-	-	-	50	64	50	64
Overall	(0)		(1)		(3)		(0)		(4)		(8)	
1 year	-	-	100	100	67	67	-	-	50	53	63	64
3 years	-	-	100	100	67	69	-	-	50	59	63	69
5 years	-	-	100	100	67	71	-	-	25	34	50	59

DENMARK

AREA	NUMBER OF CASES			PERIOD	MEAN AGE		
	Males	Females	All		Males	Females	All
Denmark	143	125	268	1985-1989	66.6	69.0	67.8

OBSERVED AND RELATIVE SURVIVAL (%) BY AGE (number of cases in parentheses)

	15-44		45-54		55-64		65-74		75-99		ALL	
	obs	rel	obs	rel	obs	rel	obs	rel	obs	rel	obs	rel
Males	(11)		(13)		(24)		(51)		(44)		(143)	
1 year	55	55	77	77	33	34	43	45	43	48	45	48
3 years	27	27	62	63	17	18	25	29	18	25	25	29
5 years	27	28	38	40	13	14	22	27	11	20	19	25
Females	(8)		(10)		(21)		(39)		(47)		(125)	
1 year	75	75	70	70	57	58	54	55	38	41	51	53
3 years	50	50	40	41	33	35	28	31	17	22	27	31
5 years	38	38	30	31	29	31	18	21	9	14	18	23
Overall	(19)		(23)		(45)		(90)		(91)		(268)	
1 year	63	63	74	74	44	45	48	49	41	44	48	50
3 years	37	37	52	53	24	26	27	30	18	23	26	30
5 years	32	32	35	36	20	22	20	24	10	17	19	24

SMALL INTESTINE   (ICD-9 152)

ENGLAND

AREA	NUMBER OF CASES			PERIOD	MEAN AGE			5-YR RELATIVE SURVIVAL (%)	
	Males	Females	All		Males	Females	All	Males	Females
East Anglia	38	46	84	1985-1989	68.1	65.7	66.8		
Mersey	39	26	65	1985-1989	64.0	72.7	67.5		
Oxford	52	44	96	1985-1989	64.7	67.4	66.0		
South Thames	72	81	153	1985-1989	66.6	66.3	66.5		
Wessex	52	52	104	1985-1989	66.0	68.2	67.1		
West Midlands	124	109	233	1985-1989	63.5	67.9	65.6		
Yorkshire	76	60	136	1985-1989	64.1	66.4	65.1		
English Registries	453	418	871		65.0	67.4	66.2		

OBSERVED AND RELATIVE SURVIVAL (%) BY AGE (number of cases in parentheses)

	AGE CLASS										ALL	
	15-44		45-54		55-64		65-74		75-99			
	obs	rel	obs	rel	obs	rel	obs	rel	obs	rel	obs	rel
Males	(29)		(58)		(113)		(145)		(108)		(453)	
1 year	55	55	64	64	57	58	54	56	38	42	52	54
3 years	38	38	48	49	36	38	33	38	20	28	33	38
5 years	31	31	41	43	29	32	21	26	15	28	25	31
Females	(21)		(37)		(107)		(121)		(132)		(418)	
1 year	81	81	59	60	59	59	58	59	41	44	54	56
3 years	62	62	30	30	40	41	30	32	30	38	34	38
5 years	52	53	22	22	30	32	22	25	19	30	25	29
Overall	(50)		(95)		(220)		(266)		(240)		(871)	
1 year	66	66	62	62	58	58	56	57	39	43	53	55
3 years	48	48	41	42	38	40	32	35	25	34	33	38
5 years	40	40	34	35	30	32	21	25	17	29	25	30

ESTONIA

AREA	NUMBER OF CASES			PERIOD	MEAN AGE		
	Males	Females	All		Males	Females	All
Estonia	11	15	26	1985-1989	64.5	63.7	64.1

OBSERVED AND RELATIVE SURVIVAL (%) BY AGE (number of cases in parentheses)

	AGE CLASS										ALL	
	15-44		45-54		55-64		65-74		75-99			
	obs	rel	obs	rel	obs	rel	obs	rel	obs	rel	obs	rel
Males	(1)		(1)		(3)		(4)		(2)		(11)	
1 year	0	0	0	0	0	0	0	0	50	56	9	10
3 years	0	0	0	0	0	0	0	0	0	0	0	0
5 years	0	0	0	0	0	0	0	0	0	0	0	0
Females	(1)		(1)		(8)		(2)		(3)		(15)	
1 year	100	100	100	100	63	63	0	0	0	0	47	48
3 years	0	0	100	100	38	39	0	0	0	0	27	30
5 years	0	0	0	0	38	41	0	0	0	0	20	24
Overall	(2)		(2)		(11)		(6)		(5)		(26)	
1 year	50	50	50	51	45	46	0	0	20	23	31	32
3 years	0	0	50	52	27	29	0	0	0	0	15	17
5 years	0	0	0	0	27	30	0	0	0	0	12	14

SMALL INTESTINE (ICD-9 152)

FINLAND

AREA	NUMBER OF CASES			PERIOD	MEAN AGE		
	Males	Females	All		Males	Females	All
Finland	116	105	221	1985-1989	62.7	65.1	63.8

OBSERVED AND RELATIVE SURVIVAL (%) BY AGE (number of cases in parentheses)

	AGE CLASS										ALL	
	15-44		45-54		55-64		65-74		75-99			
	obs	rel	obs	rel	obs	rel	obs	rel	obs	rel	obs	rel
Males	(10)		(19)		(36)		(28)		(23)		(116)	
1 year	80	80	74	74	75	77	61	63	57	63	68	71
3 years	70	71	68	70	47	50	43	49	39	54	50	56
5 years	50	51	58	60	39	43	39	50	30	55	41	50
Females	(13)		(10)		(20)		(31)		(31)		(105)	
1 year	85	85	90	90	85	86	71	72	42	47	69	71
3 years	54	54	60	61	65	66	52	55	26	36	48	53
5 years	54	54	30	31	50	52	48	54	6	12	35	43
Overall	(23)		(29)		(56)		(59)		(54)		(221)	
1 year	83	83	79	80	79	80	66	68	48	54	68	71
3 years	61	61	66	67	54	56	47	52	31	44	49	55
5 years	52	53	48	50	43	47	44	52	17	30	38	47

FRANCE

AREA	NUMBER OF CASES			PERIOD	MEAN AGE			5-YR RELATIVE SURVIVAL (%)	
	Males	Females	All		Males	Females	All	Males	Females
Somme	6	9	15	1985-1989	60.8	72.6	67.9		
Calvados	8	7	15	1985-1989	66.9	72.7	69.7		
Côte d'Or	11	13	24	1985-1989	62.2	71.6	67.3		
Doubs	13	7	20	1985-1989	68.8	71.3	69.8		
French Registries	38	36	74		65.3	72.1	68.6		

OBSERVED AND RELATIVE SURVIVAL (%) BY AGE (number of cases in parentheses)

	AGE CLASS										ALL	
	15-44		45-54		55-64		65-74		75-99			
	obs	rel	obs	rel	obs	rel	obs	rel	obs	rel	obs	rel
Males	(3)		(3)		(13)		(9)		(10)		(38)	
1 year	67	67	100	100	60	61	78	80	37	43	64	67
3 years	67	67	67	68	34	36	49	55	37	54	44	50
5 years	67	68	33	35	34	38	33	40	0	0	33	39
Females	(1)		(3)		(6)		(8)		(18)		(36)	
1 year	100	100	67	67	80	80	54	54	27	30	45	48
3 years	100	100	67	67	53	54	36	38	20	29	35	42
5 years	0	0	33	34	27	28	36	40	10	18	20	27
Overall	(4)		(6)		(19)		(17)		(28)		(74)	
1 year	75	75	83	84	65	66	68	70	30	34	55	58
3 years	75	76	67	68	39	41	45	49	25	36	40	46
5 years	50	51	33	34	32	35	36	42	9	16	26	33

<h1 style="text-align:center">SMALL INTESTINE</h1>

(ICD-9 152)

GERMANY

AREA	NUMBER OF CASES			PERIOD	MEAN AGE		
	Males	Females	All		Males	Females	All
Saarland	31	35	66	1985-1989	65.5	69.8	67.8

OBSERVED AND RELATIVE SURVIVAL (%) BY AGE (number of cases in parentheses)

	AGE CLASS										ALL	
	15-44		45-54		55-64		65-74		75-99			
	obs	rel	obs	rel	obs	rel	obs	rel	obs	rel	obs	rel
Males	(0)		(8)		(6)		(9)		(8)		(31)	
1 year	-	-	75	76	83	85	33	35	63	71	61	64
3 years	-	-	63	64	83	88	22	26	38	55	48	56
5 years	-	-	63	65	65	72	22	29	38	75	45	59
Females	(2)		(2)		(7)		(7)		(17)		(35)	
1 year	100	100	100	100	71	72	57	59	29	32	51	54
3 years	100	100	50	50	29	29	29	31	29	37	34	39
5 years	100	100	-	-	29	30	29	33	24	37	31	40
Overall	(2)		(10)		(13)		(16)		(25)		(66)	
1 year	100	100	80	80	77	78	44	45	40	44	56	59
3 years	100	100	60	61	54	56	25	28	32	42	41	47
5 years	100	100	60	62	46	49	25	31	28	47	38	49

ICELAND

AREA	NUMBER OF CASES			PERIOD	MEAN AGE		
	Males	Females	All		Males	Females	All
Iceland	9	3	12	1985-1989	63.6	68.7	64.9

OBSERVED AND RELATIVE SURVIVAL (%) BY AGE (number of cases in parentheses)

	AGE CLASS										ALL	
	15-44		45-54		55-64		65-74		75-99			
	obs	rel	obs	rel	obs	rel	obs	rel	obs	rel	obs	rel
Males	(1)		(1)		(4)		(1)		(2)		(9)	
1 year	100	100	100	100	75	76	100	100	50	55	78	80
3 years	100	100	100	100	75	78	0	0	0	0	56	61
5 years	100	100	100	100	75	81	0	0	0	0	56	65
Females	(0)		(0)		(1)		(1)		(1)		(3)	
1 year	-	-	-	-	100	100	100	100	100	100	100	100
3 years	-	-	-	-	100	100	100	100	0	0	67	74
5 years	-	-	-	-	0	0	100	100	0	0	33	40
Overall	(1)		(1)		(5)		(2)		(3)		(12)	
1 year	100	100	100	100	80	81	100	100	67	72	83	86
3 years	100	100	100	100	80	83	50	54	0	0	58	64
5 years	100	100	100	100	60	64	50	58	0	0	50	59

SMALL INTESTINE (ICD-9 152)

ITALY

AREA	NUMBER OF CASES			PERIOD	MEAN AGE			5-YR RELATIVE SURVIVAL (%)	
	Males	Females	All		Males	Females	All	Males	Females
Florence	27	32	59	1985-1989	67.1	71.1	69.3		
Genoa	4	8	12	1986-1988	65.3	68.5	67.5		
Latina	2	4	6	1985-1987	59.5	74.5	69.7		
Modena	8	5	13	1988-1989	63.8	68.6	65.7		
Parma	11	5	16	1985-1987	61.0	51.8	58.2		
Ragusa	5	2	7	1985-1989	67.4	82.0	71.7		
Romagna	10	3	13	1986-1988	67.6	65.7	67.2		
Turin	14	14	28	1985-1987	66.6	65.0	65.8		
Varese	13	13	26	1985-1989	61.1	66.8	64.0		
Italian Registries	94	86	180		65.1	68.3	66.6		

OBSERVED AND RELATIVE SURVIVAL (%) BY AGE (number of cases in parentheses)

	AGE CLASS										ALL	
	15-44		45-54		55-64		65-74		75-99			
	obs	rel	obs	rel	obs	rel	obs	rel	obs	rel	obs	rel
Males	(5)		(17)		(22)		(22)		(28)		(94)	
1 year	60	60	47	47	55	55	64	66	21	23	46	48
3 years	60	60	41	42	23	24	36	41	18	24	30	34
5 years	60	61	35	37	18	20	27	33	11	18	23	29
Females	(1)		(15)		(15)		(24)		(31)		(86)	
1 year	100	100	53	53	67	67	46	47	29	31	45	47
3 years	0	0	33	34	47	48	29	31	16	20	28	31
5 years	0	0	33	34	33	35	29	32	10	15	23	28
Overall	(6)		(32)		(37)		(46)		(59)		(180)	
1 year	67	67	50	50	59	60	54	56	25	28	46	47
3 years	50	50	38	38	32	34	33	35	17	22	29	32
5 years	50	50	34	35	24	26	28	33	10	16	23	28

NETHERLANDS

AREA	NUMBER OF CASES			PERIOD	MEAN AGE		
	Males	Females	All		Males	Females	All
Eindhoven	16	13	29	1985-1989	64.2	58.5	61.7

OBSERVED AND RELATIVE SURVIVAL (%) BY AGE (number of cases in parentheses)

	AGE CLASS										ALL	
	15-44		45-54		55-64		65-74		75-99			
	obs	rel	obs	rel	obs	rel	obs	rel	obs	rel	obs	rel
Males	(0)		(2)		(8)		(3)		(3)		(16)	
1 year	-	-	50	50	63	63	33	35	33	38	50	52
3 years	-	-	50	51	50	53	0	0	0	0	31	35
5 years	-	-	50	52	38	41	0	0	0	0	25	30
Females	(3)		(2)		(4)		(3)		(1)		(13)	
1 year	100	100	100	100	75	76	100	100	0	0	85	86
3 years	67	67	100	100	50	51	33	35	0	0	54	56
5 years	67	67	100	100	50	52	33	37	0	0	54	58
Overall	(3)		(4)		(12)		(6)		(4)		(29)	
1 year	100	100	75	75	67	68	67	68	25	28	66	67
3 years	67	67	75	76	50	52	17	18	0	0	41	45
5 years	67	67	75	77	42	45	17	20	0	0	38	43

SMALL INTESTINE (ICD-9 152)

POLAND

AREA	NUMBER OF CASES			PERIOD	MEAN AGE			5-YR RELATIVE SURVIVAL (%)	
	Males	Females	All		Males	Females	All	Males	Females
Cracow	7	7	14	1985-1989	61.7	65.6	63.7		
Warsaw	3	5	8	1988-1989	65.0	70.6	68.6		
Polish Registries	10	12	22		62.9	67.8	65.6		

OBSERVED AND RELATIVE SURVIVAL (%) BY AGE (number of cases in parentheses)

	AGE CLASS										ALL	
	15-44		45-54		55-64		65-74		75-99			
	obs	rel	obs	rel	obs	rel	obs	rel	obs	rel	obs	rel
Males	(1)		(0)		(5)		(3)		(1)		(10)	
1 year	0	0	-	-	20	20	33	35	100	100	30	31
3 years	0	0	-	-	20	22	0	0	0	0	10	11
5 years	0	0	-	-	20	23	0	0	0	0	10	13
Females	(1)		(0)		(5)		(2)		(4)		(12)	
1 year	100	100	-	-	60	61	0	0	25	28	42	44
3 years	100	100	-	-	40	41	0	0	0	0	25	29
5 years	0	0	-	-	40	43	0	0	0	0	17	21
Overall	(2)		(0)		(10)		(5)		(5)		(22)	
1 year	50	50	-	-	40	41	20	21	40	45	36	38
3 years	50	51	-	-	30	32	0	0	0	0	18	21
5 years	0	0	-	-	30	33	0	0	0	0	14	17

SCOTLAND

AREA	NUMBER OF CASES			PERIOD	MEAN AGE		
	Males	Females	All		Males	Females	All
Scotland	100	111	211	1985-1989	63.5	70.0	66.9

OBSERVED AND RELATIVE SURVIVAL (%) BY AGE (number of cases in parentheses)

	AGE CLASS										ALL	
	15-44		45-54		55-64		65-74		75-99			
	obs	rel	obs	rel	obs	rel	obs	rel	obs	rel	obs	rel
Males	(11)		(12)		(21)		(34)		(22)		(100)	
1 year	64	64	58	59	48	49	53	56	41	46	51	53
3 years	55	55	50	51	38	41	38	45	32	46	40	46
5 years	55	55	25	26	19	21	21	27	27	54	26	33
Females	(3)		(9)		(21)		(35)		(43)		(111)	
1 year	67	67	44	45	67	67	37	38	47	51	48	50
3 years	33	33	22	23	38	40	14	16	23	31	23	27
5 years	33	34	11	11	33	36	9	10	12	20	15	20
Overall	(14)		(21)		(42)		(69)		(65)		(211)	
1 year	64	64	52	53	57	58	45	47	45	49	49	52
3 years	50	50	38	39	38	40	26	30	26	36	31	36
5 years	50	50	19	20	26	29	14	18	17	30	20	26

SMALL INTESTINE (ICD-9 152)

SLOVAKIA

AREA	NUMBER OF CASES			PERIOD	MEAN AGE		
	Males	Females	All		Males	Females	All
Slovakia	64	47	111	1985-1989	58.1	62.2	59.9

OBSERVED AND RELATIVE SURVIVAL (%) BY AGE (number of cases in parentheses)

	AGE CLASS										ALL	
	15-44		45-54		55-64		65-74		75-99			
	obs	rel	obs	rel	obs	rel	obs	rel	obs	rel	obs	rel
Males	(14)		(10)		(17)		(13)		(10)		(64)	
1 year	64	65	60	61	29	30	54	57	50	56	50	52
3 years	36	36	50	52	18	19	15	18	40	58	30	33
5 years	36	37	50	54	18	21	8	10	30	58	26	32
Females	(4)		(13)		(5)		(12)		(13)		(47)	
1 year	75	75	85	85	80	81	33	34	38	42	57	59
3 years	50	50	46	47	60	62	17	18	31	42	36	40
5 years	50	50	46	47	60	64	-	-	31	54	36	44
Overall	(18)		(23)		(22)		(25)		(23)		(111)	
1 year	67	67	74	74	41	42	44	46	43	48	53	55
3 years	39	39	48	49	27	29	16	18	35	49	32	36
5 years	39	40	48	50	27	31	8	10	30	55	30	37

SLOVENIA

AREA	NUMBER OF CASES			PERIOD	MEAN AGE		
	Males	Females	All		Males	Females	All
Slovenia	15	13	28	1985-1989	55.1	63.2	58.9

OBSERVED AND RELATIVE SURVIVAL (%) BY AGE (number of cases in parentheses)

	AGE CLASS										ALL	
	15-44		45-54		55-64		65-74		75-99			
	obs	rel	obs	rel	obs	rel	obs	rel	obs	rel	obs	rel
Males	(4)		(3)		(4)		(1)		(3)		(15)	
1 year	100	100	67	67	0	0	100	100	33	37	53	55
3 years	75	76	33	34	0	0	0	0	33	47	33	37
5 years	50	51	33	35	0	0	0	0	33	61	27	31
Females	(1)		(2)		(4)		(2)		(4)		(13)	
1 year	0	0	50	50	50	50	100	100	50	53	54	55
3 years	0	0	50	51	25	26	50	53	25	31	31	33
5 years	0	0	50	51	25	26	50	56	25	38	31	36
Overall	(5)		(5)		(8)		(3)		(7)		(28)	
1 year	80	80	60	60	25	25	100	100	43	46	54	55
3 years	60	61	40	41	13	13	33	36	29	37	32	35
5 years	40	41	40	42	13	14	33	39	29	47	29	33

SMALL INTESTINE (ICD-9 152)

SPAIN

AREA	NUMBER OF CASES			PERIOD	MEAN AGE			5-YR RELATIVE SURVIVAL (%)	
	Males	Females	All		Males	Females	All	Males	Females
Basque Country	13	14	27	1986-1988	60.3	65.3	62.9		
Mallorca	2	1	3	1988-1989	71.0	39.0	60.7		
Navarra	7	5	12	1985-1989	66.3	67.2	66.8		
Tarragona	12	6	18	1985-1989	64.0	69.5	65.9		
Spanish Registries	34	26	60		63.6	65.8	64.5		

OBSERVED AND RELATIVE SURVIVAL (%) BY AGE (number of cases in parentheses)

	AGE CLASS										ALL	
	15-44		45-54		55-64		65-74		75-99			
	obs	rel	obs	rel	obs	rel	obs	rel	obs	rel	obs	rel
Males	(1)		(4)		(12)		(12)		(5)		(34)	
1 year	0	0	50	50	50	51	42	43	20	21	41	42
3 years	0	0	50	51	42	43	42	46	0	0	35	38
5 years	0	0	-	-	42	45	17	20	0	0	23	27
Females	(2)		(3)		(7)		(4)		(10)		(26)	
1 year	100	100	100	100	86	86	25	25	40	42	62	63
3 years	50	50	33	34	57	58	25	26	20	24	35	37
5 years	50	50	-	-	43	44	-	-	10	14	25	28
Overall	(3)		(7)		(19)		(16)		(15)		(60)	
1 year	67	67	71	72	63	64	38	39	33	35	50	51
3 years	33	33	43	43	47	49	38	41	13	16	35	38
5 years	33	34	-	-	41	43	15	18	7	10	24	28

SWEDEN

AREA	NUMBER OF CASES			PERIOD	MEAN AGE		
	Males	Females	All		Males	Females	All
South Sweden	53	48	101	1985-1989	65.7	72.6	69.0

OBSERVED AND RELATIVE SURVIVAL (%) BY AGE (number of cases in parentheses)

	AGE CLASS										ALL	
	15-44		45-54		55-64		65-74		75-99			
	obs	rel	obs	rel	obs	rel	obs	rel	obs	rel	obs	rel
Males	(3)		(7)		(8)		(23)		(12)		(53)	
1 year	33	33	71	72	50	51	48	49	50	56	51	53
3 years	33	33	71	73	50	52	35	38	33	47	42	47
5 years	33	34	57	59	38	40	35	42	17	31	34	42
Females	(0)		(2)		(7)		(17)		(22)		(48)	
1 year	-	-	100	100	71	72	65	66	59	64	65	67
3 years	-	-	100	100	71	73	35	37	23	30	38	43
5 years	-	-	50	51	71	74	24	26	5	7	23	29
Overall	(3)		(9)		(15)		(40)		(34)		(101)	
1 year	33	33	78	78	60	61	55	56	56	61	57	60
3 years	33	33	78	79	60	62	35	38	26	35	40	45
5 years	33	34	56	57	53	56	30	35	9	15	29	36

SMALL INTESTINE (ICD-9 152)

SWITZERLAND

AREA	NUMBER OF CASES			PERIOD	MEAN AGE		
	Males	Females	All		Males	Females	All
Geneva	10	9	19	1985-1989	64.7	68.2	66.4

OBSERVED AND RELATIVE SURVIVAL (%) BY AGE (number of cases in parentheses)

	AGE CLASS										ALL	
	15-44		45-54		55-64		65-74		75-99			
	obs	rel	obs	rel	obs	rel	obs	rel	obs	rel	obs	rel
Males	(2)		(1)		(1)		(2)		(4)		(10)	
1 year	100	100	0	0	100	100	50	52	50	54	60	63
3 years	100	100	0	0	100	100	50	57	25	33	50	57
5 years	100	100	0	0	100	100	50	64	25	41	50	63
Females	(0)		(0)		(3)		(5)		(1)		(9)	
1 year	-	-	-	-	100	100	20	20	0	0	44	45
3 years	-	-	-	-	33	34	20	21	0	0	22	24
5 years	-	-	-	-	0	0	0	0	0	0	0	0
Overall	(2)		(1)		(4)		(7)		(5)		(19)	
1 year	100	100	0	0	100	100	29	29	40	43	53	54
3 years	100	100	0	0	50	51	29	31	20	26	37	41
5 years	100	100	0	0	25	26	14	17	20	32	26	31

SMALL INTESTINE   (ICD-9 152)

EUROPE, 1985-89
Weighted analyses

COUNTRY	% COVERAGE WITH C.R.s	YEARLY NO. OF CASES (Mean No. of cases recorded)			RELATIVE SURVIVAL (%) (Age-standardized)
		Males	Females	All	
AUSTRIA	8	3	1	4	
DENMARK	100	29	25	54	
ENGLAND	50	91	84	175	
ESTONIA	100	2	3	5	
FINLAND	100	23	21	44	
FRANCE	4	8	7	15	
GERMANY	2	6	7	13	
ICELAND	100	2	1	3	
ITALY	10	27	23	50	
NETHERLANDS	6	3	3	6	
POLAND	6	4	6	10	
SCOTLAND	100	20	22	42	
SLOVAKIA	100	13	9	22	
SLOVENIA	100	3	3	6	
SPAIN	10	10	8	18	
SWEDEN	17	11	10	21	
SWITZERLAND	6	2	2	4	

□ 1 year   ■ 5 years

OBSERVED AND RELATIVE SURVIVAL (%) BY AGE

	AGE CLASS										ALL	
	15-44		45-54		55-64		65-74		75-99			
	obs	rel	obs	rel	obs	rel	obs	rel	obs	rel	obs	rel
Males												
1 year	50	51	67	67	62	63	51	53	43	47	53	55
3 years	46	46	55	56	48	50	31	35	24	34	38	43
5 years	44	45	47	48	40	44	23	29	16	30	32	40
Females												
1 year	96	96	79	79	71	71	49	50	32	34	52	54
3 years	70	70	49	50	42	43	28	30	22	28	34	38
5 years	46	46	35	36	33	35	26	29	14	22	26	32
Overall												
1 year	73	73	73	73	66	67	50	51	37	41	52	55
3 years	57	58	52	53	45	47	29	32	23	31	36	41
5 years	45	45	41	42	37	39	24	29	15	26	29	36

AGE STANDARDIZED RELATIVE SURVIVAL(%)

COUNTRY	MALES		FEMALES	
	1-year (95% C.I.)	5-years (95% C.I.)	1-year (95% C.I.)	5-years (95% C.I.)
AUSTRIA	-	-	-	-
DENMARK	47.6 (39.9 - 56.8)	23.7 (16.8 - 33.4)	54.9 (46.6 - 64.7)	23.3 (16.3 - 33.5)
ENGLAND	53.2 (48.6 - 58.3)	30.3 (25.5 - 36.0)	56.3 (51.7 - 61.4)	29.5 (24.9 - 34.9)
ESTONIA	16.1 (4.0 - 64.5)	0.0 (0.0 - 0.0)	33.3 (26.2 - 42.3)	9.5 (3.9 - 23.3)
FINLAND	68.7 (59.7 - 79.0)	51.1 (39.6 - 66.0)	70.9 (62.8 - 80.1)	38.6 (29.9 - 49.7)
FRANCE	66.2 (51.9 - 84.5)	29.0 (16.6 - 50.8)	58.0 (43.3 - 77.8)	27.1 (13.1 - 56.1)
GERMANY	-	-	61.6 (48.2 - 78.7)	-
ICELAND	81.3 (60.4 -109.3)	37.4 (28.1 - 49.8)	-	-
ITALY	48.6 (39.5 - 59.7)	27.9 (19.2 - 40.4)	51.4 (42.3 - 62.4)	25.8 (17.6 - 37.8)
NETHERLANDS	-	-	65.4 (56.1 - 76.2)	39.3 (22.8 - 67.7)
POLAND	-	-	-	-
SCOTLAND	52.1 (42.6 - 63.9)	35.3 (24.3 - 51.2)	51.5 (42.6 - 62.3)	20.8 (13.6 - 31.8)
SLOVAKIA	51.3 (38.6 - 68.2)	33.2 (19.4 - 57.0)	56.2 (43.2 - 73.0)	-
SLOVENIA	54.5 (39.0 - 76.2)	25.3 (7.9 - 80.7)	62.3 (44.7 - 86.8)	39.3 (17.4 - 88.9)
SPAIN	36.5 (23.3 - 57.0)	-	58.3 (43.7 - 77.7)	-
SWEDEN	53.0 (40.1 - 70.0)	39.7 (26.1 - 60.3)	-	-
SWITZERLAND	61.2 (39.9 - 93.7)	60.7 (35.4 -103.9)	-	-
EUROPE, 1985-89	55.0 (49.7 - 61.0)	36.3 (28.2 - 46.7)	57.0 (51.5 - 63.2)	30.2 (24.0 - 38.1)

COLON (ICD-9 153)

AUSTRIA

AREA	NUMBER OF CASES			PERIOD	MEAN AGE		
	Males	Females	All		Males	Females	All
Tirol	126	172	298	1988-1989	66.4	68.8	67.8

OBSERVED AND RELATIVE SURVIVAL (%) BY AGE (number of cases in parentheses)

	15-44		45-54		55-64		65-74		75-99		ALL	
	obs	rel	obs	rel	obs	rel	obs	rel	obs	rel	obs	rel
Males	(9)		(7)		(32)		(44)		(34)		(126)	
1 year	78	78	86	86	78	79	82	84	59	64	75	77
3 years	44	45	57	58	69	71	59	65	32	42	53	59
5 years	44	45	57	59	66	70	52	62	26	42	48	58
Females	(15)		(10)		(23)		(58)		(66)		(172)	
1 year	60	60	70	70	74	74	50	51	56	60	58	59
3 years	53	53	70	71	57	57	40	42	35	43	43	47
5 years	47	47	70	71	48	49	36	40	27	40	37	44
Overall	(24)		(17)		(55)		(102)		(100)		(298)	
1 year	67	67	76	77	76	77	64	65	57	61	65	67
3 years	50	50	65	65	64	66	48	51	34	42	47	52
5 years	46	46	65	66	58	61	43	49	27	40	42	50

DENMARK

AREA	NUMBER OF CASES			PERIOD	MEAN AGE		
	Males	Females	All		Males	Females	All
Denmark	4172	5312	9484	1985-1989	70.0	71.6	70.9

OBSERVED AND RELATIVE SURVIVAL (%) BY AGE (number of cases in parentheses)

	15-44		45-54		55-64		65-74		75-99		ALL	
	obs	rel	obs	rel	obs	rel	obs	rel	obs	rel	obs	rel
Males	(130)		(263)		(723)		(1448)		(1608)		(4172)	
1 year	65	65	74	75	70	71	63	66	50	56	60	64
3 years	44	44	56	57	46	49	41	47	28	40	38	46
5 years	39	40	51	53	37	42	30	39	19	36	29	40
Females	(136)		(341)		(808)		(1607)		(2420)		(5312)	
1 year	78	78	71	71	70	71	65	67	52	56	60	63
3 years	60	60	52	53	50	52	46	50	32	42	41	48
5 years	50	50	41	42	43	46	39	45	24	39	33	43
Overall	(266)		(604)		(1531)		(3055)		(4028)		(9484)	
1 year	71	72	72	73	70	71	65	67	51	56	60	64
3 years	52	52	54	55	48	51	44	49	30	41	40	47
5 years	45	45	45	47	40	44	35	42	22	38	31	42

COLON (ICD-9 153)

ENGLAND

AREA	NUMBER OF CASES			PERIOD	MEAN AGE			5-YR RELATIVE SURVIVAL (%)	
	Males	Females	All		Males	Females	All	Males	Females
East Anglia	1489	1791	3280	1985-1989	70.0	72.1	71.1		
Mersey	1649	1933	3582	1985-1989	68.7	72.0	70.5		
Oxford	1693	2009	3702	1985-1989	68.4	71.4	70.0		
South Thames	3596	4585	8181	1985-1989	69.9	72.4	71.3		
Wessex	2490	2857	5347	1985-1989	70.3	72.0	71.2		
West Midlands	3864	4200	8064	1985-1989	68.6	71.8	70.3		
Yorkshire	2351	2892	5243	1985-1989	69.3	72.5	71.0		
English Registries	17132	20267	37399		69.3	72.1	70.8		

5-YR RELATIVE SURVIVAL (%) chart: scale Males 100 80 60 40 20 0, Females 0 20 40 60 80 100; rows E.Angl, Mersey, Oxford, S.Tham, Wessex, W.Midl, Yorksh

OBSERVED AND RELATIVE SURVIVAL (%) BY AGE (number of cases in parentheses)

	AGE CLASS										ALL	
	15-44		45-54		55-64		65-74		75-99			
	obs	rel	obs	rel	obs	rel	obs	rel	obs	rel	obs	rel
Males	(539)		(1261)		(3351)		(5771)		(6210)		(17132)	
1 year	67	67	70	70	67	68	61	63	49	55	59	62
3 years	47	47	50	51	47	50	40	46	30	42	39	46
5 years	43	43	42	43	39	43	32	40	21	40	31	41
Females	(554)		(1184)		(3188)		(5654)		(9687)		(20267)	
1 year	73	73	71	71	68	69	63	65	46	50	56	59
3 years	54	54	49	50	48	49	46	49	30	39	39	45
5 years	47	48	43	44	41	43	38	44	23	38	32	41
Overall	(1093)		(2445)		(6539)		(11425)		(15897)		(37399)	
1 year	70	70	70	71	68	69	62	64	47	52	57	61
3 years	51	51	49	50	48	50	43	48	30	40	39	46
5 years	45	46	43	44	40	43	35	42	22	38	31	41

ESTONIA

AREA	NUMBER OF CASES			PERIOD	MEAN AGE		
	Males	Females	All		Males	Females	All
Estonia	475	700	1175	1985-1989	64.2	66.4	65.5

OBSERVED AND RELATIVE SURVIVAL (%) BY AGE (number of cases in parentheses)

	AGE CLASS										ALL	
	15-44		45-54		55-64		65-74		75-99			
	obs	rel	obs	rel	obs	rel	obs	rel	obs	rel	obs	rel
Males	(36)		(49)		(139)		(142)		(109)		(475)	
1 year	58	59	63	64	60	62	50	53	38	42	52	55
3 years	50	51	51	53	40	44	34	40	26	38	37	43
5 years	47	49	41	44	31	36	26	35	17	35	29	38
Females	(34)		(79)		(177)		(206)		(204)		(700)	
1 year	85	85	70	70	62	63	54	56	36	40	54	56
3 years	56	56	54	55	47	48	37	41	24	33	38	44
5 years	53	53	52	53	42	45	31	37	18	31	33	41
Overall	(70)		(128)		(316)		(348)		(313)		(1175)	
1 year	71	72	67	68	61	62	52	54	36	41	53	56
3 years	53	53	53	55	44	46	35	40	24	34	38	43
5 years	50	51	48	50	37	41	29	36	18	32	31	40

COLON (ICD-9 153)

FINLAND

AREA	NUMBER OF CASES			PERIOD	MEAN AGE		
	Males	Females	All		Males	Females	All
Finland	1699	2409	4108	1985-1989	65.5	69.6	67.9

OBSERVED AND RELATIVE SURVIVAL (%) BY AGE (number of cases in parentheses)

	AGE CLASS										ALL	
	15-44		45-54		55-64		65-74		75-99			
	obs	rel	obs	rel	obs	rel	obs	rel	obs	rel	obs	rel
Males	(140)		(177)		(386)		(533)		(463)		(1699)	
1 year	79	80	73	73	74	75	67	70	56	63	67	70
3 years	62	63	55	56	53	56	49	56	35	51	48	55
5 years	59	60	45	47	43	48	39	50	24	44	38	49
Females	(156)		(172)		(340)		(713)		(1028)		(2409)	
1 year	90	90	81	82	78	79	69	71	54	58	66	69
3 years	80	80	62	62	63	64	50	53	34	45	48	55
5 years	78	78	59	60	54	56	44	50	26	43	41	52
Overall	(296)		(349)		(726)		(1246)		(1491)		(4108)	
1 year	85	85	77	77	76	77	68	70	54	60	66	70
3 years	72	72	58	59	57	60	49	55	34	46	48	55
5 years	69	70	52	53	48	52	42	50	25	43	40	51

FRANCE

AREA	NUMBER OF CASES			PERIOD	MEAN AGE			5-YR RELATIVE SURVIVAL (%)	
	Males	Females	All		Males	Females	All	Males	Females
Somme	338	321	659	1985-1989	68.3	70.8	69.5		
Calvados	343	353	696	1985-1989	68.3	70.5	69.5		
Côte d'Or	420	361	781	1985-1989	68.2	71.6	69.8		
Doubs	296	290	586	1985-1989	67.5	69.0	68.2		
French Registries	1397	1325	2722		68.1	70.5	69.3		

OBSERVED AND RELATIVE SURVIVAL (%) BY AGE (number of cases in parentheses)

	AGE CLASS										ALL	
	15-44		45-54		55-64		65-74		75-99			
	obs	rel	obs	rel	obs	rel	obs	rel	obs	rel	obs	rel
Males	(57)		(102)		(329)		(461)		(448)		(1397)	
1 year	81	81	86	86	76	77	71	74	62	69	71	74
3 years	56	57	66	68	53	56	54	61	41	57	51	59
5 years	42	42	56	58	45	50	42	52	29	52	39	52
Females	(57)		(112)		(234)		(311)		(611)		(1325)	
1 year	76	76	84	84	79	80	71	72	61	67	69	72
3 years	61	61	65	66	58	60	53	56	40	53	49	57
5 years	58	59	61	62	53	55	47	52	32	53	43	55
Overall	(114)		(214)		(563)		(772)		(1059)		(2722)	
1 year	78	78	85	85	77	78	71	73	62	68	70	73
3 years	59	59	66	67	56	58	54	59	40	55	50	58
5 years	50	50	58	60	48	52	44	52	31	53	41	53

COLON   (ICD-9 153)

GERMANY

AREA	NUMBER OF CASES			PERIOD	MEAN AGE		
	Males	Females	All		Males	Females	All
Saarland	831	1115	1946	1985-1989	68.2	70.3	69.4

OBSERVED AND RELATIVE SURVIVAL (%) BY AGE (number of cases in parentheses)

	15-44		45-54		55-64		65-74		75-99		ALL	
	obs	rel	obs	rel	obs	rel	obs	rel	obs	rel	obs	rel
Males	(24)		(73)		(188)		(275)		(271)		(831)	
1 year	92	92	68	69	73	75	68	71	50	56	64	68
3 years	83	84	55	56	55	59	51	59	28	41	46	55
5 years	78	79	49	51	44	49	41	54	21	44	37	51
Females	(38)		(83)		(203)		(309)		(482)		(1115)	
1 year	89	90	80	80	77	78	71	73	56	60	67	70
3 years	71	71	65	66	61	63	50	53	35	46	47	54
5 years	66	66	61	62	55	57	44	51	25	42	40	51
Overall	(62)		(156)		(391)		(584)		(753)		(1946)	
1 year	90	90	74	75	75	76	70	72	54	59	66	69
3 years	76	76	60	61	58	61	50	56	32	44	47	55
5 years	70	71	56	57	49	53	42	52	24	43	39	51

ICELAND

AREA	NUMBER OF CASES			PERIOD	MEAN AGE		
	Males	Females	All		Males	Females	All
Iceland	144	134	278	1985-1989	69.8	70.7	70.2

OBSERVED AND RELATIVE SURVIVAL (%) BY AGE (number of cases in parentheses)

	15-44		45-54		55-64		65-74		75-99		ALL	
	obs	rel	obs	rel	obs	rel	obs	rel	obs	rel	obs	rel
Males	(5)		(11)		(31)		(38)		(59)		(144)	
1 year	60	60	91	91	74	75	66	68	41	45	59	62
3 years	40	40	82	83	52	54	45	49	27	37	42	49
5 years	40	40	82	84	39	42	39	47	20	35	35	45
Females	(4)		(11)		(24)		(37)		(58)		(134)	
1 year	100	100	64	64	75	76	70	71	53	58	64	67
3 years	100	100	27	28	63	64	57	60	38	49	49	55
5 years	100	100	27	28	50	52	49	55	31	50	41	51
Overall	(9)		(22)		(55)		(75)		(117)		(278)	
1 year	78	78	77	78	75	75	68	70	47	51	62	64
3 years	67	67	55	55	56	58	51	55	32	43	45	52
5 years	67	67	55	56	44	46	44	51	26	42	38	48

COLON (ICD-9 153)

ITALY

AREA	NUMBER OF CASES			PERIOD	MEAN AGE			5-YR RELATIVE SURVIVAL (%)	
	Males	Females	All		Males	Females	All	Males	Females
Florence	1137	1283	2420	1985-1989	67.9	70.4	69.2		
Genoa	427	458	885	1986-1988	67.6	70.5	69.1		
Latina	104	105	209	1985-1987	65.5	67.2	66.3		
Modena	328	337	665	1985-1989	67.7	70.0	68.8		
Parma	260	241	501	1985-1987	68.6	71.0	69.7		
Ragusa	92	129	221	1985-1989	70.1	67.9	68.9		
Romagna	250	289	539	1986-1988	66.6	69.6	68.2		
Turin	482	535	1017	1985-1987	66.6	69.1	67.9		
Varese	634	698	1332	1985-1989	67.0	69.8	68.5		
Italian Registries	3714	4075	7789		67.5	69.9	68.8		

OBSERVED AND RELATIVE SURVIVAL (%) BY AGE (number of cases in parentheses)

	AGE CLASS										ALL	
	15-44		45-54		55-64		65-74		75-99			
	obs	rel	obs	rel	obs	rel	obs	rel	obs	rel	obs	rel
Males	(123)		(362)		(917)		(1156)		(1156)		(3714)	
1 year	78	78	78	78	71	72	67	69	55	60	66	69
3 years	63	63	57	58	53	56	46	52	34	46	46	52
5 years	55	56	51	52	46	50	38	47	25	44	38	48
Females	(147)		(362)		(729)		(1114)		(1723)		(4075)	
1 year	76	76	81	82	76	76	72	73	54	58	66	68
3 years	57	58	65	66	57	58	54	57	33	42	47	53
5 years	53	53	58	59	49	51	46	51	25	39	39	48
Overall	(270)		(724)		(1646)		(2270)		(2879)		(7789)	
1 year	77	77	80	80	73	74	70	71	54	59	66	69
3 years	60	60	61	62	55	57	50	55	33	44	46	53
5 years	54	54	54	56	47	50	42	49	25	41	39	48

NETHERLANDS

AREA	NUMBER OF CASES			PERIOD	MEAN AGE			5-YR RELATIVE SURVIVAL (%)	
	Males	Females	All		Males	Females	All	Males	Females
Eindhoven	542	579	1121	1985-1989	67.0	68.6	67.8		
Rotterdam	602	735	1337	1987-1989	69.0	71.4	70.3		
Dutch Registries	1144	1314	2458		68.1	70.2	69.2		

OBSERVED AND RELATIVE SURVIVAL (%) BY AGE (number of cases in parentheses)

	AGE CLASS										ALL	
	15-44		45-54		55-64		65-74		75-99			
	obs	rel	obs	rel	obs	rel	obs	rel	obs	rel	obs	rel
Males	(48)		(101)		(243)		(374)		(378)		(1144)	
1 year	81	81	75	75	77	78	74	77	65	73	72	76
3 years	68	68	55	56	62	65	54	62	45	65	54	63
5 years	60	60	47	48	57	63	44	56	31	61	44	58
Females	(51)		(99)		(203)		(408)		(553)		(1314)	
1 year	92	92	80	80	75	76	74	76	60	65	70	72
3 years	80	81	62	62	58	59	58	61	45	58	54	61
5 years	76	76	58	59	48	50	50	56	35	56	45	56
Overall	(99)		(200)		(446)		(782)		(931)		(2458)	
1 year	87	87	77	78	76	77	74	76	62	68	71	74
3 years	75	75	58	59	60	62	56	62	45	61	54	62
5 years	68	68	52	54	53	57	47	56	34	57	45	57

COLON (ICD-9 153)

POLAND

AREA	NUMBER OF CASES			PERIOD	MEAN AGE			5-YR RELATIVE SURVIVAL (%)	
	Males	Females	All		Males	Females	All	Males	Females
Cracow	150	212	362	1985-1989	63.8	66.6	65.4		
Warsaw	249	308	557	1988-1989	65.8	70.2	68.2		
Polish Registries	399	520	919		65.0	68.7	67.1		

100 80 60 40 20 0   0 20 40 60 80 100

Cracow
Warsaw

OBSERVED AND RELATIVE SURVIVAL (%) BY AGE (number of cases in parentheses)

	AGE CLASS										ALL	
	15-44		45-54		55-64		65-74		75-99			
	obs	rel	obs	rel	obs	rel	obs	rel	obs	rel	obs	rel
Males	(22)		(49)		(122)		(107)		(99)		(399)	
1 year	59	59	55	56	50	51	48	50	27	31	45	47
3 years	45	46	33	34	30	33	28	34	13	19	27	31
5 years	45	47	24	26	24	28	20	27	10	19	21	27
Females	(28)		(43)		(110)		(126)		(213)		(520)	
1 year	61	61	72	72	47	47	48	50	27	29	42	44
3 years	36	36	55	56	32	33	26	28	11	14	24	27
5 years	29	29	43	44	26	28	22	26	8	13	19	24
Overall	(50)		(92)		(232)		(233)		(312)		(919)	
1 year	60	60	63	63	49	50	48	50	27	29	43	45
3 years	40	40	43	44	31	33	27	31	11	15	25	29
5 years	36	37	33	35	25	28	21	26	9	15	20	26

SCOTLAND

AREA	NUMBER OF CASES			PERIOD	MEAN AGE		
	Males	Females	All		Males	Females	All
Scotland	3886	4970	8856	1985-1989	68.8	71.7	70.4

OBSERVED AND RELATIVE SURVIVAL (%) BY AGE (number of cases in parentheses)

	AGE CLASS										ALL	
	15-44		45-54		55-64		65-74		75-99			
	obs	rel	obs	rel	obs	rel	obs	rel	obs	rel	obs	rel
Males	(126)		(273)		(794)		(1381)		(1312)		(3886)	
1 year	71	71	67	67	65	66	62	65	48	54	59	62
3 years	50	50	50	51	43	46	40	47	29	43	38	46
5 years	45	46	43	45	35	39	31	42	20	40	30	41
Females	(136)		(318)		(810)		(1351)		(2355)		(4970)	
1 year	71	71	71	71	70	70	63	65	47	51	57	60
3 years	55	55	53	53	47	49	44	48	31	42	39	46
5 years	49	50	44	45	39	42	36	43	22	38	31	41
Overall	(262)		(591)		(1604)		(2732)		(3667)		(8856)	
1 year	71	71	69	69	67	68	63	65	47	52	58	61
3 years	53	53	51	52	45	48	42	48	30	42	39	46
5 years	47	48	43	45	37	41	34	42	21	39	30	41

COLON   (ICD-9 153)

SLOVAKIA

AREA	NUMBER OF CASES			PERIOD	MEAN AGE		
	Males	Females	All		Males	Females	All
Slovakia	2318	1997	4315	1985-1989	64.3	65.9	65.1

OBSERVED AND RELATIVE SURVIVAL (%) BY AGE (number of cases in parentheses)

	AGE CLASS										ALL	
	15-44		45-54		55-64		65-74		75-99			
	obs	rel	obs	rel	obs	rel	obs	rel	obs	rel	obs	rel
Males	(140)		(278)		(695)		(715)		(490)		(2318)	
1 year	71	71	64	64	57	59	55	58	39	44	54	57
3 years	48	48	41	43	38	42	38	45	24	36	36	42
5 years	46	47	36	39	33	39	31	42	18	36	30	40
Females	(113)		(233)		(488)		(606)		(557)		(1997)	
1 year	73	74	67	67	67	68	53	55	39	43	55	57
3 years	50	51	50	51	49	51	36	39	23	31	38	43
5 years	45	46	43	45	42	45	31	38	19	33	33	41
Overall	(253)		(511)		(1183)		(1321)		(1047)		(4315)	
1 year	72	72	65	66	61	62	54	57	39	44	55	57
3 years	49	49	45	47	43	46	37	42	23	33	37	43
5 years	46	46	39	42	37	42	31	40	19	34	32	40

SLOVENIA

AREA	NUMBER OF CASES			PERIOD	MEAN AGE		
	Males	Females	All		Males	Females	All
Slovenia	674	719	1393	1985-1989	65.0	67.1	66.1

OBSERVED AND RELATIVE SURVIVAL (%) BY AGE (number of cases in parentheses)

	AGE CLASS										ALL	
	15-44		45-54		55-64		65-74		75-99			
	obs	rel	obs	rel	obs	rel	obs	rel	obs	rel	obs	rel
Males	(43)		(93)		(158)		(215)		(165)		(674)	
1 year	67	68	63	64	54	55	45	47	41	46	50	53
3 years	42	42	47	49	38	41	25	29	24	35	32	37
5 years	40	40	40	42	30	34	21	28	18	34	26	34
Females	(35)		(75)		(168)		(210)		(231)		(719)	
1 year	62	62	72	72	65	66	51	52	42	46	54	56
3 years	44	45	53	54	46	47	36	39	27	36	38	42
5 years	38	39	45	46	40	42	27	32	24	39	31	39
Overall	(78)		(168)		(326)		(425)		(396)		(1393)	
1 year	65	65	67	68	60	61	48	50	41	46	52	54
3 years	43	43	50	51	42	44	30	34	26	36	35	40
5 years	39	40	42	44	35	38	24	30	21	37	29	37

COLON (ICD-9 153)

SPAIN

AREA	NUMBER OF CASES			PERIOD	MEAN AGE			5-YR RELATIVE SURVIVAL (%)	
	Males	Females	All		Males	Females	All	Males	Females
Basque Country	574	503	1077	1986-1988	65.5	68.5	66.9		
Mallorca	288	306	594	1985-1989	68.4	67.6	68.0		
Navarra	253	274	527	1985-1989	67.9	67.7	67.8		
Tarragona	298	284	582	1985-1989	68.1	68.4	68.3		
Spanish Registries	1413	1367	2780		67.0	68.1	67.6		

OBSERVED AND RELATIVE SURVIVAL (%) BY AGE (number of cases in parentheses)

	AGE CLASS										ALL	
	15-44		45-54		55-64		65-74		75-99			
	obs	rel	obs	rel	obs	rel	obs	rel	obs	rel	obs	rel
Males	(67)		(124)		(354)		(448)		(420)		(1413)	
1 year	79	79	70	71	72	73	66	68	55	60	65	68
3 years	64	64	52	53	56	59	46	52	34	46	46	53
5 years	58	59	45	46	50	54	39	47	28	49	40	50
Females	(80)		(108)		(271)		(417)		(491)		(1367)	
1 year	74	74	75	75	77	78	66	67	54	58	65	67
3 years	55	55	59	60	58	59	50	52	37	47	48	53
5 years	49	49	55	56	54	55	43	47	32	47	42	50
Overall	(147)		(232)		(625)		(865)		(911)		(2780)	
1 year	76	76	72	73	74	75	66	68	54	59	65	68
3 years	59	59	56	56	57	59	48	52	36	47	47	53
5 years	53	53	50	51	51	54	41	47	30	48	41	50

SWEDEN

AREA	NUMBER OF CASES			PERIOD	MEAN AGE		
	Males	Females	All		Males	Females	All
South Sweden	1162	1328	2490	1985-1989	70.3	71.5	71.0

OBSERVED AND RELATIVE SURVIVAL (%) BY AGE (number of cases in parentheses)

	AGE CLASS										ALL	
	15-44		45-54		55-64		65-74		75-99			
	obs	rel	obs	rel	obs	rel	obs	rel	obs	rel	obs	rel
Males	(35)		(56)		(202)		(402)		(467)		(1162)	
1 year	86	86	79	79	72	73	71	73	60	67	67	71
3 years	60	60	61	62	56	59	50	56	41	57	48	58
5 years	57	58	59	61	47	51	42	52	28	50	38	52
Females	(49)		(68)		(182)		(409)		(620)		(1328)	
1 year	90	90	72	72	76	77	74	75	64	69	70	73
3 years	71	72	62	62	58	60	59	62	43	56	52	59
5 years	71	72	59	60	53	55	50	56	34	53	44	55
Overall	(84)		(124)		(384)		(811)		(1087)		(2490)	
1 year	88	88	75	75	74	75	72	74	62	68	69	72
3 years	67	67	61	62	57	59	55	59	42	56	50	59
5 years	65	66	59	60	50	53	46	54	31	52	41	54

COLON (ICD-9 153)

SWITZERLAND

AREA	NUMBER OF CASES			PERIOD	MEAN AGE			5-YR RELATIVE SURVIVAL (%)	
	Males	Females	All		Males	Females	All	Males	Females
Basel	255	258	513	1985-1988	69.9	71.4	70.7		
Geneva	288	288	576	1985-1989	69.3	72.7	71.0		
Swiss Registries	543	546	1089		69.6	72.1	70.8		

OBSERVED AND RELATIVE SURVIVAL (%) BY AGE (number of cases in parentheses)

	AGE CLASS										ALL	
	15-44		45-54		55-64		65-74		75-99			
	obs	rel	obs	rel	obs	rel	obs	rel	obs	rel	obs	rel
Males	(17)		(46)		(116)		(150)		(214)		(543)	
1 year	100	100	83	83	81	82	75	78	58	64	71	75
3 years	88	88	62	63	63	66	54	60	40	56	52	62
5 years	81	82	57	59	52	57	44	54	24	45	40	54
Females	(18)		(34)		(83)		(138)		(273)		(546)	
1 year	89	89	79	80	71	71	79	80	62	67	70	73
3 years	67	67	71	71	55	56	51	54	43	56	49	57
5 years	67	67	59	60	43	44	45	50	30	48	39	50
Overall	(35)		(80)		(199)		(288)		(487)		(1089)	
1 year	94	94	81	82	77	78	77	79	60	66	70	74
3 years	77	77	66	67	59	62	52	57	42	56	51	59
5 years	74	74	58	59	48	52	44	52	28	47	39	52

COLON (ICD-9 153)

EUROPE, 1985-89
Weighted analyses

COUNTRY	% COVERAGE WITH C.R.s	YEARLY NO. OF CASES (Mean No. of cases recorded)		
		Males	Females	All
AUSTRIA	8	63	86	149
DENMARK	100	834	1062	1896
ENGLAND	50	3426	4053	7479
ESTONIA	100	95	140	235
FINLAND	100	340	482	822
FRANCE	4	279	265	544
GERMANY	2	166	223	389
ICELAND	100	29	27	56
ITALY	10	946	1032	1978
NETHERLANDS	20	309	361	670
POLAND	6	155	196	351
SCOTLAND	100	777	994	1771
SLOVAKIA	100	464	399	863
SLOVENIA	100	135	144	279
SPAIN	10	359	341	700
SWEDEN	17	232	266	498
SWITZERLAND	11	121	122	243

RELATIVE SURVIVAL (%) (Age-standardized)

□ 1 year ■ 5 years

OBSERVED AND RELATIVE SURVIVAL (%) BY AGE

	AGE CLASS										ALL	
	15-44		45-54		55-64		65-74		75-99			
	obs	rel	obs	rel	obs	rel	obs	rel	obs	rel	obs	rel
Males												
1 year	79	79	74	74	71	72	66	69	53	59	64	67
3 years	63	63	55	56	52	55	47	54	32	46	45	53
5 years	56	57	48	50	44	48	38	48	24	44	36	48
Females												
1 year	79	79	78	78	73	74	68	69	53	57	63	66
3 years	61	61	61	62	55	56	49	52	34	44	45	51
5 years	56	56	55	56	48	50	42	48	26	41	38	48
Overall												
1 year	79	79	76	76	72	73	67	69	53	58	64	67
3 years	62	62	58	59	54	56	48	53	33	45	45	52
5 years	56	56	52	53	46	49	40	48	25	43	37	48

AGE STANDARDIZED RELATIVE SURVIVAL(%)

COUNTRY	MALES		FEMALES	
	1-year (95% C.I.)	5-years (95% C.I.)	1-year (95% C.I.)	5-years (95% C.I.)
AUSTRIA	75.0 (66.8 - 84.2)	54.7 (44.2 - 67.7)	60.5 (53.3 - 68.6)	44.0 (36.1 - 53.6)
DENMARK	63.7 (62.2 - 65.3)	39.2 (37.3 - 41.2)	64.0 (62.7 - 65.4)	42.7 (41.1 - 44.4)
ENGLAND	61.6 (60.8 - 62.4)	41.0 (40.0 - 42.0)	60.5 (59.9 - 61.2)	41.3 (40.5 - 42.1)
ESTONIA	51.5 (46.5 - 57.0)	36.5 (30.4 - 44.0)	52.7 (48.9 - 56.8)	38.0 (33.5 - 43.0)
FINLAND	68.6 (66.1 - 71.2)	47.6 (44.2 - 51.2)	68.8 (66.9 - 70.8)	50.0 (47.6 - 52.5)
FRANCE	73.7 (71.0 - 76.4)	51.8 (47.9 - 56.1)	72.5 (69.9 - 75.2)	54.0 (50.4 - 57.8)
GERMANY	66.4 (63.0 - 70.1)	49.6 (44.7 - 55.0)	70.0 (67.2 - 72.8)	49.9 (46.3 - 53.8)
ICELAND	61.6 (54.0 - 70.2)	43.7 (34.8 - 54.8)	67.4 (59.7 - 76.1)	51.8 (42.4 - 63.2)
ITALY	67.3 (65.6 - 69.0)	46.9 (44.8 - 49.2)	68.5 (67.0 - 70.0)	47.0 (45.2 - 48.9)
NETHERLANDS	75.7 (72.9 - 78.7)	58.7 (54.2 - 63.6)	72.4 (69.9 - 75.0)	55.7 (52.2 - 59.4)
POLAND	43.4 (38.4 - 49.2)	24.8 (19.6 - 31.4)	43.1 (38.9 - 47.7)	22.6 (18.9 - 27.2)
SCOTLAND	61.5 (59.8 - 63.2)	41.1 (39.0 - 43.3)	61.3 (59.9 - 62.8)	41.1 (39.4 - 42.8)
SLOVAKIA	53.7 (51.3 - 56.2)	38.9 (35.7 - 42.4)	54.1 (51.8 - 56.5)	38.3 (35.4 - 41.3)
SLOVENIA	50.1 (46.0 - 54.6)	33.2 (28.3 - 39.0)	53.9 (50.2 - 57.9)	38.1 (33.7 - 43.0)
SPAIN	66.6 (63.9 - 69.4)	49.5 (45.8 - 53.4)	66.5 (63.9 - 69.1)	49.4 (46.2 - 52.8)
SWEDEN	71.4 (68.6 - 74.3)	51.8 (48.0 - 55.8)	73.4 (70.9 - 76.0)	55.2 (52.0 - 58.6)
SWITZERLAND	74.6 (70.7 - 78.6)	52.3 (46.9 - 58.3)	73.7 (69.9 - 77.7)	49.4 (44.5 - 54.8)
EUROPE, 1985-89	66.3 (65.3 - 67.3)	46.8 (45.4 - 48.3)	66.4 (65.5 - 67.3)	46.7 (45.6 - 47.9)

RECTUM (ICD-9 154)

AUSTRIA

AREA	NUMBER OF CASES			PERIOD	MEAN AGE		
	Males	Females	All		Males	Females	All
Tirol	90	95	185	1988-1989	66.1	70.7	68.5

OBSERVED AND RELATIVE SURVIVAL (%) BY AGE (number of cases in parentheses)

	AGE CLASS										ALL	
	15-44		45-54		55-64		65-74		75-99			
	obs	rel	obs	rel	obs	rel	obs	rel	obs	rel	obs	rel
Males	(2)		(13)		(19)		(34)		(22)		(90)	
1 year	100	100	77	77	68	69	71	73	64	69	70	72
3 years	0	0	54	55	37	38	56	61	45	58	48	53
5 years	0	0	46	47	26	28	38	45	41	64	37	44
Females	(2)		(9)		(12)		(31)		(41)		(95)	
1 year	100	100	56	56	83	84	81	82	63	67	72	74
3 years	100	100	44	45	75	76	52	54	41	50	51	56
5 years	100	100	44	45	75	77	39	43	34	48	43	51
Overall	(4)		(22)		(31)		(65)		(63)		(185)	
1 year	100	100	68	68	74	75	75	77	63	68	71	73
3 years	50	50	50	51	52	53	54	58	43	53	49	54
5 years	50	50	45	46	45	47	38	44	37	53	40	48

DENMARK

AREA	NUMBER OF CASES			PERIOD	MEAN AGE		
	Males	Females	All		Males	Females	All
Denmark	3471	2752	6223	1985-1989	69.1	70.2	69.6

OBSERVED AND RELATIVE SURVIVAL (%) BY AGE (number of cases in parentheses)

	AGE CLASS										ALL	
	15-44		45-54		55-64		65-74		75-99			
	obs	rel	obs	rel	obs	rel	obs	rel	obs	rel	obs	rel
Males	(89)		(259)		(729)		(1199)		(1195)		(3471)	
1 year	75	75	79	79	76	78	69	72	54	60	66	70
3 years	43	43	53	54	49	52	44	50	29	41	40	48
5 years	30	31	44	46	35	39	32	41	18	33	29	39
Females	(78)		(196)		(520)		(851)		(1107)		(2752)	
1 year	85	85	80	80	78	79	71	73	53	57	66	69
3 years	55	55	58	58	55	57	51	55	28	37	43	49
5 years	44	44	48	50	45	48	39	45	20	31	33	42
Overall	(167)		(455)		(1249)		(2050)		(2302)		(6223)	
1 year	80	80	79	80	77	78	70	72	53	59	66	69
3 years	49	49	55	56	52	54	47	52	28	39	42	49
5 years	37	37	46	48	39	43	35	43	19	32	31	40

RECTUM   (ICD-9 154)

ENGLAND

AREA	NUMBER OF CASES			PERIOD	MEAN AGE			5-YR RELATIVE SURVIVAL (%)	
	Males	Females	All		Males	Females	All	Males	Females
East Anglia	1201	914	2115	1985-1989	69.1	71.9	70.3		
Mersey	1379	1086	2465	1985-1989	67.9	71.4	69.5		
Oxford	1156	927	2083	1985-1989	68.1	70.9	69.4		
South Thames	2657	2344	5001	1985-1989	69.2	71.3	70.2		
Wessex	1476	1294	2770	1985-1989	68.9	71.7	70.2		
West Midlands	3124	2065	5189	1985-1989	67.5	70.5	68.7		
Yorkshire	2025	1664	3689	1985-1989	68.3	71.4	69.7		
English Registries	13018	10294	23312		68.4	71.2	69.6		

5-YR RELATIVE SURVIVAL (%) chart:
100 80 60 40 20 0 | E.Angl | Mersey | Oxford | S.Tham | Wessex | W.Midl | Yorksh | 0 20 40 60 80 100

OBSERVED AND RELATIVE SURVIVAL (%) BY AGE (number of cases in parentheses)

	AGE CLASS										ALL	
	15-44		45-54		55-64		65-74		75-99			
	obs	rel	obs	rel	obs	rel	obs	rel	obs	rel	obs	rel
Males	(385)		(1046)		(2933)		(4525)		(4129)		(13018)	
1 year	77	77	76	77	74	76	66	69	52	58	64	68
3 years	56	56	51	52	50	52	42	48	29	41	41	48
5 years	50	50	41	43	38	42	32	41	20	36	31	41
Females	(292)		(684)		(1731)		(3061)		(4526)		(10294)	
1 year	82	82	79	79	76	77	70	71	51	56	64	67
3 years	56	56	55	56	54	56	47	51	29	39	41	48
5 years	47	47	47	48	43	46	38	43	21	34	32	41
Overall	(677)		(1730)		(4664)		(7586)		(8655)		(23312)	
1 year	79	79	77	78	75	76	67	70	51	57	64	67
3 years	56	56	53	54	51	54	44	49	29	40	41	48
5 years	48	49	44	45	40	44	34	42	20	35	31	41

ESTONIA

AREA	NUMBER OF CASES			PERIOD	MEAN AGE		
	Males	Females	All		Males	Females	All
Estonia	475	516	991	1985-1989	65.1	67.1	66.1

OBSERVED AND RELATIVE SURVIVAL (%) BY AGE (number of cases in parentheses)

	AGE CLASS										ALL	
	15-44		45-54		55-64		65-74		75-99			
	obs	rel	obs	rel	obs	rel	obs	rel	obs	rel	obs	rel
Males	(13)		(65)		(152)		(137)		(108)		(475)	
1 year	46	46	72	73	67	69	57	60	38	43	58	61
3 years	23	23	43	45	44	49	36	42	18	27	35	42
5 years	23	24	38	42	36	43	28	39	11	23	28	38
Females	(16)		(53)		(138)		(167)		(142)		(516)	
1 year	69	69	81	81	80	81	59	60	40	44	62	65
3 years	50	50	58	59	55	58	38	42	17	24	40	45
5 years	50	50	53	54	46	50	29	35	12	21	32	40
Overall	(29)		(118)		(290)		(304)		(250)		(991)	
1 year	59	59	76	77	73	75	58	60	39	44	60	63
3 years	38	38	50	52	50	53	37	42	18	25	37	43
5 years	38	39	45	48	41	46	29	37	11	22	30	39

RECTUM   (ICD-9 154)

FINLAND

AREA	NUMBER OF CASES			PERIOD	MEAN AGE		
	Males	Females	All		Males	Females	All
Finland	1409	1429	2838	1985-1989	67.9	69.6	68.7

OBSERVED AND RELATIVE SURVIVAL (%) BY AGE (number of cases in parentheses)

	AGE CLASS										ALL	
	15-44		45-54		55-64		65-74		75-99			
	obs	rel	obs	rel	obs	rel	obs	rel	obs	rel	obs	rel
Males	(42)		(119)		(341)		(495)		(412)		(1409)	
1 year	83	84	83	84	86	88	76	80	67	75	77	81
3 years	62	63	66	68	58	62	48	56	40	57	50	59
5 years	57	58	55	57	45	50	35	45	26	50	37	49
Females	(52)		(124)		(240)		(446)		(567)		(1429)	
1 year	87	87	85	85	81	81	76	78	61	66	72	75
3 years	79	79	65	66	59	61	53	57	34	44	48	55
5 years	63	64	56	57	50	52	42	47	23	37	38	47
Overall	(94)		(243)		(581)		(941)		(979)		(2838)	
1 year	85	85	84	84	84	85	76	79	64	70	74	78
3 years	71	72	66	67	59	61	51	56	36	49	49	57
5 years	61	61	55	57	47	51	38	46	24	42	37	48

FRANCE

AREA	NUMBER OF CASES			PERIOD	MEAN AGE			5-YR RELATIVE SURVIVAL (%)	
	Males	Females	All		Males	Females	All	Males	Females
Somme	249	200	449	1985-1989	68.0	69.3	68.6		
Calvados	286	236	522	1985-1989	65.2	70.4	67.5		
Côte d'Or	281	179	460	1985-1989	69.4	70.4	69.8		
Doubs	237	195	432	1985-1989	66.7	69.9	68.2		
French Registries	1053	810	1863		67.3	70.0	68.5		

OBSERVED AND RELATIVE SURVIVAL (%) BY AGE (number of cases in parentheses)

	AGE CLASS										ALL	
	15-44		45-54		55-64		65-74		75-99			
	obs	rel	obs	rel	obs	rel	obs	rel	obs	rel	obs	rel
Males	(52)		(89)		(276)		(290)		(346)		(1053)	
1 year	80	80	86	86	83	84	80	83	63	70	75	79
3 years	52	53	58	59	61	64	56	63	38	53	51	60
5 years	43	44	48	50	47	51	40	49	25	46	38	49
Females	(29)		(59)		(185)		(196)		(341)		(810)	
1 year	82	82	86	86	81	82	81	82	68	74	76	79
3 years	60	60	58	59	60	61	58	61	37	49	50	56
5 years	60	60	52	53	49	50	49	54	25	40	39	49
Overall	(81)		(148)		(461)		(486)		(687)		(1863)	
1 year	81	81	86	86	82	83	80	83	65	72	76	79
3 years	55	55	58	59	60	63	57	62	38	51	51	58
5 years	49	50	49	51	47	51	43	51	25	43	38	49

RECTUM   (ICD-9 154)

GERMANY

AREA	NUMBER OF CASES			PERIOD	MEAN AGE		
	Males	Females	All		Males	Females	All
Saarland	654	592	1246	1985-1989	66.6	69.2	67.9

OBSERVED AND RELATIVE SURVIVAL (%) BY AGE (number of cases in parentheses)

	AGE CLASS										ALL	
	15-44		45-54		55-64		65-74		75-99			
	obs	rel	obs	rel	obs	rel	obs	rel	obs	rel	obs	rel
Males	(19)		(92)		(165)		(179)		(199)		(654)	
1 year	74	74	80	81	84	86	74	78	56	63	72	76
3 years	42	42	55	57	50	53	44	51	31	45	43	51
5 years	33	33	45	46	37	41	36	47	21	42	33	44
Females	(22)		(45)		(124)		(173)		(228)		(592)	
1 year	95	96	87	87	81	81	75	77	53	57	69	72
3 years	91	91	58	58	55	56	57	61	32	41	48	54
5 years	72	72	51	52	43	45	41	46	22	35	36	45
Overall	(41)		(137)		(289)		(352)		(427)		(1246)	
1 year	85	86	82	83	83	84	75	77	55	60	71	74
3 years	68	69	56	57	52	55	50	56	31	42	45	52
5 years	54	54	47	48	40	43	38	47	21	38	34	44

ICELAND

AREA	NUMBER OF CASES			PERIOD	MEAN AGE		
	Males	Females	All		Males	Females	All
Iceland	42	46	88	1985-1989	70.7	68.6	69.6

OBSERVED AND RELATIVE SURVIVAL (%) BY AGE (number of cases in parentheses)

	AGE CLASS										ALL	
	15-44		45-54		55-64		65-74		75-99			
	obs	rel	obs	rel	obs	rel	obs	rel	obs	rel	obs	rel
Males	(0)		(2)		(10)		(15)		(15)		(42)	
1 year	-	-	100	100	90	91	80	82	60	67	76	80
3 years	-	-	100	100	60	63	60	66	40	55	55	64
5 years	-	-	50	52	50	54	60	71	27	47	45	58
Females	(1)		(3)		(11)		(13)		(18)		(46)	
1 year	100	100	67	67	100	100	92	94	56	59	78	81
3 years	0	0	67	67	73	74	77	81	33	41	57	62
5 years	0	0	67	68	64	66	62	68	22	32	46	54
Overall	(1)		(5)		(21)		(28)		(33)		(88)	
1 year	100	100	80	80	95	96	86	88	58	62	77	80
3 years	0	0	80	81	67	69	68	73	36	47	56	63
5 years	0	0	60	61	57	60	61	69	24	38	45	56

RECTUM (ICD-9 154)

ITALY

AREA	NUMBER OF CASES			PERIOD	MEAN AGE			5-YR RELATIVE SURVIVAL (%)	
	Males	Females	All		Males	Females	All	Males	Females
Florence	841	645	1486	1985-1989	68.6	70.2	69.3		
Genoa	237	228	465	1986-1988	67.4	69.2	68.3		
Latina	70	74	144	1985-1987	64.6	64.3	64.5		
Modena	221	162	383	1985-1989	66.8	69.5	68.0		
Parma	148	131	279	1985-1987	68.9	68.7	68.8		
Ragusa	115	72	187	1985-1989	66.3	69.3	67.5		
Romagna	150	107	257	1986-1988	69.0	68.3	68.7		
Turin	284	236	520	1985-1987	66.1	68.2	67.1		
Varese	372	298	670	1985-1989	65.8	68.6	67.0		
Italian Registries	2438	1953	4391		67.4	69.1	68.2		

OBSERVED AND RELATIVE SURVIVAL (%) BY AGE (number of cases in parentheses)

	AGE CLASS										ALL	
	15-44		45-54		55-64		65-74		75-99			
	obs	rel	obs	rel	obs	rel	obs	rel	obs	rel	obs	rel
Males	(83)		(252)		(621)		(714)		(768)		(2438)	
1 year	83	83	83	83	78	79	72	74	57	63	70	73
3 years	60	61	57	58	55	58	49	55	31	43	46	53
5 years	49	50	45	47	47	52	38	46	19	34	35	45
Females	(61)		(189)		(385)		(590)		(728)		(1953)	
1 year	87	87	86	86	83	84	73	74	59	63	71	74
3 years	66	66	65	65	58	59	50	53	33	41	47	52
5 years	59	59	56	57	45	47	40	45	25	38	38	45
Overall	(144)		(441)		(1006)		(1304)		(1496)		(4391)	
1 year	85	85	84	85	80	81	72	74	58	63	71	74
3 years	63	63	60	61	56	58	50	54	32	42	47	53
5 years	53	54	50	51	47	50	39	45	22	36	36	45

NETHERLANDS

AREA	NUMBER OF CASES			PERIOD	MEAN AGE			5-YR RELATIVE SURVIVAL (%)	
	Males	Females	All		Males	Females	All	Males	Females
Eindhoven	426	302	728	1985-1989	65.7	66.1	65.9		
Rotterdam	404	306	710	1987-1989	68.3	70.0	69.1		
Dutch Registries	830	608	1438		67.0	68.1	67.5		

OBSERVED AND RELATIVE SURVIVAL (%) BY AGE (number of cases in parentheses)

	AGE CLASS										ALL	
	15-44		45-54		55-64		65-74		75-99			
	obs	rel	obs	rel	obs	rel	obs	rel	obs	rel	obs	rel
Males	(41)		(87)		(205)		(247)		(250)		(830)	
1 year	83	83	81	82	83	85	77	81	65	73	76	80
3 years	70	71	61	62	61	64	50	57	37	54	51	60
5 years	52	53	50	51	53	58	39	49	27	52	41	53
Females	(22)		(65)		(137)		(178)		(206)		(608)	
1 year	91	91	78	79	84	84	82	83	69	75	78	81
3 years	81	82	57	58	59	60	62	66	44	57	55	61
5 years	71	72	49	50	53	54	54	61	29	46	46	55
Overall	(63)		(152)		(342)		(425)		(456)		(1438)	
1 year	86	86	80	80	83	84	79	82	67	74	77	80
3 years	74	75	59	60	60	62	55	61	40	55	53	60
5 years	58	59	49	51	53	56	45	54	28	49	43	54

RECTUM (ICD-9 154)

POLAND

AREA	NUMBER OF CASES			PERIOD	MEAN AGE			5-YR RELATIVE SURVIVAL (%)	
	Males	Females	All		Males	Females	All	Males	Females
Cracow	179	199	378	1985-1989	64.6	66.4	65.6		
Warsaw	195	222	417	1988-1989	64.3	67.9	66.2		
Polish Registries	374	421	795		64.5	67.2	65.9		

OBSERVED AND RELATIVE SURVIVAL (%) BY AGE (number of cases in parentheses)

	AGE CLASS										ALL	
	15-44		45-54		55-64		65-74		75-99			
	obs	rel	obs	rel	obs	rel	obs	rel	obs	rel	obs	rel
Males	(16)		(39)		(134)		(108)		(77)		(374)	
1 year	50	50	67	67	65	67	49	51	38	43	54	57
3 years	13	13	36	37	37	40	31	36	8	12	28	33
5 years	13	13	28	30	26	31	25	34	1	3	20	27
Females	(15)		(52)		(103)		(111)		(140)		(421)	
1 year	60	60	60	60	65	65	53	55	38	42	52	54
3 years	33	34	29	29	37	39	24	27	15	20	25	29
5 years	33	34	25	26	31	33	19	22	8	13	19	24
Overall	(31)		(91)		(237)		(219)		(217)		(795)	
1 year	55	55	63	63	65	66	51	53	38	42	53	55
3 years	23	23	32	33	37	39	28	31	13	17	27	31
5 years	23	23	26	28	28	32	22	28	6	9	20	25

SCOTLAND

AREA	NUMBER OF CASES			PERIOD	MEAN AGE		
	Males	Females	All		Males	Females	All
Scotland	2293	2111	4404	1985-1989	68.1	71.0	69.5

OBSERVED AND RELATIVE SURVIVAL (%) BY AGE (number of cases in parentheses)

	AGE CLASS										ALL	
	15-44		45-54		55-64		65-74		75-99			
	obs	rel	obs	rel	obs	rel	obs	rel	obs	rel	obs	rel
Males	(69)		(182)		(522)		(827)		(693)		(2293)	
1 year	70	70	71	72	72	74	69	73	46	52	63	67
3 years	43	44	46	47	49	52	43	50	24	36	39	47
5 years	36	37	39	41	37	42	29	38	15	30	28	38
Females	(71)		(147)		(382)		(583)		(928)		(2111)	
1 year	75	75	77	77	75	76	67	69	46	51	60	64
3 years	58	58	56	57	50	52	45	49	25	35	38	45
5 years	44	44	48	50	38	41	35	41	18	32	29	39
Overall	(140)		(329)		(904)		(1410)		(1621)		(4404)	
1 year	72	72	74	74	73	75	68	71	46	52	62	65
3 years	51	51	50	51	49	52	44	50	25	35	39	46
5 years	40	40	43	45	38	42	31	40	17	31	28	38

RECTUM (ICD-9 154)

SLOVAKIA

AREA	NUMBER OF CASES			PERIOD	MEAN AGE		
	Males	Females	All		Males	Females	All
Slovakia	2639	1788	4427	1985-1989	65.3	66.4	65.8

OBSERVED AND RELATIVE SURVIVAL (%) BY AGE (number of cases in parentheses)

	AGE CLASS										ALL	
	15-44		45-54		55-64		65-74		75-99			
	obs	rel	obs	rel	obs	rel	obs	rel	obs	rel	obs	rel
Males	(128)		(321)		(751)		(799)		(640)		(2639)	
1 year	78	78	70	71	66	68	58	61	44	50	59	63
3 years	49	50	41	43	40	44	32	39	22	33	34	40
5 years	40	41	33	35	33	38	25	34	17	33	27	36
Females	(92)		(218)		(410)		(533)		(535)		(1788)	
1 year	72	72	71	71	71	72	62	64	47	52	61	64
3 years	43	44	44	45	47	48	39	43	24	33	37	42
5 years	37	37	38	39	38	40	33	40	18	32	31	38
Overall	(220)		(539)		(1161)		(1332)		(1175)		(4427)	
1 year	75	76	71	71	68	69	60	62	46	51	60	63
3 years	47	47	42	44	42	45	35	40	23	33	35	41
5 years	39	39	35	37	35	39	28	37	17	33	28	37

SLOVENIA

AREA	NUMBER OF CASES			PERIOD	MEAN AGE		
	Males	Females	All		Males	Females	All
Slovenia	823	759	1582	1985-1989	65.0	66.8	65.9

OBSERVED AND RELATIVE SURVIVAL (%) BY AGE (number of cases in parentheses)

	AGE CLASS										ALL	
	15-44		45-54		55-64		65-74		75-99			
	obs	rel	obs	rel	obs	rel	obs	rel	obs	rel	obs	rel
Males	(46)		(122)		(222)		(209)		(224)		(823)	
1 year	80	81	72	72	70	72	60	63	41	46	61	64
3 years	50	51	47	49	38	41	33	38	16	23	33	38
5 years	35	36	38	41	32	36	24	32	9	17	25	32
Females	(39)		(73)		(195)		(208)		(244)		(759)	
1 year	62	62	73	73	71	71	63	64	43	47	59	62
3 years	33	33	47	47	44	45	37	40	23	32	35	40
5 years	26	26	41	42	34	36	27	32	15	26	26	33
Overall	(85)		(195)		(417)		(417)		(468)		(1582)	
1 year	72	72	72	73	71	72	61	64	42	46	60	63
3 years	42	43	47	48	41	43	35	39	20	28	34	39
5 years	31	31	39	41	33	36	26	32	12	22	25	32

RECTUM   (ICD-9 154)

SPAIN

AREA	NUMBER OF CASES			PERIOD	MEAN AGE			5-YR RELATIVE SURVIVAL (%)	
	Males	Females	All		Males	Females	All	Males	Females
Basque Country	549	309	858	1986-1988	66.3	65.4	66.0		
Mallorca	279	190	469	1985-1989	68.7	68.8	68.8		
Navarra	244	141	385	1985-1989	67.2	67.3	67.2		
Tarragona	234	166	400	1985-1989	68.6	68.2	68.4		
Spanish Registries	1306	806	2112		67.4	67.1	67.3		

OBSERVED AND RELATIVE SURVIVAL (%) BY AGE (number of cases in parentheses)

	AGE CLASS										ALL	
	15-44		45-54		55-64		65-74		75-99			
	obs	rel	obs	rel	obs	rel	obs	rel	obs	rel	obs	rel
Males	(59)		(114)		(300)		(431)		(402)		(1306)	
1 year	71	71	83	84	74	75	70	72	61	67	69	72
3 years	49	49	57	58	46	48	43	48	36	50	43	49
5 years	45	46	50	52	37	40	34	41	26	45	34	43
Females	(41)		(87)		(180)		(237)		(261)		(806)	
1 year	80	81	78	78	76	76	74	75	55	59	69	71
3 years	61	61	60	60	52	53	47	49	31	39	45	49
5 years	45	45	51	52	44	45	38	42	27	40	38	44
Overall	(100)		(201)		(480)		(668)		(663)		(2112)	
1 year	75	75	81	81	75	75	71	73	59	64	69	72
3 years	54	54	58	59	48	50	44	48	34	45	44	49
5 years	46	46	50	52	40	42	35	42	26	43	35	43

SWEDEN

AREA	NUMBER OF CASES			PERIOD	MEAN AGE		
	Males	Females	All		Males	Females	All
South Sweden	854	666	1520	1985-1989	69.6	70.5	70.0

OBSERVED AND RELATIVE SURVIVAL (%) BY AGE (number of cases in parentheses)

	AGE CLASS										ALL	
	15-44		45-54		55-64		65-74		75-99			
	obs	rel	obs	rel	obs	rel	obs	rel	obs	rel	obs	rel
Males	(18)		(54)		(172)		(306)		(304)		(854)	
1 year	100	100	81	82	75	76	77	80	63	69	72	76
3 years	78	78	65	66	52	55	53	59	37	51	48	56
5 years	72	73	56	57	43	47	40	48	27	47	37	49
Females	(25)		(53)		(110)		(190)		(288)		(666)	
1 year	92	92	85	85	81	81	79	80	69	75	76	79
3 years	76	76	66	67	57	59	62	66	41	53	53	60
5 years	72	72	64	65	48	50	49	55	28	45	42	52
Overall	(43)		(107)		(282)		(496)		(592)		(1520)	
1 year	95	95	83	84	77	78	78	80	66	72	74	77
3 years	77	77	65	66	54	56	56	61	39	52	50	58
5 years	72	73	60	61	45	48	43	51	27	46	39	51

RECTUM (ICD-9 154)

SWITZERLAND

AREA	NUMBER OF CASES			PERIOD	MEAN AGE			5-YR RELATIVE SURVIVAL (%)	
	Males	Females	All		Males	Females	All	Males	Females
Basel	190	154	344	1985-1988	69.0	72.0	70.3		
Geneva	141	147	288	1985-1989	68.1	69.7	68.9		
Swiss Registries	331	301	632		68.6	70.9	69.7		

OBSERVED AND RELATIVE SURVIVAL (%) BY AGE (number of cases in parentheses)

	AGE CLASS										ALL	
	15-44		45-54		55-64		65-74		75-99			
	obs	rel	obs	rel	obs	rel	obs	rel	obs	rel	obs	rel
Males	(13)		(28)		(65)		(115)		(110)		(331)	
1 year	85	85	86	86	83	84	71	74	62	69	72	76
3 years	68	68	46	47	71	74	50	56	38	53	50	59
5 years	42	43	46	48	55	60	43	52	28	51	40	53
Females	(12)		(23)		(47)		(78)		(141)		(301)	
1 year	91	91	78	78	89	90	85	86	71	76	79	82
3 years	73	73	52	53	66	67	53	56	42	53	50	57
5 years	64	64	52	53	60	62	45	50	29	45	41	51
Overall	(25)		(51)		(112)		(193)		(251)		(632)	
1 year	88	88	82	83	86	87	77	79	67	73	75	79
3 years	71	71	49	50	69	71	51	56	40	53	50	58
5 years	53	53	49	50	57	61	44	51	28	47	41	52

RECTUM (ICD-9 154)

EUROPE, 1985-89

Weighted analyses

COUNTRY	% COVERAGE WITH C.R.s	YEARLY NO. OF CASES (Mean No. of cases recorded)		
		Males	Females	All
AUSTRIA	8	45	48	93
DENMARK	100	694	550	1244
ENGLAND	50	2604	2059	4663
ESTONIA	100	95	103	198
FINLAND	100	282	286	568
FRANCE	4	211	162	373
GERMANY	2	131	118	249
ICELAND	100	8	9	17
ITALY	10	606	494	1100
NETHERLANDS	20	220	162	382
POLAND	6	133	151	284
SCOTLAND	100	459	422	881
SLOVAKIA	100	528	358	886
SLOVENIA	100	165	152	317
SPAIN	10	334	202	536
SWEDEN	17	171	133	304
SWITZERLAND	11	76	68	144

RELATIVE SURVIVAL (%) (Age-standardized)

□ 1 year ■ 5 years

OBSERVED AND RELATIVE SURVIVAL (%) BY AGE

	AGE CLASS										ALL	
	15-44		45-54		55-64		65-74		75-99			
	obs	rel	obs	rel	obs	rel	obs	rel	obs	rel	obs	rel
Males												
1 year	77	77	80	81	78	79	71	74	56	63	69	73
3 years	50	50	54	56	52	55	46	52	31	44	44	51
5 years	41	42	45	46	40	45	35	45	21	39	33	44
Females												
1 year	85	85	81	81	79	80	73	75	56	61	69	71
3 years	67	68	56	57	55	56	50	54	32	41	45	51
5 years	58	58	49	50	45	47	40	45	22	35	35	44
Overall												
1 year	80	81	81	81	78	79	72	74	56	62	69	72
3 years	58	58	55	56	53	55	48	53	31	43	44	51
5 years	49	49	47	48	42	46	37	45	22	37	34	44

AGE STANDARDIZED RELATIVE SURVIVAL(%)

COUNTRY	MALES		FEMALES	
	1-year (95% C.I.)	5-years (95% C.I.)	1-year (95% C.I.)	5-years (95% C.I.)
AUSTRIA	71.7 (62.1 - 82.9)	46.7 (34.7 - 62.7)	75.6 (67.2 - 85.0)	54.2 (44.1 - 66.6)
DENMARK	69.7 (68.0 - 71.3)	38.2 (36.1 - 40.3)	69.7 (68.0 - 71.5)	41.5 (39.4 - 43.7)
ENGLAND	67.4 (66.5 - 68.2)	40.1 (39.0 - 41.2)	68.2 (67.3 - 69.2)	41.0 (39.9 - 42.2)
ESTONIA	56.8 (51.9 - 62.0)	34.1 (28.6 - 40.6)	61.4 (57.1 - 65.9)	35.5 (30.9 - 40.7)
FINLAND	80.4 (78.0 - 82.8)	49.3 (45.7 - 53.1)	75.5 (73.2 - 77.9)	46.1 (43.1 - 49.2)
FRANCE	78.6 (75.9 - 81.5)	48.4 (44.1 - 53.1)	79.6 (76.6 - 82.7)	48.4 (44.2 - 53.1)
GERMANY	74.5 (70.8 - 78.4)	43.5 (38.3 - 49.3)	72.4 (68.9 - 76.2)	43.6 (39.0 - 48.8)
ICELAND	-	-	80.8 (70.8 - 92.3)	52.5 (39.1 - 70.5)
ITALY	72.4 (70.5 - 74.3)	43.0 (40.6 - 45.6)	74.0 (72.0 - 76.0)	44.2 (41.7 - 46.8)
NETHERLANDS	79.0 (75.8 - 82.2)	52.4 (47.6 - 57.8)	80.4 (77.0 - 83.9)	53.8 (48.8 - 59.3)
POLAND	52.9 (47.4 - 59.1)	21.2 (17.1 - 26.3)	53.1 (48.4 - 58.4)	21.9 (17.8 - 26.9)
SCOTLAND	65.5 (63.4 - 67.6)	36.3 (33.8 - 39.0)	65.2 (63.2 - 67.4)	38.7 (36.3 - 41.3)
SLOVAKIA	60.0 (58.0 - 62.2)	35.1 (32.5 - 38.0)	62.4 (60.1 - 64.9)	37.1 (34.3 - 40.2)
SLOVENIA	60.4 (56.8 - 64.2)	28.6 (25.0 - 32.8)	60.3 (56.8 - 64.0)	31.3 (27.6 - 35.6)
SPAIN	71.9 (69.3 - 74.6)	43.3 (39.8 - 47.0)	70.3 (67.1 - 73.7)	43.1 (39.1 - 47.4)
SWEDEN	76.1 (73.1 - 79.3)	49.2 (45.1 - 53.8)	79.5 (76.3 - 82.9)	51.9 (47.5 - 56.6)
SWITZERLAND	75.9 (71.0 - 81.1)	52.6 (45.8 - 60.4)	82.9 (78.5 - 87.6)	51.6 (45.3 - 58.9)
EUROPE, 1985-89	71.9 (70.8 - 73.0)	42.6 (41.1 - 44.2)	71.8 (70.6 - 72.9)	42.9 (41.4 - 44.4)

LIVER   (ICD-9 155)

AUSTRIA

AREA	NUMBER OF CASES			PERIOD	MEAN AGE		
	Males	Females	All		Males	Females	All
Tirol	22	10	32	1988-1989	65.7	70.9	67.3

OBSERVED AND RELATIVE SURVIVAL (%) BY AGE (number of cases in parentheses)

	AGE CLASS										ALL	
	15-44		45-54		55-64		65-74		75-99			
	obs	rel	obs	rel	obs	rel	obs	rel	obs	rel	obs	rel
Males	(2)		(2)		(4)		(7)		(7)		(22)	
1 year	50	50	0	0	50	51	14	15	0	0	18	19
3 years	50	50	0	0	25	26	0	0	0	0	9	10
5 years	50	50	0	0	25	27	0	0	0	0	9	11
Females	(0)		(0)		(2)		(4)		(4)		(10)	
1 year	-	-	-	-	0	0	0	0	25	26	10	10
3 years	-	-	-	-	0	0	0	0	25	29	10	11
5 years	-	-	-	-	0	0	0	0	25	34	10	12
Overall	(2)		(2)		(6)		(11)		(11)		(32)	
1 year	50	50	0	0	33	34	9	9	9	10	16	16
3 years	50	50	0	0	17	17	0	0	9	11	9	10
5 years	50	50	0	0	17	18	0	0	9	13	9	11

DENMARK

AREA	NUMBER OF CASES			PERIOD	MEAN AGE		
	Males	Females	All		Males	Females	All
Denmark	1112	921	2033	1985-1989	69.6	71.3	70.4

OBSERVED AND RELATIVE SURVIVAL (%) BY AGE (number of cases in parentheses)

	AGE CLASS										ALL	
	15-44		45-54		55-64		65-74		75-99			
	obs	rel	obs	rel	obs	rel	obs	rel	obs	rel	obs	rel
Males	(28)		(75)		(207)		(406)		(396)		(1112)	
1 year	11	11	11	11	3	3	4	4	6	6	5	5
3 years	0	0	4	4	2	2	0	1	1	2	1	2
5 years	0	0	4	4	2	2	0	0	1	1	1	1
Females	(24)		(53)		(168)		(261)		(415)		(921)	
1 year	21	21	9	9	12	12	8	9	4	4	7	8
3 years	8	8	4	4	3	3	3	4	1	1	2	3
5 years	8	8	0	0	3	3	1	1	0	1	1	2
Overall	(52)		(128)		(375)		(667)		(811)		(2033)	
1 year	15	15	10	10	7	7	6	6	5	5	6	6
3 years	4	4	4	4	2	3	2	2	1	2	2	2
5 years	4	4	2	2	2	3	0	1	0	1	1	1

LIVER   (ICD-9 155)

ENGLAND

AREA	NUMBER OF CASES			PERIOD	MEAN AGE			5-YR RELATIVE SURVIVAL (%)	
	Males	Females	All		Males	Females	All	Males	Females
East Anglia	60	42	102	1985-1989	67.9	64.7	66.6		
Mersey	141	78	219	1985-1989	64.4	67.1	65.3		
Oxford	130	85	215	1985-1989	67.5	70.7	68.8		
South Thames	290	176	466	1985-1989	65.1	68.5	66.4		
Wessex	188	118	306	1985-1989	66.7	69.9	67.9		
West Midlands	237	133	370	1985-1989	65.0	68.4	66.2		
Yorkshire	223	135	358	1985-1989	67.7	69.8	68.5		
English Registries	1269	767	2036		66.1	68.8	67.1		

OBSERVED AND RELATIVE SURVIVAL (%) BY AGE (number of cases in parentheses)

	AGE CLASS										ALL	
	15-44		45-54		55-64		65-74		75-99			
	obs	rel	obs	rel	obs	rel	obs	rel	obs	rel	obs	rel
Males	(72)		(118)		(302)		(451)		(326)		(1269)	
1 year	36	36	16	16	11	11	9	10	8	9	11	12
3 years	15	15	9	10	5	5	3	4	2	2	4	5
5 years	11	11	8	8	3	3	2	3	1	2	3	4
Females	(44)		(55)		(145)		(225)		(298)		(767)	
1 year	39	39	18	18	10	10	12	12	6	6	11	12
3 years	16	16	7	7	4	4	4	4	2	2	4	4
5 years	11	11	7	7	3	3	2	3	1	2	3	4
Overall	(116)		(173)		(447)		(676)		(624)		(2036)	
1 year	37	37	17	17	11	11	10	10	7	7	11	12
3 years	16	16	9	9	4	5	3	4	2	2	4	5
5 years	11	11	8	8	3	3	2	3	1	2	3	4

ESTONIA

AREA	NUMBER OF CASES			PERIOD	MEAN AGE		
	Males	Females	All		Males	Females	All
Estonia	112	90	202	1985-1989	62.8	69.1	65.6

OBSERVED AND RELATIVE SURVIVAL (%) BY AGE (number of cases in parentheses)

	AGE CLASS										ALL	
	15-44		45-54		55-64		65-74		75-99			
	obs	rel	obs	rel	obs	rel	obs	rel	obs	rel	obs	rel
Males	(5)		(10)		(49)		(39)		(9)		(112)	
1 year	0	0	10	10	6	6	8	8	22	25	8	8
3 years	0	0	0	0	2	2	5	6	0	0	3	3
5 years	0	0	0	0	2	2	3	4	0	0	2	2
Females	(2)		(5)		(18)		(35)		(30)		(90)	
1 year	0	0	20	20	17	17	11	12	7	7	11	12
3 years	0	0	0	0	6	6	3	3	3	4	3	4
5 years	0	0	0	0	0	0	0	0	3	6	1	1
Overall	(7)		(15)		(67)		(74)		(39)		(202)	
1 year	0	0	13	13	9	9	9	10	10	11	9	10
3 years	0	0	0	0	3	3	4	5	3	4	3	3
5 years	0	0	0	0	1	2	1	2	3	5	1	2

LIVER (ICD-9 155)

FINLAND

AREA	NUMBER OF CASES			PERIOD	MEAN AGE		
	Males	Females	All		Males	Females	All
Finland	581	546	1127	1985-1989	68.0	71.7	69.8

OBSERVED AND RELATIVE SURVIVAL (%) BY AGE (number of cases in parentheses)

	AGE CLASS										ALL	
	15-44		45-54		55-64		65-74		75-99			
	obs	rel	obs	rel	obs	rel	obs	rel	obs	rel	obs	rel
Males	(23)		(32)		(145)		(209)		(172)		(581)	
1 year	43	44	25	25	17	17	14	15	14	16	16	17
3 years	13	13	9	10	5	5	5	6	3	5	5	6
5 years	13	13	9	10	3	3	4	5	1	2	3	5
Females	(18)		(26)		(94)		(148)		(260)		(546)	
1 year	33	33	31	31	18	18	16	16	10	11	15	16
3 years	11	11	12	12	4	4	5	5	1	2	3	4
5 years	11	11	12	12	3	3	2	2	0	1	2	3
Overall	(41)		(58)		(239)		(357)		(432)		(1127)	
1 year	39	39	28	28	17	17	15	15	12	13	16	16
3 years	12	12	10	11	5	5	5	5	2	3	4	5
5 years	12	12	10	11	3	3	3	4	1	1	3	4

FRANCE

AREA	NUMBER OF CASES			PERIOD	MEAN AGE			5-YR RELATIVE SURVIVAL (%)	
	Males	Females	All		Males	Females	All	Males	Females
Somme	81	25	106	1985-1989	64.3	67.8	65.1		
Calvados	141	21	162	1985-1989	65.7	64.5	65.5		
Côte d'Or	114	29	143	1985-1989	66.1	71.7	67.2		
Doubs	81	20	101	1985-1989	65.5	60.2	64.5		
French Registries	417	95	512		65.5	66.7	65.7		

OBSERVED AND RELATIVE SURVIVAL (%) BY AGE (number of cases in parentheses)

	AGE CLASS										ALL	
	15-44		45-54		55-64		65-74		75-99			
	obs	rel	obs	rel	obs	rel	obs	rel	obs	rel	obs	rel
Males	(9)		(46)		(129)		(157)		(76)		(417)	
1 year	22	22	34	34	24	24	20	20	21	23	23	24
3 years	11	11	14	14	10	10	10	11	10	13	10	12
5 years	11	11	3	4	7	7	8	9	3	5	6	8
Females	(14)		(5)		(17)		(25)		(34)		(95)	
1 year	43	43	-	-	39	39	29	29	13	14	26	27
3 years	21	22	-	-	13	13	10	10	6	8	10	12
5 years	21	22	-	-	0	0	5	5	6	11	6	8
Overall	(23)		(51)		(146)		(182)		(110)		(512)	
1 year	35	35	31	31	25	26	21	21	18	20	23	24
3 years	16	16	13	13	10	10	10	11	9	12	10	12
5 years	16	16	3	3	6	6	7	9	5	8	6	8

LIVER   (ICD-9 155)

GERMANY

AREA	NUMBER OF CASES			PERIOD	MEAN AGE		
	Males	Females	All		Males	Females	All
Saarland	101	67	168	1985-1989	63.5	70.9	66.5

OBSERVED AND RELATIVE SURVIVAL (%) BY AGE (number of cases in parentheses)

	AGE CLASS										ALL	
	15-44		45-54		55-64		65-74		75-99			
	obs	rel	obs	rel	obs	rel	obs	rel	obs	rel	obs	rel
Males	(2)		(17)		(37)		(27)		(18)		(101)	
1 year	50	50	12	12	16	16	15	15	11	12	15	15
3 years	50	50	6	6	8	9	4	4	0	0	6	7
5 years	-	-	6	6	8	9	0	0	0	0	5	6
Females	(2)		(1)		(16)		(23)		(25)		(67)	
1 year	50	50	0	0	13	13	13	13	12	13	13	14
3 years	0	0	0	0	0	0	9	9	4	5	4	5
5 years	0	0	0	0	0	0	9	10	4	7	4	6
Overall	(4)		(18)		(53)		(50)		(43)		(168)	
1 year	50	50	11	11	15	15	14	14	12	13	14	15
3 years	25	25	6	6	6	6	6	7	2	3	5	6
5 years	-	-	6	6	6	6	4	5	2	4	5	6

ICELAND

AREA	NUMBER OF CASES			PERIOD	MEAN AGE		
	Males	Females	All		Males	Females	All
Iceland	17	15	32	1985-1989	74.6	69.5	72.3

OBSERVED AND RELATIVE SURVIVAL (%) BY AGE (number of cases in parentheses)

	AGE CLASS										ALL	
	15-44		45-54		55-64		65-74		75-99			
	obs	rel	obs	rel	obs	rel	obs	rel	obs	rel	obs	rel
Males	(1)		(0)		(2)		(5)		(9)		(17)	
1 year	100	100	-	-	0	0	0	0	11	13	12	13
3 years	100	100	-	-	0	0	0	0	0	0	6	8
5 years	100	100	-	-	0	0	0	0	0	0	6	9
Females	(0)		(3)		(2)		(4)		(6)		(15)	
1 year	-	-	0	0	0	0	25	25	17	18	13	14
3 years	-	-	0	0	0	0	25	26	0	0	7	8
5 years	-	-	0	0	0	0	25	28	0	0	7	8
Overall	(1)		(3)		(4)		(9)		(15)		(32)	
1 year	100	100	0	0	0	0	11	11	13	15	13	13
3 years	100	100	0	0	0	0	11	12	0	0	6	8
5 years	100	100	0	0	0	0	11	13	0	0	6	9

LIVER

(ICD-9 155)

ITALY

AREA	NUMBER OF CASES			PERIOD	MEAN AGE			5-YR RELATIVE SURVIVAL (%)	
	Males	Females	All		Males	Females	All	Males	Females
Florence	258	167	425	1985-1989	69.0	70.9	69.8		
Genoa	145	70	215	1986-1988	67.5	71.0	68.6		
Latina	40	32	72	1985-1987	67.4	67.7	67.6		
Modena	88	53	141	1988-1989	67.6	74.5	70.2		
Parma	91	45	136	1985-1987	67.1	73.6	69.2		
Ragusa	96	39	135	1985-1989	68.3	70.4	68.9		
Romagna	78	28	106	1986-1988	66.0	72.9	67.8		
Turin	212	96	308	1985-1987	65.9	70.0	67.2		
Varese	281	129	410	1985-1989	67.4	71.4	68.7		
Italian Registries	1289	659	1948		67.5	71.3	68.8		

OBSERVED AND RELATIVE SURVIVAL (%) BY AGE (number of cases in parentheses)

	AGE CLASS										ALL	
	15-44		45-54		55-64		65-74		75-99			
	obs	rel	obs	rel	obs	rel	obs	rel	obs	rel	obs	rel
Males	(12)		(103)		(370)		(470)		(334)		(1289)	
1 year	14	14	17	18	18	18	20	21	9	10	16	17
3 years	0	0	5	5	6	6	6	7	2	3	5	6
5 years	0	0	4	4	4	4	3	4	1	2	3	4
Females	(15)		(40)		(100)		(219)		(285)		(659)	
1 year	33	33	25	25	28	28	25	25	9	10	19	20
3 years	7	7	8	8	9	9	10	11	1	2	6	7
5 years	7	7	5	5	6	6	5	6	0	1	3	4
Overall	(27)		(143)		(470)		(689)		(619)		(1948)	
1 year	25	25	20	20	20	20	22	22	9	10	17	18
3 years	4	4	6	6	7	7	7	8	2	3	5	6
5 years	4	4	4	4	4	4	4	5	1	1	3	4

NETHERLANDS

AREA	NUMBER OF CASES			PERIOD	MEAN AGE		
	Males	Females	All		Males	Females	All
Eindhoven	31	8	39	1985-1989	65.4	62.6	64.8

OBSERVED AND RELATIVE SURVIVAL (%) BY AGE (number of cases in parentheses)

	AGE CLASS										ALL	
	15-44		45-54		55-64		65-74		75-99			
	obs	rel	obs	rel	obs	rel	obs	rel	obs	rel	obs	rel
Males	(2)		(3)		(6)		(13)		(7)		(31)	
1 year	0	0	0	0	0	0	15	16	14	16	10	10
3 years	0	0	0	0	0	0	8	9	0	0	3	4
5 years	0	0	0	0	0	0	0	0	0	0	0	0
Females	(1)		(0)		(3)		(3)		(1)		(8)	
1 year	100	100	-	-	0	0	0	0	0	0	13	13
3 years	0	0	-	-	0	0	0	0	0	0	0	0
5 years	0	0	-	-	0	0	0	0	0	0	0	0
Overall	(3)		(3)		(9)		(16)		(8)		(39)	
1 year	33	33	0	0	0	0	13	13	13	14	10	11
3 years	0	0	0	0	0	0	6	7	0	0	3	3
5 years	0	0	0	0	0	0	0	0	0	0	0	0

LIVER   (ICD-9 155)

POLAND

AREA	NUMBER OF CASES			PERIOD	MEAN AGE			5-YR RELATIVE SURVIVAL (%)	
	Males	Females	All		Males	Females	All	Males	Females
Cracow	74	78	152	1985-1989	61.4	67.4	64.5		
Warsaw	78	60	138	1988-1989	67.8	68.5	68.1		
Polish Registries	152	138	290		64.7	67.9	66.2		

OBSERVED AND RELATIVE SURVIVAL (%) BY AGE (number of cases in parentheses)

	AGE CLASS										ALL	
	15-44		45-54		55-64		65-74		75-99			
	obs	rel	obs	rel	obs	rel	obs	rel	obs	rel	obs	rel
Males	(6)		(21)		(50)		(40)		(35)		(152)	
1 year	17	17	14	14	4	4	3	3	6	6	6	6
3 years	17	17	5	5	0	0	0	0	0	0	1	2
5 years	17	17	5	5	0	0	0	0	0	0	1	2
Females	(7)		(8)		(39)		(35)		(49)		(138)	
1 year	29	29	25	25	0	0	11	12	6	7	8	9
3 years	14	14	25	25	0	0	3	3	2	3	4	4
5 years	14	14	13	13	0	0	3	3	2	3	3	4
Overall	(13)		(29)		(89)		(75)		(84)		(290)	
1 year	23	23	17	17	2	2	7	7	6	7	7	7
3 years	15	15	10	11	0	0	1	2	1	2	2	3
5 years	15	16	7	7	0	0	1	2	1	2	2	3

SCOTLAND

AREA	NUMBER OF CASES			PERIOD	MEAN AGE		
	Males	Females	All		Males	Females	All
Scotland	460	274	734	1985-1989	68.2	71.6	69.5

OBSERVED AND RELATIVE SURVIVAL (%) BY AGE (number of cases in parentheses)

	AGE CLASS										ALL	
	15-44		45-54		55-64		65-74		75-99			
	obs	rel	obs	rel	obs	rel	obs	rel	obs	rel	obs	rel
Males	(18)		(23)		(108)		(187)		(124)		(460)	
1 year	17	17	17	18	9	9	9	9	4	5	8	9
3 years	6	6	9	9	1	1	2	2	0	0	2	2
5 years	0	0	4	5	1	1	1	1	0	0	1	1
Females	(8)		(15)		(50)		(69)		(132)		(274)	
1 year	50	50	7	7	12	12	13	13	6	7	10	11
3 years	13	13	7	7	4	4	6	6	2	3	4	5
5 years	0	0	7	7	4	4	4	5	2	3	3	4
Overall	(26)		(38)		(158)		(256)		(256)		(734)	
1 year	27	27	13	13	10	10	10	10	5	6	9	10
3 years	8	8	8	8	2	2	3	3	1	2	2	3
5 years	0	0	5	5	2	2	2	2	1	1	1	2

LIVER (ICD-9 155)

SLOVAKIA

AREA	NUMBER OF CASES			PERIOD	MEAN AGE		
	Males	Females	All		Males	Females	All
Slovakia	407	274	681	1985-1989	63.9	66.1	64.8

OBSERVED AND RELATIVE SURVIVAL (%) BY AGE (number of cases in parentheses)

	AGE CLASS										ALL	
	15-44		45-54		55-64		65-74		75-99			
	obs	rel	obs	rel	obs	rel	obs	rel	obs	rel	obs	rel
Males	(20)		(48)		(144)		(113)		(82)		(407)	
1 year	15	15	6	6	6	6	6	7	4	4	6	6
3 years	10	10	6	7	1	2	4	5	2	4	3	4
5 years	-	-	3	3	1	2	4	6	2	5	3	4
Females	(17)		(24)		(74)		(84)		(75)		(274)	
1 year	24	24	13	13	11	11	2	2	7	7	8	8
3 years	18	18	4	4	7	7	0	0	7	9	5	6
5 years	11	11	-	-	7	7	0	0	7	11	5	6
Overall	(37)		(72)		(218)		(197)		(157)		(681)	
1 year	19	19	8	8	7	8	5	5	5	6	7	7
3 years	14	14	6	6	3	3	3	3	4	6	4	5
5 years	6	6	3	3	3	4	3	3	4	8	4	5

SLOVENIA

AREA	NUMBER OF CASES			PERIOD	MEAN AGE		
	Males	Females	All		Males	Females	All
Slovenia	90	58	148	1985-1989	61.9	65.3	63.2

OBSERVED AND RELATIVE SURVIVAL (%) BY AGE (number of cases in parentheses)

	AGE CLASS										ALL	
	15-44		45-54		55-64		65-74		75-99			
	obs	rel	obs	rel	obs	rel	obs	rel	obs	rel	obs	rel
Males	(7)		(8)		(38)		(29)		(8)		(90)	
1 year	14	14	0	0	16	16	7	7	13	14	11	11
3 years	0	0	0	0	3	3	-	-	0	0	2	2
5 years	0	0	0	0	0	0	-	-	0	0	0	0
Females	(4)		(3)		(17)		(21)		(13)		(58)	
1 year	71	72	33	33	18	18	10	10	8	8	16	17
3 years	36	36	0	0	0	0	0	0	0	0	2	2
5 years	0	0	0	0	0	0	0	0	0	0	0	0
Overall	(11)		(11)		(55)		(50)		(21)		(148)	
1 year	32	32	9	9	16	17	8	8	10	10	13	14
3 years	11	11	0	0	2	2	-	-	0	0	2	2
5 years	0	0	0	0	0	0	-	-	0	0	0	0

LIVER (ICD-9 155)

SPAIN

AREA	NUMBER OF CASES			PERIOD	MEAN AGE			5-YR RELATIVE SURVIVAL (%)	
	Males	Females	All		Males	Females	All	Males	Females
Basque Country	200	63	263	1986-1988	65.4	64.7	65.3		
Mallorca	42	19	61	1988-1989	64.9	72.4	67.2		
Navarra	123	44	167	1985-1989	65.5	71.4	67.0		
Tarragona	67	36	103	1985-1989	66.1	69.1	67.2		
Spanish Registries	432	162	594		65.5	68.5	66.3		

5-YR RELATIVE SURVIVAL (%) chart scale: Males 100 80 60 40 20 0, Females 0 20 40 60 80 100; bars labelled Basque, Mallor, Navarr, Tarrag.

OBSERVED AND RELATIVE SURVIVAL (%) BY AGE (number of cases in parentheses)

	AGE CLASS									ALL	
	15-44		45-54		55-64		65-74		75-99			
	obs	rel	obs	rel	obs	rel	obs	rel	obs	rel	obs	rel
Males	(17)		(42)		(125)		(158)		(90)		(432)	
1 year	47	47	21	22	22	23	17	18	17	18	20	21
3 years	18	18	12	12	11	12	10	11	9	12	11	12
5 years	18	18	12	12	11	12	6	8	6	10	9	11
Females	(7)		(8)		(35)		(57)		(55)		(162)	
1 year	43	43	38	38	20	20	18	18	9	10	17	18
3 years	29	29	0	0	9	9	9	9	5	7	8	9
5 years	29	29	0	0	3	3	9	10	5	8	7	8
Overall	(24)		(50)		(160)		(215)		(145)		(594)	
1 year	46	46	24	24	22	22	17	18	14	15	19	20
3 years	21	21	10	10	11	11	10	11	8	10	10	11
5 years	21	21	10	10	9	10	7	8	6	9	8	10

SWEDEN

AREA	NUMBER OF CASES			PERIOD	MEAN AGE		
	Males	Females	All		Males	Females	All
South Sweden	178	141	319	1985-1989	70.2	69.9	70.1

OBSERVED AND RELATIVE SURVIVAL (%) BY AGE (number of cases in parentheses)

	AGE CLASS									ALL	
	15-44		45-54		55-64		65-74		75-99			
	obs	rel	obs	rel	obs	rel	obs	rel	obs	rel	obs	rel
Males	(7)		(9)		(29)		(62)		(71)		(178)	
1 year	0	0	22	22	17	17	11	12	6	6	10	11
3 years	0	0	11	11	3	4	6	7	1	2	4	5
5 years	0	0	11	11	3	4	5	6	0	0	3	4
Females	(7)		(16)		(17)		(37)		(64)		(141)	
1 year	14	14	19	19	6	6	19	19	11	12	13	14
3 years	0	0	13	13	0	0	8	9	6	8	6	7
5 years	0	0	6	6	0	0	5	6	5	7	4	5
Overall	(14)		(25)		(46)		(99)		(135)		(319)	
1 year	7	7	20	20	13	13	14	15	8	9	12	12
3 years	0	0	12	12	2	2	7	8	4	5	5	6
5 years	0	0	8	8	2	2	5	6	2	4	3	4

LIVER

(ICD-9 155)

SWITZERLAND

AREA	NUMBER OF CASES			PERIOD	MEAN AGE			5-YR RELATIVE SURVIVAL (%)	
	Males	Females	All		Males	Females	All	Males	Females
Basel	66	21	87	1985-1988	68.1	76.5	70.1		
Geneva	91	27	118	1985-1989	68.2	72.0	69.1		
Swiss Registries	157	48	205		68.2	74.0	69.5		

OBSERVED AND RELATIVE SURVIVAL (%) BY AGE (number of cases in parentheses)

	AGE CLASS										ALL	
	15-44		45-54		55-64		65-74		75-99			
	obs	rel	obs	rel	obs	rel	obs	rel	obs	rel	obs	rel
Males	(2)		(14)		(46)		(42)		(53)		(157)	
1 year	50	50	36	36	23	23	26	27	9	10	21	22
3 years	0	0	7	7	2	2	2	3	0	0	2	2
5 years	0	0	7	7	2	2	2	3	0	0	2	2
Females	(0)		(3)		(4)		(17)		(24)		(48)	
1 year	-	-	67	67	50	50	35	36	8	9	25	26
3 years	-	-	33	34	25	25	18	19	0	0	10	12
5 years	-	-	0	0	0	0	12	13	0	0	4	5
Overall	(2)		(17)		(50)		(59)		(77)		(205)	
1 year	50	50	41	41	25	25	29	30	9	10	22	23
3 years	0	0	12	12	4	4	7	7	0	0	4	5
5 years	0	0	6	6	2	2	5	6	0	0	2	3

LIVER

(ICD-9 155)

EUROPE, 1985-89

Weighted analyses

COUNTRY	% COVERAGE WITH C.R.s	YEARLY NO. OF CASES (Mean No. of cases recorded) Males	Females	All
AUSTRIA	8	11	5	16
DENMARK	100	222	184	406
ENGLAND	50	254	153	407
ESTONIA	100	22	18	40
FINLAND	100	116	109	225
FRANCE	4	83	19	102
GERMANY	2	20	13	33
ICELAND	100	3	3	6
ITALY	10	360	184	544
NETHERLANDS	6	6	2	8
POLAND	6	54	46	100
SCOTLAND	100	92	55	147
SLOVAKIA	100	81	55	136
SLOVENIA	100	18	12	30
SPAIN	10	126	47	173
SWEDEN	17	36	28	64
SWITZERLAND	11	35	11	46

RELATIVE SURVIVAL (%) (Age-standardized)

□ 1 year ■ 5 years

OBSERVED AND RELATIVE SURVIVAL (%) BY AGE

	AGE CLASS 15-44 obs rel	45-54 obs rel	55-64 obs rel	65-74 obs rel	75-99 obs rel	ALL obs rel
Males						
1 year	26 26	20 20	18 18	17 17	12 13	16 17
3 years	13 13	8 8	7 7	6 7	4 5	6 7
5 years	8 8	5 6	5 6	4 5	2 3	4 5
Females						
1 year	37 37	21 22	19 19	19 19	9 10	16 16
3 years	11 11	9 9	6 6	8 8	3 4	6 7
5 years	10 10	5 5	3 3	5 6	3 4	4 5
Overall						
1 year	29 30	21 21	18 18	17 18	11 12	16 17
3 years	12 12	8 8	7 7	7 7	4 5	6 7
5 years	9 9	5 5	4 5	4 5	2 3	4 5

AGE STANDARDIZED RELATIVE SURVIVAL(%)

COUNTRY	MALES 1-year (95% C.I.)	5-years (95% C.I.)	FEMALES 1-year (95% C.I.)	5-years (95% C.I.)
AUSTRIA	18.5 (8.3 - 41.2)	8.1 (2.1 - 31.2)	-	-
DENMARK	5.3 (4.1 - 6.9)	1.2 (0.7 - 2.3)	8.4 (6.7 - 10.6)	1.6 (0.9 - 2.8)
ENGLAND	11.1 (9.5 - 13.0)	3.3 (2.4 - 4.6)	11.1 (9.1 - 13.6)	3.2 (2.1 - 4.9)
ESTONIA	13.1 (5.8 - 29.5)	1.7 (0.4 - 7.5)	11.7 (6.5 - 20.9)	1.8 (0.3 - 12.8)
FINLAND	17.3 (14.4 - 20.8)	4.3 (2.8 - 6.6)	16.8 (13.7 - 20.5)	3.0 (1.8 - 5.3)
FRANCE	23.2 (18.9 - 28.4)	7.1 (4.2 - 11.8)	-	-
GERMANY	15.7 (9.4 - 26.1)	-	13.4 (7.4 - 24.2)	5.5 (1.8 - 16.7)
ICELAND	-	-	-	-
ITALY	16.4 (14.4 - 18.6)	3.2 (2.3 - 4.5)	21.3 (18.2 - 24.9)	4.1 (2.7 - 6.3)
NETHERLANDS	10.5 (3.5 - 31.6)	0.0 (0.0 - 0.0)	-	-
POLAND	5.6 (2.8 - 11.2)	1.0 (0.2 - 4.1)	9.0 (5.1 - 15.7)	3.7 (1.4 - 9.8)
SCOTLAND	8.6 (6.3 - 11.7)	0.8 (0.2 - 2.7)	11.8 (8.3 - 16.6)	4.1 (2.1 - 8.1)
SLOVAKIA	5.9 (3.9 - 8.9)	-	7.5 (5.0 - 11.4)	-
SLOVENIA	11.1 (4.9 - 25.5)	-	15.2 (8.4 - 27.5)	0.0 (0.0 - 0.0)
SPAIN	20.4 (16.7 - 24.8)	10.4 (7.3 - 14.8)	18.1 (13.0 - 25.2)	7.4 (4.2 - 13.2)
SWEDEN	11.7 (7.5 - 18.0)	3.7 (1.6 - 8.7)	13.5 (8.7 - 20.9)	4.8 (2.1 - 10.6)
SWITZERLAND	22.2 (16.3 - 30.3)	2.1 (0.7 - 6.8)	-	-
EUROPE, 1985-89	16.7 (15.1 - 18.4)	4.6 (3.5 - 6.0)	17.1 (15.0 - 19.4)	4.7 (3.4 - 6.6)

BILIARY TRACT (ICD-9 156)

AUSTRIA

AREA	NUMBER OF CASES			PERIOD	MEAN AGE		
	Males	Females	All		Males	Females	All
Tirol	19	36	55	1988-1989	65.5	73.7	70.9

OBSERVED AND RELATIVE SURVIVAL (%) BY AGE (number of cases in parentheses)

	15-44		45-54		55-64		65-74		75-99		ALL	
	obs	rel	obs	rel	obs	rel	obs	rel	obs	rel	obs	rel
Males	(0)		(3)		(4)		(8)		(4)		(19)	
1 year	-	-	67	67	50	51	38	38	50	53	47	49
3 years	-	-	67	67	25	26	0	0	0	0	16	17
5 years	-	-	67	68	25	27	0	0	0	0	16	18
Females	(0)		(1)		(5)		(12)		(18)		(36)	
1 year	-	-	100	100	40	40	33	34	39	41	39	40
3 years	-	-	100	100	0	0	17	18	28	34	22	25
5 years	-	-	100	100	0	0	17	18	17	23	17	20
Overall	(0)		(4)		(9)		(20)		(22)		(55)	
1 year	-	-	75	75	44	45	35	36	41	44	42	43
3 years	-	-	75	76	11	11	10	11	23	28	20	22
5 years	-	-	75	77	11	12	10	11	14	19	16	20

DENMARK

AREA	NUMBER OF CASES			PERIOD	MEAN AGE		
	Males	Females	All		Males	Females	All
Denmark	373	737	1110	1985-1989	68.9	72.3	71.2

OBSERVED AND RELATIVE SURVIVAL (%) BY AGE (number of cases in parentheses)

	15-44		45-54		55-64		65-74		75-99		ALL	
	obs	rel	obs	rel	obs	rel	obs	rel	obs	rel	obs	rel
Males	(17)		(28)		(66)		(135)		(127)		(373)	
1 year	41	41	50	50	29	29	18	19	8	9	20	21
3 years	24	24	14	15	14	14	2	3	3	5	6	8
5 years	12	12	11	11	8	8	2	3	2	3	4	5
Females	(15)		(24)		(126)		(226)		(346)		(737)	
1 year	53	53	33	33	21	22	19	19	14	15	18	19
3 years	20	20	4	4	10	10	6	6	5	6	6	7
5 years	7	7	0	0	7	8	3	3	2	4	3	4
Overall	(32)		(52)		(192)		(361)		(473)		(1110)	
1 year	47	47	42	43	24	24	19	19	12	14	19	20
3 years	22	22	10	10	11	11	4	5	4	6	6	7
5 years	9	9	6	6	7	8	2	3	2	4	4	5

BILIARY TRACT (ICD-9 156)

ENGLAND

AREA	NUMBER OF CASES			PERIOD	MEAN AGE			5-YR RELATIVE SURVIVAL (%)	
	Males	Females	All		Males	Females	All	Males	Females
East Anglia	126	158	284	1985-1989	70.8	73.2	72.2		
Mersey	99	129	228	1985-1989	67.7	72.0	70.2		
Oxford	85	128	213	1985-1989	68.0	72.0	70.4		
South Thames	226	331	557	1985-1989	70.1	73.8	72.3		
Wessex	97	152	249	1985-1989	69.9	73.5	72.1		
West Midlands	274	419	693	1985-1989	69.3	70.9	70.3		
Yorkshire	136	240	376	1985-1989	69.9	72.5	71.6		
English Registries	1043	1557	2600		69.5	72.5	71.3		

5-YR RELATIVE SURVIVAL (%) chart scale: Males 100 80 60 40 20 0; Females 0 20 40 60 80 100. Registries listed: E.Angl, Mersey, Oxford, S.Tham, Wessex, W.Midl, Yorksh

OBSERVED AND RELATIVE SURVIVAL (%) BY AGE (number of cases in parentheses)

	AGE CLASS										ALL	
	15-44		45-54		55-64		65-74		75-99			
	obs	rel	obs	rel	obs	rel	obs	rel	obs	rel	obs	rel
Males	(27)		(79)		(190)		(379)		(368)		(1043)	
1 year	51	51	51	51	38	39	25	26	15	16	26	28
3 years	31	31	28	28	16	17	11	13	5	7	12	14
5 years	31	31	25	26	12	13	8	10	3	5	9	12
Females	(29)		(78)		(227)		(461)		(762)		(1557)	
1 year	52	52	42	42	28	28	26	26	15	17	22	23
3 years	31	31	22	22	15	16	11	12	7	9	11	12
5 years	24	24	21	21	11	12	9	11	4	7	8	10
Overall	(56)		(157)		(417)		(840)		(1130)		(2600)	
1 year	51	51	46	47	33	33	25	26	15	17	24	25
3 years	31	31	25	25	16	16	11	13	6	8	11	13
5 years	27	28	23	23	12	12	9	11	4	7	8	11

ESTONIA

AREA	NUMBER OF CASES			PERIOD	MEAN AGE		
	Males	Females	All		Males	Females	All
Estonia	44	109	153	1985-1989	59.0	68.0	65.4

OBSERVED AND RELATIVE SURVIVAL (%) BY AGE (number of cases in parentheses)

	AGE CLASS										ALL	
	15-44		45-54		55-64		65-74		75-99			
	obs	rel	obs	rel	obs	rel	obs	rel	obs	rel	obs	rel
Males	(5)		(5)		(22)		(7)		(5)		(44)	
1 year	40	40	40	40	23	23	14	15	0	0	23	24
3 years	40	41	40	42	14	15	0	0	0	0	16	18
5 years	40	41	0	0	5	5	0	0	0	0	7	8
Females	(1)		(8)		(37)		(22)		(41)		(109)	
1 year	100	100	50	50	5	5	14	14	17	19	16	16
3 years	100	100	25	25	3	3	5	5	0	0	5	5
5 years	0	0	13	13	0	0	5	5	0	0	2	2
Overall	(6)		(13)		(59)		(29)		(46)		(153)	
1 year	50	50	46	46	12	12	14	14	15	17	18	18
3 years	50	51	31	31	7	7	3	4	0	0	8	9
5 years	33	34	8	8	2	2	3	4	0	0	3	4

BILIARY TRACT   (ICD-9 156)

FINLAND

AREA	NUMBER OF CASES			PERIOD	MEAN AGE		
	Males	Females	All		Males	Females	All
Finland	324	886	1210	1985-1989	67.9	72.3	71.1

OBSERVED AND RELATIVE SURVIVAL (%) BY AGE (number of cases in parentheses)

	AGE CLASS										ALL	
	15-44		45-54		55-64		65-74		75-99			
	obs	rel	obs	rel	obs	rel	obs	rel	obs	rel	obs	rel
Males	(11)		(21)		(94)		(93)		(105)		(324)	
1 year	27	27	33	34	36	37	22	22	13	15	24	25
3 years	18	18	0	0	15	16	9	10	2	3	8	10
5 years	18	19	0	0	12	13	6	8	1	2	6	8
Females	(16)		(45)		(152)		(257)		(416)		(886)	
1 year	63	63	33	33	28	29	21	21	13	14	20	21
3 years	31	31	13	13	15	15	9	9	5	6	8	10
5 years	25	25	9	9	14	14	5	6	3	5	6	8
Overall	(27)		(66)		(246)		(350)		(521)		(1210)	
1 year	48	48	33	33	31	32	21	22	13	14	21	22
3 years	26	26	9	9	15	16	9	9	4	6	8	10
5 years	22	22	6	6	13	14	6	7	3	5	6	8

FRANCE

AREA	NUMBER OF CASES			PERIOD	MEAN AGE			5-YR RELATIVE SURVIVAL (%)	
	Males	Females	All		Males	Females	All	Males	Females
Somme	25	61	86	1985-1989	70.9	70.5	70.7		
Calvados	35	44	79	1985-1989	70.5	74.1	72.5		
Côte d'Or	34	57	91	1985-1989	72.7	73.1	73.0		
Doubs	18	41	59	1985-1989	66.6	68.5	67.9		
French Registries	112	203	315		70.7	71.6	71.3		

OBSERVED AND RELATIVE SURVIVAL (%) BY AGE (number of cases in parentheses)

	AGE CLASS										ALL	
	15-44		45-54		55-64		65-74		75-99			
	obs	rel	obs	rel	obs	rel	obs	rel	obs	rel	obs	rel
Males	(3)		(1)		(24)		(34)		(50)		(112)	
1 year	33	33	100	100	42	43	34	35	27	30	33	35
3 years	33	34	100	100	12	13	15	17	16	22	16	20
5 years	33	34	100	100	6	7	11	14	3	5	8	11
Females	(5)		(14)		(41)		(45)		(98)		(203)	
1 year	80	80	70	70	49	49	39	40	24	26	37	39
3 years	-	-	39	39	30	30	25	26	7	9	18	21
5 years	-	-	23	24	26	27	22	24	5	9	14	18
Overall	(8)		(15)		(65)		(79)		(148)		(315)	
1 year	63	63	72	72	46	47	37	38	25	27	35	37
3 years	23	23	43	44	24	24	21	22	10	13	17	20
5 years	23	23	29	29	19	20	17	20	4	7	12	16

BILIARY TRACT   (ICD-9 156)

GERMANY

AREA	NUMBER OF CASES			PERIOD	MEAN AGE		
	Males	Females	All		Males	Females	All
Saarland	117	347	464	1985-1989	69.3	72.6	71.8

OBSERVED AND RELATIVE SURVIVAL (%) BY AGE (number of cases in parentheses)

	AGE CLASS									ALL	
	15-44		45-54		55-64		65-74		75-99			
	obs	rel	obs	rel	obs	rel	obs	rel	obs	rel	obs	rel
Males	(3)		(12)		(23)		(30)		(49)		(117)	
1 year	67	67	75	76	35	35	27	28	18	21	31	33
3 years	33	34	25	26	17	18	13	15	14	21	16	20
5 years	33	34	25	26	-	-	10	12	10	21	11	16
Females	(1)		(13)		(56)		(120)		(157)		(347)	
1 year	100	100	23	23	21	22	33	33	25	27	27	28
3 years	0	0	8	8	11	11	21	22	12	16	15	17
5 years	0	0	-	-	9	9	19	22	9	15	12	16
Overall	(4)		(25)		(79)		(150)		(206)		(464)	
1 year	75	75	48	48	25	26	31	32	23	26	28	29
3 years	25	25	16	16	13	13	19	21	13	17	15	18
5 years	25	25	16	16	9	9	17	20	9	16	12	16

ICELAND

AREA	NUMBER OF CASES			PERIOD	MEAN AGE		
	Males	Females	All		Males	Females	All
Iceland	11	17	28	1985-1989	68.6	74.3	72.1

OBSERVED AND RELATIVE SURVIVAL (%) BY AGE (number of cases in parentheses)

	AGE CLASS									ALL	
	15-44		45-54		55-64		65-74		75-99			
	obs	rel	obs	rel	obs	rel	obs	rel	obs	rel	obs	rel
Males	(0)		(0)		(5)		(3)		(3)		(11)	
1 year	-	-	-	-	20	20	33	34	33	38	27	29
3 years	-	-	-	-	0	0	33	37	0	0	9	10
5 years	-	-	-	-	0	0	33	40	0	0	9	12
Females	(0)		(0)		(4)		(5)		(8)		(17)	
1 year	-	-	-	-	75	76	20	20	38	41	41	43
3 years	-	-	-	-	25	26	20	22	25	34	24	28
5 years	-	-	-	-	25	26	20	23	13	21	18	23
Overall	(0)		(0)		(9)		(8)		(11)		(28)	
1 year	-	-	-	-	44	45	25	26	36	40	36	37
3 years	-	-	-	-	11	11	25	27	18	25	18	21
5 years	-	-	-	-	11	12	25	29	9	16	14	19

BILIARY TRACT (ICD-9 156)

ITALY

AREA	NUMBER OF CASES			PERIOD	MEAN AGE			5-YR RELATIVE SURVIVAL (%)	
	Males	Females	All		Males	Females	All	Males	Females
Florence	133	242	375	1985-1989	71.2	72.6	72.1		
Genoa	59	119	178	1986-1988	69.8	72.0	71.3		
Latina	16	35	51	1985-1987	71.0	72.1	71.8		
Modena	16	42	58	1988-1989	71.9	73.1	72.8		
Parma	28	44	72	1985-1987	70.0	68.9	69.3		
Ragusa	39	54	93	1985-1989	69.9	70.9	70.5		
Romagna	25	39	64	1986-1988	71.0	75.1	73.5		
Turin	55	111	166	1985-1987	67.9	72.2	70.8		
Varese	66	158	224	1985-1989	67.5	70.7	69.8		
Italian Registries	437	844	1281		69.9	71.9	71.2		

5-YR RELATIVE SURVIVAL (%) scale — Males: 100 80 60 40 20 0; Females: 0 20 40 60 80 100. Registries listed: Floren, Genoa, Latina, Modena, Parma, Ragusa, Romagn, Turin, Varese.

OBSERVED AND RELATIVE SURVIVAL (%) BY AGE (number of cases in parentheses)

	AGE CLASS										ALL	
	15-44		45-54		55-64		65-74		75-99			
	obs	rel	obs	rel	obs	rel	obs	rel	obs	rel	obs	rel
Males	(4)		(27)		(93)		(158)		(155)		(437)	
1 year	75	75	33	33	24	24	27	28	20	22	25	26
3 years	50	50	15	15	10	10	12	13	6	8	10	12
5 years	50	51	7	8	7	7	5	7	4	7	6	7
Females	(9)		(39)		(172)		(238)		(386)		(844)	
1 year	56	56	38	39	30	30	25	25	17	19	23	24
3 years	33	33	26	26	15	15	11	12	8	11	11	13
5 years	22	22	18	18	12	12	7	8	6	10	8	10
Overall	(13)		(66)		(265)		(396)		(541)		(1281)	
1 year	62	62	36	36	28	28	26	26	18	20	24	25
3 years	38	39	21	21	13	13	11	12	8	10	11	13
5 years	31	31	14	14	10	11	6	7	6	9	7	9

NETHERLANDS

AREA	NUMBER OF CASES			PERIOD	MEAN AGE		
	Males	Females	All		Males	Females	All
Eindhoven	62	120	182	1985-1989	66.0	72.7	70.4

OBSERVED AND RELATIVE SURVIVAL (%) BY AGE (number of cases in parentheses)

	AGE CLASS										ALL	
	15-44		45-54		55-64		65-74		75-99			
	obs	rel	obs	rel	obs	rel	obs	rel	obs	rel	obs	rel
Males	(3)		(5)		(18)		(23)		(13)		(62)	
1 year	33	33	80	80	72	73	26	27	15	17	42	44
3 years	33	34	20	20	22	23	0	0	0	0	10	11
5 years	33	34	20	21	6	6	0	0	0	0	5	6
Females	(0)		(6)		(20)		(38)		(56)		(120)	
1 year	-	-	33	33	35	35	18	19	21	23	23	24
3 years	-	-	17	17	20	20	8	8	7	9	10	12
5 years	-	-	17	17	20	21	5	6	4	6	8	10
Overall	(3)		(11)		(38)		(61)		(69)		(182)	
1 year	33	33	55	55	53	53	21	22	20	22	30	31
3 years	33	34	18	18	21	22	5	5	6	8	10	11
5 years	33	34	18	19	13	14	3	4	3	5	7	8

BILIARY TRACT (ICD-9 156)

POLAND

AREA	NUMBER OF CASES			PERIOD	MEAN AGE			5-YR RELATIVE SURVIVAL (%)	
	Males	Females	All		Males	Females	All	Males	Females
Cracow	48	169	217	1985-1989	65.8	70.0	69.1		
Warsaw	73	269	342	1988-1989	66.7	71.7	70.6		
Polish Registries	121	438	559		66.4	71.0	70.0		

OBSERVED AND RELATIVE SURVIVAL (%) BY AGE (number of cases in parentheses)

	AGE CLASS										ALL	
	15-44		45-54		55-64		65-74		75-99			
	obs	rel	obs	rel	obs	rel	obs	rel	obs	rel	obs	rel
Males	(7)		(11)		(36)		(27)		(40)		(121)	
1 year	43	43	9	9	19	20	19	20	5	6	15	16
3 years	14	15	9	9	14	15	7	9	0	0	7	9
5 years	0	0	9	10	11	13	4	5	0	0	5	7
Females	(4)		(22)		(105)		(115)		(192)		(438)	
1 year	0	0	23	23	16	16	18	18	5	5	12	13
3 years	0	0	9	9	6	6	11	12	2	2	5	6
5 years	0	0	9	9	4	4	10	12	1	1	4	5
Overall	(11)		(33)		(141)		(142)		(232)		(559)	
1 year	27	27	18	18	17	17	18	19	5	5	13	13
3 years	9	9	9	9	8	8	10	11	1	2	6	7
5 years	0	0	9	9	6	6	9	11	0	1	4	6

SCOTLAND

AREA	NUMBER OF CASES			PERIOD	MEAN AGE		
	Males	Females	All		Males	Females	All
Scotland	238	408	646	1985-1989	70.1	73.8	72.4

OBSERVED AND RELATIVE SURVIVAL (%) BY AGE (number of cases in parentheses)

	AGE CLASS										ALL	
	15-44		45-54		55-64		65-74		75-99			
	obs	rel	obs	rel	obs	rel	obs	rel	obs	rel	obs	rel
Males	(7)		(8)		(46)		(92)		(85)		(238)	
1 year	86	86	13	13	30	31	25	26	15	17	24	26
3 years	29	29	0	0	15	16	10	11	5	7	9	11
5 years	14	15	0	0	11	12	5	7	2	5	5	8
Females	(6)		(15)		(66)		(103)		(218)		(408)	
1 year	0	0	53	54	27	28	25	26	13	14	20	21
3 years	0	0	27	27	14	14	9	10	6	8	8	10
5 years	0	0	27	27	8	8	8	9	3	6	6	8
Overall	(13)		(23)		(112)		(195)		(303)		(646)	
1 year	46	46	39	39	29	29	25	26	14	15	21	23
3 years	15	15	17	18	14	15	9	10	5	7	9	11
5 years	8	8	17	18	9	10	7	8	3	5	6	8

BILIARY TRACT (ICD-9 156)

SLOVAKIA

AREA	NUMBER OF CASES			PERIOD	MEAN AGE		
	Males	Females	All		Males	Females	All
Slovakia	399	1042	1441	1985-1989	66.8	68.7	68.2

OBSERVED AND RELATIVE SURVIVAL (%) BY AGE (number of cases in parentheses)

	15-44		45-54		55-64		65-74		75-99		ALL	
	obs	rel	obs	rel	obs	rel	obs	rel	obs	rel	obs	rel
Males	(10)		(42)		(106)		(138)		(103)		(399)	
1 year	40	40	29	29	31	32	22	23	12	13	23	24
3 years	20	20	12	12	18	20	14	16	8	11	13	16
5 years	20	21	12	13	13	15	13	18	5	10	11	15
Females	(12)		(64)		(284)		(348)		(334)		(1042)	
1 year	25	25	27	27	20	21	19	19	11	12	17	18
3 years	17	17	14	14	10	11	10	11	6	9	9	10
5 years	17	17	14	14	8	9	8	9	5	9	8	10
Overall	(22)		(106)		(390)		(486)		(437)		(1441)	
1 year	32	32	27	28	23	24	19	20	11	13	19	20
3 years	18	18	13	14	12	13	11	12	7	9	10	12
5 years	18	18	13	14	9	10	9	12	5	9	8	11

SLOVENIA

AREA	NUMBER OF CASES			PERIOD	MEAN AGE		
	Males	Females	All		Males	Females	All
Slovenia	114	327	441	1985-1989	67.3	70.2	69.5

OBSERVED AND RELATIVE SURVIVAL (%) BY AGE (number of cases in parentheses)

	15-44		45-54		55-64		65-74		75-99		ALL	
	obs	rel	obs	rel	obs	rel	obs	rel	obs	rel	obs	rel
Males	(5)		(7)		(30)		(38)		(34)		(114)	
1 year	20	20	29	29	20	20	21	22	9	10	18	19
3 years	0	0	0	0	7	7	5	6	0	0	4	4
5 years	0	0	0	0	7	8	5	7	0	0	4	5
Females	(4)		(23)		(69)		(102)		(129)		(327)	
1 year	25	25	22	22	12	12	17	17	7	8	12	13
3 years	0	0	17	18	7	7	4	4	5	7	6	7
5 years	0	0	17	18	4	5	2	2	3	5	4	5
Overall	(9)		(30)		(99)		(140)		(163)		(441)	
1 year	22	22	23	23	14	14	18	19	7	8	14	14
3 years	0	0	13	14	7	7	4	5	4	6	5	6
5 years	0	0	13	14	5	5	3	4	2	4	4	5

BILIARY TRACT (ICD-9 156)

SPAIN

AREA	NUMBER OF CASES			PERIOD	MEAN AGE			5-YR RELATIVE SURVIVAL (%)	
	Males	Females	All		Males	Females	All	Males	Females
Basque Country	80	171	251	1986-1988	66.0	71.7	69.9		
Mallorca	14	41	55	1988-1989	68.9	74.0	72.7		
Navarra	64	108	172	1985-1989	69.2	73.1	71.6		
Tarragona	31	71	102	1985-1989	73.5	73.3	73.4		
Spanish Registries	189	391	580		68.6	72.6	71.3		

OBSERVED AND RELATIVE SURVIVAL (%) BY AGE (number of cases in parentheses)

	AGE CLASS										ALL	
	15-44		45-54		55-64		65-74		75-99			
	obs	rel	obs	rel	obs	rel	obs	rel	obs	rel	obs	rel
Males	(7)		(10)		(49)		(60)		(63)		(189)	
1 year	71	72	40	40	55	56	45	47	23	25	41	43
3 years	57	58	20	20	47	49	28	32	5	7	26	30
5 years	57	58	20	21	34	37	17	21	5	9	20	25
Females	(6)		(10)		(57)		(136)		(182)		(391)	
1 year	67	67	70	70	28	28	27	28	16	17	24	25
3 years	33	33	50	50	14	14	15	16	8	10	13	15
5 years	17	17	38	38	14	14	13	14	6	9	10	13
Overall	(13)		(20)		(106)		(196)		(245)		(580)	
1 year	69	69	55	55	41	41	33	33	18	19	29	31
3 years	46	46	35	35	29	30	19	21	7	10	17	20
5 years	35	35	28	29	24	25	15	17	6	9	13	17

SWEDEN

AREA	NUMBER OF CASES			PERIOD	MEAN AGE		
	Males	Females	All		Males	Females	All
South Sweden	146	329	475	1985-1989	68.3	72.0	70.9

OBSERVED AND RELATIVE SURVIVAL (%) BY AGE (number of cases in parentheses)

	AGE CLASS										ALL	
	15-44		45-54		55-64		65-74		75-99			
	obs	rel	obs	rel	obs	rel	obs	rel	obs	rel	obs	rel
Males	(4)		(5)		(37)		(62)		(38)		(146)	
1 year	50	50	40	40	27	27	26	27	21	23	26	27
3 years	0	0	20	20	19	20	10	11	13	18	13	15
5 years	0	0	20	21	19	20	5	6	13	23	11	14
Females	(2)		(20)		(47)		(107)		(153)		(329)	
1 year	100	100	35	35	19	19	20	20	16	17	19	20
3 years	0	0	10	10	11	11	7	8	6	7	7	8
5 years	0	0	5	5	6	7	6	6	4	6	5	6
Overall	(6)		(25)		(84)		(169)		(191)		(475)	
1 year	67	67	36	36	23	23	22	22	17	18	21	22
3 years	0	0	12	12	14	15	8	9	7	9	9	10
5 years	0	0	8	8	12	13	5	6	6	9	7	8

BILIARY TRACT

(ICD-9 156)

SWITZERLAND

AREA	NUMBER OF CASES			PERIOD	MEAN AGE			5-YR RELATIVE SURVIVAL (%)	
	Males	Females	All		Males	Females	All	Males	Females
Basel	17	51	68	1985-1988	71.1	74.9	73.9		
Geneva	25	39	64	1985-1989	70.8	78.5	75.5		
Swiss Registries	42	90	132		71.0	76.5	74.7		

OBSERVED AND RELATIVE SURVIVAL (%) BY AGE (number of cases in parentheses)

	AGE CLASS										ALL	
	15-44		45-54		55-64		65-74		75-99			
	obs	rel	obs	rel	obs	rel	obs	rel	obs	rel	obs	rel
Males	(2)		(1)		(5)		(17)		(17)		(42)	
1 year	100	100	0	0	60	61	12	12	29	33	29	30
3 years	100	100	0	0	40	42	6	7	18	25	19	23
5 years	100	100	0	0	40	43	6	7	0	0	11	15
Females	(1)		(6)		(4)		(23)		(56)		(90)	
1 year	0	0	33	33	50	50	48	49	14	16	26	27
3 years	0	0	17	17	25	25	30	32	7	10	14	18
5 years	0	0	0	0	0	0	22	24	4	6	8	11
Overall	(3)		(7)		(9)		(40)		(73)		(132)	
1 year	67	67	29	29	56	56	33	33	18	20	27	28
3 years	67	67	14	14	33	34	20	22	10	13	16	19
5 years	67	67	0	0	22	24	15	17	3	5	9	12

BILIARY TRACT (ICD-9 156)

EUROPE, 1985-89

Weighted analyses

COUNTRY	% COVERAGE WITH C.R.s	YEARLY NO. OF CASES (Mean No. of cases recorded)		
		Males	Females	All
AUSTRIA	8	10	18	28
DENMARK	100	75	147	222
ENGLAND	50	209	311	520
ESTONIA	100	9	22	31
FINLAND	100	65	177	242
FRANCE	4	22	41	63
GERMANY	2	23	69	92
ICELAND	100	2	3	5
ITALY	10	117	228	345
NETHERLANDS	6	12	24	36
POLAND	6	46	168	214
SCOTLAND	100	48	82	130
SLOVAKIA	100	80	208	288
SLOVENIA	100	23	65	88
SPAIN	10	53	113	166
SWEDEN	17	29	66	95
SWITZERLAND	11	9	21	30

RELATIVE SURVIVAL (%) (Age-standardized)
Males   Females

□ 1 year   ■ 5 years

OBSERVED AND RELATIVE SURVIVAL (%) BY AGE

	AGE CLASS										ALL	
	15-44		45-54		55-64		65-74		75-99			
	obs	rel	obs	rel	obs	rel	obs	rel	obs	rel	obs	rel
Males												
1 year	59	59	51	51	35	36	28	29	18	21	28	30
3 years	36	36	28	28	18	19	12	14	8	11	14	16
5 years	34	34	26	26	13	14	8	10	5	9	9	12
Females												
1 year	60	60	36	37	26	26	27	27	18	19	23	24
3 years	12	12	20	20	13	13	15	16	8	10	12	13
5 years	8	8	19	19	10	11	13	15	6	9	9	12
Overall												
1 year	60	60	41	41	28	29	27	28	18	19	25	26
3 years	19	19	22	22	14	15	14	16	8	11	12	14
5 years	15	15	21	21	11	12	12	13	5	9	9	12

AGE STANDARDIZED RELATIVE SURVIVAL(%)

COUNTRY	MALES		FEMALES	
	1-year (95% C.I.)	5-years (95% C.I.)	1-year (95% C.I.)	5-years (95% C.I.)
AUSTRIA	-	-	-	-
DENMARK	18.9 (15.4 - 23.2)	4.7 (2.7 - 8.0)	19.7 (16.9 - 22.9)	4.2 (2.8 - 6.2)
ENGLAND	26.6 (24.0 - 29.4)	10.1 (8.2 - 12.4)	24.2 (22.1 - 26.5)	10.2 (8.6 - 12.1)
ESTONIA	12.4 (5.7 - 26.9)	1.9 (0.6 - 6.2)	17.9 (11.9 - 27.1)	2.4 (0.6 - 10.5)
FINLAND	23.0 (18.7 - 28.2)	6.3 (4.0 - 10.0)	21.2 (18.6 - 24.1)	8.0 (6.2 - 10.3)
FRANCE	37.9 (29.8 - 48.0)	13.9 (8.7 - 22.2)	38.5 (32.0 - 46.3)	-
GERMANY	29.9 (22.5 - 39.6)	-	29.1 (24.7 - 34.2)	-
ICELAND	-	-	-	-
ITALY	26.2 (22.3 - 30.8)	7.7 (5.2 - 11.5)	24.7 (21.9 - 27.9)	10.4 (8.3 - 13.0)
NETHERLANDS	35.4 (25.3 - 49.4)	3.0 (1.0 - 8.9)	-	-
POLAND	13.8 (8.6 - 22.0)	4.7 (2.0 - 11.1)	12.5 (9.7 - 16.2)	5.4 (3.4 - 8.4)
SCOTLAND	23.9 (19.0 - 30.2)	7.0 (4.0 - 12.2)	22.5 (18.6 - 27.2)	8.4 (5.7 - 12.3)
SLOVAKIA	21.4 (17.6 - 26.0)	13.7 (9.9 - 19.0)	17.2 (15.0 - 19.8)	9.6 (7.6 - 12.2)
SLOVENIA	17.1 (11.3 - 25.8)	3.7 (1.4 - 9.8)	12.7 (9.5 - 16.9)	4.9 (2.8 - 8.6)
SPAIN	39.8 (33.3 - 47.6)	19.9 (14.1 - 28.0)	26.6 (22.5 - 31.4)	13.5 (10.0 - 18.1)
SWEDEN	26.6 (19.8 - 35.8)	16.7 (9.8 - 28.3)	20.9 (17.0 - 25.7)	6.0 (3.7 - 9.7)
SWITZERLAND	31.3 (20.0 - 49.1)	12.8 (5.8 - 28.4)	33.6 (23.0 - 49.0)	10.2 (5.2 - 20.0)
EUROPE, 1985-89	28.6 (26.0 - 31.5)	11.8 (9.2 - 15.2)	24.9 (23.1 - 26.7)	11.8 (10.3 - 13.6)

PANCREAS (ICD-9 157)

AUSTRIA

AREA	NUMBER OF CASES			PERIOD	MEAN AGE		
	Males	Females	All		Males	Females	All
Tirol	41	59	100	1988-1989	67.4	73.3	70.9

OBSERVED AND RELATIVE SURVIVAL (%) BY AGE (number of cases in parentheses)

	15-44		45-54		55-64		65-74		75-99		ALL	
	obs	rel	obs	rel	obs	rel	obs	rel	obs	rel	obs	rel
Males	(1)		(5)		(9)		(14)		(12)		(41)	
1 year	100	100	0	0	22	22	21	22	17	18	20	20
3 years	100	100	0	0	22	23	7	8	0	0	10	11
5 years	0	0	0	0	11	12	7	8	0	0	5	6
Females	(0)		(2)		(9)		(13)		(35)		(59)	
1 year	-	-	50	50	0	0	23	23	23	24	20	21
3 years	-	-	50	50	0	0	15	16	11	14	12	13
5 years	-	-	50	51	0	0	8	8	9	12	8	10
Overall	(1)		(7)		(18)		(27)		(47)		(100)	
1 year	100	100	14	14	11	11	22	23	21	23	20	21
3 years	100	100	14	14	11	11	11	12	9	10	11	12
5 years	0	0	14	15	6	6	7	8	6	9	7	9

DENMARK

AREA	NUMBER OF CASES			PERIOD	MEAN AGE		
	Males	Females	All		Males	Females	All
Denmark	1613	1644	3257	1985-1989	68.8	71.3	70.1

OBSERVED AND RELATIVE SURVIVAL (%) BY AGE (number of cases in parentheses)

	15-44		45-54		55-64		65-74		75-99		ALL	
	obs	rel	obs	rel	obs	rel	obs	rel	obs	rel	obs	rel
Males	(44)		(124)		(342)		(583)		(520)		(1613)	
1 year	16	16	15	15	15	15	11	12	7	8	11	12
3 years	7	7	2	2	4	4	2	3	1	2	2	3
5 years	5	5	2	2	3	4	1	2	1	2	2	2
Females	(36)		(94)		(278)		(523)		(713)		(1644)	
1 year	31	31	13	13	10	10	13	13	6	6	10	10
3 years	11	11	3	3	3	3	3	4	0	1	2	2
5 years	11	11	2	2	2	2	2	2	0	1	2	2
Overall	(80)		(218)		(620)		(1106)		(1233)		(3257)	
1 year	23	23	14	14	13	13	12	12	6	7	10	11
3 years	9	9	2	2	3	4	3	3	1	1	2	3
5 years	8	8	2	2	3	3	2	2	1	1	2	2

PANCREAS   (ICD-9 157)

ENGLAND

AREA	NUMBER OF CASES			PERIOD	MEAN AGE			5-YR RELATIVE SURVIVAL (%)	
	Males	Females	All		Males	Females	All	Males	Females
East Anglia	529	546	1075	1985-1989	69.2	73.3	71.3		
Mersey	600	666	1266	1985-1989	68.1	72.9	70.7		
Oxford	621	669	1290	1985-1989	68.3	72.6	70.5		
South Thames	1426	1483	2909	1985-1989	69.2	73.0	71.1		
Wessex	739	794	1533	1985-1989	69.9	72.8	71.4		
West Midlands	1285	1269	2554	1985-1989	68.8	72.4	70.6		
Yorkshire	894	936	1830	1985-1989	68.6	72.9	70.8		
English Registries	6094	6363	12457		68.9	72.8	70.9		

OBSERVED AND RELATIVE SURVIVAL (%) BY AGE (number of cases in parentheses)

	AGE CLASS										ALL	
	15-44		45-54		55-64		65-74		75-99			
	obs	rel	obs	rel	obs	rel	obs	rel	obs	rel	obs	rel
Males	(159)		(431)		(1341)		(2148)		(2015)		(6094)	
1 year	14	14	19	19	14	14	11	12	9	10	12	12
3 years	8	8	6	6	5	5	3	4	2	3	4	4
5 years	8	8	4	4	3	4	2	3	1	3	3	3
Females	(105)		(296)		(977)		(1853)		(3132)		(6363)	
1 year	19	19	18	18	13	13	13	13	8	8	10	11
3 years	11	11	6	6	4	4	3	3	2	3	3	3
5 years	10	10	4	5	3	4	2	2	2	3	2	3
Overall	(264)		(727)		(2318)		(4001)		(5147)		(12457)	
1 year	16	16	18	19	14	14	12	12	8	9	11	12
3 years	9	9	6	6	4	5	3	3	2	3	3	4
5 years	9	9	4	4	3	4	2	3	2	3	2	3

ESTONIA

AREA	NUMBER OF CASES			PERIOD	MEAN AGE		
	Males	Females	All		Males	Females	All
Estonia	373	355	728	1985-1989	63.8	69.4	66.5

OBSERVED AND RELATIVE SURVIVAL (%) BY AGE (number of cases in parentheses)

	AGE CLASS										ALL	
	15-44		45-54		55-64		65-74		75-99			
	obs	rel	obs	rel	obs	rel	obs	rel	obs	rel	obs	rel
Males	(8)		(70)		(113)		(114)		(68)		(373)	
1 year	13	13	19	19	7	7	12	13	13	15	12	13
3 years	0	0	4	4	0	0	3	3	7	10	3	3
5 years	0	0	3	3	0	0	3	4	3	7	2	3
Females	(10)		(26)		(63)		(129)		(127)		(355)	
1 year	10	10	12	12	14	14	9	9	9	10	10	11
3 years	0	0	4	4	5	5	2	2	3	4	3	3
5 years	0	0	0	0	2	2	0	0	0	0	0	0
Overall	(18)		(96)		(176)		(243)		(195)		(728)	
1 year	11	11	17	17	10	10	10	11	11	12	11	12
3 years	0	0	4	4	2	2	2	2	4	6	3	3
5 years	0	0	2	2	1	1	1	2	1	2	1	1

PANCREAS

(ICD-9 157)

FINLAND

AREA	NUMBER OF CASES			PERIOD	MEAN AGE		
	Males	Females	All		Males	Females	All
Finland	1328	1522	2850	1985-1989	66.1	71.7	69.1

OBSERVED AND RELATIVE SURVIVAL (%) BY AGE (number of cases in parentheses)

	AGE CLASS										ALL	
	15-44		45-54		55-64		65-74		75-99			
	obs	rel	obs	rel	obs	rel	obs	rel	obs	rel	obs	rel
Males	(56)		(157)		(342)		(449)		(324)		(1328)	
1 year	18	18	17	17	18	18	12	13	10	11	14	14
3 years	9	9	3	3	5	5	2	2	2	3	3	4
5 years	9	9	1	1	3	4	1	1	1	2	2	2
Females	(34)		(75)		(248)		(493)		(672)		(1522)	
1 year	32	32	24	24	18	18	14	14	11	12	14	15
3 years	21	21	9	9	7	7	2	2	2	3	3	4
5 years	21	21	8	8	3	3	1	1	2	3	2	3
Overall	(90)		(232)		(590)		(942)		(996)		(2850)	
1 year	23	23	19	19	18	18	13	13	11	12	14	15
3 years	13	13	5	5	6	6	2	2	2	3	3	4
5 years	13	14	3	3	3	3	1	1	1	2	2	3

FRANCE

AREA	NUMBER OF CASES			PERIOD	MEAN AGE			5-YR RELATIVE SURVIVAL (%)	
	Males	Females	All		Males	Females	All	Males	Females
Somme	96	70	166	1985-1989	65.9	72.3	68.6		
Calvados	92	74	166	1985-1989	69.7	70.6	70.1		
Côte d'Or	101	89	190	1985-1989	65.9	71.0	68.3		
Doubs	61	46	107	1985-1989	62.2	66.3	64.0		
French Registries	350	279	629		66.2	70.5	68.1		

OBSERVED AND RELATIVE SURVIVAL (%) BY AGE (number of cases in parentheses)

	AGE CLASS										ALL	
	15-44		45-54		55-64		65-74		75-99			
	obs	rel	obs	rel	obs	rel	obs	rel	obs	rel	obs	rel
Males	(17)		(34)		(108)		(93)		(98)		(350)	
1 year	24	24	25	25	23	23	21	22	14	15	20	21
3 years	6	6	4	4	11	12	14	15	2	3	8	10
5 years	-	-	0	0	6	7	12	15	2	4	6	8
Females	(9)		(20)		(58)		(66)		(126)		(279)	
1 year	78	78	46	46	20	20	20	20	15	16	21	22
3 years	66	66	17	17	5	6	5	5	4	5	8	9
5 years	66	66	17	17	4	4	5	5	3	5	6	8
Overall	(26)		(54)		(166)		(159)		(224)		(629)	
1 year	42	42	32	32	22	22	21	21	14	16	21	22
3 years	26	26	9	10	9	9	10	11	3	4	8	9
5 years	26	26	6	7	5	6	9	11	3	4	6	8

PANCREAS   (ICD-9 157)

GERMANY

AREA	NUMBER OF CASES			PERIOD	MEAN AGE		
	Males	Females	All		Males	Females	All
Saarland	230	226	456	1985-1989	65.7	71.8	68.8

OBSERVED AND RELATIVE SURVIVAL (%) BY AGE (number of cases in parentheses)

	AGE CLASS										ALL	
	15-44		45-54		55-64		65-74		75-99			
	obs	rel	obs	rel	obs	rel	obs	rel	obs	rel	obs	rel
Males	(7)		(35)		(64)		(58)		(66)		(230)	
1 year	14	14	23	23	17	17	22	23	9	10	17	18
3 years	14	14	9	9	6	7	3	4	0	0	4	5
5 years	-	-	9	9	5	5	3	4	0	0	4	5
Females	(6)		(11)		(41)		(62)		(106)		(226)	
1 year	33	33	36	36	15	15	15	15	8	9	13	14
3 years	33	34	9	9	0	0	5	5	2	3	4	4
5 years	33	34	0	0	0	0	3	4	0	0	2	3
Overall	(13)		(46)		(105)		(120)		(172)		(456)	
1 year	23	23	26	26	16	16	18	19	9	10	15	16
3 years	23	23	9	9	4	4	4	5	1	2	4	5
5 years	23	23	7	7	3	3	3	4	0	0	3	4

ICELAND

AREA	NUMBER OF CASES			PERIOD	MEAN AGE		
	Males	Females	All		Males	Females	All
Iceland	64	54	118	1985-1989	68.3	71.1	69.6

OBSERVED AND RELATIVE SURVIVAL (%) BY AGE (number of cases in parentheses)

	AGE CLASS										ALL	
	15-44		45-54		55-64		65-74		75-99			
	obs	rel	obs	rel	obs	rel	obs	rel	obs	rel	obs	rel
Males	(4)		(7)		(12)		(19)		(22)		(64)	
1 year	50	50	14	14	42	42	21	22	14	15	23	25
3 years	25	25	14	15	17	17	5	6	0	0	8	9
5 years	25	25	0	0	8	9	5	6	0	0	5	6
Females	(0)		(2)		(16)		(10)		(26)		(54)	
1 year	-	-	0	0	6	6	10	10	12	13	9	10
3 years	-	-	0	0	0	0	0	0	0	0	0	0
5 years	-	-	0	0	0	0	0	0	0	0	0	0
Overall	(4)		(9)		(28)		(29)		(48)		(118)	
1 year	50	50	11	11	21	22	17	18	13	14	17	18
3 years	25	25	11	11	7	7	3	4	0	0	4	5
5 years	25	25	0	0	4	4	3	4	0	0	3	3

PANCREAS (ICD-9 157)

ITALY

AREA	NUMBER OF CASES			PERIOD	MEAN AGE			5-YR RELATIVE SURVIVAL (%)	
	Males	Females	All		Males	Females	All	Males	Females
Florence	342	333	675	1985-1989	67.5	71.6	69.5		
Genoa	141	146	287	1986-1988	66.3	72.3	69.3		
Latina	31	28	59	1985-1987	66.1	69.3	67.6		
Modena	87	76	163	1988-1989	67.6	71.6	69.5		
Parma	107	64	171	1985-1987	65.7	72.5	68.2		
Ragusa	71	51	122	1985-1989	67.5	69.9	68.5		
Romagna	79	86	165	1986-1988	66.5	71.3	69.0		
Turin	149	153	302	1985-1987	67.9	70.6	69.3		
Varese	206	204	410	1985-1989	66.8	72.0	69.4		
Italian Registries	1213	1141	2354		67.0	71.5	69.2		

5-YR RELATIVE SURVIVAL (%) chart legend: Floren, Genoa, Latina, Modena, Parma, Ragusa, Romagn, Turin, Varese

OBSERVED AND RELATIVE SURVIVAL (%) BY AGE (number of cases in parentheses)

	AGE CLASS										ALL	
	15-44		45-54		55-64		65-74		75-99			
	obs	rel	obs	rel	obs	rel	obs	rel	obs	rel	obs	rel
Males	(29)		(126)		(331)		(394)		(333)		(1213)	
1 year	21	21	19	19	22	22	14	14	12	13	16	17
3 years	3	3	8	8	5	5	4	4	4	6	5	5
5 years	3	3	6	6	4	4	3	4	3	5	3	4
Females	(17)		(71)		(196)		(343)		(514)		(1141)	
1 year	41	41	24	24	22	22	17	18	16	17	18	19
3 years	35	35	10	10	3	3	5	5	3	4	4	5
5 years	29	30	8	9	1	1	3	3	1	2	3	3
Overall	(46)		(197)		(527)		(737)		(847)		(2354)	
1 year	28	28	21	21	22	22	15	16	14	16	17	18
3 years	15	15	9	9	4	4	4	5	4	5	5	5
5 years	13	13	7	7	3	3	3	3	2	3	3	4

NETHERLANDS

AREA	NUMBER OF CASES			PERIOD	MEAN AGE		
	Males	Females	All		Males	Females	All
Eindhoven	152	142	294	1985-1989	66.0	66.8	66.4

OBSERVED AND RELATIVE SURVIVAL (%) BY AGE (number of cases in parentheses)

	AGE CLASS										ALL	
	15-44		45-54		55-64		65-74		75-99			
	obs	rel	obs	rel	obs	rel	obs	rel	obs	rel	obs	rel
Males	(7)		(13)		(43)		(55)		(34)		(152)	
1 year	0	0	15	15	26	26	7	8	12	13	14	14
3 years	0	0	0	0	2	2	2	2	3	4	2	2
5 years	0	0	0	0	0	0	2	2	3	6	1	2
Females	(6)		(13)		(44)		(37)		(42)		(142)	
1 year	0	0	0	0	11	11	24	25	7	8	12	12
3 years	0	0	0	0	2	2	7	7	0	0	2	3
5 years	0	0	0	0	2	2	7	7	0	0	2	3
Overall	(13)		(26)		(87)		(92)		(76)		(294)	
1 year	0	0	8	8	18	19	14	15	9	10	13	13
3 years	0	0	0	0	2	2	4	4	1	2	2	2
5 years	0	0	0	0	1	1	4	5	1	2	2	2

PANCREAS

(ICD-9 157)

POLAND

AREA	NUMBER OF CASES			PERIOD	MEAN AGE			5-YR RELATIVE SURVIVAL (%)	
	Males	Females	All		Males	Females	All	Males	Females
Cracow	155	138	293	1985-1989	62.2	69.4	65.6		
Warsaw	169	174	343	1988-1989	64.5	70.0	67.3		
Polish Registries	324	312	636		63.4	69.7	66.5		

100 80 60 40 20 0   0 20 40 60 80 100

Cracow
Warsaw

OBSERVED AND RELATIVE SURVIVAL (%) BY AGE (number of cases in parentheses)

	AGE CLASS										ALL	
	15-44		45-54		55-64		65-74		75-99			
	obs	rel	obs	rel	obs	rel	obs	rel	obs	rel	obs	rel
Males	(22)		(33)		(127)		(85)		(57)		(324)	
1 year	32	32	6	6	13	14	12	12	4	4	12	12
3 years	23	23	3	3	2	3	5	6	0	0	4	5
5 years	18	19	0	0	2	2	5	7	0	0	3	4
Females	(7)		(26)		(73)		(85)		(121)		(312)	
1 year	29	29	19	19	16	16	9	9	8	9	11	12
3 years	0	0	4	4	7	7	4	4	3	4	4	5
5 years	0	0	4	4	7	8	2	3	2	4	4	5
Overall	(29)		(59)		(200)		(170)		(178)		(636)	
1 year	31	31	12	12	14	14	10	11	7	7	12	12
3 years	17	17	3	3	4	4	4	5	2	3	4	5
5 years	14	14	2	2	4	4	4	5	2	3	3	4

SCOTLAND

AREA	NUMBER OF CASES			PERIOD	MEAN AGE		
	Males	Females	All		Males	Females	All
Scotland	1336	1441	2777	1985-1989	68.8	71.8	70.3

OBSERVED AND RELATIVE SURVIVAL (%) BY AGE (number of cases in parentheses)

	AGE CLASS										ALL	
	15-44		45-54		55-64		65-74		75-99			
	obs	rel	obs	rel	obs	rel	obs	rel	obs	rel	obs	rel
Males	(30)		(86)		(318)		(454)		(448)		(1336)	
1 year	30	30	17	18	14	14	10	10	11	12	12	13
3 years	20	20	6	6	5	5	4	4	2	3	4	5
5 years	17	17	6	6	4	5	3	4	1	2	3	4
Females	(25)		(76)		(245)		(459)		(636)		(1441)	
1 year	28	28	20	20	12	12	12	12	7	8	11	11
3 years	8	8	9	9	2	3	3	3	2	2	3	3
5 years	8	8	8	8	2	2	3	3	1	2	2	3
Overall	(55)		(162)		(563)		(913)		(1084)		(2777)	
1 year	29	29	19	19	13	13	11	11	9	10	11	12
3 years	15	15	7	8	4	4	3	4	2	2	3	4
5 years	13	13	7	7	3	3	3	3	1	2	3	4

PANCREAS (ICD-9 157)

SLOVAKIA

AREA	NUMBER OF CASES			PERIOD	MEAN AGE		
	Males	Females	All		Males	Females	All
Slovakia	1093	798	1891	1985-1989	63.6	68.4	65.6

OBSERVED AND RELATIVE SURVIVAL (%) BY AGE (number of cases in parentheses)

	AGE CLASS										ALL	
	15-44		45-54		55-64		65-74		75-99			
	obs	rel	obs	rel	obs	rel	obs	rel	obs	rel	obs	rel
Males	(87)		(137)		(323)		(331)		(215)		(1093)	
1 year	25	25	15	16	13	14	13	14	13	15	15	15
3 years	16	16	11	11	6	7	7	8	7	11	8	9
5 years	13	14	10	11	5	6	5	7	6	12	6	8
Females	(22)		(61)		(180)		(275)		(260)		(798)	
1 year	41	41	13	13	14	14	16	17	12	13	15	15
3 years	32	32	7	7	5	5	9	10	6	8	8	9
5 years	26	26	7	7	4	4	8	9	6	10	7	8
Overall	(109)		(198)		(503)		(606)		(475)		(1891)	
1 year	28	29	15	15	14	14	15	15	12	14	15	15
3 years	19	20	10	10	6	6	8	9	7	10	8	9
5 years	16	16	9	10	4	5	6	8	6	11	7	8

SLOVENIA

AREA	NUMBER OF CASES			PERIOD	MEAN AGE		
	Males	Females	All		Males	Females	All
Slovenia	342	339	681	1985-1989	65.1	70.0	67.6

OBSERVED AND RELATIVE SURVIVAL (%) BY AGE (number of cases in parentheses)

	AGE CLASS										ALL	
	15-44		45-54		55-64		65-74		75-99			
	obs	rel	obs	rel	obs	rel	obs	rel	obs	rel	obs	rel
Males	(11)		(46)		(117)		(86)		(82)		(342)	
1 year	18	18	13	13	13	13	10	11	11	12	12	13
3 years	9	9	4	4	1	1	2	3	1	2	2	2
5 years	9	9	4	5	1	1	0	0	1	2	1	2
Females	(9)		(16)		(81)		(98)		(135)		(339)	
1 year	11	11	27	27	17	17	11	12	7	8	12	12
3 years	0	0	7	7	4	4	5	6	6	8	5	6
5 years	0	0	0	0	1	1	3	4	4	7	3	4
Overall	(20)		(62)		(198)		(184)		(217)		(681)	
1 year	15	15	17	17	15	15	11	11	9	10	12	12
3 years	5	5	5	5	2	2	4	4	4	5	3	4
5 years	5	5	3	3	1	1	2	2	3	5	2	3

PANCREAS (ICD-9 157)

SPAIN

AREA	NUMBER OF CASES			PERIOD	MEAN AGE			5-YR RELATIVE SURVIVAL (%)	
	Males	Females	All		Males	Females	All	Males	Females
Basque Country	175	144	319	1986-1988	64.3	70.2	66.9		
Mallorca	47	30	77	1988-1989	65.3	69.7	67.1		
Navarra	100	77	177	1985-1989	66.2	71.7	68.6		
Tarragona	78	65	143	1985-1989	66.3	68.2	67.2		
Spanish Registries	400	316	716		65.3	70.1	67.4		

5-YR RELATIVE SURVIVAL (%) Males scale: 100 80 60 40 20 0 ; Females scale: 0 20 40 60 80 100 — Basque, Mallor, Navarr, Tarrag

OBSERVED AND RELATIVE SURVIVAL (%) BY AGE (number of cases in parentheses)

	AGE CLASS										ALL	
	15-44		45-54		55-64		65-74		75-99			
	obs	rel	obs	rel	obs	rel	obs	rel	obs	rel	obs	rel
Males	(21)		(57)		(105)		(117)		(100)		(400)	
1 year	43	43	18	18	13	14	17	18	9	10	16	16
3 years	24	24	4	4	2	2	3	3	4	6	4	5
5 years	17	17	4	4	2	2	2	2	4	7	3	4
Females	(6)		(27)		(57)		(104)		(122)		(316)	
1 year	0	0	22	22	19	19	14	14	11	12	14	15
3 years	0	0	10	10	9	9	4	4	3	4	5	6
5 years	0	0	10	10	9	9	1	2	3	5	4	5
Overall	(27)		(84)		(162)		(221)		(222)		(716)	
1 year	33	33	19	19	15	16	16	16	10	11	15	16
3 years	19	19	6	6	4	4	3	4	4	5	5	5
5 years	13	13	6	6	4	5	2	2	4	6	4	5

SWEDEN

AREA	NUMBER OF CASES			PERIOD	MEAN AGE		
	Males	Females	All		Males	Females	All
South Sweden	460	443	903	1985-1989	67.8	71.4	69.6

OBSERVED AND RELATIVE SURVIVAL (%) BY AGE (number of cases in parentheses)

	AGE CLASS										ALL	
	15-44		45-54		55-64		65-74		75-99			
	obs	rel	obs	rel	obs	rel	obs	rel	obs	rel	obs	rel
Males	(20)		(42)		(102)		(151)		(145)		(460)	
1 year	30	30	29	29	21	21	14	14	8	8	15	16
3 years	20	20	7	7	3	3	4	4	1	1	4	4
5 years	20	20	5	5	3	3	1	2	0	0	2	3
Females	(8)		(36)		(54)		(159)		(186)		(443)	
1 year	0	0	25	25	19	19	14	15	8	9	13	13
3 years	0	0	14	14	2	2	4	4	2	2	3	4
5 years	0	0	14	14	2	2	3	3	2	3	3	4
Overall	(28)		(78)		(156)		(310)		(331)		(903)	
1 year	21	21	27	27	20	20	14	15	8	9	14	15
3 years	14	14	10	10	3	3	4	4	1	2	4	4
5 years	14	14	9	9	3	3	2	2	1	2	3	3

PANCREAS (ICD-9 157)

SWITZERLAND

AREA	NUMBER OF CASES			PERIOD	MEAN AGE			5-YR RELATIVE SURVIVAL (%)	
	Males	Females	All		Males	Females	All	Males	Females
Basel	76	81	157	1985-1988	67.8	72.0	70.0		
Geneva	106	112	218	1985-1989	67.5	72.3	70.0		
Swiss Registries	182	193	375		67.7	72.2	70.0		

OBSERVED AND RELATIVE SURVIVAL (%) BY AGE (number of cases in parentheses)

	AGE CLASS										ALL	
	15-44		45-54		55-64		65-74		75-99			
	obs	rel	obs	rel	obs	rel	obs	rel	obs	rel	obs	rel
Males	(9)		(16)		(40)		(53)		(64)		(182)	
1 year	40	40	17	17	33	33	23	23	9	10	20	21
3 years	13	13	0	0	3	3	4	4	2	2	3	3
5 years	0	0	0	0	3	3	0	0	2	3	1	1
Females	(2)		(16)		(30)		(50)		(95)		(193)	
1 year	50	50	25	25	23	23	14	14	2	2	11	11
3 years	0	0	13	13	3	3	8	9	0	0	4	4
5 years	0	0	13	13	3	3	4	4	0	0	3	3
Overall	(11)		(32)		(70)		(103)		(159)		(375)	
1 year	41	41	21	21	29	29	18	19	5	5	15	16
3 years	10	10	7	7	3	3	6	6	1	1	3	4
5 years	0	0	7	7	3	3	2	2	1	1	2	2

PANCREAS (ICD-9 157)

EUROPE, 1985-89

Weighted analyses

COUNTRY	% COVERAGE WITH C.R.s	YEARLY NO. OF CASES (Mean No. of cases recorded) Males	Females	All
AUSTRIA	8	21	30	51
DENMARK	100	323	329	652
ENGLAND	50	1219	1273	2492
ESTONIA	100	75	71	146
FINLAND	100	266	304	570
FRANCE	4	70	56	126
GERMANY	2	46	45	91
ICELAND	100	13	11	24
ITALY	10	336	315	651
NETHERLANDS	6	30	28	58
POLAND	6	116	115	231
SCOTLAND	100	267	288	555
SLOVAKIA	100	219	160	379
SLOVENIA	100	68	68	136
SPAIN	10	117	91	208
SWEDEN	17	92	89	181
SWITZERLAND	11	40	43	83

RELATIVE SURVIVAL (%) (Age-standardized)

□ 1 year ■ 5 years

OBSERVED AND RELATIVE SURVIVAL (%) BY AGE

	AGE CLASS										ALL	
	15-44		45-54		55-64		65-74		75-99			
	obs	rel	obs	rel	obs	rel	obs	rel	obs	rel	obs	rel
Males												
1 year	23	23	18	18	18	19	16	16	10	11	15	16
3 years	13	13	6	6	5	6	5	5	2	3	5	5
5 years	9	9	4	4	4	4	4	5	2	3	3	4
Females												
1 year	32	32	26	26	16	17	15	15	11	12	14	15
3 years	23	23	10	10	4	4	4	5	3	4	4	5
5 years	21	21	8	8	3	3	3	3	2	3	3	4
Overall												
1 year	28	28	22	22	17	18	15	16	10	11	15	16
3 years	17	18	8	8	4	5	5	5	2	3	4	5
5 years	15	15	6	6	3	4	4	4	2	3	3	4

AGE STANDARDIZED RELATIVE SURVIVAL(%)

COUNTRY	MALES 1-year (95% C.I.)	5-years (95% C.I.)	FEMALES 1-year (95% C.I.)	5-years (95% C.I.)
AUSTRIA	21.2 (11.7 - 38.2)	5.1 (1.4 - 19.4)	-	-
DENMARK	11.3 (9.8 - 13.0)	2.2 (1.5 - 3.3)	10.5 (9.1 - 12.1)	2.0 (1.3 - 2.9)
ENGLAND	12.2 (11.4 - 13.1)	3.2 (2.8 - 3.8)	11.7 (10.9 - 12.6)	3.1 (2.6 - 3.6)
ESTONIA	12.9 (9.4 - 17.9)	3.9 (1.5 - 9.7)	10.8 (7.9 - 14.7)	0.4 (0.0 - 3.8)
FINLAND	13.5 (11.7 - 15.6)	2.1 (1.3 - 3.3)	15.4 (13.6 - 17.4)	3.2 (2.4 - 4.4)
FRANCE	20.0 (15.8 - 25.1)	-	22.1 (17.5 - 27.9)	7.1 (4.4 - 11.5)
GERMANY	17.0 (12.5 - 23.0)	-	14.8 (10.7 - 20.6)	2.1 (0.8 - 5.4)
ICELAND	23.8 (15.2 - 37.1)	4.5 (1.4 - 14.6)	-	-
ITALY	16.1 (14.0 - 18.4)	4.3 (3.1 - 6.0)	19.3 (17.1 - 21.9)	3.4 (2.4 - 4.8)
NETHERLANDS	13.9 (9.0 - 21.3)	2.8 (0.6 - 12.7)	13.2 (8.5 - 20.5)	2.9 (0.9 - 8.7)
POLAND	9.6 (6.7 - 13.7)	3.0 (1.4 - 6.1)	11.7 (8.6 - 15.9)	4.4 (2.4 - 7.9)
SCOTLAND	12.9 (11.1 - 14.9)	3.9 (2.8 - 5.3)	11.7 (10.1 - 13.5)	3.1 (2.2 - 4.3)
SLOVAKIA	14.8 (12.5 - 17.5)	9.0 (6.6 - 12.1)	15.1 (12.8 - 17.8)	8.7 (6.6 - 11.5)
SLOVENIA	12.3 (8.9 - 16.9)	1.7 (0.5 - 5.3)	12.6 (9.4 - 16.8)	4.1 (2.1 - 7.8)
SPAIN	14.6 (11.4 - 18.7)	4.5 (2.4 - 8.5)	14.7 (11.2 - 19.2)	5.1 (2.9 - 8.7)
SWEDEN	15.0 (12.1 - 18.6)	2.1 (1.1 - 3.8)	13.7 (10.7 - 17.5)	3.3 (1.9 - 5.6)
SWITZERLAND	20.5 (15.4 - 27.3)	1.6 (0.4 - 6.6)	13.4 (9.1 - 19.8)	3.1 (1.3 - 7.4)
EUROPE, 1985-89	15.1 (13.9 - 16.4)	4.1 (3.3 - 5.1)	15.4 (14.2 - 16.7)	3.9 (3.1 - 4.8)

NASAL CAVITIES (ICD-9 160)

AUSTRIA

AREA	NUMBER OF CASES			PERIOD	MEAN AGE		
	Males	Females	All		Males	Females	All
Tirol	1	7	8	1988-1989	80.0	63.4	65.6

OBSERVED AND RELATIVE SURVIVAL (%) BY AGE (number of cases in parentheses)

	AGE CLASS										ALL	
	15-44		45-54		55-64		65-74		75-99			
	obs	rel	obs	rel	obs	rel	obs	rel	obs	rel	obs	rel
Males	(0)		(0)		(0)		(0)		(1)		(1)	
1 year	-	-	-	-	-	-	-	-	0	0	0	0
3 years	-	-	-	-	-	-	-	-	0	0	0	0
5 years	-	-	-	-	-	-	-	-	0	0	0	0
Females	(1)		(2)		(0)		(1)		(3)		(7)	
1 year	100	100	100	100	-	-	0	0	100	100	86	88
3 years	0	0	50	50	-	-	0	0	67	78	43	46
5 years	0	0	50	51	-	-	0	0	0	0	14	17
Overall	(1)		(2)		(0)		(1)		(4)		(8)	
1 year	100	100	100	100	-	-	0	0	75	79	75	77
3 years	0	0	50	50	-	-	0	0	50	60	38	42
5 years	0	0	50	51	-	-	0	0	0	0	13	15

DENMARK

AREA	NUMBER OF CASES			PERIOD	MEAN AGE		
	Males	Females	All		Males	Females	All
Denmark	171	103	274	1985-1989	64.8	66.9	65.6

OBSERVED AND RELATIVE SURVIVAL (%) BY AGE (number of cases in parentheses)

	AGE CLASS										ALL	
	15-44		45-54		55-64		65-74		75-99			
	obs	rel	obs	rel	obs	rel	obs	rel	obs	rel	obs	rel
Males	(11)		(26)		(42)		(57)		(35)		(171)	
1 year	100	100	81	81	71	73	75	79	57	65	73	76
3 years	64	64	58	59	50	53	54	62	26	38	49	56
5 years	64	65	54	56	38	42	49	62	23	47	43	54
Females	(8)		(8)		(26)		(29)		(32)		(103)	
1 year	75	75	75	75	85	85	90	92	75	82	82	85
3 years	50	50	63	63	65	68	52	56	50	66	55	62
5 years	38	38	50	51	62	65	41	48	38	62	46	55
Overall	(19)		(34)		(68)		(86)		(67)		(274)	
1 year	89	90	79	80	76	78	80	83	66	73	76	79
3 years	58	58	59	60	56	59	53	60	37	53	51	58
5 years	53	53	53	55	47	52	47	57	30	55	44	54

NASAL CAVITIES   (ICD-9 160)

ENGLAND

AREA	NUMBER OF CASES			PERIOD	MEAN AGE			5-YR RELATIVE SURVIVAL (%)	
	Males	Females	All		Males	Females	All	Males	Females
East Anglia	56	29	85	1985-1989	66.1	70.9	67.7		
Mersey	45	39	84	1985-1989	65.5	69.6	67.4		
Oxford	62	30	92	1985-1989	67.3	67.3	67.3		
South Thames	122	85	207	1985-1989	64.1	68.0	65.7		
Wessex	69	48	117	1985-1989	63.1	68.2	65.2		
West Midlands	88	77	165	1985-1989	62.2	68.8	65.3		
Yorkshire	69	36	105	1985-1989	65.1	63.5	64.6		
English Registries	511	344	855		64.5	68.1	66.0		

OBSERVED AND RELATIVE SURVIVAL (%) BY AGE (number of cases in parentheses)

	AGE CLASS										ALL	
	15-44		45-54		55-64		65-74		75-99			
	obs	rel	obs	rel	obs	rel	obs	rel	obs	rel	obs	rel
Males	(31)		(66)		(138)		(171)		(105)		(511)	
1 year	77	78	80	81	69	70	62	65	53	60	65	68
3 years	65	65	55	56	53	56	38	44	30	43	44	50
5 years	55	55	47	49	48	53	27	34	21	39	36	44
Females	(26)		(24)		(70)		(95)		(129)		(344)	
1 year	65	65	83	84	76	76	79	81	45	49	65	68
3 years	50	50	54	55	53	54	49	53	24	32	41	47
5 years	46	46	50	51	44	47	39	44	18	30	33	42
Overall	(57)		(90)		(208)		(266)		(234)		(855)	
1 year	72	72	81	82	71	72	68	70	49	54	65	68
3 years	58	58	54	55	53	55	42	47	27	37	43	49
5 years	51	51	48	49	47	51	31	38	19	33	35	43

ESTONIA

AREA	NUMBER OF CASES			PERIOD	MEAN AGE		
	Males	Females	All		Males	Females	All
Estonia	28	20	48	1985-1989	54.8	65.0	59.1

OBSERVED AND RELATIVE SURVIVAL (%) BY AGE (number of cases in parentheses)

	AGE CLASS										ALL	
	15-44		45-54		55-64		65-74		75-99			
	obs	rel	obs	rel	obs	rel	obs	rel	obs	rel	obs	rel
Males	(7)		(7)		(6)		(6)		(2)		(28)	
1 year	29	29	57	58	83	86	67	71	100	100	61	63
3 years	14	14	14	15	33	36	33	41	50	79	25	28
5 years	14	15	14	15	33	39	17	24	50	100	21	26
Females	(2)		(3)		(1)		(7)		(7)		(20)	
1 year	100	100	67	67	0	0	71	73	57	63	65	68
3 years	50	50	0	0	0	0	14	16	29	39	20	23
5 years	50	50	0	0	0	0	14	17	0	0	10	13
Overall	(9)		(10)		(7)		(13)		(9)		(48)	
1 year	44	45	60	61	71	73	69	72	67	74	63	65
3 years	22	22	10	10	29	31	23	27	33	47	23	26
5 years	22	23	10	11	29	33	15	20	11	21	17	20

NASAL CAVITIES (ICD-9 160)

FINLAND

AREA	NUMBER OF CASES			PERIOD	MEAN AGE		
	Males	Females	All		Males	Females	All
Finland	77	55	132	1985-1989	62.1	70.2	65.5

OBSERVED AND RELATIVE SURVIVAL (%) BY AGE (number of cases in parentheses)

	AGE CLASS										ALL	
	15-44		45-54		55-64		65-74		75-99			
	obs	rel	obs	rel	obs	rel	obs	rel	obs	rel	obs	rel
Males	(6)		(16)		(23)		(21)		(11)		(77)	
1 year	100	100	100	100	74	75	67	70	55	61	77	79
3 years	50	51	75	77	39	42	52	61	27	39	49	55
5 years	17	17	69	72	22	24	48	62	9	17	36	44
Females	(1)		(4)		(9)		(21)		(20)		(55)	
1 year	100	100	50	50	100	100	90	92	75	82	84	87
3 years	0	0	25	25	67	68	48	51	45	60	47	54
5 years	0	0	25	25	56	58	33	38	20	34	31	39
Overall	(7)		(20)		(32)		(42)		(31)		(132)	
1 year	100	100	90	91	81	83	79	81	68	75	80	83
3 years	43	43	65	66	47	49	50	56	39	53	48	55
5 years	14	15	60	62	31	34	40	49	16	28	34	42

FRANCE

AREA	NUMBER OF CASES			PERIOD	MEAN AGE			5-YR RELATIVE SURVIVAL (%)	
	Males	Females	All		Males	Females	All	Males	Females
Somme	19	10	29	1985-1989	58.3	68.5	61.9		
Calvados	30	7	37	1985-1989	62.9	65.4	63.4		
Doubs	7	1	8	1985-1989	68.4	53.0	66.6		
French Registries	56	18	74		62.1	66.6	63.2		

OBSERVED AND RELATIVE SURVIVAL (%) BY AGE (number of cases in parentheses)

	AGE CLASS										ALL	
	15-44		45-54		55-64		65-74		75-99			
	obs	rel	obs	rel	obs	rel	obs	rel	obs	rel	obs	rel
Males	(2)		(16)		(16)		(10)		(12)		(56)	
1 year	100	100	69	69	81	83	70	73	58	64	71	74
3 years	50	50	25	26	54	57	47	53	33	44	39	44
5 years	0	0	25	26	54	60	23	29	33	57	34	41
Females	(1)		(5)		(1)		(4)		(7)		(18)	
1 year	100	100	80	80	100	100	75	76	86	91	83	86
3 years	100	100	60	61	100	100	25	27	86	100	67	74
5 years	100	100	60	61	100	100	25	28	33	49	49	58
Overall	(3)		(21)		(17)		(14)		(19)		(74)	
1 year	100	100	71	72	82	84	71	74	68	74	74	77
3 years	67	67	33	34	57	60	40	44	53	69	46	51
5 years	33	34	33	35	57	63	26	32	35	56	38	45

NASAL CAVITIES

(ICD-9 160)

GERMANY

AREA	NUMBER OF CASES			PERIOD	MEAN AGE		
	Males	Females	All		Males	Females	All
Saarland	7	13	20	1985-1989	59.0	64.5	62.7

OBSERVED AND RELATIVE SURVIVAL (%) BY AGE (number of cases in parentheses)

	AGE CLASS										ALL	
	15-44		45-54		55-64		65-74		75-99			
	obs	rel	obs	rel	obs	rel	obs	rel	obs	rel	obs	rel
Males	(2)		(0)		(3)		(1)		(1)		(7)	
1 year	100	100	-	-	67	68	100	100	0	0	71	73
3 years	50	51	-	-	0	0	0	0	0	0	14	16
5 years	-	-	-	-	0	0	0	0	0	0	-	-
Females	(1)		(3)		(3)		(0)		(6)		(13)	
1 year	100	100	0	0	100	100	-	-	33	36	46	48
3 years	100	100	0	0	67	68	-	-	33	42	38	43
5 years	100	100	0	0	67	70	-	-	0	0	23	28
Overall	(3)		(3)		(6)		(1)		(7)		(20)	
1 year	100	100	0	0	83	84	100	100	29	31	55	57
3 years	67	67	0	0	33	35	0	0	29	36	30	33
5 years	67	68	0	0	33	36	0	0	0	0	20	24

ICELAND

AREA	NUMBER OF CASES			PERIOD	MEAN AGE		
	Males	Females	All		Males	Females	All
Iceland	10	3	13	1985-1989	67.3	68.3	67.6

OBSERVED AND RELATIVE SURVIVAL (%) BY AGE (number of cases in parentheses)

	AGE CLASS										ALL	
	15-44		45-54		55-64		65-74		75-99			
	obs	rel	obs	rel	obs	rel	obs	rel	obs	rel	obs	rel
Males	(1)		(1)		(1)		(2)		(5)		(10)	
1 year	100	100	100	100	100	100	50	51	80	87	80	84
3 years	100	100	0	0	100	100	50	53	40	54	50	59
5 years	100	100	0	0	100	100	50	56	40	67	50	65
Females	(0)		(0)		(2)		(0)		(1)		(3)	
1 year	-	-	-	-	50	50	-	-	100	100	67	71
3 years	-	-	-	-	50	51	-	-	100	100	67	79
5 years	-	-	-	-	50	52	-	-	100	100	67	88
Overall	(1)		(1)		(3)		(2)		(6)		(13)	
1 year	100	100	100	100	67	67	50	51	83	92	77	81
3 years	100	100	0	0	67	68	50	53	50	70	54	63
5 years	100	100	0	0	67	69	50	56	50	91	54	70

NASAL CAVITIES (ICD-9 160)

ITALY

AREA	NUMBER OF CASES			PERIOD	MEAN AGE			5-YR RELATIVE SURVIVAL (%)	
	Males	Females	All		Males	Females	All	Males	Females
Florence	31	11	42	1985-1989	63.9	60.5	63.0		
Genoa	11	8	19	1986-1988	66.8	67.0	66.9		
Latina	3	0	3	1985-1987	58.0	-	58.0		
Modena	2	1	3	1988-1989	74.5	24.0	58.0		
Parma	8	1	9	1985-1987	59.5	52.0	58.8		
Ragusa	1	2	3	1985-1989	73.0	65.0	68.0		
Romagna	4	1	5	1986-1988	72.8	60.0	70.4		
Turin	18	6	24	1985-1987	62.3	40.2	56.8		
Varese	20	7	27	1985-1989	60.1	63.0	60.9		
Italian Registries	98	37	135		63.4	58.3	62.0		

OBSERVED AND RELATIVE SURVIVAL (%) BY AGE (number of cases in parentheses)

	AGE CLASS										ALL	
	15-44		45-54		55-64		65-74		75-99			
	obs	rel	obs	rel	obs	rel	obs	rel	obs	rel	obs	rel
Males	(7)		(12)		(30)		(32)		(17)		(98)	
1 year	86	86	92	92	77	78	78	80	71	76	78	81
3 years	57	57	67	68	50	52	55	62	47	60	54	59
5 years	57	58	42	43	43	47	42	52	35	56	42	50
Females	(7)		(7)		(7)		(8)		(8)		(37)	
1 year	100	100	86	86	86	86	100	100	50	54	84	86
3 years	57	57	57	58	57	58	75	79	25	32	54	58
5 years	57	57	43	44	57	59	63	69	25	39	49	54
Overall	(14)		(19)		(37)		(40)		(25)		(135)	
1 year	93	93	89	90	78	79	82	85	64	69	80	82
3 years	57	57	63	64	51	53	59	65	40	51	54	59
5 years	57	58	42	43	46	49	46	55	32	50	44	51

NETHERLANDS

AREA	NUMBER OF CASES			PERIOD	MEAN AGE		
	Males	Females	All		Males	Females	All
Eindhoven	14	8	22	1985-1989	67.9	61.8	65.7

OBSERVED AND RELATIVE SURVIVAL (%) BY AGE (number of cases in parentheses)

	AGE CLASS										ALL	
	15-44		45-54		55-64		65-74		75-99			
	obs	rel	obs	rel	obs	rel	obs	rel	obs	rel	obs	rel
Males	(0)		(1)		(3)		(7)		(3)		(14)	
1 year	-	-	100	100	100	100	100	100	100	100	100	100
3 years	-	-	100	100	67	70	71	83	0	0	57	66
5 years	-	-	100	100	67	72	57	74	0	0	50	64
Females	(2)		(1)		(0)		(2)		(3)		(8)	
1 year	100	100	100	100	-	-	50	51	67	72	75	77
3 years	50	50	100	100	-	-	50	53	0	0	38	41
5 years	50	50	100	100	-	-	50	57	0	0	38	44
Overall	(2)		(2)		(3)		(9)		(6)		(22)	
1 year	100	100	100	100	100	100	89	92	83	90	91	95
3 years	50	50	100	100	67	70	67	76	0	0	50	57
5 years	50	50	100	100	67	72	56	70	0	0	45	56

NASAL CAVITIES (ICD-9 160)

POLAND

AREA	NUMBER OF CASES			PERIOD	MEAN AGE			5-YR RELATIVE SURVIVAL (%)	
	Males	Females	All		Males	Females	All	Males	Females
Cracow	18	6	24	1985-1989	57.8	63.8	59.3		
Warsaw	5	1	6	1988-1989	73.0	49.0	69.2		
Polish Registries	23	7	30		61.2	62.0	61.4		

OBSERVED AND RELATIVE SURVIVAL (%) BY AGE (number of cases in parentheses)

	AGE CLASS										ALL	
	15-44		45-54		55-64		65-74		75-99			
	obs	rel	obs	rel	obs	rel	obs	rel	obs	rel	obs	rel
Males	(1)		(7)		(4)		(5)		(6)		(23)	
1 year	100	100	86	87	75	76	80	83	33	37	70	73
3 years	0	0	29	30	50	53	40	46	33	47	35	40
5 years	0	0	29	30	50	57	20	26	17	30	26	33
Females	(0)		(2)		(3)		(1)		(1)		(7)	
1 year	-	-	50	50	100	100	100	100	0	0	71	73
3 years	-	-	50	51	67	69	100	100	0	0	57	62
5 years	-	-	50	51	67	71	100	100	0	0	57	65
Overall	(1)		(9)		(7)		(6)		(7)		(30)	
1 year	100	100	78	78	86	87	83	87	29	32	70	73
3 years	0	0	33	34	57	60	50	57	29	40	40	45
5 years	0	0	33	35	57	63	33	43	14	26	33	41

SCOTLAND

AREA	NUMBER OF CASES			PERIOD	MEAN AGE		
	Males	Females	All		Males	Females	All
Scotland	78	60	138	1985-1989	61.7	66.4	63.7

OBSERVED AND RELATIVE SURVIVAL (%) BY AGE (number of cases in parentheses)

	AGE CLASS										ALL	
	15-44		45-54		55-64		65-74		75-99			
	obs	rel	obs	rel	obs	rel	obs	rel	obs	rel	obs	rel
Males	(5)		(13)		(28)		(24)		(8)		(78)	
1 year	60	60	77	78	68	69	58	61	50	56	64	66
3 years	60	60	38	39	54	57	54	63	25	36	49	54
5 years	40	40	31	32	46	52	38	49	25	49	38	46
Females	(8)		(4)		(7)		(20)		(21)		(60)	
1 year	88	88	50	50	86	87	70	72	29	31	58	61
3 years	88	88	0	0	57	59	45	49	14	19	38	44
5 years	88	88	0	0	57	61	40	47	10	16	35	44
Overall	(13)		(17)		(35)		(44)		(29)		(138)	
1 year	77	77	71	71	71	73	64	66	34	38	62	64
3 years	77	77	29	30	54	58	50	56	17	24	44	50
5 years	69	70	24	25	49	54	39	48	14	24	37	45

NASAL CAVITIES

(ICD-9 160)

SLOVAKIA

AREA	NUMBER OF CASES			PERIOD	MEAN AGE		
	Males	Females	All		Males	Females	All
Slovakia	86	44	130	1985-1989	61.0	65.3	62.4

OBSERVED AND RELATIVE SURVIVAL (%) BY AGE (number of cases in parentheses)

	AGE CLASS										ALL	
	15-44		45-54		55-64		65-74		75-99			
	obs	rel	obs	rel	obs	rel	obs	rel	obs	rel	obs	rel
Males	(13)		(16)		(18)		(25)		(14)		(86)	
1 year	85	85	75	76	61	63	44	47	36	41	58	61
3 years	38	39	31	33	28	30	8	10	29	46	24	28
5 years	30	31	0	0	14	16	8	11	21	50	14	18
Females	(4)		(3)		(13)		(11)		(13)		(44)	
1 year	50	50	67	67	69	70	55	56	31	34	52	55
3 years	50	50	67	68	54	56	18	20	8	11	32	36
5 years	50	50	67	69	21	22	9	11	-	-	21	26
Overall	(17)		(19)		(31)		(36)		(27)		(130)	
1 year	76	77	74	75	65	66	47	50	33	38	56	59
3 years	41	42	37	38	39	41	11	13	19	28	27	31
5 years	35	36	15	16	16	18	8	11	15	31	16	21

SLOVENIA

AREA	NUMBER OF CASES			PERIOD	MEAN AGE		
	Males	Females	All		Males	Females	All
Slovenia	39	26	65	1985-1989	59.4	68.2	62.9

OBSERVED AND RELATIVE SURVIVAL (%) BY AGE (number of cases in parentheses)

	AGE CLASS										ALL	
	15-44		45-54		55-64		65-74		75-99			
	obs	rel	obs	rel	obs	rel	obs	rel	obs	rel	obs	rel
Males	(7)		(7)		(8)		(11)		(6)		(39)	
1 year	43	43	57	58	50	51	73	76	50	56	56	59
3 years	0	0	57	59	38	40	27	32	33	48	30	34
5 years	0	0	57	60	25	28	18	24	17	33	22	27
Females	(3)		(2)		(5)		(3)		(13)		(26)	
1 year	100	100	100	100	40	40	67	68	69	80	68	73
3 years	50	50	50	51	40	41	0	0	23	35	28	35
5 years	50	50	50	51	20	21	0	0	8	16	16	23
Overall	(10)		(9)		(13)		(14)		(19)		(65)	
1 year	56	56	67	67	46	47	71	75	63	72	61	64
3 years	11	11	56	57	38	40	21	25	26	40	29	34
5 years	11	11	56	58	23	25	14	18	11	22	20	25

NASAL CAVITIES   (ICD-9 160)

SPAIN

AREA	NUMBER OF CASES			PERIOD	MEAN AGE			5-YR RELATIVE SURVIVAL (%)	
	Males	Females	All		Males	Females	All	Males	Females
Basque Country	33	16	49	1986-1988	61.8	66.1	63.2		
Mallorca	4	1	5	1988-1989	53.3	68.0	56.4		
Navarra	9	4	13	1985-1989	64.0	65.0	64.4		
Tarragona	11	2	13	1985-1989	60.9	75.0	63.2		
Spanish Registries	57	23	80		61.5	66.9	63.0		

OBSERVED AND RELATIVE SURVIVAL (%) BY AGE (number of cases in parentheses)

	AGE CLASS										ALL	
	15-44		45-54		55-64		65-74		75-99			
	obs	rel	obs	rel	obs	rel	obs	rel	obs	rel	obs	rel
Males	(7)		(6)		(21)		(13)		(10)		(57)	
1 year	86	86	83	84	71	72	62	64	40	44	67	69
3 years	71	72	67	68	48	50	38	43	40	55	49	54
5 years	71	72	67	69	42	45	23	28	27	48	40	47
Females	(1)		(2)		(9)		(5)		(6)		(23)	
1 year	100	100	50	50	78	78	60	61	50	54	65	67
3 years	100	100	0	0	44	45	40	43	50	65	43	47
5 years	100	100	0	0	44	46	40	45	-	-	43	50
Overall	(8)		(8)		(30)		(18)		(16)		(80)	
1 year	88	88	75	75	73	74	61	63	44	48	66	68
3 years	75	75	50	51	47	48	39	43	44	59	48	52
5 years	75	76	50	51	43	46	28	33	36	62	41	48

SWEDEN

AREA	NUMBER OF CASES			PERIOD	MEAN AGE		
	Males	Females	All		Males	Females	All
South Sweden	37	23	60	1985-1989	67.8	71.2	69.1

OBSERVED AND RELATIVE SURVIVAL (%) BY AGE (number of cases in parentheses)

	AGE CLASS										ALL	
	15-44		45-54		55-64		65-74		75-99			
	obs	rel	obs	rel	obs	rel	obs	rel	obs	rel	obs	rel
Males	(2)		(1)		(10)		(13)		(11)		(37)	
1 year	100	100	100	100	100	100	92	96	55	60	84	88
3 years	100	100	100	100	80	84	54	60	18	25	54	62
5 years	100	100	100	100	50	54	38	47	9	16	38	48
Females	(2)		(0)		(6)		(2)		(13)		(23)	
1 year	100	100	-	-	83	84	100	100	69	75	78	82
3 years	50	50	-	-	67	68	100	100	38	51	52	61
5 years	50	50	-	-	50	52	100	100	23	38	39	52
Overall	(4)		(1)		(16)		(15)		(24)		(60)	
1 year	100	100	100	100	94	95	93	96	63	68	82	86
3 years	75	75	100	100	75	78	60	67	29	39	53	62
5 years	75	76	100	100	50	53	47	56	17	28	38	49

NASAL CAVITIES   (ICD-9 160)

SWITZERLAND

AREA	NUMBER OF CASES			PERIOD	MEAN AGE		
	Males	Females	All		Males	Females	All
Geneva	5	2	7	1985-1989	57.2	76.0	62.7

OBSERVED AND RELATIVE SURVIVAL (%) BY AGE (number of cases in parentheses)

	15-44		45-54		55-64		65-74		75-99		ALL	
	obs	rel	obs	rel	obs	rel	obs	rel	obs	rel	obs	rel
Males	(1)		(1)		(2)		(0)		(1)		(5)	
1 year	100	100	100	100	100	100	-	-	100	100	100	100
3 years	100	100	100	100	100	100	-	-	0	0	75	81
5 years	100	100	0	0	100	100	-	-	0	0	50	57
Females	(0)		(0)		(0)		(0)		(2)		(2)	
1 year	-	-	-	-	-	-	-	-	100	100	100	100
3 years	-	-	-	-	-	-	-	-	100	100	100	100
5 years	-	-	-	-	-	-	-	-	100	100	100	100
Overall	(1)		(1)		(2)		(0)		(3)		(7)	
1 year	100	100	100	100	100	100	-	-	100	100	100	100
3 years	100	100	100	100	100	100	-	-	67	79	83	91
5 years	100	100	0	0	100	100	-	-	67	91	67	79

NASAL CAVITIES (ICD-9 160)

EUROPE, 1985-89

Weighted analyses

COUNTRY	% COVERAGE WITH C.R.s	Males	Females	All		
		YEARLY NO. OF CASES (Mean No. of cases recorded)			RELATIVE SURVIVAL (%) (Age-standardized)	
AUSTRIA	8	1	4	5		A
DENMARK	100	34	21	55		DK
ENGLAND	50	102	69	171		ENG
ESTONIA	100	6	4	10		EST
FINLAND	100	15	11	26		FIN
FRANCE	3	12	4	16		F
GERMANY	2	1	3	4		D
ICELAND	100	2	1	3		IS
ITALY	10	27	10	37		I
NETHERLANDS	6	3	2	5		NL
POLAND	6	9	2	11		PL
SCOTLAND	100	16	12	28		SCO
SLOVAKIA	100	17	9	26		SK
SLOVENIA	100	8	5	13		SLO
SPAIN	10	17	7	24		E
SWEDEN	17	7	5	12		S
SWITZERLAND	6	1	1	2		CH
						EUR

□ 1 year ■ 5 years

OBSERVED AND RELATIVE SURVIVAL (%) BY AGE

	15-44 obs rel	45-54 obs rel	55-64 obs rel	65-74 obs rel	75-99 obs rel	ALL obs rel
Males						
1 year	91 91	82 82	77 78	73 76	53 58	72 75
3 years	54 54	51 52	50 53	43 49	32 43	44 49
5 years	37 37	43 44	46 50	28 35	24 42	37 44
Females						
1 year	92 92	62 62	88 89	74 75	55 58	70 72
3 years	71 71	39 40	65 66	48 51	40 50	48 53
5 years	70 70	36 37	62 64	43 47	16 25	38 44
Overall						
1 year	91 91	75 75	81 82	74 76	54 58	71 74
3 years	60 60	47 48	56 58	45 50	35 45	45 50
5 years	49 49	40 42	52 55	33 39	22 36	37 44

AGE STANDARDIZED RELATIVE SURVIVAL(%)

COUNTRY	MALES 1-year (95% C.I.)	MALES 5-years (95% C.I.)	FEMALES 1-year (95% C.I.)	FEMALES 5-years (95% C.I.)
AUSTRIA	-	-	-	-
DENMARK	75.7 (69.0 - 83.1)	52.8 (43.6 - 64.0)	84.2 (76.8 - 92.4)	55.4 (44.8 - 68.5)
ENGLAND	67.7 (63.5 - 72.2)	43.5 (38.4 - 49.3)	70.8 (66.1 - 75.8)	42.2 (36.5 - 48.7)
ESTONIA	76.9 (63.3 - 93.4)	45.4 (17.8 -115.9)	54.0 (40.2 - 72.5)	9.0 (2.8 - 29.1)
FINLAND	75.3 (64.8 - 87.5)	38.8 (27.7 - 54.4)	86.9 (78.3 - 96.3)	37.1 (25.3 - 54.3)
FRANCE	74.7 (62.9 - 88.7)	41.1 (25.9 - 65.3)	88.5 (74.6 -104.9)	61.2 (43.1 - 86.8)
GERMANY	-	-	-	-
ICELAND	82.5 (62.7 -108.7)	66.0 (42.6 -102.4)	-	-
ITALY	80.6 (72.3 - 90.0)	50.9 (39.5 - 65.5)	83.1 (71.9 - 95.9)	54.6 (38.3 - 77.7)
NETHERLANDS	-	-	-	-
POLAND	71.6 (55.1 - 93.1)	32.9 (16.0 - 67.7)	-	-
SCOTLAND	63.8 (51.9 - 78.5)	47.0 (32.0 - 69.0)	63.7 (52.6 - 77.2)	39.8 (28.5 - 55.6)
SLOVAKIA	56.1 (45.6 - 68.9)	22.3 (11.5 - 43.6)	54.9 (41.6 - 72.3)	-
SLOVENIA	59.9 (44.8 - 80.0)	30.1 (15.5 - 58.3)	70.9 (53.1 - 94.6)	19.8 (8.9 - 44.3)
SPAIN	65.2 (53.1 - 80.0)	46.1 (31.4 - 67.7)	65.3 (48.0 - 88.9)	-
SWEDEN	88.6 (79.7 - 98.4)	52.0 (39.2 - 68.9)	-	-
SWITZERLAND	-	-	-	-
EUROPE, 1985-89	73.9 (69.3 - 78.7)	42.0 (35.5 - 49.8)	73.9 (69.2 - 79.0)	46.3 (39.1 - 54.7)

LARYNX (ICD-9 161)

AUSTRIA

AREA	NUMBER OF CASES			PERIOD	MEAN AGE		
	Males	Females	All		Males	Females	All
Tirol	50	3	53	1988-1989	60.3	58.0	60.2

OBSERVED AND RELATIVE SURVIVAL (%) BY AGE (number of cases in parentheses)

	15-44		45-54		55-64		65-74		75-99		ALL	
	obs	rel	obs	rel	obs	rel	obs	rel	obs	rel	obs	rel
Males	(3)		(11)		(23)		(6)		(7)		(50)	
1 year	67	67	82	82	87	88	100	100	71	76	84	86
3 years	33	34	64	65	70	72	67	73	29	36	60	64
5 years	33	34	55	56	65	69	50	58	29	43	54	60
Females	(0)		(2)		(0)		(1)		(0)		(3)	
1 year	-	-	0	0	-	-	100	100	-	-	33	34
3 years	-	-	0	0	-	-	100	100	-	-	33	34
5 years	-	-	0	0	-	-	0	0	-	-	0	0
Overall	(3)		(13)		(23)		(7)		(7)		(53)	
1 year	67	67	69	70	87	88	100	100	71	76	81	83
3 years	33	34	54	55	70	72	71	78	29	36	58	62
5 years	33	34	46	47	65	69	43	50	29	43	51	56

DENMARK

AREA	NUMBER OF CASES			PERIOD	MEAN AGE		
	Males	Females	All		Males	Females	All
Denmark	985	240	1225	1985-1989	64.4	62.6	64.1

OBSERVED AND RELATIVE SURVIVAL (%) BY AGE (number of cases in parentheses)

	15-44		45-54		55-64		65-74		75-99		ALL	
	obs	rel	obs	rel	obs	rel	obs	rel	obs	rel	obs	rel
Males	(37)		(130)		(296)		(346)		(176)		(985)	
1 year	89	89	85	85	82	84	82	86	73	80	81	84
3 years	78	79	65	66	63	67	61	70	46	63	60	68
5 years	76	77	53	55	54	60	48	60	33	57	49	60
Females	(16)		(35)		(87)		(67)		(35)		(240)	
1 year	88	88	97	98	86	87	79	81	71	77	84	85
3 years	81	82	74	75	70	73	61	66	34	43	64	68
5 years	75	76	71	73	56	60	45	51	31	48	53	60
Overall	(53)		(165)		(383)		(413)		(211)		(1225)	
1 year	89	89	87	88	83	84	82	85	73	79	82	84
3 years	79	80	67	68	65	68	61	69	44	59	61	68
5 years	75	76	57	59	54	60	47	59	33	55	50	60

LARYNX

(ICD-9 161)

ENGLAND

AREA	NUMBER OF CASES			PERIOD	MEAN AGE			5-YR RELATIVE SURVIVAL (%)	
	Males	Females	All		Males	Females	All	Males	Females
East Anglia	244	55	299	1985-1989	67.5	68.1	67.6		
Mersey	403	117	520	1985-1989	64.0	65.9	64.4		
Oxford	280	66	346	1985-1989	65.8	68.9	66.4		
South Thames	796	177	973	1985-1989	66.3	67.7	66.6		
Wessex	412	77	489	1985-1989	66.6	68.7	67.0		
West Midlands	767	153	920	1985-1989	64.6	64.4	64.6		
Yorkshire	577	135	712	1985-1989	64.5	65.7	64.7		
English Registries	3479	780	4259		65.5	66.7	65.7		

OBSERVED AND RELATIVE SURVIVAL (%) BY AGE (number of cases in parentheses)

	AGE CLASS										ALL	
	15-44		45-54		55-64		65-74		75-99			
	obs	rel	obs	rel	obs	rel	obs	rel	obs	rel	obs	rel
Males	(110)		(382)		(1065)		(1245)		(677)		(3479)	
1 year	89	89	81	81	86	87	82	85	68	76	81	84
3 years	78	79	68	70	70	74	62	71	49	68	63	71
5 years	73	73	62	64	61	68	50	64	37	67	53	66
Females	(31)		(74)		(215)		(268)		(192)		(780)	
1 year	90	90	91	91	86	86	80	82	60	66	78	80
3 years	87	87	77	78	70	72	60	64	38	49	60	65
5 years	84	84	72	73	65	68	52	59	27	43	52	62
Overall	(141)		(456)		(1280)		(1513)		(869)		(4259)	
1 year	89	90	82	83	86	87	82	85	66	73	80	83
3 years	80	81	70	71	70	73	62	69	46	64	62	70
5 years	75	76	63	65	62	68	51	63	35	61	53	65

ESTONIA

AREA	NUMBER OF CASES			PERIOD	MEAN AGE		
	Males	Females	All		Males	Females	All
Estonia	300	17	317	1985-1989	57.5	57.6	57.5

OBSERVED AND RELATIVE SURVIVAL (%) BY AGE (number of cases in parentheses)

	AGE CLASS										ALL	
	15-44		45-54		55-64		65-74		75-99			
	obs	rel	obs	rel	obs	rel	obs	rel	obs	rel	obs	rel
Males	(27)		(81)		(126)		(57)		(9)		(300)	
1 year	96	97	89	90	79	81	70	74	22	25	80	82
3 years	63	64	68	71	54	59	46	54	11	16	56	61
5 years	63	65	54	59	39	46	35	48	0	0	44	51
Females	(2)		(4)		(6)		(4)		(1)		(17)	
1 year	100	100	100	100	100	100	50	51	0	0	82	84
3 years	50	50	100	100	100	100	50	55	0	0	76	80
5 years	50	51	100	100	100	100	25	29	0	0	71	77
Overall	(29)		(85)		(132)		(61)		(10)		(317)	
1 year	97	97	89	91	80	82	69	72	20	22	80	82
3 years	62	63	69	72	56	61	46	54	10	14	57	62
5 years	62	64	56	61	42	49	34	46	0	0	45	53

LARYNX (ICD-9 161)

FINLAND

AREA	NUMBER OF CASES			PERIOD	MEAN AGE		
	Males	Females	All		Males	Females	All
Finland	523	51	574	1985-1989	63.7	63.4	63.6

OBSERVED AND RELATIVE SURVIVAL (%) BY AGE (number of cases in parentheses)

	AGE CLASS										ALL	
	15-44		45-54		55-64		65-74		75-99			
	obs	rel	obs	rel	obs	rel	obs	rel	obs	rel	obs	rel
Males	(23)		(64)		(189)		(166)		(81)		(523)	
1 year	91	92	86	87	90	92	83	87	57	64	82	86
3 years	83	84	70	72	68	72	57	65	33	48	60	67
5 years	83	84	64	67	59	66	41	52	25	47	50	61
Females	(5)		(4)		(17)		(18)		(7)		(51)	
1 year	80	80	100	100	88	89	89	91	29	31	80	82
3 years	40	40	50	51	71	72	67	72	29	38	59	63
5 years	40	40	50	51	59	61	56	63	14	24	49	55
Overall	(28)		(68)		(206)		(184)		(88)		(574)	
1 year	89	90	87	87	90	92	84	87	55	61	82	85
3 years	75	76	69	71	68	72	58	66	33	47	60	67
5 years	75	76	63	66	59	65	42	53	24	45	50	60

FRANCE

AREA	NUMBER OF CASES			PERIOD	MEAN AGE			5-YR RELATIVE SURVIVAL (%)
	Males	Females	All		Males	Females	All	Males / Females
Somme	209	13	222	1985-1989	59.7	57.9	59.6	
Calvados	207	10	217	1985-1989	60.2	65.5	60.5	
Doubs	177	12	189	1985-1989	60.9	61.8	61.0	
French Registries	593	35	628		60.3	61.5	60.3	

OBSERVED AND RELATIVE SURVIVAL (%) BY AGE (number of cases in parentheses)

	AGE CLASS										ALL	
	15-44		45-54		55-64		65-74		75-99			
	obs	rel	obs	rel	obs	rel	obs	rel	obs	rel	obs	rel
Males	(37)		(127)		(236)		(134)		(59)		(593)	
1 year	83	84	84	84	84	85	78	81	81	89	82	84
3 years	58	59	60	62	54	57	54	61	44	59	55	59
5 years	51	52	51	53	48	52	40	48	29	50	45	52
Females	(3)		(7)		(9)		(9)		(7)		(35)	
1 year	100	100	71	72	100	100	76	77	57	61	80	81
3 years	67	67	29	29	88	90	76	80	38	47	60	63
5 years	67	67	0	0	63	65	76	82	38	57	46	51
Overall	(40)		(134)		(245)		(143)		(66)		(628)	
1 year	85	85	83	84	84	86	78	81	79	86	82	84
3 years	59	59	58	60	56	59	55	62	43	58	55	60
5 years	52	53	48	51	48	53	41	50	30	51	45	52

LARYNX (ICD-9 161)

GERMANY

AREA	NUMBER OF CASES			PERIOD	MEAN AGE		
	Males	Females	All		Males	Females	All
Saarland	283	33	316	1985-1989	59.8	63.9	60.3

OBSERVED AND RELATIVE SURVIVAL (%) BY AGE (number of cases in parentheses)

	15-44		45-54		55-64		65-74		75-99		ALL	
	obs	rel	obs	rel	obs	rel	obs	rel	obs	rel	obs	rel
Males	(20)		(72)		(101)		(59)		(31)		(283)	
1 year	100	100	88	88	91	93	88	92	77	86	89	91
3 years	80	81	68	70	70	74	68	78	68	95	70	76
5 years	73	75	58	61	59	65	57	74	52	100	59	69
Females	(1)		(8)		(8)		(7)		(9)		(33)	
1 year	100	100	88	88	75	76	100	100	67	72	82	84
3 years	100	100	50	50	75	77	100	100	44	57	67	73
5 years	100	100	38	38	75	78	100	100	20	32	56	65
Overall	(21)		(80)		(109)		(66)		(40)		(316)	
1 year	100	100	88	88	90	91	89	93	75	83	88	90
3 years	81	82	66	68	71	74	71	81	63	86	69	76
5 years	75	76	56	58	61	66	61	78	45	82	58	68

ICELAND

AREA	NUMBER OF CASES			PERIOD	MEAN AGE		
	Males	Females	All		Males	Females	All
Iceland	16	3	19	1985-1989	62.2	70.0	63.5

OBSERVED AND RELATIVE SURVIVAL (%) BY AGE (number of cases in parentheses)

	15-44		45-54		55-64		65-74		75-99		ALL	
	obs	rel	obs	rel	obs	rel	obs	rel	obs	rel	obs	rel
Males	(1)		(2)		(8)		(2)		(3)		(16)	
1 year	100	100	100	100	88	88	100	100	33	36	81	83
3 years	100	100	100	100	88	91	100	100	33	42	81	87
5 years	100	100	100	100	63	67	100	100	0	0	63	71
Females	(0)		(0)		(1)		(1)		(1)		(3)	
1 year	-	-	-	-	100	100	100	100	100	100	100	100
3 years	-	-	-	-	100	100	100	100	100	100	100	100
5 years	-	-	-	-	100	100	100	100	100	100	100	100
Overall	(1)		(2)		(9)		(3)		(4)		(19)	
1 year	100	100	100	100	89	90	100	100	50	54	84	86
3 years	100	100	100	100	89	92	100	100	50	63	84	91
5 years	100	100	100	100	67	71	100	100	25	38	68	78

LARYNX   (ICD-9 161)

ITALY

AREA	NUMBER OF CASES			PERIOD	MEAN AGE			5-YR RELATIVE SURVIVAL (%)	
	Males	Females	All		Males	Females	All	Males	Females
Florence	644	60	704	1985-1989	63.3	63.9	63.4		
Genoa	234	19	253	1986-1988	62.4	60.5	62.3		
Latina	60	4	64	1985-1987	62.0	63.3	62.1		
Modena	120	7	127	1988-1989	64.5	63.1	64.4		
Parma	129	12	141	1985-1987	64.0	54.8	63.2		
Ragusa	73	2	75	1985-1989	63.6	74.5	63.9		
Romagna	119	9	128	1986-1988	62.8	64.4	63.0		
Turin	314	15	329	1985-1987	61.5	66.7	61.8		
Varese	317	20	337	1985-1989	61.6	69.4	62.1		
Italian Registries	2010	148	2158		62.7	63.9	62.8		

OBSERVED AND RELATIVE SURVIVAL (%) BY AGE (number of cases in parentheses)

	AGE CLASS										ALL	
	15-44		45-54		55-64		65-74		75-99			
	obs	rel	obs	rel	obs	rel	obs	rel	obs	rel	obs	rel
Males	(69)		(325)		(791)		(559)		(266)		(2010)	
1 year	96	96	91	91	89	90	87	90	71	78	87	89
3 years	83	83	77	78	73	76	67	75	47	62	69	75
5 years	78	79	70	72	65	70	54	65	31	52	58	68
Females	(10)		(18)		(48)		(41)		(31)		(148)	
1 year	90	90	94	95	81	82	85	87	47	50	78	79
3 years	90	90	94	95	71	72	68	72	37	45	67	71
5 years	80	80	89	90	65	67	54	59	27	38	58	64
Overall	(79)		(343)		(839)		(600)		(297)		(2158)	
1 year	95	95	91	92	89	90	87	89	69	75	86	88
3 years	84	84	78	79	73	76	67	75	46	60	69	75
5 years	78	79	71	73	65	70	54	65	31	50	58	68

NETHERLANDS

AREA	NUMBER OF CASES			PERIOD	MEAN AGE		
	Males	Females	All		Males	Females	All
Eindhoven	165	15	180	1985-1989	62.8	57.1	62.3

OBSERVED AND RELATIVE SURVIVAL (%) BY AGE (number of cases in parentheses)

	AGE CLASS										ALL	
	15-44		45-54		55-64		65-74		75-99			
	obs	rel	obs	rel	obs	rel	obs	rel	obs	rel	obs	rel
Males	(4)		(30)		(58)		(53)		(20)		(165)	
1 year	75	75	97	97	91	93	91	94	90	99	91	94
3 years	50	50	93	95	77	81	77	88	60	82	77	85
5 years	50	51	90	93	68	74	56	70	45	79	65	76
Females	(2)		(4)		(7)		(1)		(1)		(15)	
1 year	100	100	100	100	100	100	100	100	100	100	100	100
3 years	100	100	100	100	100	100	100	100	100	100	100	100
5 years	100	100	100	100	100	100	100	100	100	100	100	100
Overall	(6)		(34)		(65)		(54)		(21)		(180)	
1 year	83	83	97	98	92	93	91	94	90	100	92	95
3 years	67	67	94	96	79	83	78	88	62	84	79	87
5 years	67	67	91	94	71	77	57	71	48	83	67	79

LARYNX (ICD-9 161)

POLAND

AREA	NUMBER OF CASES			PERIOD	MEAN AGE			5-YR RELATIVE SURVIVAL (%)	
	Males	Females	All		Males	Females	All	Males	Females
Cracow	203	19	222	1985-1989	58.8	59.7	58.9		
Warsaw	173	30	203	1988-1989	59.0	60.3	59.2		
Polish Registries	376	49	425		58.9	60.1	59.0		

OBSERVED AND RELATIVE SURVIVAL (%) BY AGE (number of cases in parentheses)

	AGE CLASS										ALL	
	15-44		45-54		55-64		65-74		75-99			
	obs	rel	obs	rel	obs	rel	obs	rel	obs	rel	obs	rel
Males	(36)		(78)		(164)		(78)		(20)		(376)	
1 year	83	84	73	74	74	76	60	63	60	68	71	73
3 years	64	65	52	54	48	52	44	53	30	44	48	54
5 years	61	63	40	44	38	45	31	42	20	40	39	46
Females	(7)		(6)		(19)		(11)		(6)		(49)	
1 year	100	100	100	100	89	90	64	65	67	72	83	85
3 years	71	72	83	85	61	64	36	40	50	63	58	62
5 years	71	72	83	86	56	60	27	32	50	75	54	61
Overall	(43)		(84)		(183)		(89)		(26)		(425)	
1 year	86	86	75	76	75	77	60	63	62	69	72	75
3 years	65	66	54	57	49	53	43	51	35	49	50	55
5 years	63	65	44	47	40	46	31	41	27	50	40	48

SCOTLAND

AREA	NUMBER OF CASES			PERIOD	MEAN AGE		
	Males	Females	All		Males	Females	All
Scotland	905	227	1132	1985-1989	63.3	64.3	63.5

OBSERVED AND RELATIVE SURVIVAL (%) BY AGE (number of cases in parentheses)

	AGE CLASS										ALL	
	15-44		45-54		55-64		65-74		75-99			
	obs	rel	obs	rel	obs	rel	obs	rel	obs	rel	obs	rel
Males	(27)		(160)		(302)		(287)		(129)		(905)	
1 year	96	97	88	88	87	89	81	85	71	80	83	86
3 years	85	86	72	74	67	72	58	68	50	71	63	71
5 years	81	83	64	67	56	63	45	59	36	68	52	64
Females	(10)		(32)		(72)		(71)		(42)		(227)	
1 year	90	90	88	88	85	86	75	77	69	74	79	81
3 years	60	60	78	79	63	65	56	62	50	64	60	66
5 years	60	61	78	80	53	57	44	51	33	52	50	58
Overall	(37)		(192)		(374)		(358)		(171)		(1132)	
1 year	95	95	88	88	87	88	80	83	71	78	82	85
3 years	78	79	73	75	66	71	58	66	50	69	63	70
5 years	76	77	66	69	55	62	45	57	35	63	51	62

LARYNX   (ICD-9 161)

SLOVAKIA

AREA	NUMBER OF CASES			PERIOD	MEAN AGE		
	Males	Females	All		Males	Females	All
Slovakia	1387	69	1456	1985-1989	57.9	56.7	57.8

OBSERVED AND RELATIVE SURVIVAL (%) BY AGE (number of cases in parentheses)

	AGE CLASS										ALL	
	15-44		45-54		55-64		65-74		75-99			
	obs	rel	obs	rel	obs	rel	obs	rel	obs	rel	obs	rel
Males	(144)		(383)		(509)		(255)		(96)		(1387)	
1 year	71	71	76	77	71	73	65	68	60	69	71	73
3 years	42	43	49	51	43	47	45	54	40	60	45	49
5 years	37	38	43	46	38	44	40	54	29	61	39	46
Females	(10)		(20)		(22)		(11)		(6)		(69)	
1 year	80	80	80	80	77	78	73	75	50	54	75	77
3 years	80	80	60	61	64	66	45	50	17	22	58	61
5 years	80	81	53	54	52	55	32	38	17	27	50	55
Overall	(154)		(403)		(531)		(266)		(102)		(1456)	
1 year	71	72	76	77	71	73	65	69	60	68	71	73
3 years	45	46	49	51	44	48	45	53	38	57	45	50
5 years	40	41	43	46	38	44	40	54	28	58	39	47

SLOVENIA

AREA	NUMBER OF CASES			PERIOD	MEAN AGE		
	Males	Females	All		Males	Females	All
Slovenia	452	33	485	1985-1989	59.3	56.0	59.0

OBSERVED AND RELATIVE SURVIVAL (%) BY AGE (number of cases in parentheses)

	AGE CLASS										ALL	
	15-44		45-54		55-64		65-74		75-99			
	obs	rel	obs	rel	obs	rel	obs	rel	obs	rel	obs	rel
Males	(27)		(112)		(196)		(73)		(44)		(452)	
1 year	85	85	87	88	79	80	74	77	61	68	79	81
3 years	58	59	63	65	53	57	53	61	39	55	54	60
5 years	58	59	53	56	44	49	43	56	23	43	45	52
Females	(7)		(6)		(15)		(3)		(2)		(33)	
1 year	71	72	83	84	80	81	67	68	100	100	79	80
3 years	71	72	67	68	67	69	33	36	100	100	67	69
5 years	71	72	50	51	67	70	33	39	100	100	64	68
Overall	(34)		(118)		(211)		(76)		(46)		(485)	
1 year	82	82	87	88	79	80	74	77	63	70	79	81
3 years	61	61	63	65	54	58	52	60	41	58	55	60
5 years	61	62	53	56	45	51	43	56	26	49	46	54

LARYNX (ICD-9 161)

SPAIN

AREA	NUMBER OF CASES			PERIOD	MEAN AGE			5-YR RELATIVE SURVIVAL (%)	
	Males	Females	All		Males	Females	All	Males	Females
Basque Country	724	12	736	1986-1988	59.2	63.3	59.3		
Mallorca	88	3	91	1988-1989	59.6	58.3	59.5		
Navarra	257	5	262	1985-1989	59.8	62.0	59.8		
Tarragona	201	5	206	1985-1989	62.2	55.2	62.1		
Spanish Registries	1270	25	1295		59.9	61.0	59.9		

OBSERVED AND RELATIVE SURVIVAL (%) BY AGE (number of cases in parentheses)

	15-44		45-54		55-64		65-74		75-99		ALL	
	obs	rel	obs	rel	obs	rel	obs	rel	obs	rel	obs	rel
Males	(98)		(285)		(469)		(318)		(100)		(1270)	
1 year	95	95	88	89	86	87	81	83	70	77	84	86
3 years	84	84	68	70	67	70	59	66	53	70	66	70
5 years	77	78	60	62	60	64	51	61	46	76	58	65
Females	(5)		(3)		(5)		(9)		(3)		(25)	
1 year	100	100	67	67	60	60	100	100	67	73	84	86
3 years	80	80	67	67	40	41	56	59	67	87	60	63
5 years	80	80	67	67	-	-	56	62	67	100	60	66
Overall	(103)		(288)		(474)		(327)		(103)		(1295)	
1 year	95	95	88	89	85	86	81	84	70	76	84	86
3 years	83	84	68	70	67	70	59	66	53	71	66	70
5 years	77	78	60	62	59	64	51	61	47	77	58	65

SWEDEN

AREA	NUMBER OF CASES			PERIOD	MEAN AGE		
	Males	Females	All		Males	Females	All
South Sweden	202	20	222	1985-1989	66.7	57.0	65.8

OBSERVED AND RELATIVE SURVIVAL (%) BY AGE (number of cases in parentheses)

	15-44		45-54		55-64		65-74		75-99		ALL	
	obs	rel	obs	rel	obs	rel	obs	rel	obs	rel	obs	rel
Males	(11)		(9)		(54)		(79)		(49)		(202)	
1 year	91	91	100	100	94	96	85	88	84	91	88	91
3 years	73	73	89	90	76	79	71	79	67	90	72	81
5 years	64	64	67	69	70	76	57	69	51	86	60	74
Females	(4)		(5)		(5)		(3)		(3)		(20)	
1 year	100	100	80	80	100	100	100	100	100	100	95	96
3 years	100	100	60	61	80	82	100	100	67	79	80	83
5 years	100	100	60	61	40	42	67	75	67	91	65	70
Overall	(15)		(14)		(59)		(82)		(52)		(222)	
1 year	93	93	93	93	95	96	85	88	85	92	89	92
3 years	80	80	79	80	76	79	72	80	67	89	73	82
5 years	73	74	64	66	68	73	57	69	52	87	60	73

LARYNX (ICD-9 161)

SWITZERLAND

AREA	NUMBER OF CASES			PERIOD	MEAN AGE			5-YR RELATIVE SURVIVAL (%)	
	Males	Females	All		Males	Females	All	Males	Females
Basel	61	4	65	1985-1988	62.8	54.3	62.3		
Geneva	106	11	117	1985-1989	60.7	61.4	60.8		
Swiss Registries	167	15	182		61.5	59.6	61.3		

OBSERVED AND RELATIVE SURVIVAL (%) BY AGE (number of cases in parentheses)

	AGE CLASS										ALL	
	15-44		45-54		55-64		65-74		75-99			
	obs	rel	obs	rel	obs	rel	obs	rel	obs	rel	obs	rel
Males	(10)		(36)		(64)		(34)		(23)		(167)	
1 year	90	90	94	95	92	93	85	88	83	92	90	92
3 years	60	60	80	81	59	62	65	72	57	79	65	70
5 years	60	61	69	71	54	59	53	65	22	40	53	61
Females	(0)		(4)		(8)		(2)		(1)		(15)	
1 year	-	-	100	100	100	100	100	100	100	100	100	100
3 years	-	-	100	100	88	89	100	100	0	0	87	89
5 years	-	-	75	76	74	76	100	100	0	0	73	76
Overall	(10)		(40)		(72)		(36)		(24)		(182)	
1 year	90	90	95	95	93	94	86	89	83	92	91	93
3 years	60	60	82	83	63	65	67	74	54	75	66	72
5 years	60	61	69	71	57	61	56	68	21	37	55	63

LARYNX (ICD-9 161)

EUROPE, 1985-89
Weighted analyses

COUNTRY	% COVERAGE WITH C.R.s	Males	Females	All
AUSTRIA	8	25	2	27
DENMARK	100	197	48	245
ENGLAND	50	696	156	852
ESTONIA	100	60	3	63
FINLAND	100	105	10	115
FRANCE	3	119	7	126
GERMANY	2	57	7	64
ICELAND	100	3	1	4
ITALY	10	552	40	592
NETHERLANDS	6	33	3	36
POLAND	6	127	19	146
SCOTLAND	100	181	45	226
SLOVAKIA	100	277	14	291
SLOVENIA	100	90	7	97
SPAIN	10	377	8	385
SWEDEN	17	40	4	44
SWITZERLAND	11	37	3	40

YEARLY NO. OF CASES (Mean No. of cases recorded); RELATIVE SURVIVAL (%) (Age-standardized)

□ 1 year ■ 5 years

OBSERVED AND RELATIVE SURVIVAL (%) BY AGE

	15-44 obs	rel	45-54 obs	rel	55-64 obs	rel	65-74 obs	rel	75-99 obs	rel	ALL obs	rel
Males												
1 year	91	91	86	87	86	87	81	84	73	80	84	86
3 years	73	74	68	70	65	68	61	69	49	67	63	69
5 years	68	69	60	62	57	62	48	60	36	63	53	62
Females												
1 year	95	95	88	89	85	85	84	85	62	66	81	83
3 years	84	85	70	70	72	74	70	73	44	54	64	68
5 years	82	82	61	62	65	68	62	67	34	50	55	62
Overall												
1 year	91	92	87	87	86	87	82	84	72	79	84	86
3 years	74	75	68	70	66	69	62	69	49	66	63	69
5 years	69	70	60	62	57	63	50	61	36	62	53	62

AGE STANDARDIZED RELATIVE SURVIVAL(%)

COUNTRY	MALES 1-year (95% C.I.)	MALES 5-years (95% C.I.)	FEMALES 1-year (95% C.I.)	FEMALES 5-years (95% C.I.)
AUSTRIA	87.7 (79.5 - 96.6)	58.4 (43.0 - 79.2)	-	-
DENMARK	84.2 (81.8 - 86.8)	59.7 (56.0 - 63.6)	85.6 (81.1 - 90.4)	58.8 (52.2 - 66.2)
ENGLAND	84.1 (82.8 - 85.5)	66.0 (64.0 - 68.1)	83.0 (80.3 - 85.8)	63.6 (59.8 - 67.6)
ESTONIA	73.2 (67.2 - 79.8)	43.2 (37.3 - 50.0)	71.7 (58.7 - 87.7)	62.8 (49.6 - 79.6)
FINLAND	85.6 (82.4 - 88.9)	60.2 (55.3 - 65.5)	82.6 (74.2 - 91.9)	53.6 (40.1 - 71.7)
FRANCE	84.3 (80.9 - 87.7)	51.0 (45.8 - 56.8)	83.1 (72.4 - 95.5)	58.1 (40.9 - 82.4)
GERMANY	91.1 (87.0 - 95.3)	72.4 (64.5 - 81.3)	85.4 (74.0 - 98.5)	72.2 (59.7 - 87.4)
ICELAND	86.8 (76.0 - 99.2)	74.1 (62.6 - 87.6)	-	-
ITALY	88.8 (87.3 - 90.4)	66.9 (64.4 - 69.5)	81.3 (75.4 - 87.5)	65.2 (57.6 - 73.8)
NETHERLANDS	93.8 (89.2 - 98.7)	75.6 (66.9 - 85.4)	100.0 (100.0 -100.0)	100.0 (100.0 -100.0)
POLAND	71.0 (65.6 - 76.9)	44.1 (37.3 - 52.2)	82.6 (71.9 - 94.8)	59.2 (45.1 - 77.6)
SCOTLAND	86.7 (84.2 - 89.2)	64.1 (60.1 - 68.3)	82.1 (77.1 - 87.5)	58.6 (51.8 - 66.3)
SLOVAKIA	71.6 (68.8 - 74.6)	49.3 (45.3 - 53.7)	74.1 (63.0 - 87.3)	47.4 (34.3 - 65.5)
SLOVENIA	79.3 (74.9 - 84.0)	52.1 (46.1 - 58.9)	80.0 (63.8 -100.2)	62.5 (44.5 - 87.8)
SPAIN	85.0 (82.7 - 87.3)	65.4 (61.8 - 69.2)	76.7 (59.6 - 98.8)	-
SWEDEN	93.2 (89.6 - 97.0)	73.6 (65.3 - 82.9)	96.7 (90.9 -102.8)	64.7 (43.0 - 97.5)
SWITZERLAND	91.8 (86.7 - 97.1)	60.0 (51.4 - 70.0)	-	-
EUROPE, 1985-89	85.6 (84.5 - 86.8)	62.2 (60.2 - 64.2)	83.5 (80.0 - 87.3)	65.0 (60.2 - 70.3)

253

LUNG (ICD-9 162)

AUSTRIA

AREA	NUMBER OF CASES			PERIOD	MEAN AGE		
	Males	Females	All		Males	Females	All
Tirol	391	96	487	1988-1989	66.1	64.7	65.8

OBSERVED AND RELATIVE SURVIVAL (%) BY AGE (number of cases in parentheses)

	AGE CLASS										ALL	
	15-44		45-54		55-64		65-74		75-99			
	obs	rel	obs	rel	obs	rel	obs	rel	obs	rel	obs	rel
Males	(12)		(39)		(127)		(107)		(106)		(391)	
1 year	67	67	41	41	37	37	38	39	20	21	34	35
3 years	42	42	23	23	15	16	14	15	5	6	14	15
5 years	33	34	21	21	11	12	7	8	4	6	9	11
Females	(6)		(21)		(15)		(24)		(30)		(96)	
1 year	67	67	24	24	40	40	38	38	23	25	32	33
3 years	50	50	19	19	27	27	17	17	7	8	18	19
5 years	50	50	14	14	20	21	17	18	0	0	14	15
Overall	(18)		(60)		(142)		(131)		(136)		(487)	
1 year	67	67	35	35	37	38	38	39	21	22	34	35
3 years	44	45	22	22	16	17	15	16	5	6	14	16
5 years	39	39	18	19	12	13	8	10	3	4	10	12

DENMARK

AREA	NUMBER OF CASES			PERIOD	MEAN AGE		
	Males	Females	All		Males	Females	All
Denmark	10466	4929	15395	1985-1989	67.6	65.3	66.9

OBSERVED AND RELATIVE SURVIVAL (%) BY AGE (number of cases in parentheses)

	AGE CLASS										ALL	
	15-44		45-54		55-64		65-74		75-99			
	obs	rel	obs	rel	obs	rel	obs	rel	obs	rel	obs	rel
Males	(204)		(777)		(2679)		(4183)		(2623)		(10466)	
1 year	35	35	31	31	29	29	24	25	13	14	23	24
3 years	17	17	10	11	10	11	7	8	2	3	7	8
5 years	13	13	8	8	7	8	4	5	1	2	5	6
Females	(169)		(622)		(1415)		(1701)		(1022)		(4929)	
1 year	37	37	34	34	30	30	23	23	16	17	25	26
3 years	18	18	12	12	11	11	7	8	4	5	9	9
5 years	12	12	10	11	7	8	4	5	2	4	6	7
Overall	(373)		(1399)		(4094)		(5884)		(3645)		(15395)	
1 year	36	36	32	33	29	29	24	24	14	15	24	25
3 years	17	18	11	11	10	11	7	8	3	4	8	9
5 years	13	13	9	9	7	8	4	5	1	2	5	6

LUNG (ICD-9 162)

ENGLAND

AREA	NUMBER OF CASES			PERIOD	MEAN AGE			5-YR RELATIVE SURVIVAL (%)	
	Males	Females	All		Males	Females	All	Males	Females
East Anglia	4417	1717	6134	1985-1989	70.4	69.9	70.3		
Mersey	6308	3044	9352	1985-1989	68.1	67.7	67.9		
Oxford	5036	2115	7151	1985-1989	69.4	69.0	69.3		
South Thames	12032	5506	17538	1985-1989	69.2	69.4	69.3		
Wessex	5941	2579	8520	1985-1989	69.7	69.1	69.5		
West Midlands	12221	4258	16479	1985-1989	68.3	68.4	68.4		
Yorkshire	8589	3663	12252	1985-1989	68.7	68.5	68.7		
English Registries	54544	22882	77426		69.0	68.8	68.9		

5-YR RELATIVE SURVIVAL (%) chart: scale 100 80 60 40 20 0 (Males) and 0 20 40 60 80 100 (Females) for E.Angl, Mersey, Oxford, S.Tham, Wessex, W.Midl, Yorksh

OBSERVED AND RELATIVE SURVIVAL (%) BY AGE (number of cases in parentheses)

	AGE CLASS										ALL	
	15-44		45-54		55-64		65-74		75-99			
	obs	rel	obs	rel	obs	rel	obs	rel	obs	rel	obs	rel
Males	(715)		(3216)		(12737)		(21470)		(16406)		(54544)	
1 year	33	34	29	29	27	27	21	22	14	15	21	22
3 years	16	16	14	14	11	12	7	8	3	4	7	9
5 years	15	15	11	12	8	9	5	6	2	3	5	7
Females	(458)		(1435)		(5500)		(8472)		(7017)		(22882)	
1 year	40	40	30	30	26	27	21	22	13	14	21	22
3 years	21	21	14	14	11	12	8	8	3	4	8	9
5 years	20	20	12	12	9	9	5	6	2	3	6	7
Overall	(1173)		(4651)		(18237)		(29942)		(23423)		(77426)	
1 year	36	36	29	30	27	27	21	22	14	15	21	22
3 years	18	18	14	14	11	12	7	8	3	4	7	9
5 years	17	17	12	12	8	9	5	6	2	3	5	7

ESTONIA

AREA	NUMBER OF CASES			PERIOD	MEAN AGE		
	Males	Females	All		Males	Females	All
Estonia	2613	483	3096	1985-1989	61.8	65.8	62.4

OBSERVED AND RELATIVE SURVIVAL (%) BY AGE (number of cases in parentheses)

	AGE CLASS										ALL	
	15-44		45-54		55-64		65-74		75-99			
	obs	rel	obs	rel	obs	rel	obs	rel	obs	rel	obs	rel
Males	(73)		(459)		(1139)		(636)		(306)		(2613)	
1 year	34	34	32	32	30	31	26	28	21	24	29	30
3 years	15	16	12	12	8	9	7	8	4	6	8	9
5 years	14	14	7	7	6	7	4	5	1	2	5	7
Females	(16)		(41)		(161)		(155)		(110)		(483)	
1 year	69	69	37	37	32	32	31	32	24	26	32	33
3 years	56	56	24	24	13	14	16	18	12	16	16	18
5 years	49	49	16	17	9	10	13	16	6	11	12	14
Overall	(89)		(500)		(1300)		(791)		(416)		(3096)	
1 year	40	40	32	32	31	31	27	29	22	24	29	30
3 years	23	23	13	13	9	10	9	10	6	9	9	11
5 years	20	21	8	8	7	8	6	8	2	5	6	8

LUNG (ICD-9 162)

FINLAND

AREA	NUMBER OF CASES			PERIOD	MEAN AGE		
	Males	Females	All		Males	Females	All
Finland	8017	1492	9509	1985-1989	66.5	67.5	66.7

OBSERVED AND RELATIVE SURVIVAL (%) BY AGE (number of cases in parentheses)

	AGE CLASS										ALL	
	15-44		45-54		55-64		65-74		75-99			
	obs	rel	obs	rel	obs	rel	obs	rel	obs	rel	obs	rel
Males	(134)		(627)		(2569)		(3005)		(1682)		(8017)	
1 year	41	41	41	41	43	44	40	42	29	32	39	40
3 years	17	17	19	20	16	17	14	16	6	9	13	15
5 years	13	14	16	17	11	12	8	10	2	4	9	11
Females	(54)		(131)		(363)		(521)		(423)		(1492)	
1 year	50	50	47	47	51	52	39	40	26	28	39	41
3 years	30	30	21	22	22	23	15	16	6	7	15	17
5 years	26	26	17	17	16	16	9	11	2	3	10	12
Overall	(188)		(758)		(2932)		(3526)		(2105)		(9509)	
1 year	44	44	42	42	44	45	40	41	28	31	39	40
3 years	21	21	20	20	17	18	14	16	6	8	14	16
5 years	17	17	16	17	12	13	8	10	2	4	9	11

FRANCE

AREA	NUMBER OF CASES			PERIOD	MEAN AGE			5-YR RELATIVE SURVIVAL (%)	
	Males	Females	All		Males	Females	All	Males	Females
Somme	979	84	1063	1985-1989	64.2	65.4	64.3		
Calvados	862	75	937	1985-1989	62.7	62.6	62.7		
Doubs	753	92	845	1985-1989	63.6	60.3	63.2		
French Registries	2594	251	2845		63.5	62.7	63.4		

OBSERVED AND RELATIVE SURVIVAL (%) BY AGE (number of cases in parentheses)

	AGE CLASS										ALL	
	15-44		45-54		55-64		65-74		75-99			
	obs	rel	obs	rel	obs	rel	obs	rel	obs	rel	obs	rel
Males	(125)		(359)		(915)		(752)		(443)		(2594)	
1 year	46	47	52	52	41	42	40	41	27	30	40	41
3 years	20	20	20	21	16	17	15	17	8	11	15	17
5 years	14	15	15	16	13	14	10	12	4	7	11	13
Females	(29)		(25)		(74)		(76)		(47)		(251)	
1 year	55	55	40	40	45	45	43	44	29	31	42	43
3 years	41	42	20	20	23	23	30	32	5	5	24	25
5 years	41	42	16	16	17	18	20	22	2	3	18	20
Overall	(154)		(384)		(989)		(828)		(490)		(2845)	
1 year	48	48	51	51	41	42	40	41	28	30	40	42
3 years	24	24	20	21	17	18	16	18	8	10	16	18
5 years	20	20	15	16	13	14	11	13	4	6	11	14

LUNG (ICD-9 162)

GERMANY

AREA	NUMBER OF CASES			PERIOD	MEAN AGE		
	Males	Females	All		Males	Females	All
Saarland	2202	372	2574	1985-1989	64.9	66.1	65.0

OBSERVED AND RELATIVE SURVIVAL (%) BY AGE (number of cases in parentheses)

	AGE CLASS										ALL	
	15-44		45-54		55-64		65-74		75-99			
	obs	rel	obs	rel	obs	rel	obs	rel	obs	rel	obs	rel
Males	(54)		(327)		(718)		(655)		(448)		(2202)	
1 year	43	43	39	39	35	35	28	29	20	22	30	32
3 years	19	19	16	16	12	13	9	10	4	5	10	12
5 years	16	17	12	13	9	11	7	8	3	5	8	10
Females	(14)		(30)		(123)		(102)		(103)		(372)	
1 year	64	64	40	40	40	40	31	32	19	21	33	34
3 years	50	50	17	17	20	20	17	18	5	6	16	17
5 years	50	50	13	14	18	19	13	15	3	4	13	15
Overall	(68)		(357)		(841)		(757)		(551)		(2574)	
1 year	47	47	39	39	35	36	28	29	20	22	31	32
3 years	25	25	16	16	13	14	10	11	4	6	11	12
5 years	23	24	13	13	11	12	7	9	3	5	9	11

ICELAND

AREA	NUMBER OF CASES			PERIOD	MEAN AGE		
	Males	Females	All		Males	Females	All
Iceland	215	169	384	1985-1989	67.8	66.0	67.0

OBSERVED AND RELATIVE SURVIVAL (%) BY AGE (number of cases in parentheses)

	AGE CLASS										ALL	
	15-44		45-54		55-64		65-74		75-99			
	obs	rel	obs	rel	obs	rel	obs	rel	obs	rel	obs	rel
Males	(2)		(11)		(65)		(88)		(49)		(215)	
1 year	50	50	18	18	43	44	38	39	24	27	35	37
3 years	50	50	9	9	18	19	19	21	6	8	16	18
5 years	50	50	9	9	12	13	9	11	6	10	10	12
Females	(3)		(30)		(44)		(49)		(43)		(169)	
1 year	67	67	43	43	45	46	37	37	26	27	38	39
3 years	67	67	20	20	11	12	14	15	14	17	15	17
5 years	67	67	17	17	9	9	8	9	9	14	11	13
Overall	(5)		(41)		(109)		(137)		(92)		(384)	
1 year	60	60	37	37	44	44	37	38	25	27	36	38
3 years	60	60	17	17	16	16	18	19	10	13	16	17
5 years	60	60	15	15	11	12	9	10	8	12	10	12

LUNG (ICD-9 162)

ITALY

AREA	NUMBER OF CASES			PERIOD	MEAN AGE		
	Males	Females	All		Males	Females	All
Florence	2907	556	3463	1985-1989	65.5	66.9	65.7
Genoa	1456	251	1707	1986-1988	66.3	69.1	66.7
Latina	430	48	478	1985-1987	65.1	62.9	64.8
Modena	679	106	785	1988-1989	65.1	67.9	65.5
Parma	613	116	729	1985-1987	65.4	68.1	65.9
Ragusa	356	43	399	1985-1989	65.5	70.0	66.0
Romagna	769	142	911	1986-1988	65.9	68.8	66.4
Turin	1403	335	1738	1985-1987	64.5	66.1	64.8
Varese	1974	286	2260	1985-1989	64.4	67.4	64.8
Italian Registries	10587	1883	12470		65.3	67.4	65.6

5-YR RELATIVE SURVIVAL (%)

Males — Females

Floren, Genoa, Latina, Modena, Parma, Ragusa, Romagn, Turin, Varese

OBSERVED AND RELATIVE SURVIVAL (%) BY AGE (number of cases in parentheses)

	AGE CLASS										ALL	
	15-44		45-54		55-64		65-74		75-99			
	obs	rel	obs	rel	obs	rel	obs	rel	obs	rel	obs	rel
Males	(233)		(1240)		(3571)		(3476)		(2067)		(10587)	
1 year	38	38	42	42	36	36	31	32	21	23	32	33
3 years	18	18	17	17	14	15	10	11	5	7	11	13
5 years	14	14	13	14	11	12	6	8	3	4	8	10
Females	(73)		(184)		(473)		(571)		(582)		(1883)	
1 year	42	43	43	44	37	37	30	31	19	21	30	31
3 years	23	23	22	22	17	18	11	12	6	8	13	14
5 years	21	21	18	18	13	14	7	8	4	5	9	11
Overall	(306)		(1424)		(4044)		(4047)		(2649)		(12470)	
1 year	39	39	42	42	36	36	31	32	21	22	32	33
3 years	19	19	18	18	15	15	10	11	6	7	12	13
5 years	16	16	14	14	11	12	6	8	3	5	8	10

NETHERLANDS

AREA	NUMBER OF CASES			PERIOD	MEAN AGE		
	Males	Females	All		Males	Females	All
Eindhoven	2057	276	2333	1985-1989	66.6	61.6	66.0

OBSERVED AND RELATIVE SURVIVAL (%) BY AGE (number of cases in parentheses)

	AGE CLASS										ALL	
	15-44		45-54		55-64		65-74		75-99			
	obs	rel	obs	rel	obs	rel	obs	rel	obs	rel	obs	rel
Males	(34)		(198)		(594)		(781)		(450)		(2057)	
1 year	44	44	43	44	44	44	39	40	26	29	38	40
3 years	24	24	19	20	17	18	15	17	7	9	14	16
5 years	24	24	14	15	13	14	9	11	4	7	10	12
Females	(25)		(51)		(88)		(68)		(44)		(276)	
1 year	40	40	57	57	50	50	43	43	11	12	42	43
3 years	12	12	35	36	22	22	13	14	2	3	18	19
5 years	12	12	25	26	16	16	7	8	2	3	13	14
Overall	(59)		(249)		(682)		(849)		(494)		(2333)	
1 year	42	42	46	46	44	45	39	41	25	28	38	40
3 years	19	19	22	23	18	19	15	17	6	9	15	17
5 years	19	19	16	17	13	15	9	11	4	7	10	13

LUNG   (ICD-9 162)

POLAND

AREA	NUMBER OF CASES			PERIOD	MEAN AGE			5-YR RELATIVE SURVIVAL (%)	
	Males	Females	All		Males	Females	All	Males	Females
Cracow	1315	365	1680	1985-1989	62.1	64.2	62.6		
Warsaw	1168	476	1644	1988-1989	63.3	66.4	64.2		
Polish Registries	2483	841	3324		62.7	65.4	63.4		

OBSERVED AND RELATIVE SURVIVAL (%) BY AGE (number of cases in parentheses)

	AGE CLASS										ALL	
	15-44		45-54		55-64		65-74		75-99			
	obs	rel	obs	rel	obs	rel	obs	rel	obs	rel	obs	rel
Males	(97)		(376)		(996)		(656)		(358)		(2483)	
1 year	45	45	33	33	30	31	22	23	14	16	27	28
3 years	16	16	14	15	11	11	5	6	3	4	9	10
5 years	14	14	9	10	6	7	4	5	1	3	6	7
Females	(33)		(87)		(284)		(252)		(185)		(841)	
1 year	53	53	41	42	33	34	24	25	12	13	27	28
3 years	22	22	17	17	12	13	8	9	6	7	10	11
5 years	22	22	15	15	9	10	8	9	2	4	8	10
Overall	(130)		(463)		(1280)		(908)		(543)		(3324)	
1 year	47	47	35	35	31	32	23	24	13	15	27	28
3 years	17	17	15	15	11	12	6	7	4	5	9	10
5 years	16	16	10	11	7	8	5	6	2	3	6	8

SCOTLAND

AREA	NUMBER OF CASES			PERIOD	MEAN AGE		
	Males	Females	All		Males	Females	All
Scotland	14086	6895	20981	1985-1989	68.2	68.1	68.1

OBSERVED AND RELATIVE SURVIVAL (%) BY AGE (number of cases in parentheses)

	AGE CLASS										ALL	
	15-44		45-54		55-64		65-74		75-99			
	obs	rel	obs	rel	obs	rel	obs	rel	obs	rel	obs	rel
Males	(209)		(963)		(3679)		(5354)		(3881)		(14086)	
1 year	30	30	30	30	28	28	21	22	13	15	21	23
3 years	14	14	12	12	10	11	7	8	3	4	7	8
5 years	12	13	10	10	8	8	4	6	1	2	5	6
Females	(122)		(526)		(1787)		(2553)		(1907)		(6895)	
1 year	34	34	31	31	27	28	21	22	13	14	22	22
3 years	18	18	13	13	11	12	7	8	3	4	8	9
5 years	17	17	11	12	8	8	5	5	2	3	5	7
Overall	(331)		(1489)		(5466)		(7907)		(5788)		(20981)	
1 year	31	31	30	30	28	28	21	22	13	14	21	23
3 years	15	16	12	13	11	11	7	8	3	4	7	9
5 years	14	14	10	11	8	8	4	5	1	2	5	6

LUNG

(ICD-9 162)

SLOVAKIA

AREA	NUMBER OF CASES			PERIOD	MEAN AGE		
	Males	Females	All		Males	Females	All
Slovakia	9360	1152	10512	1985-1989	62.4	65.7	62.8

OBSERVED AND RELATIVE SURVIVAL (%) BY AGE (number of cases in parentheses)

	AGE CLASS										ALL	
	15-44		45-54		55-64		65-74		75-99			
	obs	rel	obs	rel	obs	rel	obs	rel	obs	rel	obs	rel
Males	(388)		(1603)		(3612)		(2468)		(1289)		(9360)	
1 year	39	39	38	39	35	36	26	28	24	27	32	33
3 years	21	21	16	17	13	14	9	11	10	15	12	14
5 years	17	17	13	14	10	12	7	9	8	15	10	12
Females	(62)		(137)		(293)		(367)		(293)		(1152)	
1 year	47	47	45	45	31	32	30	31	27	30	32	34
3 years	34	34	25	25	18	19	17	19	15	21	19	21
5 years	28	29	20	21	16	17	14	17	13	23	16	19
Overall	(450)		(1740)		(3905)		(2835)		(1582)		(10512)	
1 year	40	40	39	39	34	35	27	28	25	28	32	33
3 years	22	23	17	18	13	15	10	12	11	16	13	15
5 years	18	19	14	15	10	12	8	10	9	17	10	13

SLOVENIA

AREA	NUMBER OF CASES			PERIOD	MEAN AGE		
	Males	Females	All		Males	Females	All
Slovenia	3170	572	3742	1985-1989	61.9	64.1	62.3

OBSERVED AND RELATIVE SURVIVAL (%) BY AGE (number of cases in parentheses)

	AGE CLASS										ALL	
	15-44		45-54		55-64		65-74		75-99			
	obs	rel	obs	rel	obs	rel	obs	rel	obs	rel	obs	rel
Males	(139)		(566)		(1272)		(765)		(428)		(3170)	
1 year	33	33	35	35	34	35	26	28	14	16	30	31
3 years	14	15	12	13	12	13	7	9	3	4	10	11
5 years	11	11	10	10	8	9	4	5	2	3	6	8
Females	(42)		(79)		(160)		(159)		(132)		(572)	
1 year	31	31	35	36	32	32	25	25	12	13	26	27
3 years	17	17	14	14	10	10	9	10	8	10	10	11
5 years	10	10	10	10	4	5	4	4	7	11	6	7
Overall	(181)		(645)		(1432)		(924)		(560)		(3742)	
1 year	33	33	35	35	34	35	26	27	14	15	29	30
3 years	15	15	12	13	12	13	8	9	4	6	10	11
5 years	10	11	10	10	7	8	4	5	3	5	6	8

LUNG (ICD-9 162)

SPAIN

AREA	NUMBER OF CASES			PERIOD	MEAN AGE			5-YR RELATIVE SURVIVAL (%)	
	Males	Females	All		Males	Females	All	Males	Females
Basque Country	1842	148	1990	1986-1988	63.8	64.6	63.9		
Granada	487	33	520	1985-1989	65.0	61.9	64.8		
Mallorca	433	39	472	1988-1989	65.4	67.0	65.6		
Navarra	642	60	702	1985-1989	65.2	65.6	65.3		
Tarragona	742	53	795	1985-1989	65.1	64.6	65.1		
Spanish Registries	4146	333	4479		64.6	64.8	64.6		

OBSERVED AND RELATIVE SURVIVAL (%) BY AGE (number of cases in parentheses)

	AGE CLASS										ALL	
	15-44		45-54		55-64		65-74		75-99			
	obs	rel	obs	rel	obs	rel	obs	rel	obs	rel	obs	rel
Males	(189)		(486)		(1285)		(1452)		(734)		(4146)	
1 year	36	36	38	38	34	34	28	29	21	23	30	31
3 years	19	19	17	18	15	15	12	13	8	10	13	14
5 years	18	18	15	16	12	13	9	11	6	10	11	13
Females	(22)		(53)		(70)		(104)		(84)		(333)	
1 year	32	32	45	45	33	33	27	27	24	25	31	31
3 years	18	18	28	29	20	20	12	12	8	10	16	17
5 years	-	-	20	21	19	19	11	12	7	9	13	15
Overall	(211)		(539)		(1355)		(1556)		(818)		(4479)	
1 year	36	36	39	39	34	34	28	29	21	23	30	31
3 years	19	19	18	19	15	16	12	13	8	10	13	15
5 years	17	18	16	16	12	13	9	11	6	10	11	13

SWEDEN

AREA	NUMBER OF CASES			PERIOD	MEAN AGE		
	Males	Females	All		Males	Females	All
South Sweden	1609	579	2188	1985-1989	67.6	63.7	66.5

OBSERVED AND RELATIVE SURVIVAL (%) BY AGE (number of cases in parentheses)

	AGE CLASS										ALL	
	15-44		45-54		55-64		65-74		75-99			
	obs	rel	obs	rel	obs	rel	obs	rel	obs	rel	obs	rel
Males	(35)		(131)		(381)		(653)		(409)		(1609)	
1 year	51	52	41	41	38	39	27	28	23	25	30	32
3 years	17	17	18	18	15	15	8	9	6	8	10	12
5 years	17	17	15	16	11	12	6	7	3	5	7	9
Females	(37)		(95)		(168)		(164)		(115)		(579)	
1 year	38	38	45	45	32	32	37	38	17	18	33	33
3 years	14	14	26	27	10	10	13	14	5	7	13	14
5 years	14	14	23	24	8	9	8	9	4	7	10	11
Overall	(72)		(226)		(549)		(817)		(524)		(2188)	
1 year	44	45	43	43	36	36	29	30	22	24	31	32
3 years	15	15	21	22	13	14	9	10	6	8	11	12
5 years	15	15	19	19	10	11	6	7	3	6	8	10

LUNG   (ICD-9 162)

SWITZERLAND

AREA	NUMBER OF CASES			PERIOD	MEAN AGE			5-YR RELATIVE SURVIVAL (%)	
	Males	Females	All		Males	Females	All	Males	Females
Basel	644	154	798	1985-1988	66.4	66.1	66.3		
Geneva	641	223	864	1985-1989	66.0	67.0	66.3		
Swiss Registries	1285	377	1662		66.2	66.6	66.3		

OBSERVED AND RELATIVE SURVIVAL (%) BY AGE (number of cases in parentheses)

	AGE CLASS										ALL	
	15-44		45-54		55-64		65-74		75-99			
	obs	rel	obs	rel	obs	rel	obs	rel	obs	rel	obs	rel
Males	(32)		(162)		(364)		(411)		(316)		(1285)	
1 year	49	49	56	56	47	48	35	36	22	25	38	40
3 years	29	29	31	31	19	20	14	15	4	6	15	17
5 years	25	26	23	24	12	13	7	8	2	4	10	12
Females	(20)		(41)		(92)		(113)		(111)		(377)	
1 year	53	53	49	49	43	43	35	35	31	33	38	39
3 years	27	27	29	30	20	20	12	13	9	11	16	17
5 years	21	21	27	27	12	13	6	7	5	7	10	12
Overall	(52)		(203)		(456)		(524)		(427)		(1662)	
1 year	50	50	54	55	46	47	35	36	24	27	38	40
3 years	28	28	30	31	19	20	14	15	5	7	15	17
5 years	24	24	24	25	12	13	7	8	3	5	10	12

LUNG (ICD-9 162)

EUROPE, 1985-89

Weighted analyses

COUNTRY	% COVERAGE WITH C.R.s	YEARLY NO. OF CASES (Mean No. of cases recorded) Males	Females	All
AUSTRIA	8	196	48	244
DENMARK	100	2093	986	3079
ENGLAND	50	10909	4576	15485
ESTONIA	100	523	97	620
FINLAND	100	1603	298	1901
FRANCE	3	519	50	569
GERMANY	2	440	74	514
ICELAND	100	43	34	77
ITALY	10	2944	527	3471
NETHERLANDS	6	411	55	466
POLAND	6	847	311	1158
SCOTLAND	100	2817	1379	4196
SLOVAKIA	100	1872	230	2102
SLOVENIA	100	634	114	748
SPAIN	11	1270	102	1372
SWEDEN	17	322	116	438
SWITZERLAND	11	289	83	372

RELATIVE SURVIVAL (%) (Age-standardized)

□ 1 year ■ 5 years

OBSERVED AND RELATIVE SURVIVAL (%) BY AGE

	15-44 obs	15-44 rel	45-54 obs	45-54 rel	55-64 obs	55-64 rel	65-74 obs	65-74 rel	75-99 obs	75-99 rel	ALL obs	ALL rel
Males												
1 year	41	41	39	39	35	35	29	30	20	22	30	32
3 years	19	19	17	17	13	14	10	11	5	7	11	12
5 years	16	16	13	14	10	11	7	8	3	5	8	10
Females												
1 year	47	47	38	38	34	34	28	28	17	18	28	29
3 years	27	27	18	18	15	16	11	12	5	6	12	13
5 years	26	26	15	15	12	13	8	9	3	4	9	11
Overall												
1 year	42	42	39	39	34	35	29	30	19	21	30	31
3 years	20	20	17	17	14	14	10	11	5	7	11	13
5 years	18	18	13	14	10	11	7	8	3	5	8	10

AGE STANDARDIZED RELATIVE SURVIVAL(%)

COUNTRY	MALES 1-year (95% C.I.)	MALES 5-years (95% C.I.)	FEMALES 1-year (95% C.I.)	FEMALES 5-years (95% C.I.)
AUSTRIA	35.0 (30.5 - 40.2)	10.1 (7.3 - 13.8)	34.6 (25.3 - 47.3)	14.6 (8.2 - 25.9)
DENMARK	24.2 (23.3 - 25.0)	5.6 (5.2 - 6.1)	25.0 (23.9 - 26.3)	5.9 (5.3 - 6.7)
ENGLAND	22.7 (22.4 - 23.1)	7.0 (6.8 - 7.3)	22.4 (21.8 - 22.9)	7.1 (6.7 - 7.4)
ESTONIA	28.1 (26.1 - 30.2)	5.4 (4.4 - 6.6)	32.0 (28.0 - 36.5)	13.9 (10.7 - 18.0)
FINLAND	39.7 (38.6 - 40.9)	10.0 (9.3 - 10.7)	41.0 (38.5 - 43.6)	11.2 (9.6 - 13.0)
FRANCE	39.5 (37.5 - 41.6)	11.5 (10.1 - 13.1)	40.9 (34.9 - 47.9)	15.9 (11.8 - 21.5)
GERMANY	30.1 (28.1 - 32.2)	8.7 (7.4 - 10.3)	32.8 (28.3 - 38.1)	13.8 (10.5 - 18.2)
ICELAND	35.4 (29.5 - 42.6)	12.0 (7.9 - 18.1)	38.4 (31.5 - 46.8)	12.5 (8.1 - 19.3)
ITALY	31.9 (31.0 - 32.8)	8.6 (8.1 - 9.2)	31.3 (29.3 - 33.5)	10.1 (8.8 - 11.7)
NETHERLANDS	39.0 (36.9 - 41.2)	11.7 (10.2 - 13.4)	38.5 (33.0 - 44.9)	10.8 (7.6 - 15.5)
POLAND	25.0 (23.2 - 26.9)	5.7 (4.7 - 6.9)	26.2 (23.4 - 29.4)	8.8 (6.9 - 11.3)
SCOTLAND	22.8 (22.1 - 23.6)	6.1 (5.7 - 6.6)	22.6 (21.7 - 23.7)	6.3 (5.7 - 7.0)
SLOVAKIA	31.0 (29.9 - 32.1)	12.0 (11.1 - 13.0)	32.5 (29.8 - 35.4)	19.1 (16.6 - 22.1)
SLOVENIA	27.5 (25.8 - 29.3)	6.2 (5.3 - 7.3)	25.3 (21.9 - 29.3)	6.9 (4.8 - 9.9)
SPAIN	30.0 (28.5 - 31.5)	11.9 (10.8 - 13.2)	30.1 (25.3 - 35.7)	-
SWEDEN	32.0 (29.8 - 34.4)	8.8 (7.4 - 10.5)	31.7 (28.0 - 35.9)	9.6 (7.3 - 12.5)
SWITZERLAND	38.4 (35.8 - 41.2)	10.3 (8.6 - 12.2)	38.3 (33.6 - 43.8)	10.5 (7.7 - 14.3)
EUROPE, 1985-89	30.5 (30.0 - 31.1)	8.9 (8.5 - 9.3)	28.6 (27.7 - 29.7)	9.9 (9.1 - 10.6)

PLEURA   (ICD-9 163)

AUSTRIA

AREA	NUMBER OF CASES			PERIOD	MEAN AGE		
	Males	Females	All		Males	Females	All
Tirol	4	1	5	1988-1989	65.0	69.0	66.0

OBSERVED AND RELATIVE SURVIVAL (%) BY AGE (number of cases in parentheses)

	15-44		45-54		55-64		65-74		75-99		ALL	
	obs	rel	obs	rel	obs	rel	obs	rel	obs	rel	obs	rel
Males	(0)		(0)		(3)		(1)		(0)		(4)	
1 year	-	-	-	-	33	34	0	0	-	-	25	25
3 years	-	-	-	-	0	0	0	0	-	-	0	0
5 years	-	-	-	-	0	0	0	0	-	-	0	0
Females	(0)		(0)		(0)		(1)		(0)		(1)	
1 year	-	-	-	-	-	-	0	0	-	-	0	0
3 years	-	-	-	-	-	-	0	0	-	-	0	0
5 years	-	-	-	-	-	-	0	0	-	-	0	0
Overall	(0)		(0)		(3)		(2)		(0)		(5)	
1 year	-	-	-	-	33	34	0	0	-	-	20	20
3 years	-	-	-	-	0	0	0	0	-	-	0	0
5 years	-	-	-	-	0	0	0	0	-	-	0	0

DENMARK

AREA	NUMBER OF CASES			PERIOD	MEAN AGE		
	Males	Females	All		Males	Females	All
Denmark	286	141	427	1985-1989	65.8	70.3	67.3

OBSERVED AND RELATIVE SURVIVAL (%) BY AGE (number of cases in parentheses)

	15-44		45-54		55-64		65-74		75-99		ALL	
	obs	rel	obs	rel	obs	rel	obs	rel	obs	rel	obs	rel
Males	(18)		(31)		(75)		(88)		(74)		(286)	
1 year	44	45	26	26	24	24	19	20	19	21	23	24
3 years	6	6	10	10	3	3	3	4	3	4	4	4
5 years	0	0	0	0	0	0	2	3	0	0	1	1
Females	(6)		(8)		(21)		(46)		(60)		(141)	
1 year	50	50	13	13	29	29	26	27	17	18	23	24
3 years	33	34	0	0	5	5	7	7	0	0	4	5
5 years	17	17	0	0	0	0	7	7	0	0	3	4
Overall	(24)		(39)		(96)		(134)		(134)		(427)	
1 year	46	46	23	23	25	25	22	22	18	20	23	24
3 years	13	13	8	8	3	3	4	5	1	2	4	5
5 years	4	4	0	0	0	0	4	5	0	0	1	2

PLEURA   (ICD-9 163)

ENGLAND

AREA	NUMBER OF CASES			PERIOD	MEAN AGE			5-YR RELATIVE SURVIVAL (%)	
	Males	Females	All		Males	Females	All	Males	Females
East Anglia	95	19	114	1985-1989	64.9	67.1	65.3		
Mersey	161	30	191	1985-1989	64.9	65.9	65.0		
Oxford	111	23	134	1985-1989	61.3	66.2	62.2		
South Thames	343	73	416	1985-1989	64.9	66.9	65.3		
Wessex	326	37	363	1985-1989	66.8	67.2	66.9		
West Midlands	139	32	171	1985-1989	63.5	65.4	63.9		
Yorkshire	174	50	224	1985-1989	61.9	65.9	62.8		
English Registries	1349	264	1613		64.6	66.4	64.9		

OBSERVED AND RELATIVE SURVIVAL (%) BY AGE (number of cases in parentheses)

	15-44 obs rel	45-54 obs rel	55-64 obs rel	65-74 obs rel	75-99 obs rel	ALL obs rel
Males	(56)	(189)	(415)	(421)	(268)	(1349)
1 year	40 40	38 38	29 29	24 25	16 17	26 28
3 years	18 18	7 8	6 6	5 5	2 3	5 6
5 years	11 11	5 5	5 5	3 3	1 2	4 4
Females	(15)	(20)	(74)	(89)	(66)	(264)
1 year	47 47	65 65	39 40	22 23	20 21	31 32
3 years	20 20	25 25	11 11	3 4	6 8	9 10
5 years	7 7	15 15	8 9	1 1	5 7	5 6
Overall	(71)	(209)	(489)	(510)	(334)	(1613)
1 year	42 42	40 40	30 31	24 25	16 18	27 28
3 years	19 19	9 9	7 7	5 5	3 4	6 7
5 years	10 10	6 6	5 6	2 3	2 3	4 5

ESTONIA

AREA	NUMBER OF CASES			PERIOD	MEAN AGE		
	Males	Females	All		Males	Females	All
Estonia	17	17	34	1985-1989	56.8	59.6	58.2

OBSERVED AND RELATIVE SURVIVAL (%) BY AGE (number of cases in parentheses)

	15-44 obs rel	45-54 obs rel	55-64 obs rel	65-74 obs rel	75-99 obs rel	ALL obs rel
Males	(3)	(6)	(5)	(1)	(2)	(17)
1 year	33 34	33 34	40 41	0 0	0 0	29 30
3 years	- -	0 0	40 44	0 0	0 0	15 16
5 years	- -	0 0	20 24	0 0	0 0	7 9
Females	(1)	(6)	(4)	(4)	(2)	(17)
1 year	100 100	17 17	50 51	50 52	50 53	41 42
3 years	0 0	0 0	50 52	0 0	50 62	18 19
5 years	0 0	0 0	- -	0 0	50 76	11 12
Overall	(4)	(12)	(9)	(5)	(4)	(34)
1 year	50 50	25 25	44 45	40 42	25 27	35 36
3 years	0 0	0 0	44 47	0 0	25 32	16 18
5 years	0 0	0 0	20 23	0 0	25 40	9 11

PLEURA (ICD-9 163)

FINLAND

AREA	NUMBER OF CASES			PERIOD	MEAN AGE		
	Males	Females	All		Males	Females	All
Finland	161	75	236	1985-1989	62.1	67.5	63.8

OBSERVED AND RELATIVE SURVIVAL (%) BY AGE (number of cases in parentheses)

	15-44		45-54		55-64		65-74		75-99		ALL	
	obs	rel	obs	rel	obs	rel	obs	rel	obs	rel	obs	rel
Males	(13)		(32)		(51)		(36)		(29)		(161)	
1 year	46	46	41	41	35	36	31	32	24	27	34	35
3 years	8	8	6	6	8	8	3	3	7	10	6	7
5 years	8	8	6	7	4	4	3	4	7	12	5	6
Females	(6)		(5)		(16)		(25)		(23)		(75)	
1 year	67	67	60	60	50	50	28	29	13	14	33	35
3 years	33	33	60	61	13	13	12	13	9	12	16	18
5 years	0	0	20	20	6	7	8	9	4	7	7	8
Overall	(19)		(37)		(67)		(61)		(52)		(236)	
1 year	53	53	43	44	39	39	30	31	19	21	34	35
3 years	16	16	14	14	9	9	7	7	8	10	9	10
5 years	5	5	8	8	4	5	5	6	6	10	6	7

FRANCE

AREA	NUMBER OF CASES			PERIOD	MEAN AGE			5-YR RELATIVE SURVIVAL (%)	
	Males	Females	All		Males	Females	All	Males	Females
Somme	24	7	31	1985-1989	61.9	57.7	61.0		
Calvados	25	8	33	1985-1989	60.1	68.1	62.1		
Doubs	18	5	23	1985-1989	64.5	64.0	64.4		
French Registries	67	20	87		62.0	63.6	62.3		

OBSERVED AND RELATIVE SURVIVAL (%) BY AGE (number of cases in parentheses)

	15-44		45-54		55-64		65-74		75-99		ALL	
	obs	rel	obs	rel	obs	rel	obs	rel	obs	rel	obs	rel
Males	(9)		(12)		(16)		(15)		(15)		(67)	
1 year	44	45	18	18	61	62	42	43	4	4	34	35
3 years	22	22	0	0	20	22	8	9	-	-	10	11
5 years	22	23	0	0	7	8	-	-	-	-	7	8
Females	(2)		(4)		(3)		(4)		(7)		(20)	
1 year	100	100	75	75	100	100	25	25	14	15	48	49
3 years	100	100	25	25	33	34	0	0	-	-	21	22
5 years	100	100	25	25	-	-	0	0	-	-	21	24
Overall	(11)		(16)		(19)		(19)		(22)		(87)	
1 year	51	51	33	34	67	69	38	39	7	8	37	38
3 years	30	31	7	7	22	24	6	7	-	-	12	14
5 years	30	31	7	7	11	12	-	-	-	-	10	12

PLEURA (ICD-9 163)

GERMANY

AREA	NUMBER OF CASES			PERIOD	MEAN AGE		
	Males	Females	All		Males	Females	All
Saarland	24	12	36	1985-1989	69.5	72.1	70.4

OBSERVED AND RELATIVE SURVIVAL (%) BY AGE (number of cases in parentheses)

	AGE CLASS										ALL	
	15-44		45-54		55-64		65-74		75-99			
	obs	rel	obs	rel	obs	rel	obs	rel	obs	rel	obs	rel
Males	(1)		(0)		(8)		(4)		(11)		(24)	
1 year	100	100	-	-	0	0	25	26	0	0	8	9
3 years	100	100	-	-	0	0	25	28	0	0	8	10
5 years	100	100	-	-	0	0	25	31	0	0	8	12
Females	(0)		(1)		(0)		(6)		(5)		(12)	
1 year	-	-	100	100	-	-	17	17	0	0	17	17
3 years	-	-	0	0	-	-	0	0	0	0	0	0
5 years	-	-	0	0	-	-	0	0	0	0	0	0
Overall	(1)		(1)		(8)		(10)		(16)		(36)	
1 year	100	100	100	100	0	0	20	21	0	0	11	12
3 years	100	100	0	0	0	0	10	11	0	0	6	7
5 years	100	100	0	0	0	0	10	12	0	0	6	8

ICELAND

AREA	NUMBER OF CASES			PERIOD	MEAN AGE		
	Males	Females	All		Males	Females	All
Iceland	6	1	7	1985-1989	66.2	62.0	65.7

OBSERVED AND RELATIVE SURVIVAL (%) BY AGE (number of cases in parentheses)

	AGE CLASS										ALL	
	15-44		45-54		55-64		65-74		75-99			
	obs	rel	obs	rel	obs	rel	obs	rel	obs	rel	obs	rel
Males	(1)		(1)		(0)		(1)		(3)		(6)	
1 year	0	0	100	100	-	-	0	0	33	35	33	35
3 years	0	0	0	0	-	-	0	0	0	0	0	0
5 years	0	0	0	0	-	-	0	0	0	0	0	0
Females	(0)		(0)		(1)		(0)		(0)		(1)	
1 year	-	-	-	-	0	0	-	-	-	-	0	0
3 years	-	-	-	-	0	0	-	-	-	-	0	0
5 years	-	-	-	-	0	0	-	-	-	-	0	0
Overall	(1)		(1)		(1)		(1)		(3)		(7)	
1 year	0	0	100	100	0	0	0	0	33	35	29	30
3 years	0	0	0	0	0	0	0	0	0	0	0	0
5 years	0	0	0	0	0	0	0	0	0	0	0	0

PLEURA (ICD-9 163)

ITALY

AREA	NUMBER OF CASES			PERIOD	MEAN AGE			5-YR RELATIVE SURVIVAL (%)	
	Males	Females	All		Males	Females	All	Males	Females
Florence	26	9	35	1985-1989	63.5	65.4	64.1		
Genoa	73	30	103	1986-1988	65.4	71.5	67.2		
Latina	2	2	4	1985-1987	62.5	72.0	67.5		
Modena	8	2	10	1988-1989	59.0	74.5	62.2		
Parma	11	7	18	1985-1987	66.7	68.7	67.6		
Ragusa	5	0	5	1985-1989	58.8	-	58.8		
Romagna	9	2	11	1986-1988	63.2	79.5	66.3		
Turin	21	17	38	1985-1987	65.7	68.2	66.8		
Varese	18	6	24	1985-1989	63.4	63.0	63.4		
Italian Registries	173	75	248		64.5	69.5	66.0		

OBSERVED AND RELATIVE SURVIVAL (%) BY AGE (number of cases in parentheses)

	15-44		45-54		55-64		65-74		75-99		ALL	
	obs	rel	obs	rel	obs	rel	obs	rel	obs	rel	obs	rel
Males	(6)		(35)		(40)		(58)		(34)		(173)	
1 year	50	50	43	43	35	36	47	48	26	29	39	41
3 years	0	0	11	12	5	5	10	12	6	8	8	9
5 years	0	0	3	3	0	0	3	4	3	5	2	3
Females	(2)		(9)		(10)		(25)		(29)		(75)	
1 year	50	50	56	56	40	40	28	29	7	7	25	26
3 years	0	0	22	22	10	10	8	8	0	0	7	7
5 years	0	0	22	23	0	0	4	4	0	0	4	5
Overall	(8)		(44)		(50)		(83)		(63)		(248)	
1 year	50	50	45	46	36	37	41	42	17	19	35	36
3 years	0	0	14	14	6	6	10	11	3	4	8	9
5 years	0	0	7	7	0	0	4	4	2	3	3	3

NETHERLANDS

AREA	NUMBER OF CASES			PERIOD	MEAN AGE		
	Males	Females	All		Males	Females	All
Eindhoven	21	8	29	1985-1989	59.4	64.0	60.7

OBSERVED AND RELATIVE SURVIVAL (%) BY AGE (number of cases in parentheses)

	15-44		45-54		55-64		65-74		75-99		ALL	
	obs	rel	obs	rel	obs	rel	obs	rel	obs	rel	obs	rel
Males	(4)		(3)		(5)		(6)		(3)		(21)	
1 year	25	25	33	34	20	20	33	35	33	37	29	29
3 years	0	0	0	0	0	0	0	0	33	44	5	5
5 years	0	0	0	0	0	0	0	0	-	-	-	-
Females	(1)		(1)		(1)		(2)		(3)		(8)	
1 year	0	0	0	0	0	0	50	51	33	35	25	26
3 years	0	0	0	0	0	0	0	0	0	0	0	0
5 years	0	0	0	0	0	0	0	0	0	0	0	0
Overall	(5)		(4)		(6)		(8)		(6)		(29)	
1 year	20	20	25	25	17	17	38	39	33	36	28	28
3 years	0	0	0	0	0	0	0	0	17	20	3	4
5 years	0	0	0	0	0	0	0	0	-	-	-	-

PLEURA (ICD-9 163)

POLAND

AREA	NUMBER OF CASES			PERIOD	MEAN AGE			5-YR RELATIVE SURVIVAL (%)	
	Males	Females	All		Males	Females	All	Males	Females
Cracow	9	5	14	1985-1989	55.9	55.2	55.7		
Warsaw	8	4	12	1988-1989	63.8	68.5	65.4		
Polish Registries	17	9	26		59.7	61.3	60.3		

OBSERVED AND RELATIVE SURVIVAL (%) BY AGE (number of cases in parentheses)

	AGE CLASS										ALL	
	15-44		45-54		55-64		65-74		75-99			
	obs	rel	obs	rel	obs	rel	obs	rel	obs	rel	obs	rel
Males	(1)		(4)		(7)		(3)		(2)		(17)	
1 year	0	0	0	0	29	29	67	70	0	0	24	24
3 years	0	0	0	0	14	16	33	40	0	0	12	13
5 years	0	0	0	0	14	17	33	45	0	0	12	14
Females	(1)		(0)		(4)		(2)		(2)		(9)	
1 year	0	0	-	-	25	25	50	51	0	0	22	23
3 years	0	0	-	-	25	26	0	0	0	0	11	12
5 years	0	0	-	-	25	27	0	0	0	0	11	13
Overall	(2)		(4)		(11)		(5)		(4)		(26)	
1 year	0	0	0	0	27	28	60	63	0	0	23	24
3 years	0	0	0	0	18	20	20	23	0	0	12	13
5 years	0	0	0	0	18	21	20	25	0	0	12	14

SCOTLAND

AREA	NUMBER OF CASES			PERIOD	MEAN AGE		
	Males	Females	All		Males	Females	All
Scotland	460	65	525	1985-1989	66.1	69.1	66.5

OBSERVED AND RELATIVE SURVIVAL (%) BY AGE (number of cases in parentheses)

	AGE CLASS										ALL	
	15-44		45-54		55-64		65-74		75-99			
	obs	rel	obs	rel	obs	rel	obs	rel	obs	rel	obs	rel
Males	(7)		(53)		(139)		(157)		(104)		(460)	
1 year	57	57	40	40	22	22	20	21	11	12	21	22
3 years	14	14	11	12	2	2	4	5	3	4	4	5
5 years	14	15	4	4	1	1	2	3	2	4	2	3
Females	(0)		(7)		(14)		(23)		(21)		(65)	
1 year	-	-	57	57	14	14	13	13	19	21	20	21
3 years	-	-	14	14	0	0	4	5	0	0	3	4
5 years	-	-	14	15	0	0	0	0	0	0	2	2
Overall	(7)		(60)		(153)		(180)		(125)		(525)	
1 year	57	57	42	42	21	21	19	20	12	13	21	22
3 years	14	14	12	12	2	2	4	5	2	3	4	5
5 years	14	15	5	5	1	1	2	2	2	3	2	2

PLEURA (ICD-9 163)

SLOVAKIA

AREA	NUMBER OF CASES			PERIOD	MEAN AGE		
	Males	Females	All		Males	Females	All
Slovakia	24	23	47	1985-1989	65.0	64.3	64.7

OBSERVED AND RELATIVE SURVIVAL (%) BY AGE (number of cases in parentheses)

	AGE CLASS										ALL	
	15-44		45-54		55-64		65-74		75-99			
	obs	rel	obs	rel	obs	rel	obs	rel	obs	rel	obs	rel
Males	(2)		(2)		(6)		(9)		(5)		(24)	
1 year	100	100	0	0	17	17	0	0	0	0	13	13
3 years	50	51	0	0	0	0	0	0	0	0	4	5
5 years	50	51	0	0	0	0	0	0	0	0	4	6
Females	(2)		(2)		(7)		(7)		(5)		(23)	
1 year	0	0	50	50	29	29	29	29	20	22	26	27
3 years	0	0	0	0	14	15	14	16	20	26	13	14
5 years	0	0	0	0	0	0	14	17	20	32	9	10
Overall	(4)		(4)		(13)		(16)		(10)		(47)	
1 year	50	50	25	25	23	24	13	13	10	11	19	20
3 years	25	25	0	0	8	8	6	7	10	14	9	10
5 years	25	25	0	0	0	0	6	8	10	17	6	8

SLOVENIA

AREA	NUMBER OF CASES			PERIOD	MEAN AGE		
	Males	Females	All		Males	Females	All
Slovenia	43	18	61	1985-1989	57.3	61.1	58.5

OBSERVED AND RELATIVE SURVIVAL (%) BY AGE (number of cases in parentheses)

	AGE CLASS										ALL	
	15-44		45-54		55-64		65-74		75-99			
	obs	rel	obs	rel	obs	rel	obs	rel	obs	rel	obs	rel
Males	(6)		(14)		(10)		(5)		(8)		(43)	
1 year	17	17	14	14	20	20	56	58	13	14	19	20
3 years	17	17	7	7	0	0	28	32	0	0	7	8
5 years	17	17	7	7	0	0	0	0	0	0	5	6
Females	(3)		(2)		(6)		(5)		(2)		(18)	
1 year	33	33	50	50	17	17	0	0	0	0	17	17
3 years	33	34	0	0	0	0	0	0	0	0	6	6
5 years	33	34	0	0	0	0	0	0	0	0	6	6
Overall	(9)		(16)		(16)		(10)		(10)		(61)	
1 year	22	22	19	19	19	19	25	25	10	11	19	19
3 years	22	22	6	6	0	0	12	14	0	0	7	7
5 years	22	23	6	7	0	0	0	0	0	0	5	6

PLEURA (ICD-9 163)

SPAIN

AREA	NUMBER OF CASES			PERIOD	MEAN AGE			5-YR RELATIVE SURVIVAL (%)	
	Males	Females	All		Males	Females	All	Males	Females
Basque Country	15	8	23	1986-1988	59.1	58.3	58.8		
Mallorca	4	2	6	1988-1989	60.3	71.5	64.2		
Navarra	9	10	19	1985-1989	60.0	67.9	64.2		
Tarragona	6	3	9	1985-1989	60.3	64.7	61.9		
Spanish Registries	34	23	57		59.8	64.6	61.7		

OBSERVED AND RELATIVE SURVIVAL (%) BY AGE (number of cases in parentheses)

	AGE CLASS										ALL	
	15-44		45-54		55-64		65-74		75-99			
	obs	rel	obs	rel	obs	rel	obs	rel	obs	rel	obs	rel
Males	(3)		(4)		(16)		(11)		(0)		(34)	
1 year	0	0	50	50	38	38	36	38	-	-	35	36
3 years	0	0	0	0	0	0	18	20	-	-	6	6
5 years	0	0	0	0	0	0	18	22	-	-	6	6
Females	(3)		(1)		(5)		(8)		(6)		(23)	
1 year	33	33	100	100	40	40	50	51	33	35	43	44
3 years	33	33	100	100	20	20	25	26	17	20	26	28
5 years	-	-	100	100	20	21	25	27	17	24	26	30
Overall	(6)		(5)		(21)		(19)		(6)		(57)	
1 year	17	17	60	60	38	39	42	43	33	35	39	39
3 years	17	17	20	20	5	5	21	23	17	20	14	15
5 years	-	-	20	21	5	5	21	24	17	24	14	16

SWEDEN

AREA	NUMBER OF CASES			PERIOD	MEAN AGE		
	Males	Females	All		Males	Females	All
South Sweden	80	11	91	1985-1989	64.8	72.6	65.8

OBSERVED AND RELATIVE SURVIVAL (%) BY AGE (number of cases in parentheses)

	AGE CLASS										ALL	
	15-44		45-54		55-64		65-74		75-99			
	obs	rel	obs	rel	obs	rel	obs	rel	obs	rel	obs	rel
Males	(6)		(11)		(15)		(23)		(25)		(80)	
1 year	50	50	55	55	47	47	39	40	24	26	39	40
3 years	17	17	9	9	13	14	13	14	4	5	10	11
5 years	17	17	9	9	7	7	9	10	4	6	8	9
Females	(0)		(1)		(1)		(4)		(5)		(11)	
1 year	-	-	0	0	0	0	25	25	40	45	27	29
3 years	-	-	0	0	0	0	0	0	20	28	9	11
5 years	-	-	0	0	0	0	0	0	0	0	0	0
Overall	(6)		(12)		(16)		(27)		(30)		(91)	
1 year	50	50	50	50	44	44	37	38	27	29	37	39
3 years	17	17	8	8	13	13	11	12	7	9	10	11
5 years	17	17	8	9	6	7	7	9	3	5	7	8

PLEURA   (ICD-9 163)

SWITZERLAND

AREA	NUMBER OF CASES			PERIOD	MEAN AGE		
	Males	Females	All		Males	Females	All
Geneva	8	8	16	1985-1989	59.5	71.9	65.8

OBSERVED AND RELATIVE SURVIVAL (%) BY AGE (number of cases in parentheses)

	15-44		45-54		55-64		65-74		75-99		ALL	
	obs	rel	obs	rel	obs	rel	obs	rel	obs	rel	obs	rel
Males	(0)		(0)		(7)		(1)		(0)		(8)	
1 year	-	-	-	-	14	14	0	0	-	-	13	13
3 years	-	-	-	-	0	0	0	0	-	-	0	0
5 years	-	-	-	-	0	0	0	0	-	-	0	0
Females	(0)		(1)		(0)		(5)		(2)		(8)	
1 year	-	-	0	0	-	-	20	20	50	55	25	26
3 years	-	-	0	0	-	-	0	0	50	69	13	14
5 years	-	-	0	0	-	-	0	0	0	0	0	0
Overall	(0)		(1)		(7)		(6)		(2)		(16)	
1 year	-	-	0	0	14	14	17	17	50	55	19	19
3 years	-	-	0	0	0	0	0	0	50	69	6	7
5 years	-	-	0	0	0	0	0	0	0	0	0	0

PLEURA (ICD-9 163)

EUROPE, 1985-89

Weighted analyses

COUNTRY	% COVERAGE WITH C.R.s	YEARLY NO. OF CASES (Mean No. of cases recorded) Males	Females	All
AUSTRIA	8	2	1	3
DENMARK	100	57	28	85
ENGLAND	50	270	53	323
ESTONIA	100	4	4	8
FINLAND	100	32	15	47
FRANCE	3	13	4	17
GERMANY	2	5	2	7
ICELAND	100	2	0	2
ITALY	10	53	23	76
NETHERLANDS	6	5	2	7
POLAND	6	10	5	15
SCOTLAND	100	92	13	105
SLOVAKIA	100	5	5	10
SLOVENIA	100	9	4	13
SPAIN	10	10	6	16
SWEDEN	17	16	2	18
SWITZERLAND	6	2	2	4

RELATIVE SURVIVAL (%) (Age-standardized) — Males / Females

□ 1 year ■ 5 years

OBSERVED AND RELATIVE SURVIVAL (%) BY AGE

	15-44 obs rel	45-54 obs rel	55-64 obs rel	65-74 obs rel	75-99 obs rel	ALL obs rel
Males						
1 year	46 47	33 33	33 33	35 37	14 15	29 30
3 years	21 21	6 6	8 8	11 13	4 6	8 9
5 years	20 20	3 3	3 4	9 12	2 3	5 6
Females						
1 year	50 50	64 64	46 46	29 29	13 14	29 30
3 years	27 27	23 23	16 16	5 5	5 7	10 11
5 years	23 23	21 21	7 7	3 4	2 4	8 9
Overall						
1 year	47 47	41 42	36 37	34 35	14 15	29 30
3 years	23 23	10 10	10 10	10 11	4 6	8 9
5 years	20 20	7 8	4 5	8 9	2 3	6 7

AGE STANDARDIZED RELATIVE SURVIVAL(%)

COUNTRY	MALES 1-year (95% C.I.)	5-years (95% C.I.)	FEMALES 1-year (95% C.I.)	5-years (95% C.I.)
AUSTRIA	-	-	-	-
DENMARK	23.5 (19.0 - 29.1)	0.9 (0.2 - 3.8)	24.6 (17.7 - 34.0)	3.2 (1.2 - 8.1)
ENGLAND	26.9 (24.7 - 29.5)	4.1 (3.1 - 5.5)	33.9 (28.7 - 40.1)	6.8 (4.0 - 11.3)
ESTONIA	17.5 (8.1 - 37.9)	-	49.7 (28.7 - 86.1)	-
FINLAND	33.8 (26.8 - 42.5)	6.5 (3.0 - 13.8)	37.4 (27.7 - 50.4)	9.0 (3.8 - 21.0)
FRANCE	36.2 (26.2 - 50.1)	-	54.0 (40.3 - 72.4)	-
GERMANY	-	-	-	-
ICELAND	-	-	-	-
ITALY	39.7 (32.8 - 48.1)	2.9 (1.0 - 8.1)	31.5 (21.7 - 45.8)	4.3 (1.5 - 12.2)
NETHERLANDS	30.4 (14.8 - 62.6)	-	23.8 (8.2 - 68.9)	0.0 (0.0 - 0.0)
POLAND	29.9 (15.4 - 58.0)	18.7 (5.2 - 67.4)	-	-
SCOTLAND	23.6 (19.8 - 28.1)	3.1 (1.6 - 6.2)	-	-
SLOVAKIA	9.8 (4.1 - 23.4)	2.6 (0.6 - 10.4)	28.8 (14.8 - 55.8)	12.9 (3.6 - 45.9)
SLOVENIA	29.6 (16.3 - 53.8)	1.8 (0.5 - 7.0)	12.9 (4.9 - 34.4)	1.7 (0.3 - 8.6)
SPAIN	-	-	49.9 (34.2 - 72.8)	-
SWEDEN	41.3 (31.4 - 54.3)	8.8 (4.0 - 19.3)	-	-
SWITZERLAND	-	-	-	-
EUROPE, 1985-89	30.9 (27.3 - 35.0)	6.7 (3.8 - 11.7)	36.0 (30.6 - 42.4)	7.9 (3.5 - 17.8)

BONE (ICD-9 170)

AUSTRIA

AREA	NUMBER OF CASES			PERIOD	MEAN AGE		
	Males	Females	All		Males	Females	All
Tirol	5	3	8	1988-1989	53.2	50.0	52.1

OBSERVED AND RELATIVE SURVIVAL (%) BY AGE (number of cases in parentheses)

	20-44		45-54		55-64		65-74		75-99			ALL	
	obs	rel	obs	rel	obs	rel	obs	rel	obs	rel		obs	rel
Males	(1)		(1)		(2)		(0)		(1)			(5)	
1 year	0	0	100	100	100	100	-	-	0	0		60	61
3 years	0	0	100	100	100	100	-	-	0	0		60	63
5 years	0	0	100	100	100	100	-	-	0	0		60	65
Females	(1)		(0)		(1)		(1)		(0)			(3)	
1 year	100	100	-	-	0	0	100	100	-	-		67	67
3 years	100	100	-	-	0	0	0	0	-	-		33	34
5 years	100	100	-	-	0	0	0	0	-	-		33	34
Overall	(2)		(1)		(3)		(1)		(1)			(8)	
1 year	50	50	100	100	67	67	100	100	0	0		63	63
3 years	50	50	100	100	67	68	0	0	0	0		50	52
5 years	50	50	100	100	67	69	0	0	0	0		50	53

DENMARK

AREA	NUMBER OF CASES			PERIOD	MEAN AGE		
	Males	Females	All		Males	Females	All
Denmark	153	136	289	1985-1989	59.6	67.7	63.4

OBSERVED AND RELATIVE SURVIVAL (%) BY AGE (number of cases in parentheses)

	20-44		45-54		55-64		65-74		75-99			ALL	
	obs	rel	obs	rel	obs	rel	obs	rel	obs	rel		obs	rel
Males	(38)		(17)		(23)		(30)		(45)			(153)	
1 year	71	71	65	65	74	75	33	35	27	30		50	53
3 years	58	58	53	54	48	51	20	23	11	16		35	40
5 years	47	48	53	55	39	43	17	21	9	18		29	37
Females	(16)		(11)		(17)		(35)		(57)			(136)	
1 year	94	94	64	64	65	65	40	41	47	52		54	57
3 years	88	88	55	55	35	36	20	22	23	30		34	39
5 years	88	88	45	47	29	31	17	20	18	30		29	37
Overall	(54)		(28)		(40)		(65)		(102)			(289)	
1 year	78	78	64	65	70	71	37	38	38	42		52	55
3 years	67	67	54	55	43	45	20	22	18	24		34	39
5 years	59	60	50	52	35	38	17	20	14	25		29	37

BONE   (ICD-9 170)

ENGLAND

AREA	NUMBER OF CASES			PERIOD	MEAN AGE			5-YR RELATIVE SURVIVAL (%)	
	Males	Females	All		Males	Females	All	Males	Females
East Anglia	31	15	46	1985-1989	63.7	58.1	61.9		
Mersey	28	27	55	1985-1989	51.2	61.0	56.1		
Oxford	45	27	72	1985-1989	52.7	55.7	53.8		
South Thames	113	111	224	1985-1989	52.4	54.2	53.3		
Wessex	67	53	120	1985-1989	58.9	59.2	59.0		
West Midlands	64	60	124	1985-1989	50.1	56.8	53.3		
Yorkshire	49	38	87	1985-1989	53.9	59.2	56.2		
English Registries	397	331	728		54.2	56.9	55.4		

OBSERVED AND RELATIVE SURVIVAL (%) BY AGE (number of cases in parentheses)

	AGE CLASS										ALL	
	20-44		45-54		55-64		65-74		75-99			
	obs	rel	obs	rel	obs	rel	obs	rel	obs	rel	obs	rel
Males	(131)		(41)		(76)		(85)		(64)		(397)	
1 year	86	86	76	76	64	66	51	53	38	42	65	67
3 years	72	72	59	60	54	57	38	43	25	36	52	57
5 years	67	68	51	53	42	46	32	40	13	23	44	51
Females	(103)		(29)		(53)		(62)		(84)		(331)	
1 year	94	94	93	93	72	72	60	61	44	48	71	73
3 years	80	80	72	73	60	62	45	48	35	44	58	63
5 years	74	74	66	67	51	54	32	37	21	34	48	55
Overall	(234)		(70)		(129)		(147)		(148)		(728)	
1 year	90	90	83	83	67	68	54	56	41	45	68	70
3 years	75	75	64	65	57	59	41	45	30	41	55	60
5 years	70	70	57	59	46	49	32	38	18	30	46	53

ESTONIA

AREA	NUMBER OF CASES			PERIOD	MEAN AGE		
	Males	Females	All		Males	Females	All
Estonia	24	22	46	1985-1989	52.9	52.7	52.8

OBSERVED AND RELATIVE SURVIVAL (%) BY AGE (number of cases in parentheses)

	AGE CLASS										ALL	
	20-44		45-54		55-64		65-74		75-99			
	obs	rel	obs	rel	obs	rel	obs	rel	obs	rel	obs	rel
Males	(6)		(7)		(4)		(4)		(3)		(24)	
1 year	50	50	57	58	25	26	25	26	33	37	42	43
3 years	33	34	43	45	0	0	25	30	33	45	29	32
5 years	33	34	43	46	0	0	25	35	33	58	29	34
Females	(7)		(4)		(6)		(3)		(2)		(22)	
1 year	86	86	50	50	67	67	33	34	100	100	68	69
3 years	57	57	50	51	50	52	33	37	50	65	50	53
5 years	43	43	50	52	33	36	0	0	0	0	32	35
Overall	(13)		(11)		(10)		(7)		(5)		(46)	
1 year	69	69	55	55	50	51	29	30	60	66	54	56
3 years	46	46	45	47	30	32	29	33	40	53	39	42
5 years	38	39	45	48	20	22	14	19	20	34	30	35

BONE

(ICD-9 170)

FINLAND

AREA	NUMBER OF CASES			PERIOD	MEAN AGE		
	Males	Females	All		Males	Females	All
Finland	72	68	140	1985-1989	49.4	51.9	50.6

OBSERVED AND RELATIVE SURVIVAL (%) BY AGE (number of cases in parentheses)

	AGE CLASS										ALL	
	20-44		45-54		55-64		65-74		75-99			
	obs	rel	obs	rel	obs	rel	obs	rel	obs	rel	obs	rel
Males	(29)		(10)		(15)		(12)		(6)		(72)	
1 year	97	97	90	91	73	75	67	69	33	37	81	82
3 years	69	69	80	82	67	70	42	47	17	22	61	65
5 years	59	59	80	83	53	58	42	52	17	28	54	60
Females	(25)		(7)		(15)		(13)		(8)		(68)	
1 year	92	92	100	100	87	87	46	47	75	82	81	82
3 years	80	80	71	72	87	88	31	33	13	17	63	66
5 years	76	76	71	73	67	69	23	26	13	20	56	61
Overall	(54)		(17)		(30)		(25)		(14)		(140)	
1 year	94	95	94	95	80	81	56	58	57	63	81	82
3 years	74	74	76	78	77	79	36	40	14	19	62	66
5 years	67	67	76	79	60	64	32	38	14	24	55	60

FRANCE

AREA	NUMBER OF CASES			PERIOD	MEAN AGE			5-YR RELATIVE SURVIVAL (%)	
	Males	Females	All		Males	Females	All	Males	Females
Somme	4	5	9	1985-1989	57.5	55.4	56.4		
Calvados	12	9	21	1985-1989	41.0	45.4	43.0		
Doubs	8	2	10	1985-1989	39.9	67.0	45.4		
French Registries	24	16	40		43.5	51.4	46.7		

OBSERVED AND RELATIVE SURVIVAL (%) BY AGE (number of cases in parentheses)

	AGE CLASS										ALL	
	20-44		45-54		55-64		65-74		75-99			
	obs	rel	obs	rel	obs	rel	obs	rel	obs	rel	obs	rel
Males	(16)		(1)		(5)		(1)		(1)		(24)	
1 year	88	88	100	100	80	81	100	100	0	0	83	84
3 years	69	69	100	100	80	85	100	100	0	0	71	73
5 years	69	70	100	100	80	89	100	100	0	0	71	75
Females	(6)		(2)		(4)		(2)		(2)		(16)	
1 year	67	67	100	100	75	75	100	100	50	52	74	75
3 years	50	50	50	50	50	51	100	100	50	57	54	56
5 years	50	50	50	51	50	52	100	100	50	65	54	57
Overall	(22)		(3)		(9)		(3)		(3)		(40)	
1 year	82	82	100	100	78	79	100	100	33	35	80	81
3 years	64	64	67	68	67	69	100	100	33	39	64	66
5 years	64	64	67	69	67	72	100	100	33	46	64	68

BONE   (ICD-9 170)

GERMANY

AREA	NUMBER OF CASES			PERIOD	MEAN AGE		
	Males	Females	All		Males	Females	All
Saarland	24	14	38	1985-1989	43.3	57.4	48.5

OBSERVED AND RELATIVE SURVIVAL (%) BY AGE (number of cases in parentheses)

	AGE CLASS										ALL	
	20-44		45-54		55-64		65-74		75-99			
	obs	rel	obs	rel	obs	rel	obs	rel	obs	rel	obs	rel
Males	(12)		(6)		(3)		(3)		(0)		(24)	
1 year	67	67	100	100	100	100	67	70	-	-	79	80
3 years	67	67	67	68	100	100	67	77	-	-	71	73
5 years	46	47	33	35	100	100	33	44	-	-	47	50
Females	(5)		(0)		(1)		(5)		(3)		(14)	
1 year	60	60	-	-	100	100	40	41	33	36	50	51
3 years	40	40	-	-	100	100	40	44	0	0	36	39
5 years	40	40	-	-	-	-	40	47	0	0	36	41
Overall	(17)		(6)		(4)		(8)		(3)		(38)	
1 year	65	65	100	100	100	100	50	52	33	36	68	69
3 years	59	59	67	68	100	100	50	56	0	0	58	61
5 years	45	45	33	35	100	100	33	41	0	0	43	47

ICELAND

AREA	NUMBER OF CASES			PERIOD	MEAN AGE		
	Males	Females	All		Males	Females	All
Iceland	7	3	10	1985-1989	48.4	50.3	49.1

OBSERVED AND RELATIVE SURVIVAL (%) BY AGE (number of cases in parentheses)

	AGE CLASS										ALL	
	20-44		45-54		55-64		65-74		75-99			
	obs	rel	obs	rel	obs	rel	obs	rel	obs	rel	obs	rel
Males	(3)		(1)		(1)		(1)		(1)		(7)	
1 year	100	100	100	100	100	100	100	100	0	0	86	87
3 years	100	100	0	0	100	100	100	100	0	0	71	76
5 years	100	100	0	0	100	100	0	0	0	0	57	63
Females	(1)		(1)		(0)		(1)		(0)		(3)	
1 year	100	100	100	100	-	-	100	100	-	-	100	100
3 years	0	0	100	100	-	-	0	0	-	-	33	34
5 years	0	0	100	100	-	-	0	0	-	-	33	34
Overall	(4)		(2)		(1)		(2)		(1)		(10)	
1 year	100	100	100	100	100	100	100	100	0	0	90	91
3 years	75	75	50	50	100	100	50	54	0	0	60	63
5 years	75	75	50	51	100	100	0	0	0	0	50	54

BONE (ICD-9 170)

ITALY

AREA	Males	Females	All	PERIOD	Males	Females	All
	NUMBER OF CASES				**MEAN AGE**		
Florence	42	17	59	1985-1989	57.2	57.4	57.2
Genoa	3	7	10	1986-1988	68.0	61.7	63.7
Latina	4	6	10	1985-1987	47.8	51.8	50.3
Modena	2	2	4	1988-1989	56.5	68.0	62.5
Parma	1	0	1	1985-1987	71.0	-	71.0
Ragusa	13	6	19	1985-1989	51.9	55.7	53.2
Romagna	9	3	12	1986-1988	52.8	34.7	48.3
Turin	13	10	23	1985-1987	55.5	58.5	56.8
Varese	15	29	44	1985-1989	53.7	59.3	57.4
Italian Registries	102	80	182		55.5	57.6	56.4

5-YR RELATIVE SURVIVAL (%)

OBSERVED AND RELATIVE SURVIVAL (%) BY AGE (number of cases in parentheses)

	20-44 obs rel	45-54 obs rel	55-64 obs rel	65-74 obs rel	75-99 obs rel	ALL obs rel
Males	(27)	(11)	(21)	(27)	(16)	(102)
1 year	77 77	64 64	71 72	56 58	44 48	63 65
3 years	46 46	64 65	57 59	22 25	25 33	41 44
5 years	38 38	55 56	57 61	15 18	13 20	34 39
Females	(18)	(11)	(19)	(19)	(13)	(80)
1 year	83 83	90 90	79 79	74 75	46 49	75 76
3 years	72 72	70 70	58 59	58 61	23 28	57 60
5 years	72 72	60 61	53 55	47 53	23 34	52 57
Overall	(45)	(22)	(40)	(46)	(29)	(182)
1 year	80 80	76 77	75 76	63 65	45 48	68 70
3 years	57 57	67 68	58 59	37 41	24 31	48 51
5 years	52 52	57 58	55 58	28 33	17 27	42 47

NETHERLANDS

AREA	Males	Females	All	PERIOD	Males	Females	All
	NUMBER OF CASES				**MEAN AGE**		
Eindhoven	12	13	25	1985-1989	44.4	61.8	53.5

OBSERVED AND RELATIVE SURVIVAL (%) BY AGE (number of cases in parentheses)

	20-44 obs rel	45-54 obs rel	55-64 obs rel	65-74 obs rel	75-99 obs rel	ALL obs rel
Males	(6)	(3)	(2)	(0)	(1)	(12)
1 year	100 100	67 67	100 100	- -	100 100	92 94
3 years	67 67	33 34	100 100	- -	100 100	67 70
5 years	67 67	33 34	50 55	- -	100 100	58 64
Females	(2)	(0)	(4)	(3)	(4)	(13)
1 year	100 100	- -	100 100	100 100	75 79	92 94
3 years	50 50	- -	75 76	67 70	25 30	54 58
5 years	50 50	- -	50 52	67 75	25 34	46 52
Overall	(8)	(3)	(6)	(3)	(5)	(25)
1 year	100 100	67 67	100 100	100 100	80 87	92 94
3 years	63 63	33 34	83 86	67 70	40 51	60 64
5 years	63 63	33 34	48 50	67 75	40 61	52 58

BONE   (ICD-9 170)

POLAND

AREA	NUMBER OF CASES			PERIOD	MEAN AGE			5-YR RELATIVE SURVIVAL (%)	
	Males	Females	All		Males	Females	All	Males	Females
Cracow	13	6	19	1985-1989	44.9	71.3	53.3		
Warsaw	16	12	28	1988-1989	54.3	41.3	48.8		
Polish Registries	29	18	47		50.2	51.4	50.7		

OBSERVED AND RELATIVE SURVIVAL (%) BY AGE (number of cases in parentheses)

	AGE CLASS										ALL	
	20-44		45-54		55-64		65-74		75-99			
	obs	rel	obs	rel	obs	rel	obs	rel	obs	rel	obs	rel
Males	(13)		(3)		(4)		(5)		(4)		(29)	
1 year	46	46	67	67	25	26	20	21	25	28	38	39
3 years	46	47	0	0	0	0	20	24	25	36	28	30
5 years	46	47	0	0	0	0	20	27	25	49	28	32
Females	(7)		(3)		(2)		(4)		(2)		(18)	
1 year	43	43	67	67	100	100	50	52	0	0	50	51
3 years	43	43	33	34	50	52	25	29	0	0	33	35
5 years	43	43	33	34	50	54	25	32	0	0	33	37
Overall	(20)		(6)		(6)		(9)		(6)		(47)	
1 year	45	45	67	67	50	51	33	35	17	18	43	44
3 years	45	45	17	17	17	18	22	26	17	23	30	32
5 years	45	46	17	17	17	19	22	29	17	29	30	34

SCOTLAND

AREA	NUMBER OF CASES			PERIOD	MEAN AGE		
	Males	Females	All		Males	Females	All
Scotland	71	72	143	1985-1989	50.0	59.8	54.9

OBSERVED AND RELATIVE SURVIVAL (%) BY AGE (number of cases in parentheses)

	AGE CLASS										ALL	
	20-44		45-54		55-64		65-74		75-99			
	obs	rel	obs	rel	obs	rel	obs	rel	obs	rel	obs	rel
Males	(30)		(5)		(17)		(12)		(7)		(71)	
1 year	87	87	80	81	65	66	42	44	43	50	69	71
3 years	73	74	60	61	35	38	8	10	0	0	45	49
5 years	63	64	40	42	24	27	8	11	0	0	37	42
Females	(21)		(2)		(11)		(18)		(20)		(72)	
1 year	86	86	100	100	55	55	50	51	40	44	60	62
3 years	57	57	100	100	27	28	50	55	20	28	42	47
5 years	57	57	100	100	18	20	39	46	15	27	36	44
Overall	(51)		(7)		(28)		(30)		(27)		(143)	
1 year	86	86	86	86	61	62	47	48	41	46	64	66
3 years	67	67	71	73	32	34	33	37	15	21	43	48
5 years	61	61	57	59	21	24	27	33	11	21	36	43

BONE

(ICD-9 170)

SLOVAKIA

AREA	NUMBER OF CASES			PERIOD	MEAN AGE		
	Males	Females	All		Males	Females	All
Slovakia	76	60	136	1985-1989	49.4	53.0	51.0

OBSERVED AND RELATIVE SURVIVAL (%) BY AGE (number of cases in parentheses)

	AGE CLASS										ALL	
	20-44		45-54		55-64		65-74		75-99			
	obs	rel	obs	rel	obs	rel	obs	rel	obs	rel	obs	rel
Males	(31)		(12)		(16)		(13)		(4)		(76)	
1 year	74	74	67	67	19	19	31	32	0	0	50	51
3 years	61	62	50	52	19	20	8	9	0	0	38	41
5 years	46	46	50	53	19	22	8	10	0	0	32	37
Females	(20)		(10)		(13)		(8)		(9)		(60)	
1 year	70	70	60	60	46	47	38	39	22	25	52	53
3 years	45	45	40	41	38	40	38	42	11	16	37	39
5 years	45	45	40	41	38	41	38	46	11	22	37	42
Overall	(51)		(22)		(29)		(21)		(13)		(136)	
1 year	73	73	64	64	31	32	33	35	15	18	51	52
3 years	55	55	45	47	28	29	19	22	8	12	38	40
5 years	45	46	45	48	28	31	19	25	8	16	34	39

SLOVENIA

AREA	NUMBER OF CASES			PERIOD	MEAN AGE		
	Males	Females	All		Males	Females	All
Slovenia	27	20	47	1985-1989	43.4	51.2	46.7

OBSERVED AND RELATIVE SURVIVAL (%) BY AGE (number of cases in parentheses)

	AGE CLASS										ALL	
	20-44		45-54		55-64		65-74		75-99			
	obs	rel	obs	rel	obs	rel	obs	rel	obs	rel	obs	rel
Males	(15)		(6)		(3)		(1)		(2)		(27)	
1 year	87	87	80	81	67	68	0	0	50	54	77	78
3 years	53	54	60	62	0	0	0	0	50	64	46	48
5 years	40	40	60	64	0	0	0	0	0	0	35	37
Females	(7)		(3)		(3)		(4)		(3)		(20)	
1 year	86	86	67	67	33	34	25	26	33	36	55	56
3 years	86	86	33	34	33	34	25	27	33	44	50	53
5 years	57	57	33	34	33	35	0	0	0	0	30	33
Overall	(22)		(9)		(6)		(5)		(5)		(47)	
1 year	86	87	76	76	50	51	20	21	40	43	68	69
3 years	64	64	50	52	17	18	20	22	40	52	48	50
5 years	45	46	50	53	17	18	0	0	0	0	33	36

BONE (ICD-9 170)

SPAIN

AREA	NUMBER OF CASES			PERIOD	MEAN AGE			5-YR RELATIVE SURVIVAL (%)	
	Males	Females	All		Males	Females	All	Males	Females
Basque Country	15	20	35	1986-1988	41.7	50.0	46.4		
Mallorca	1	2	3	1988-1989	79.0	39.0	52.7		
Navarra	6	11	17	1985-1989	52.3	52.5	52.5		
Tarragona	10	12	22	1985-1989	50.8	51.0	51.0		
Spanish Registries	32	45	77		47.8	50.4	49.4		

OBSERVED AND RELATIVE SURVIVAL (%) BY AGE (number of cases in parentheses)

	AGE CLASS										ALL	
	20-44		45-54		55-64		65-74		75-99			
	obs	rel	obs	rel	obs	rel	obs	rel	obs	rel	obs	rel
Males	(13)		(7)		(4)		(4)		(4)		(32)	
1 year	77	77	86	86	50	51	75	78	50	54	72	73
3 years	46	46	71	73	50	52	50	55	50	65	53	56
5 years	46	47	71	73	25	27	0	0	50	80	42	46
Females	(17)		(6)		(10)		(8)		(4)		(45)	
1 year	88	88	83	83	90	90	75	76	75	81	84	85
3 years	82	83	50	50	90	92	75	79	50	65	76	78
5 years	82	83	33	34	79	82	60	67	25	39	65	70
Overall	(30)		(13)		(14)		(12)		(8)		(77)	
1 year	83	83	85	85	79	79	75	77	63	67	79	80
3 years	67	67	62	62	79	80	67	72	50	65	66	69
5 years	67	67	53	54	64	67	36	42	38	60	55	60

SWEDEN

AREA	NUMBER OF CASES			PERIOD	MEAN AGE		
	Males	Females	All		Males	Females	All
South Sweden	36	15	51	1985-1989	56.5	61.8	58.1

OBSERVED AND RELATIVE SURVIVAL (%) BY AGE (number of cases in parentheses)

	AGE CLASS										ALL	
	20-44		45-54		55-64		65-74		75-99			
	obs	rel	obs	rel	obs	rel	obs	rel	obs	rel	obs	rel
Males	(9)		(4)		(5)		(12)		(6)		(36)	
1 year	100	100	100	100	100	100	75	77	33	36	81	83
3 years	78	78	75	76	80	84	50	55	17	21	58	63
5 years	67	67	75	77	80	87	42	50	17	26	53	61
Females	(5)		(1)		(1)		(3)		(5)		(15)	
1 year	100	100	0	0	100	100	67	68	60	64	73	75
3 years	100	100	0	0	100	100	67	71	20	24	60	65
5 years	100	100	0	0	100	100	67	75	20	29	60	69
Overall	(14)		(5)		(6)		(15)		(11)		(51)	
1 year	100	100	80	80	100	100	73	75	45	49	78	80
3 years	86	86	60	61	83	87	53	59	18	23	59	64
5 years	79	79	60	62	83	90	47	55	18	27	55	63

BONE

(ICD-9 170)

SWITZERLAND

AREA	NUMBER OF CASES			PERIOD	MEAN AGE		
	Males	Females	All		Males	Females	All
Geneva	6	5	11	1985-1989	47.3	63.0	54.5

OBSERVED AND RELATIVE SURVIVAL (%) BY AGE (number of cases in parentheses)

	AGE CLASS										ALL	
	20-44		45-54		55-64		65-74		75-99			
	obs	rel	obs	rel	obs	rel	obs	rel	obs	rel	obs	rel
Males	(3)		(1)		(1)		(1)		(0)		(6)	
1 year	100	100	100	100	100	100	100	100	-	-	100	100
3 years	100	100	0	0	100	100	100	100	-	-	83	85
5 years	100	100	0	0	0	0	0	0	-	-	42	44
Females	(2)		(0)		(0)		(0)		(3)		(5)	
1 year	100	100	-	-	-	-	-	-	100	100	100	100
3 years	50	50	-	-	-	-	-	-	67	95	60	73
5 years	50	50	-	-	-	-	-	-	0	0	20	28
Overall	(5)		(1)		(1)		(1)		(3)		(11)	
1 year	100	100	100	100	100	100	100	100	100	100	100	100
3 years	80	80	0	0	100	100	100	100	67	95	73	81
5 years	80	81	0	0	0	0	0	0	0	0	31	37

BONE (ICD-9 170)

EUROPE, 1985-89

Weighted analyses

COUNTRY	% COVERAGE WITH C.R.s	YEARLY NO. OF CASES (Mean No. of cases recorded) Males	Females	All
AUSTRIA	8	3	2	5
DENMARK	100	31	27	58
ENGLAND	50	79	66	145
ESTONIA	100	5	4	9
FINLAND	100	14	14	28
FRANCE	3	5	3	8
GERMANY	2	5	3	8
ICELAND	100	2	1	3
ITALY	10	26	20	46
NETHERLANDS	6	2	3	5
POLAND	6	11	7	18
SCOTLAND	100	14	14	28
SLOVAKIA	100	15	12	27
SLOVENIA	100	5	4	9
SPAIN	10	9	12	21
SWEDEN	17	7	3	10
SWITZERLAND	6	1	1	2

RELATIVE SURVIVAL (%)
(Age-standardized)

□ 1 year ■ 5 years

OBSERVED AND RELATIVE SURVIVAL (%) BY AGE

	AGE CLASS										ALL	
	20-44		45-54		55-64		65-74		75-99			
	obs	rel	obs	rel	obs	rel	obs	rel	obs	rel	obs	rel
Males												
1 year	73	73	82	82	73	73	60	62	33	35	68	70
3 years	59	59	59	60	63	65	48	52	24	31	54	57
5 years	51	52	49	51	57	60	32	38	19	30	44	49
Females												
1 year	77	77	84	84	83	84	66	67	45	48	69	70
3 years	63	63	57	57	67	68	53	57	25	31	51	55
5 years	62	62	50	51	54	56	47	52	18	27	46	51
Overall												
1 year	75	75	83	83	77	78	62	64	38	41	68	70
3 years	61	61	58	59	65	66	50	54	24	31	53	56
5 years	56	56	50	51	55	58	39	44	18	28	45	50

AGE STANDARDIZED RELATIVE SURVIVAL(%)

COUNTRY	MALES 1-year (95% C.I.)	5-years (95% C.I.)	FEMALES 1-year (95% C.I.)	5-years (95% C.I.)
AUSTRIA	-	-	-	-
DENMARK	56.2 (49.0 - 64.3)	36.8 (29.3 - 46.2)	66.9 (59.6 - 75.1)	48.5 (40.7 - 57.9)
ENGLAND	66.3 (61.9 - 71.0)	48.1 (43.0 - 53.8)	74.8 (70.5 - 79.2)	54.4 (49.1 - 60.3)
ESTONIA	39.4 (23.0 - 67.4)	34.0 (16.3 - 70.8)	71.1 (56.5 - 89.4)	26.0 (14.6 - 46.3)
FINLAND	75.2 (65.1 - 86.9)	54.5 (41.8 - 71.0)	81.3 (72.3 - 91.4)	54.0 (43.3 - 67.2)
FRANCE	73.7 (65.9 - 82.4)	69.2 (59.8 - 80.2)	75.8 (58.4 - 98.5)	63.3 (42.9 - 93.4)
GERMANY	-	-	-	-
ICELAND	81.0 (80.8 - 81.2)	50.0 (49.7 - 50.2)	-	56.6 (46.0 - 69.7)
ITALY	65.3 (56.5 - 75.5)	37.1 (28.3 - 48.6)	75.3 (66.3 - 85.5)	56.6 (46.0 - 69.7)
NETHERLANDS	-	-	-	-
POLAND	36.5 (22.5 - 59.1)	29.6 (14.9 - 58.8)	49.5 (35.4 - 69.2)	33.7 (17.6 - 64.2)
SCOTLAND	66.8 (55.7 - 80.1)	32.0 (23.9 - 43.0)	67.2 (58.2 - 77.6)	47.3 (37.4 - 59.7)
SLOVAKIA	41.2 (33.5 - 50.8)	26.8 (19.2 - 37.3)	49.9 (38.8 - 64.2)	39.6 (27.5 - 57.1)
SLOVENIA	59.3 (43.4 - 81.1)	20.1 (12.5 - 32.3)	53.0 (36.4 - 77.1)	28.5 (15.9 - 51.1)
SPAIN	69.0 (53.3 - 89.4)	43.1 (27.4 - 67.8)	84.3 (72.6 - 97.9)	65.7 (50.5 - 85.5)
SWEDEN	83.3 (74.6 - 93.0)	60.5 (45.6 - 80.1)	75.6 (62.9 - 90.7)	70.2 (56.5 - 87.2)
SWITZERLAND	-	-	-	-
EUROPE, 1985-89	64.8 (60.0 - 70.1)	46.1 (39.8 - 53.2)	71.5 (66.4 - 77.0)	51.2 (44.8 - 58.4)

SOFT TISSUES   (ICD-9 171)

AUSTRIA

AREA	NUMBER OF CASES			PERIOD	MEAN AGE		
	Males	Females	All		Males	Females	All
Tirol	17	22	39	1988-1989	62.3	57.4	59.6

OBSERVED AND RELATIVE SURVIVAL (%) BY AGE (number of cases in parentheses)

	AGE CLASS										ALL	
	15-44		45-54		55-64		65-74		75-99			
	obs	rel	obs	rel	obs	rel	obs	rel	obs	rel	obs	rel
Males	(2)		(3)		(5)		(3)		(4)		(17)	
1 year	100	100	33	33	60	61	100	100	75	85	71	73
3 years	50	50	33	34	60	63	67	72	50	74	53	59
5 years	50	50	33	34	60	65	67	76	50	100	53	64
Females	(7)		(1)		(3)		(5)		(6)		(22)	
1 year	100	100	100	100	100	100	40	41	83	88	82	83
3 years	86	86	100	100	33	34	20	21	33	40	50	53
5 years	86	86	100	100	33	34	20	22	33	48	50	56
Overall	(9)		(4)		(8)		(8)		(10)		(39)	
1 year	100	100	50	50	75	76	63	64	80	87	77	79
3 years	78	78	50	51	50	52	38	40	40	52	51	56
5 years	78	78	50	51	50	53	38	42	40	64	51	59

DENMARK

AREA	NUMBER OF CASES			PERIOD	MEAN AGE		
	Males	Females	All		Males	Females	All
Denmark	282	228	510	1985-1989	54.4	54.0	54.2

OBSERVED AND RELATIVE SURVIVAL (%) BY AGE (number of cases in parentheses)

	AGE CLASS										ALL	
	15-44		45-54		55-64		65-74		75-99			
	obs	rel	obs	rel	obs	rel	obs	rel	obs	rel	obs	rel
Males	(104)		(23)		(43)		(61)		(51)		(282)	
1 year	88	89	87	87	79	81	84	87	55	63	80	83
3 years	72	73	83	84	65	69	59	68	39	60	63	70
5 years	64	65	78	81	56	62	51	66	22	45	54	64
Females	(74)		(37)		(36)		(43)		(38)		(228)	
1 year	97	97	92	92	89	90	79	81	68	74	87	89
3 years	92	92	81	82	67	69	65	70	42	55	73	78
5 years	89	90	76	78	64	68	56	64	32	51	67	75
Overall	(178)		(60)		(79)		(104)		(89)		(510)	
1 year	92	92	90	90	84	85	82	85	61	68	83	85
3 years	80	81	82	83	66	69	62	69	40	58	67	74
5 years	75	75	77	79	59	65	53	65	26	48	60	69

SOFT TISSUES (ICD-9 171)

ENGLAND

AREA	NUMBER OF CASES			PERIOD	MEAN AGE			5-YR RELATIVE SURVIVAL (%)	
	Males	Females	All		Males	Females	All	Males	Females
East Anglia	104	97	201	1985-1989	60.4	63.0	61.7		
Mersey	92	99	191	1985-1989	61.9	58.3	60.0		
Oxford	122	104	226	1985-1989	59.2	59.1	59.1		
South Thames	237	204	441	1985-1989	54.5	58.7	56.5		
Wessex	185	168	353	1985-1989	60.6	61.8	61.2		
West Midlands	239	216	455	1985-1989	57.8	59.5	58.6		
Yorkshire	173	173	346	1985-1989	56.5	60.1	58.3		
English Registries	1152	1061	2213		58.1	60.0	59.0		

OBSERVED AND RELATIVE SURVIVAL (%) BY AGE (number of cases in parentheses)

	AGE CLASS										ALL	
	15-44		45-54		55-64		65-74		75-99			
	obs	rel	obs	rel	obs	rel	obs	rel	obs	rel	obs	rel
Males	(291)		(135)		(221)		(280)		(225)		(1152)	
1 year	82	83	81	81	74	75	68	71	55	62	72	74
3 years	61	61	58	59	60	63	50	57	37	53	53	59
5 years	55	56	53	55	55	60	41	52	29	54	46	55
Females	(251)		(124)		(177)		(217)		(292)		(1061)	
1 year	85	85	81	82	68	68	67	69	55	60	70	72
3 years	72	73	71	72	54	56	50	54	33	44	54	59
5 years	70	70	65	67	49	52	40	45	23	39	47	55
Overall	(542)		(259)		(398)		(497)		(517)		(2213)	
1 year	84	84	81	81	71	72	68	70	55	61	71	73
3 years	66	67	64	65	57	60	50	55	35	48	53	59
5 years	62	62	59	61	52	56	40	49	26	45	47	55

ESTONIA

AREA	NUMBER OF CASES			PERIOD	MEAN AGE		
	Males	Females	All		Males	Females	All
Estonia	64	85	149	1985-1989	54.0	61.1	58.1

OBSERVED AND RELATIVE SURVIVAL (%) BY AGE (number of cases in parentheses)

	AGE CLASS										ALL	
	15-44		45-54		55-64		65-74		75-99			
	obs	rel	obs	rel	obs	rel	obs	rel	obs	rel	obs	rel
Males	(18)		(9)		(20)		(10)		(7)		(64)	
1 year	50	50	89	90	55	56	50	53	57	65	58	60
3 years	33	34	67	69	30	33	40	49	14	21	36	40
5 years	33	34	67	72	25	29	40	57	0	0	33	39
Females	(12)		(12)		(23)		(20)		(18)		(85)	
1 year	92	92	75	75	78	79	55	57	50	56	68	70
3 years	67	67	58	59	43	45	35	39	33	47	45	49
5 years	58	59	58	60	30	32	25	30	28	52	36	43
Overall	(30)		(21)		(43)		(30)		(25)		(149)	
1 year	67	67	81	82	67	69	53	55	52	58	64	66
3 years	47	47	62	64	37	39	37	42	28	40	41	45
5 years	43	44	62	65	28	31	30	38	20	39	35	42

SOFT TISSUES   (ICD-9 171)

FINLAND

AREA	NUMBER OF CASES			PERIOD	MEAN AGE		
	Males	Females	All		Males	Females	All
Finland	253	251	504	1985-1989	56.7	59.6	58.2

OBSERVED AND RELATIVE SURVIVAL (%) BY AGE (number of cases in parentheses)

	AGE CLASS										ALL	
	15-44		45-54		55-64		65-74		75-99			
	obs	rel	obs	rel	obs	rel	obs	rel	obs	rel	obs	rel
Males	(72)		(37)		(52)		(45)		(47)		(253)	
1 year	89	89	78	79	67	69	60	63	66	74	74	76
3 years	72	73	57	58	50	53	29	33	40	59	52	58
5 years	69	70	46	48	46	51	22	29	26	50	45	53
Females	(61)		(23)		(47)		(57)		(63)		(251)	
1 year	87	87	91	92	70	71	61	63	57	63	71	73
3 years	69	69	65	66	55	57	44	47	29	39	50	55
5 years	61	61	61	62	47	49	37	42	17	31	42	49
Overall	(133)		(60)		(99)		(102)		(110)		(504)	
1 year	88	88	83	84	69	70	61	63	61	68	72	75
3 years	71	71	60	61	53	55	37	41	34	47	51	56
5 years	65	66	52	53	46	50	30	36	21	38	43	51

FRANCE

AREA	NUMBER OF CASES			PERIOD	MEAN AGE			5-YR RELATIVE SURVIVAL (%)
	Males	Females	All		Males	Females	All	Males Females
Somme	21	12	33	1985-1989	56.1	56.6	56.3	
Calvados	29	25	54	1985-1989	52.0	65.1	58.1	
Doubs	16	18	34	1985-1989	52.9	58.5	55.9	
French Registries	66	55	121		53.6	61.1	57.0	

OBSERVED AND RELATIVE SURVIVAL (%) BY AGE (number of cases in parentheses)

	AGE CLASS										ALL	
	15-44		45-54		55-64		65-74		75-99			
	obs	rel	obs	rel	obs	rel	obs	rel	obs	rel	obs	rel
Males	(23)		(9)		(13)		(13)		(8)		(66)	
1 year	77	78	88	89	67	68	54	56	71	80	71	73
3 years	48	49	88	90	50	53	23	26	57	83	49	53
5 years	42	42	88	92	50	56	23	29	43	86	45	52
Females	(13)		(8)		(8)		(10)		(16)		(55)	
1 year	83	83	100	100	100	100	89	90	59	65	82	85
3 years	56	56	88	88	50	51	63	67	27	37	54	59
5 years	46	46	88	89	50	52	63	70	27	47	51	60
Overall	(36)		(17)		(21)		(23)		(24)		(121)	
1 year	80	80	94	94	79	80	68	70	63	70	76	78
3 years	51	51	87	88	51	53	39	43	38	52	51	56
5 years	43	44	87	90	51	55	39	46	32	59	48	55

SOFT TISSUES   (ICD-9 171)

GERMANY

AREA	NUMBER OF CASES			PERIOD	MEAN AGE		
	Males	Females	All		Males	Females	All
Saarland	69	54	123	1985-1989	53.4	56.3	54.7

OBSERVED AND RELATIVE SURVIVAL (%) BY AGE (number of cases in parentheses)

	AGE CLASS										ALL	
	15-44		45-54		55-64		65-74		75-99			
	obs	rel	obs	rel	obs	rel	obs	rel	obs	rel	obs	rel
Males	(19)		(17)		(18)		(7)		(8)		(69)	
1 year	89	90	59	59	72	73	100	100	88	100	78	80
3 years	74	74	47	48	61	65	43	50	50	78	58	63
5 years	74	74	41	43	56	62	43	57	50	100	55	63
Females	(14)		(8)		(9)		(11)		(12)		(54)	
1 year	86	86	100	100	89	90	82	83	67	72	83	85
3 years	86	86	75	76	78	80	73	77	58	73	74	79
5 years	86	86	75	76	44	46	73	80	50	78	66	74
Overall	(33)		(25)		(27)		(18)		(20)		(123)	
1 year	88	88	72	72	78	79	89	91	75	83	80	82
3 years	79	79	56	57	67	70	61	67	55	75	65	70
5 years	79	79	52	54	52	56	61	72	50	88	60	68

ICELAND

AREA	NUMBER OF CASES			PERIOD	MEAN AGE		
	Males	Females	All		Males	Females	All
Iceland	12	7	19	1985-1989	53.8	42.7	49.8

OBSERVED AND RELATIVE SURVIVAL (%) BY AGE (number of cases in parentheses)

	AGE CLASS										ALL	
	15-44		45-54		55-64		65-74		75-99			
	obs	rel	obs	rel	obs	rel	obs	rel	obs	rel	obs	rel
Males	(5)		(2)		(0)		(1)		(4)		(12)	
1 year	100	100	50	50	-	-	100	100	25	28	67	69
3 years	80	80	50	51	-	-	100	100	25	34	58	65
5 years	80	80	50	52	-	-	100	100	25	41	58	69
Females	(3)		(4)		(0)		(0)		(0)		(7)	
1 year	100	100	75	75	-	-	-	-	-	-	86	86
3 years	100	100	50	50	-	-	-	-	-	-	71	72
5 years	100	100	50	51	-	-	-	-	-	-	71	72
Overall	(8)		(6)		(0)		(1)		(4)		(19)	
1 year	100	100	67	67	-	-	100	100	25	28	74	75
3 years	88	88	50	51	-	-	100	100	25	34	63	67
5 years	88	88	50	51	-	-	100	100	25	41	63	70

SOFT TISSUES (ICD-9 171)

ITALY

AREA	NUMBER OF CASES			PERIOD	MEAN AGE			5-YR RELATIVE SURVIVAL (%)	
	Males	Females	All		Males	Females	All	Males	Females
Florence	64	52	116	1985-1989	58.8	59.2	59.0		
Genoa	24	24	48	1986-1988	61.8	61.6	61.7		
Latina	16	22	38	1985-1987	48.9	54.4	52.1		
Modena	21	5	26	1988-1989	61.5	63.6	61.9		
Parma	20	15	35	1985-1987	63.7	60.7	62.4		
Ragusa	7	6	13	1985-1989	73.9	52.3	64.0		
Romagna	22	12	34	1986-1988	63.2	60.3	62.2		
Turin	29	25	54	1985-1987	51.2	55.2	53.0		
Varese	29	30	59	1985-1989	56.3	55.5	55.9		
Italian Registries	232	191	423		58.7	58.0	58.4		

OBSERVED AND RELATIVE SURVIVAL (%) BY AGE (number of cases in parentheses)

	AGE CLASS										ALL	
	15-44		45-54		55-64		65-74		75-99			
	obs	rel	obs	rel	obs	rel	obs	rel	obs	rel	obs	rel
Males	(47)		(38)		(56)		(34)		(57)		(232)	
1 year	89	89	89	90	73	74	71	73	67	73	77	79
3 years	79	79	63	64	44	46	56	62	39	51	55	60
5 years	74	75	58	60	40	44	50	61	32	51	49	58
Females	(39)		(29)		(43)		(47)		(33)		(191)	
1 year	84	84	86	86	84	84	74	76	55	59	77	78
3 years	65	65	72	73	67	69	60	63	36	46	60	64
5 years	60	60	69	70	63	65	49	54	27	41	53	59
Overall	(86)		(67)		(99)		(81)		(90)		(423)	
1 year	87	87	88	88	78	78	73	75	62	67	77	79
3 years	73	73	67	68	54	56	58	63	38	49	57	62
5 years	68	68	63	64	50	53	49	57	30	47	51	58

NETHERLANDS

AREA	NUMBER OF CASES			PERIOD	MEAN AGE		
	Males	Females	All		Males	Females	All
Eindhoven	45	31	76	1985-1989	56.5	54.1	55.5

OBSERVED AND RELATIVE SURVIVAL (%) BY AGE (number of cases in parentheses)

	AGE CLASS										ALL	
	15-44		45-54		55-64		65-74		75-99			
	obs	rel	obs	rel	obs	rel	obs	rel	obs	rel	obs	rel
Males	(12)		(9)		(9)		(8)		(7)		(45)	
1 year	58	58	89	89	44	45	88	91	71	87	69	72
3 years	50	50	78	79	22	23	38	43	57	100	49	55
5 years	33	34	56	57	11	12	38	48	43	100	36	43
Females	(9)		(4)		(9)		(3)		(6)		(31)	
1 year	78	78	100	100	89	89	67	68	83	95	84	86
3 years	56	56	100	100	78	79	33	35	33	50	61	66
5 years	42	42	100	100	66	68	0	0	33	67	51	58
Overall	(21)		(13)		(18)		(11)		(13)		(76)	
1 year	67	67	92	93	67	67	82	85	77	91	75	78
3 years	52	52	85	86	50	52	36	41	46	78	54	60
5 years	37	37	69	71	38	41	27	33	38	94	42	49

SOFT TISSUES   (ICD-9 171)

POLAND

AREA	NUMBER OF CASES			PERIOD	MEAN AGE			5-YR RELATIVE SURVIVAL (%)	
	Males	Females	All		Males	Females	All	Males	Females
Cracow	23	22	45	1985-1989	52.8	56.9	54.8		
Warsaw	26	25	51	1988-1989	48.1	57.0	52.5		
Polish Registries	49	47	96		50.4	57.0	53.6		

OBSERVED AND RELATIVE SURVIVAL (%) BY AGE (number of cases in parentheses)

	AGE CLASS										ALL	
	15-44		45-54		55-64		65-74		75-99			
	obs	rel	obs	rel	obs	rel	obs	rel	obs	rel	obs	rel
Males	(18)		(9)		(11)		(6)		(5)		(49)	
1 year	78	78	78	79	45	47	67	70	60	67	67	69
3 years	44	45	22	23	45	49	50	60	20	29	39	42
5 years	39	39	11	12	45	53	17	23	20	38	30	35
Females	(11)		(7)		(12)		(6)		(11)		(47)	
1 year	82	82	86	86	83	84	83	86	27	30	70	72
3 years	64	64	43	44	75	78	17	19	9	12	45	48
5 years	64	64	29	29	75	80	17	21	9	14	43	49
Overall	(29)		(16)		(23)		(12)		(16)		(96)	
1 year	79	79	81	82	65	66	75	78	38	41	69	71
3 years	52	52	31	32	61	64	33	39	13	17	42	45
5 years	48	49	19	20	61	68	17	22	13	20	36	42

SCOTLAND

AREA	NUMBER OF CASES			PERIOD	MEAN AGE		
	Males	Females	All		Males	Females	All
Scotland	233	209	442	1985-1989	57.6	58.2	57.9

OBSERVED AND RELATIVE SURVIVAL (%) BY AGE (number of cases in parentheses)

	AGE CLASS										ALL	
	15-44		45-54		55-64		65-74		75-99			
	obs	rel	obs	rel	obs	rel	obs	rel	obs	rel	obs	rel
Males	(58)		(24)		(53)		(56)		(42)		(233)	
1 year	84	85	71	71	70	71	71	75	45	51	70	72
3 years	62	62	54	55	51	55	61	71	24	36	52	58
5 years	55	56	42	43	42	47	50	66	17	34	42	52
Females	(50)		(30)		(33)		(39)		(57)		(209)	
1 year	86	86	67	67	70	71	74	76	58	63	71	73
3 years	72	72	47	47	48	50	54	59	33	44	51	56
5 years	66	66	43	44	39	42	38	45	28	47	43	51
Overall	(108)		(54)		(86)		(95)		(99)		(442)	
1 year	85	85	69	69	70	71	73	76	53	58	70	73
3 years	67	67	50	51	50	53	58	66	29	41	51	57
5 years	60	61	43	44	41	45	45	57	23	42	43	51

SOFT TISSUES   (ICD-9 171)

SLOVAKIA

AREA	NUMBER OF CASES			PERIOD	MEAN AGE		
	Males	Females	All		Males	Females	All
Slovakia	207	199	406	1985-1989	52.5	58.0	55.2

OBSERVED AND RELATIVE SURVIVAL (%) BY AGE (number of cases in parentheses)

	AGE CLASS										ALL	
	15-44		45-54		55-64		65-74		75-99			
	obs	rel	obs	rel	obs	rel	obs	rel	obs	rel	obs	rel
Males	(68)		(33)		(53)		(33)		(20)		(207)	
1 year	69	69	73	74	62	64	52	54	65	75	65	67
3 years	43	43	48	50	36	39	42	51	25	39	40	44
5 years	41	41	48	52	31	37	31	42	13	27	36	42
Females	(44)		(33)		(39)		(45)		(38)		(199)	
1 year	82	82	67	67	77	78	64	66	55	61	69	71
3 years	64	64	58	58	59	61	51	56	32	42	53	57
5 years	57	57	58	59	50	53	49	58	26	43	48	55
Overall	(112)		(66)		(92)		(78)		(58)		(406)	
1 year	74	74	70	70	68	70	59	61	59	65	67	69
3 years	51	51	53	54	46	49	47	54	29	41	46	51
5 years	47	47	53	56	39	44	41	52	23	41	42	48

SLOVENIA

AREA	NUMBER OF CASES			PERIOD	MEAN AGE		
	Males	Females	All		Males	Females	All
Slovenia	73	46	119	1985-1989	50.5	56.4	52.8

OBSERVED AND RELATIVE SURVIVAL (%) BY AGE (number of cases in parentheses)

	AGE CLASS										ALL	
	15-44		45-54		55-64		65-74		75-99			
	obs	rel	obs	rel	obs	rel	obs	rel	obs	rel	obs	rel
Males	(27)		(10)		(15)		(12)		(9)		(73)	
1 year	93	93	80	81	80	82	58	61	67	74	79	82
3 years	81	82	40	41	53	57	42	49	33	48	57	63
5 years	78	79	30	32	40	45	42	55	22	43	50	58
Females	(14)		(4)		(9)		(7)		(12)		(46)	
1 year	86	86	100	100	89	90	57	59	42	46	72	74
3 years	79	79	75	76	67	69	43	47	8	12	52	57
5 years	64	65	50	51	44	47	43	50	8	15	41	49
Overall	(41)		(14)		(24)		(19)		(21)		(119)	
1 year	90	90	86	86	83	85	58	60	52	58	76	79
3 years	80	81	50	51	58	61	42	48	19	27	55	61
5 years	73	74	36	37	42	46	42	53	14	26	47	55

SOFT TISSUES   (ICD-9 171)

SPAIN

AREA	NUMBER OF CASES			PERIOD	MEAN AGE			5-YR RELATIVE SURVIVAL (%)	
	Males	Females	All		Males	Females	All	Males	Females
Basque Country	51	57	108	1986-1988	54.2	57.6	56.0		
Mallorca	7	10	17	1988-1989	65.0	49.1	55.7		
Navarra	21	14	35	1985-1989	61.0	53.1	57.8		
Tarragona	36	27	63	1985-1989	56.8	63.1	59.5		
Spanish Registries	115	108	223		56.9	57.6	57.3		

OBSERVED AND RELATIVE SURVIVAL (%) BY AGE (number of cases in parentheses)

	AGE CLASS										ALL	
	15-44		45-54		55-64		65-74		75-99			
	obs	rel	obs	rel	obs	rel	obs	rel	obs	rel	obs	rel
Males	(35)		(13)		(16)		(23)		(28)		(115)	
1 year	89	89	77	77	81	82	70	72	50	55	73	76
3 years	83	83	69	70	56	59	65	72	39	54	63	70
5 years	79	80	52	54	56	60	65	78	35	62	60	71
Females	(28)		(13)		(26)		(19)		(22)		(108)	
1 year	79	79	77	77	73	73	84	85	55	60	73	75
3 years	64	64	69	70	69	70	58	61	32	42	58	62
5 years	47	48	69	70	53	54	53	58	26	42	48	53
Overall	(63)		(26)		(42)		(42)		(50)		(223)	
1 year	84	84	77	77	76	77	76	78	52	57	73	75
3 years	75	75	69	70	64	66	62	67	36	49	61	66
5 years	65	66	61	62	55	58	59	68	31	53	54	62

SWEDEN

AREA	NUMBER OF CASES			PERIOD	MEAN AGE		
	Males	Females	All		Males	Females	All
South Sweden	107	92	199	1985-1989	61.9	63.0	62.5

OBSERVED AND RELATIVE SURVIVAL (%) BY AGE (number of cases in parentheses)

	AGE CLASS										ALL	
	15-44		45-54		55-64		65-74		75-99			
	obs	rel	obs	rel	obs	rel	obs	rel	obs	rel	obs	rel
Males	(20)		(9)		(19)		(33)		(26)		(107)	
1 year	90	90	89	89	74	75	73	75	81	89	79	82
3 years	80	80	67	68	53	55	52	57	54	73	59	66
5 years	80	81	67	69	53	56	42	52	38	65	52	63
Females	(18)		(10)		(9)		(24)		(31)		(92)	
1 year	89	89	100	100	78	78	83	85	58	63	77	80
3 years	78	78	90	91	56	57	71	75	48	63	65	72
5 years	72	73	80	81	44	47	67	74	35	56	57	67
Overall	(38)		(19)		(28)		(57)		(57)		(199)	
1 year	89	90	95	95	75	76	77	79	68	75	78	81
3 years	79	79	79	80	54	55	60	65	51	67	62	69
5 years	76	77	74	75	50	53	53	62	37	60	54	65

SOFT TISSUES (ICD-9 171)

SWITZERLAND

AREA	NUMBER OF CASES			PERIOD	MEAN AGE		
	Males	Females	All		Males	Females	All
Geneva	25	18	43	1985-1989	49.5	60.5	54.1

OBSERVED AND RELATIVE SURVIVAL (%) BY AGE (number of cases in parentheses)

	AGE CLASS										ALL	
	15-44		45-54		55-64		65-74		75-99			
	obs	rel	obs	rel	obs	rel	obs	rel	obs	rel	obs	rel
Males	(13)		(3)		(2)		(5)		(2)		(25)	
1 year	60	60	33	33	50	51	80	83	100	100	63	64
3 years	20	20	0	0	50	52	40	45	100	100	32	33
5 years	20	20	0	0	50	54	40	50	50	81	27	30
Females	(6)		(2)		(0)		(3)		(7)		(18)	
1 year	100	100	100	100	-	-	67	68	43	49	71	75
3 years	100	100	100	100	-	-	33	35	29	43	59	70
5 years	100	100	100	100	-	-	33	37	14	28	53	69
Overall	(19)		(5)		(2)		(8)		(9)		(43)	
1 year	72	72	60	60	50	51	75	77	56	63	66	68
3 years	46	46	40	41	50	52	38	41	44	64	43	48
5 years	46	46	40	41	50	54	38	45	22	42	38	45

SOFT TISSUES (ICD-9 171)

EUROPE, 1985-89

Weighted analyses

COUNTRY	% COVERAGE WITH C.R.s	YEARLY NO. OF CASES (Mean No. of cases recorded)			RELATIVE SURVIVAL (%) (Age-standardized)
		Males	Females	All	
AUSTRIA	8	9	11	20	
DENMARK	100	56	46	102	
ENGLAND	50	230	212	442	
ESTONIA	100	13	17	30	
FINLAND	100	51	50	101	
FRANCE	3	13	11	24	
GERMANY	2	14	11	25	
ICELAND	100	2	1	3	
ITALY	10	68	54	122	
NETHERLANDS	6	9	6	15	
POLAND	6	18	17	35	
SCOTLAND	100	47	42	89	
SLOVAKIA	100	41	40	81	
SLOVENIA	100	15	9	24	
SPAIN	10	32	32	64	
SWEDEN	17	21	18	39	
SWITZERLAND	6	5	4	9	

□ 1 year ■ 5 years

OBSERVED AND RELATIVE SURVIVAL (%) BY AGE

	AGE CLASS										ALL	
	15-44		45-54		55-64		65-74		75-99			
	obs	rel	obs	rel	obs	rel	obs	rel	obs	rel	obs	rel
Males												
1 year	84	84	76	76	69	70	76	78	70	78	74	76
3 years	65	66	57	59	52	55	47	54	44	64	53	58
5 years	61	62	51	53	49	54	42	53	37	70	48	56
Females												
1 year	85	85	90	91	84	84	76	78	58	63	77	79
3 years	71	72	74	75	64	66	54	57	36	47	59	64
5 years	66	66	71	72	53	55	49	54	30	48	53	60
Overall												
1 year	85	85	83	83	76	76	76	78	64	71	75	77
3 years	68	68	65	66	58	60	51	55	41	56	56	61
5 years	63	64	60	62	51	54	45	53	34	60	50	58

AGE STANDARDIZED RELATIVE SURVIVAL(%)

COUNTRY	MALES		FEMALES	
	1-year (95% C.I.)	5-years (95% C.I.)	1-year (95% C.I.)	5-years (95% C.I.)
AUSTRIA	80.7 (67.2 - 97.0)	67.0 (41.3 -108.7)	85.2 (74.6 - 97.2)	56.4 (40.5 - 78.5)
DENMARK	81.2 (76.2 - 86.5)	62.4 (55.3 - 70.4)	87.0 (82.2 - 92.1)	70.3 (63.3 - 78.1)
ENGLAND	74.1 (71.4 - 76.8)	55.2 (51.7 - 58.9)	72.8 (70.1 - 75.6)	54.3 (51.0 - 57.7)
ESTONIA	60.2 (48.0 - 75.5)	35.5 (25.1 - 50.2)	72.2 (63.4 - 82.3)	46.5 (35.1 - 61.7)
FINLAND	75.3 (69.8 - 81.2)	50.8 (43.7 - 59.0)	74.3 (69.2 - 79.9)	48.3 (42.0 - 55.6)
FRANCE	73.3 (61.9 - 86.8)	57.8 (41.7 - 80.2)	86.2 (77.4 - 95.9)	57.7 (43.4 - 76.7)
GERMANY	87.0 (79.0 - 95.8)	69.7 (51.7 - 93.9)	84.7 (75.4 - 95.3)	74.3 (61.3 - 90.1)
ICELAND	-			
ITALY	79.6 (74.2 - 85.3)	59.1 (52.0 - 67.2)	77.3 (71.3 - 83.7)	56.8 (49.3 - 65.4)
NETHERLANDS	72.7 (59.9 - 88.3)	49.6 (29.0 - 84.8)	84.5 (70.2 -101.7)	50.9 (34.8 - 74.5)
POLAND	68.2 (54.2 - 85.7)	34.7 (20.1 - 60.0)	72.6 (61.7 - 85.5)	42.9 (31.2 - 59.1)
SCOTLAND	71.3 (65.5 - 77.6)	49.9 (42.6 - 58.5)	73.8 (67.9 - 80.2)	50.3 (43.1 - 58.6)
SLOVAKIA	66.8 (59.6 - 75.0)	38.9 (29.0 - 52.1)	71.4 (65.2 - 78.2)	53.8 (46.2 - 62.7)
SLOVENIA	78.6 (68.3 - 90.5)	53.7 (40.2 - 71.9)	74.3 (63.2 - 87.2)	45.9 (32.7 - 64.4)
SPAIN	75.4 (67.8 - 84.0)	68.7 (58.6 - 80.6)	74.8 (66.9 - 83.7)	52.8 (42.8 - 65.1)
SWEDEN	83.6 (76.4 - 91.5)	65.2 (55.0 - 77.3)	82.0 (74.2 - 90.6)	65.5 (54.9 - 78.1)
SWITZERLAND	68.0 (51.9 - 89.0)	43.2 (21.2 - 88.0)	-	-
EUROPE, 1985-89	77.8 (74.8 - 80.9)	58.9 (53.4 - 65.1)	79.3 (76.4 - 82.3)	58.6 (54.4 - 63.0)

MELANOMA OF SKIN   (ICD-9 172)

AUSTRIA

AREA	NUMBER OF CASES			PERIOD	MEAN AGE		
	Males	Females	All		Males	Females	All
Tirol	70	135	205	1988-1989	51.8	52.2	52.1

OBSERVED AND RELATIVE SURVIVAL (%) BY AGE (number of cases in parentheses)

	AGE CLASS										ALL	
	15-44		45-54		55-64		65-74		75-99			
	obs	rel	obs	rel	obs	rel	obs	rel	obs	rel	obs	rel
Males	(25)		(15)		(14)		(5)		(11)		(70)	
1 year	100	100	100	100	100	100	100	100	100	100	100	100
3 years	92	92	100	100	93	97	80	87	91	100	93	98
5 years	92	93	100	100	93	100	80	93	82	100	91	100
Females	(48)		(26)		(20)		(25)		(16)		(135)	
1 year	100	100	96	96	95	95	84	85	88	92	94	95
3 years	100	100	92	93	80	81	84	88	63	73	88	91
5 years	94	94	88	90	80	82	72	79	56	75	82	87
Overall	(73)		(41)		(34)		(30)		(27)		(205)	
1 year	100	100	98	98	97	98	87	88	93	99	96	97
3 years	97	98	95	96	85	88	83	88	74	91	90	93
5 years	93	94	93	94	85	89	73	81	67	96	85	92

DENMARK

AREA	NUMBER OF CASES			PERIOD	MEAN AGE		
	Males	Females	All		Males	Females	All
Denmark	1309	1813	3122	1985-1989	55.9	55.0	55.4

OBSERVED AND RELATIVE SURVIVAL (%) BY AGE (number of cases in parentheses)

	AGE CLASS										ALL	
	15-44		45-54		55-64		65-74		75-99			
	obs	rel	obs	rel	obs	rel	obs	rel	obs	rel	obs	rel
Males	(358)		(246)		(263)		(271)		(171)		(1309)	
1 year	94	94	93	93	91	93	87	90	80	89	90	92
3 years	87	87	76	78	79	83	65	74	49	69	74	80
5 years	79	80	69	72	66	73	53	67	32	59	63	73
Females	(581)		(319)		(310)		(322)		(281)		(1813)	
1 year	98	98	95	96	95	96	97	99	84	91	94	96
3 years	93	93	90	91	87	90	80	87	58	77	84	89
5 years	88	89	87	89	79	84	72	82	40	66	76	84
Overall	(939)		(565)		(573)		(593)		(452)		(3122)	
1 year	96	96	94	95	93	94	92	95	82	90	92	95
3 years	90	91	84	85	83	87	74	81	55	74	80	85
5 years	85	86	79	81	73	79	63	76	37	64	71	80

MELANOMA OF SKIN (ICD-9 172)

ENGLAND

AREA	NUMBER OF CASES			PERIOD	MEAN AGE			5-YR RELATIVE SURVIVAL (%)	
	Males	Females	All		Males	Females	All	Males	Females
East Anglia	291	536	827	1985-1989	54.6	56.2	55.6		
Mersey	203	369	572	1985-1989	53.7	54.7	54.4		
Oxford	341	644	985	1985-1989	53.6	52.8	53.1		
South Thames	720	1357	2077	1985-1989	54.1	54.8	54.5		
Wessex	536	936	1472	1985-1989	56.0	56.0	56.0		
West Midlands	582	1005	1587	1985-1989	54.3	54.0	54.1		
Yorkshire	379	712	1091	1985-1989	54.9	55.1	55.0		
English Registries	3052	5559	8611		54.5	54.8	54.7		

OBSERVED AND RELATIVE SURVIVAL (%) BY AGE (number of cases in parentheses)

	AGE CLASS										ALL	
	15-44		45-54		55-64		65-74		75-99			
	obs	rel	obs	rel	obs	rel	obs	rel	obs	rel	obs	rel
Males	(939)		(534)		(661)		(514)		(404)		(3052)	
1 year	93	93	93	94	91	92	86	89	75	84	89	91
3 years	80	81	77	78	73	77	66	74	49	69	72	77
5 years	74	75	68	70	64	70	53	67	33	61	62	71
Females	(1776)		(972)		(979)		(993)		(839)		(5559)	
1 year	98	98	96	97	96	97	92	94	82	90	94	96
3 years	92	93	89	90	86	88	77	82	58	75	83	87
5 years	89	89	85	87	80	84	69	78	45	71	76	84
Overall	(2715)		(1506)		(1640)		(1507)		(1243)		(8611)	
1 year	96	96	95	96	94	95	90	92	80	88	92	94
3 years	88	88	85	86	81	84	73	80	55	73	79	84
5 years	84	84	79	81	73	78	64	74	41	68	71	79

ESTONIA

AREA	NUMBER OF CASES			PERIOD	MEAN AGE		
	Males	Females	All		Males	Females	All
Estonia	117	218	335	1985-1989	53.2	56.9	55.6

OBSERVED AND RELATIVE SURVIVAL (%) BY AGE (number of cases in parentheses)

	AGE CLASS										ALL	
	15-44		45-54		55-64		65-74		75-99			
	obs	rel	obs	rel	obs	rel	obs	rel	obs	rel	obs	rel
Males	(33)		(24)		(26)		(27)		(7)		(117)	
1 year	97	97	88	89	73	75	89	94	43	50	85	87
3 years	79	80	63	66	38	42	59	70	14	24	58	64
5 years	70	71	58	64	27	32	44	60	14	34	49	58
Females	(51)		(49)		(43)		(35)		(40)		(218)	
1 year	90	90	94	94	93	94	91	94	70	78	88	90
3 years	84	85	80	81	72	75	51	56	40	56	67	73
5 years	73	73	73	75	60	64	40	47	40	73	59	68
Overall	(84)		(73)		(69)		(62)		(47)		(335)	
1 year	93	93	92	92	86	87	90	94	66	74	87	89
3 years	82	83	74	76	59	63	55	62	36	52	64	70
5 years	71	72	68	72	48	53	42	52	36	68	56	64

MELANOMA OF SKIN (ICD-9 172)

FINLAND

AREA	NUMBER OF CASES			PERIOD	MEAN AGE		
	Males	Females	All		Males	Females	All
Finland	1043	1089	2132	1985-1989	54.4	56.1	55.3

OBSERVED AND RELATIVE SURVIVAL (%) BY AGE (number of cases in parentheses)

	AGE CLASS										ALL	
	15-44		45-54		55-64		65-74		75-99			
	obs	rel	obs	rel	obs	rel	obs	rel	obs	rel	obs	rel
Males	(288)		(231)		(243)		(172)		(109)		(1043)	
1 year	95	96	95	96	91	92	89	93	81	90	92	94
3 years	86	87	87	89	79	83	73	83	47	67	78	84
5 years	80	81	81	85	68	75	60	77	29	55	69	78
Females	(324)		(174)		(193)		(200)		(198)		(1089)	
1 year	98	98	97	97	94	95	94	95	87	95	94	96
3 years	95	95	91	92	87	88	79	84	59	77	83	89
5 years	92	92	87	89	82	86	70	79	44	72	77	85
Overall	(612)		(405)		(436)		(372)		(307)		(2132)	
1 year	97	97	96	96	92	93	91	94	85	93	93	95
3 years	91	91	89	90	82	85	76	84	55	74	81	87
5 years	86	87	84	86	74	80	65	78	39	67	73	82

FRANCE

AREA	NUMBER OF CASES			PERIOD	MEAN AGE		
	Males	Females	All		Males	Females	All
Somme	36	56	92	1985-1989	53.1	59.0	56.7
Calvados	66	116	182	1985-1989	53.8	54.6	54.3
Doubs	54	96	150	1985-1989	53.9	54.2	54.1
French Registries	156	268	424		53.7	55.4	54.8

5-YR RELATIVE SURVIVAL (%)

OBSERVED AND RELATIVE SURVIVAL (%) BY AGE (number of cases in parentheses)

	AGE CLASS										ALL	
	15-44		45-54		55-64		65-74		75-99			
	obs	rel	obs	rel	obs	rel	obs	rel	obs	rel	obs	rel
Males	(53)		(27)		(38)		(17)		(21)		(156)	
1 year	98	98	92	93	89	91	88	91	75	85	91	93
3 years	84	85	72	74	59	62	75	85	48	71	70	76
5 years	79	80	64	67	50	55	69	86	30	59	62	70
Females	(85)		(39)		(58)		(45)		(41)		(268)	
1 year	98	98	92	92	95	95	93	95	88	96	94	96
3 years	94	94	84	85	89	91	86	91	55	73	84	89
5 years	86	86	72	73	81	83	81	90	40	67	74	82
Overall	(138)		(66)		(96)		(62)		(62)		(424)	
1 year	98	98	92	93	92	93	92	94	83	93	93	95
3 years	90	90	79	81	77	80	83	89	53	73	79	84
5 years	83	84	69	71	68	73	78	89	37	65	70	78

MELANOMA OF SKIN   (ICD-9 172)

GERMANY

AREA	NUMBER OF CASES			PERIOD	MEAN AGE		
	Males	Females	All		Males	Females	All
Saarland	194	252	446	1985-1989	53.2	56.1	54.9

OBSERVED AND RELATIVE SURVIVAL (%) BY AGE (number of cases in parentheses)

	AGE CLASS										ALL	
	15-44		45-54		55-64		65-74		75-99			
	obs	rel	obs	rel	obs	rel	obs	rel	obs	rel	obs	rel
Males	(55)		(45)		(47)		(28)		(19)		(194)	
1 year	89	89	100	100	87	89	89	93	58	64	88	90
3 years	75	75	89	91	70	74	68	77	32	45	72	77
5 years	68	68	89	92	60	66	55	70	17	32	64	72
Females	(55)		(63)		(47)		(48)		(39)		(252)	
1 year	95	95	98	99	96	97	81	83	82	89	91	93
3 years	85	86	90	91	83	85	73	78	69	91	81	86
5 years	85	86	83	84	76	80	65	74	55	92	74	83
Overall	(110)		(108)		(94)		(76)		(58)		(446)	
1 year	92	92	99	99	91	93	84	87	74	81	90	92
3 years	80	80	90	91	77	80	71	78	57	77	77	82
5 years	76	77	85	87	68	73	61	72	43	74	69	78

ICELAND

AREA	NUMBER OF CASES			PERIOD	MEAN AGE		
	Males	Females	All		Males	Females	All
Iceland	15	35	50	1985-1989	55.4	59.7	58.4

OBSERVED AND RELATIVE SURVIVAL (%) BY AGE (number of cases in parentheses)

	AGE CLASS										ALL	
	15-44		45-54		55-64		65-74		75-99			
	obs	rel	obs	rel	obs	rel	obs	rel	obs	rel	obs	rel
Males	(6)		(3)		(2)		(2)		(2)		(15)	
1 year	100	100	67	67	100	100	50	51	50	59	80	82
3 years	100	100	67	68	50	53	50	55	50	76	73	79
5 years	100	100	67	69	50	55	50	59	0	0	67	75
Females	(9)		(3)		(11)		(2)		(10)		(35)	
1 year	100	100	100	100	100	100	100	100	90	100	97	100
3 years	100	100	67	67	82	84	100	100	60	82	80	88
5 years	100	100	67	68	64	66	100	100	30	52	66	76
Overall	(15)		(6)		(13)		(4)		(12)		(50)	
1 year	100	100	83	84	100	100	75	77	83	93	92	95
3 years	100	100	67	68	77	79	75	81	58	81	78	85
5 years	100	100	67	68	62	64	75	86	25	44	66	76

MELANOMA OF SKIN (ICD-9 172)

ITALY

AREA	NUMBER OF CASES			PERIOD	MEAN AGE			5-YR RELATIVE SURVIVAL (%)	
	Males	Females	All		Males	Females	All	Males	Females
Florence	187	230	417	1985-1989	55.3	57.1	56.3		
Genoa	63	73	136	1986-1988	55.0	55.6	55.4		
Latina	21	18	39	1985-1987	53.3	49.6	51.6		
Modena	38	42	80	1988-1989	56.5	58.8	57.7		
Parma	27	45	72	1985-1987	60.6	58.9	59.5		
Ragusa	30	25	55	1985-1989	57.7	53.0	55.6		
Romagna	36	54	90	1986-1988	56.5	55.9	56.2		
Turin	74	98	172	1985-1987	54.0	61.2	58.1		
Varese	98	128	226	1985-1989	53.8	56.9	55.5		
Italian Registries	574	713	1287		55.3	57.3	56.4		

OBSERVED AND RELATIVE SURVIVAL (%) BY AGE (number of cases in parentheses)

	15-44		45-54		55-64		65-74		75-99		ALL	
	obs	rel	obs	rel	obs	rel	obs	rel	obs	rel	obs	rel
Males	(143)		(121)		(149)		(102)		(59)		(574)	
1 year	88	88	87	87	85	86	79	82	64	71	83	85
3 years	77	77	70	71	62	64	48	54	22	30	61	65
5 years	69	70	58	59	51	55	38	47	15	26	51	57
Females	(179)		(132)		(146)		(116)		(140)		(713)	
1 year	97	97	98	99	95	96	88	89	81	87	92	94
3 years	91	91	92	92	80	81	68	72	55	70	78	83
5 years	85	85	89	91	76	78	62	68	40	61	71	79
Overall	(322)		(253)		(295)		(218)		(199)		(1287)	
1 year	93	93	93	93	90	91	84	86	76	82	88	90
3 years	85	85	81	82	71	73	59	64	45	59	70	75
5 years	78	78	74	76	63	67	51	59	33	52	62	69

NETHERLANDS

AREA	NUMBER OF CASES			PERIOD	MEAN AGE		
	Males	Females	All		Males	Females	All
Eindhoven	110	176	286	1985-1989	51.5	47.4	49.0

OBSERVED AND RELATIVE SURVIVAL (%) BY AGE (number of cases in parentheses)

	15-44		45-54		55-64		65-74		75-99		ALL	
	obs	rel	obs	rel	obs	rel	obs	rel	obs	rel	obs	rel
Males	(41)		(25)		(22)		(10)		(12)		(110)	
1 year	98	98	96	96	86	88	100	100	65	74	92	94
3 years	80	80	84	85	77	81	90	100	37	57	77	82
5 years	77	78	70	72	77	84	68	86	28	58	70	77
Females	(80)		(42)		(25)		(20)		(9)		(176)	
1 year	100	100	100	100	100	100	100	100	89	95	99	100
3 years	92	92	100	100	92	94	80	85	33	42	89	92
5 years	88	88	93	94	92	95	70	78	33	50	84	88
Overall	(121)		(67)		(47)		(30)		(21)		(286)	
1 year	99	99	99	99	94	95	100	100	75	84	96	98
3 years	88	88	94	95	85	88	83	91	35	49	85	88
5 years	84	85	84	86	85	90	69	80	29	52	79	84

MELANOMA OF SKIN (ICD-9 172)

POLAND

AREA	NUMBER OF CASES			PERIOD	MEAN AGE			5-YR RELATIVE SURVIVAL (%)	
	Males	Females	All		Males	Females	All	Males	Females
Cracow	67	93	160	1985-1989	55.0	52.4	53.5		
Warsaw	57	95	152	1988-1989	57.9	56.8	57.2		
Polish Registries	124	188	312		56.3	54.7	55.3		

OBSERVED AND RELATIVE SURVIVAL (%) BY AGE (number of cases in parentheses)

	AGE CLASS										ALL	
	15-44		45-54		55-64		65-74		75-99			
	obs	rel	obs	rel	obs	rel	obs	rel	obs	rel	obs	rel
Males	(29)		(23)		(34)		(24)		(14)		(124)	
1 year	79	80	100	100	71	73	79	83	64	73	79	82
3 years	62	63	52	54	41	45	58	68	29	42	50	55
5 years	55	56	39	42	32	38	21	29	21	41	36	43
Females	(61)		(30)		(47)		(22)		(28)		(188)	
1 year	85	85	93	94	79	79	81	83	73	80	83	84
3 years	68	68	62	63	69	72	57	62	43	54	62	66
5 years	64	65	54	56	62	66	52	61	31	47	56	61
Overall	(90)		(53)		(81)		(46)		(42)		(312)	
1 year	83	83	96	97	75	76	80	83	70	77	81	83
3 years	66	66	58	59	57	60	57	65	38	50	57	62
5 years	61	62	48	50	49	54	35	45	28	46	47	54

SCOTLAND

AREA	NUMBER OF CASES			PERIOD	MEAN AGE		
	Males	Females	All		Males	Females	All
Scotland	805	1348	2153	1985-1989	55.1	55.5	55.3

OBSERVED AND RELATIVE SURVIVAL (%) BY AGE (number of cases in parentheses)

	AGE CLASS										ALL	
	15-44		45-54		55-64		65-74		75-99			
	obs	rel	obs	rel	obs	rel	obs	rel	obs	rel	obs	rel
Males	(238)		(134)		(169)		(154)		(110)		(805)	
1 year	96	96	93	94	87	89	88	93	78	89	90	93
3 years	89	89	79	81	70	74	66	77	54	81	74	81
5 years	80	81	69	71	62	69	54	72	35	71	63	74
Females	(429)		(214)		(224)		(241)		(240)		(1348)	
1 year	98	98	97	98	96	98	94	96	82	90	94	96
3 years	93	93	92	93	86	90	82	90	66	89	85	91
5 years	91	91	86	88	81	87	74	87	48	82	78	88
Overall	(667)		(348)		(393)		(395)		(350)		(2153)	
1 year	97	98	96	96	92	94	92	95	81	90	92	95
3 years	91	92	87	88	79	83	76	85	62	87	81	88
5 years	87	88	79	82	73	80	66	82	44	79	72	83

MELANOMA OF SKIN   (ICD-9 172)

SLOVAKIA

AREA	NUMBER OF CASES			PERIOD	MEAN AGE		
	Males	Females	All		Males	Females	All
Slovakia	556	673	1229	1985-1989	55.2	54.5	54.8

OBSERVED AND RELATIVE SURVIVAL (%) BY AGE (number of cases in parentheses)

	AGE CLASS										ALL	
	15-44		45-54		55-64		65-74		75-99			
	obs	rel	obs	rel	obs	rel	obs	rel	obs	rel	obs	rel
Males	(146)		(108)		(144)		(99)		(59)		(556)	
1 year	85	85	85	86	78	81	86	91	66	74	81	84
3 years	61	62	55	57	57	62	58	68	31	44	55	61
5 years	54	55	46	50	47	55	47	65	26	50	46	55
Females	(206)		(134)		(139)		(98)		(96)		(673)	
1 year	93	93	90	90	88	89	82	84	72	80	87	89
3 years	78	78	78	79	75	78	50	55	47	65	69	74
5 years	72	73	74	76	67	72	40	48	41	74	62	70
Overall	(352)		(242)		(283)		(197)		(155)		(1229)	
1 year	90	90	88	88	83	85	84	87	70	78	84	87
3 years	71	71	68	70	66	70	54	61	41	57	63	68
5 years	65	65	61	64	56	63	44	56	35	65	55	63

SLOVENIA

AREA	NUMBER OF CASES			PERIOD	MEAN AGE		
	Males	Females	All		Males	Females	All
Slovenia	231	293	524	1985-1989	54.1	53.7	53.9

OBSERVED AND RELATIVE SURVIVAL (%) BY AGE (number of cases in parentheses)

	AGE CLASS										ALL	
	15-44		45-54		55-64		65-74		75-99			
	obs	rel	obs	rel	obs	rel	obs	rel	obs	rel	obs	rel
Males	(64)		(46)		(56)		(45)		(20)		(231)	
1 year	83	83	83	83	77	78	89	93	55	63	80	82
3 years	67	68	63	65	52	55	53	61	25	39	56	61
5 years	56	57	50	53	36	40	33	43	20	43	42	49
Females	(96)		(49)		(56)		(53)		(39)		(293)	
1 year	93	93	86	86	89	90	89	91	77	83	88	90
3 years	80	80	71	72	70	71	70	75	56	73	71	75
5 years	75	75	65	66	64	67	62	72	36	57	64	70
Overall	(160)		(95)		(112)		(98)		(59)		(524)	
1 year	89	89	84	85	83	84	89	92	69	77	84	86
3 years	75	75	67	68	61	64	62	69	46	63	65	69
5 years	67	68	57	60	50	54	49	59	31	53	54	61

MELANOMA OF SKIN (ICD-9 172)

SPAIN

AREA	NUMBER OF CASES			PERIOD	MEAN AGE			5-YR RELATIVE SURVIVAL (%)	
	Males	Females	All		Males	Females	All	Males	Females
Basque Country	92	163	255	1986-1988	57.8	56.4	56.9		
Mallorca	22	32	54	1988-1989	56.5	58.0	57.4		
Navarra	42	65	107	1985-1989	57.2	54.9	55.8		
Tarragona	49	51	100	1985-1989	55.9	57.5	56.7		
Spanish Registries	205	311	516		57.1	56.5	56.7		

OBSERVED AND RELATIVE SURVIVAL (%) BY AGE (number of cases in parentheses)

	AGE CLASS										ALL	
	15-44		45-54		55-64		65-74		75-99			
	obs	rel	obs	rel	obs	rel	obs	rel	obs	rel	obs	rel
Males	(55)		(25)		(38)		(54)		(33)		(205)	
1 year	84	84	88	88	95	96	87	90	85	94	87	90
3 years	69	70	68	69	82	85	65	72	70	97	70	77
5 years	63	64	68	70	73	79	43	51	54	97	58	67
Females	(94)		(37)		(66)		(51)		(63)		(311)	
1 year	97	97	97	98	91	91	96	98	84	91	93	95
3 years	91	92	81	82	85	86	80	85	60	77	81	86
5 years	89	89	78	79	83	86	76	84	50	78	76	85
Overall	(149)		(62)		(104)		(105)		(96)		(516)	
1 year	92	92	94	94	92	93	91	94	84	92	91	93
3 years	83	84	76	77	84	86	72	78	64	84	77	82
5 years	79	80	74	76	79	83	58	67	51	84	69	78

SWEDEN

AREA	NUMBER OF CASES			PERIOD	MEAN AGE		
	Males	Females	All		Males	Females	All
South Sweden	560	658	1218	1985-1989	58.2	57.8	58.0

OBSERVED AND RELATIVE SURVIVAL (%) BY AGE (number of cases in parentheses)

	AGE CLASS										ALL	
	15-44		45-54		55-64		65-74		75-99			
	obs	rel	obs	rel	obs	rel	obs	rel	obs	rel	obs	rel
Males	(124)		(83)		(130)		(141)		(82)		(560)	
1 year	98	99	99	99	94	95	93	96	82	91	94	96
3 years	92	92	89	90	86	90	82	91	60	84	83	90
5 years	90	90	84	86	79	85	71	86	40	73	74	86
Females	(183)		(102)		(114)		(132)		(127)		(658)	
1 year	98	98	97	97	96	97	96	98	87	95	95	97
3 years	96	96	97	98	94	96	86	91	57	77	86	93
5 years	93	93	95	97	88	91	80	89	43	71	80	90
Overall	(307)		(185)		(244)		(273)		(209)		(1218)	
1 year	98	98	98	98	95	96	95	97	85	94	94	97
3 years	94	95	94	95	90	93	84	91	58	80	85	91
5 years	92	92	90	92	83	88	75	87	42	72	78	88

MELANOMA OF SKIN   (ICD-9 172)

SWITZERLAND

AREA	NUMBER OF CASES			PERIOD	MEAN AGE			5-YR RELATIVE SURVIVAL (%)	
	Males	Females	All		Males	Females	All	Males	Females
Basel	128	124	252	1985-1988	56.8	58.6	57.7		
Geneva	102	131	233	1985-1989	56.4	52.1	54.0		
Swiss Registries	230	255	485		56.6	55.3	55.9		

OBSERVED AND RELATIVE SURVIVAL (%) BY AGE (number of cases in parentheses)

	AGE CLASS										ALL	
	15-44		45-54		55-64		65-74		75-99			
	obs	rel	obs	rel	obs	rel	obs	rel	obs	rel	obs	rel
Males	(57)		(38)		(54)		(43)		(38)		(230)	
1 year	96	97	100	100	98	99	98	100	79	86	95	97
3 years	93	93	92	93	85	89	84	93	58	75	83	90
5 years	83	84	87	89	81	88	70	85	39	65	74	84
Females	(73)		(60)		(41)		(39)		(42)		(255)	
1 year	100	100	100	100	100	100	97	99	90	97	98	100
3 years	94	95	93	94	89	91	92	97	78	97	90	95
5 years	93	93	93	95	81	84	90	99	68	100	87	94
Overall	(130)		(98)		(95)		(82)		(80)		(485)	
1 year	98	99	100	100	99	100	98	100	85	92	96	98
3 years	94	94	93	94	87	90	88	95	68	87	87	92
5 years	89	89	91	92	81	86	79	92	55	86	80	89

MELANOMA OF SKIN $\quad$ (ICD-9 172)

EUROPE, 1985-89

Weighted analyses

COUNTRY	% COVERAGE WITH C.R.s	YEARLY NO. OF CASES (Mean No. of cases recorded)			RELATIVE SURVIVAL (%) (Age-standardized)
		Males	Females	All	
AUSTRIA	8	35	68	103	
DENMARK	100	262	363	625	
ENGLAND	50	610	1112	1722	
ESTONIA	100	23	44	67	
FINLAND	100	209	218	427	
FRANCE	3	31	54	85	
GERMANY	2	39	50	89	
ICELAND	100	3	7	10	
ITALY	10	156	194	350	
NETHERLANDS	6	22	35	57	
POLAND	6	42	66	108	
SCOTLAND	100	161	270	431	
SLOVAKIA	100	111	135	246	
SLOVENIA	100	46	59	105	
SPAIN	10	60	94	154	
SWEDEN	17	112	132	244	
SWITZERLAND	11	52	57	109	

□ 1 year ■ 5 years

OBSERVED AND RELATIVE SURVIVAL (%) BY AGE

	AGE CLASS										ALL	
	15-44		45-54		55-64		65-74		75-99			
	obs	rel	obs	rel	obs	rel	obs	rel	obs	rel	obs	rel
Males												
1 year	91	92	95	95	88	90	88	91	71	79	88	91
3 years	79	79	79	80	70	74	67	76	43	59	71	76
5 years	73	74	72	75	61	67	54	67	29	52	62	70
Females												
1 year	96	96	97	97	94	95	89	91	83	90	93	94
3 years	90	90	88	89	84	86	76	81	58	76	81	86
5 years	86	86	82	84	78	82	69	78	46	73	75	82
Overall												
1 year	94	94	96	96	92	93	89	91	78	85	91	93
3 years	85	86	84	85	78	81	73	79	52	69	77	82
5 years	81	81	78	80	71	76	63	73	39	64	69	77

AGE STANDARDIZED RELATIVE SURVIVAL(%)

COUNTRY	MALES		FEMALES	
	1-year (95% C.I.)	5-years (95% C.I.)	1-year (95% C.I.)	5-years (95% C.I.)
AUSTRIA	100.0 (100.0 -100.0)	96.5 (87.0 -107.0)	94.7 (90.5 - 99.0)	85.6 (78.4 - 93.4)
DENMARK	92.2 (90.5 - 94.0)	71.8 (68.8 - 75.1)	96.2 (95.1 - 97.3)	83.4 (81.2 - 85.6)
ENGLAND	91.1 (90.0 - 92.3)	69.6 (67.6 - 71.7)	95.5 (94.9 - 96.2)	82.9 (81.7 - 84.2)
ESTONIA	83.8 (76.1 - 92.3)	54.7 (43.6 - 68.7)	90.5 (86.4 - 94.9)	67.1 (60.0 - 75.0)
FINLAND	93.7 (91.8 - 95.6)	76.0 (72.5 - 79.7)	96.4 (95.1 - 97.7)	85.0 (82.4 - 87.7)
FRANCE	92.7 (87.6 - 98.1)	70.9 (61.5 - 81.6)	95.4 (92.4 - 98.5)	81.1 (75.2 - 87.5)
GERMANY	88.1 (83.0 - 93.5)	67.1 (59.0 - 76.3)	92.8 (89.4 - 96.4)	83.1 (76.8 - 90.0)
ICELAND	79.4 (61.8 -102.0)	63.6 (44.2 - 91.5)	100.0 (97.0 -103.1)	80.5 (68.1 - 95.0)
ITALY	84.1 (80.8 - 87.4)	54.5 (50.1 - 59.2)	94.3 (92.5 - 96.2)	78.3 (74.9 - 81.8)
NETHERLANDS	92.4 (86.7 - 98.5)	76.4 (64.9 - 89.9)	99.3 (96.1 -102.6)	83.0 (74.9 - 92.1)
POLAND	81.5 (74.3 - 89.3)	43.0 (33.6 - 55.1)	84.3 (78.9 - 90.2)	60.2 (52.4 - 69.3)
SCOTLAND	92.6 (90.5 - 94.8)	73.8 (69.7 - 78.1)	96.5 (95.3 - 97.7)	87.7 (85.2 - 90.3)
SLOVAKIA	83.8 (80.4 - 87.3)	54.9 (49.6 - 60.8)	88.3 (85.6 - 91.0)	68.9 (64.5 - 73.5)
SLOVENIA	81.0 (75.5 - 86.9)	48.4 (40.8 - 57.6)	89.2 (85.4 - 93.2)	68.7 (62.7 - 75.3)
SPAIN	89.6 (85.0 - 94.5)	70.4 (62.6 - 79.2)	95.2 (92.6 - 97.8)	84.1 (79.1 - 89.5)
SWEDEN	96.4 (94.5 - 98.3)	85.3 (81.2 - 89.6)	97.4 (95.9 - 99.0)	89.5 (86.4 - 92.6)
SWITZERLAND	96.8 (94.1 - 99.6)	83.0 (76.9 - 89.6)	99.3 (97.7 -101.0)	93.7 (88.8 - 98.8)
EUROPE, 1985-89	89.8 (88.3 - 91.4)	68.2 (65.7 - 70.9)	94.3 (93.3 - 95.3)	81.4 (79.6 - 83.2)

BREAST   (ICD-9 174-175)

AUSTRIA

AREA	NUMBER OF CASES			PERIOD	MEAN AGE		
	Males	Females	All		Males	Females	All
Tirol	1	520	521	1988-1989	47.0	63.3	63.3

OBSERVED AND RELATIVE SURVIVAL (%) BY AGE (number of cases in parentheses)

	15-44		45-54		55-64		65-74		75-99		ALL	
	obs	rel	obs	rel	obs	rel	obs	rel	obs	rel	obs	rel
Males	(0)		(1)		(0)		(0)		(0)		(1)	
1 year	-	-	0	0	-	-	-	-	-	-	0	0
3 years	-	-	0	0	-	-	-	-	-	-	0	0
5 years	-	-	0	0	-	-	-	-	-	-	0	0
Females	(60)		(96)		(104)		(131)		(129)		(520)	
1 year	92	92	88	88	85	85	89	90	75	80	85	86
3 years	78	79	73	73	71	72	73	77	60	73	70	75
5 years	67	67	61	62	63	64	56	62	43	62	56	63
Overall	(60)		(97)		(104)		(131)		(129)		(521)	
1 year	92	92	87	87	85	85	89	90	75	80	84	86
3 years	78	79	72	73	71	72	73	77	60	73	70	75
5 years	67	67	61	62	63	64	56	62	43	62	56	63

DENMARK

AREA	NUMBER OF CASES			PERIOD	MEAN AGE		
	Males	Females	All		Males	Females	All
Denmark	82	13912	13994	1985-1989	69.2	61.9	61.9

OBSERVED AND RELATIVE SURVIVAL (%) BY AGE (number of cases in parentheses)

	15-44		45-54		55-64		65-74		75-99		ALL	
	obs	rel	obs	rel	obs	rel	obs	rel	obs	rel	obs	rel
Males	(3)		(6)		(20)		(21)		(32)		(82)	
1 year	100	100	100	100	90	92	95	99	81	91	89	94
3 years	100	100	67	68	80	85	57	66	47	66	61	73
5 years	67	68	50	52	60	67	33	43	31	59	41	57
Females	(2004)		(2704)		(2958)		(3098)		(3148)		(13912)	
1 year	98	98	95	96	92	93	90	92	77	83	90	92
3 years	85	85	83	84	78	80	74	79	54	70	73	80
5 years	74	75	74	76	67	71	62	71	38	61	62	71
Overall	(2007)		(2710)		(2978)		(3119)		(3180)		(13994)	
1 year	98	98	95	96	92	93	90	92	77	83	90	92
3 years	85	85	83	84	78	80	74	79	54	70	73	80
5 years	74	75	74	76	67	71	62	71	38	61	62	71

BREAST   (ICD-9 174-175)

ENGLAND

AREA	NUMBER OF CASES			PERIOD	MEAN AGE			5-YR RELATIVE SURVIVAL (%)	
	Males	Females	All		Males	Females	All	Males	Females
East Anglia	46	5404	5450	1985-1989	69.4	63.4	63.4		
Mersey	30	5897	5927	1985-1989	69.0	61.6	61.7		
Oxford	48	6171	6219	1985-1989	63.2	61.2	61.2		
South Thames	136	15144	15280	1985-1989	68.9	62.5	62.6		
Wessex	66	7963	8029	1985-1989	71.5	63.3	63.3		
West Midlands	90	12212	12302	1985-1989	67.9	62.4	62.5		
Yorkshire	63	8417	8480	1985-1989	67.3	62.4	62.5		
English Registries	479	61208	61688		68.4	62.4	62.5		

OBSERVED AND RELATIVE SURVIVAL (%) BY AGE (number of cases in parentheses)

	AGE CLASS										ALL	
	15-44		45-54		55-64		65-74		75-99			
	obs	rel	obs	rel	obs	rel	obs	rel	obs	rel	obs	rel
Males	(20)		(38)		(108)		(142)		(171)		(479)	
1 year	100	100	87	87	86	88	86	90	72	80	82	86
3 years	80	80	76	78	79	83	69	79	51	73	66	78
5 years	65	66	66	68	65	71	54	69	36	67	52	69
Females	(7982)		(10896)		(13863)		(14324)		(14143)		(61208)	
1 year	95	95	94	94	91	92	87	89	73	80	87	89
3 years	80	80	80	80	76	78	71	76	50	66	70	76
5 years	70	70	71	72	66	69	59	67	36	57	59	67
Overall	(8002)		(10934)		(13971)		(14466)		(14314)		(61687)	
1 year	95	95	94	94	91	92	87	89	73	80	87	89
3 years	80	80	79	80	76	78	71	76	50	66	70	76
5 years	70	70	71	72	66	69	59	67	36	57	59	67

ESTONIA

AREA	NUMBER OF CASES			PERIOD	MEAN AGE		
	Males	Females	All		Males	Females	All
Estonia	14	1946	1960	1985-1989	60.9	57.5	57.5

OBSERVED AND RELATIVE SURVIVAL (%) BY AGE (number of cases in parentheses)

	AGE CLASS										ALL	
	15-44		45-54		55-64		65-74		75-99			
	obs	rel	obs	rel	obs	rel	obs	rel	obs	rel	obs	rel
Males	(1)		(3)		(4)		(4)		(2)		(14)	
1 year	100	100	67	68	100	100	100	100	100	100	93	97
3 years	100	100	33	35	100	100	100	100	50	70	77	88
5 years	100	100	33	36	33	40	100	100	0	0	54	68
Females	(317)		(539)		(503)		(337)		(250)		(1946)	
1 year	94	94	94	95	87	88	81	83	71	78	87	89
3 years	73	73	74	75	66	69	62	68	43	58	66	70
5 years	63	63	66	68	55	59	48	57	31	53	55	62
Overall	(318)		(542)		(507)		(341)		(252)		(1960)	
1 year	94	94	94	95	87	88	81	84	71	78	87	89
3 years	73	73	74	75	67	69	63	69	43	58	66	70
5 years	63	63	66	68	55	58	49	58	31	52	55	62

BREAST $\qquad$ (ICD-9 174-175)

FINLAND

AREA	NUMBER OF CASES			PERIOD	MEAN AGE		
	Males	Females	All		Males	Females	All
Finland	42	10558	10600	1985-1989	63.3	60.5	60.5

OBSERVED AND RELATIVE SURVIVAL (%) BY AGE (number of cases in parentheses)

	AGE CLASS										ALL	
	15-44		45-54		55-64		65-74		75-99			
	obs	rel	obs	rel	obs	rel	obs	rel	obs	rel	obs	rel
Males	(5)		(8)		(5)		(14)		(10)		(42)	
1 year	80	80	100	100	100	100	86	89	80	90	88	92
3 years	60	61	100	100	80	84	64	73	50	72	69	79
5 years	60	61	100	100	80	88	50	63	20	38	57	72
Females	(1568)		(2277)		(2464)		(2161)		(2088)		(10558)	
1 year	98	98	98	98	95	96	92	94	83	90	93	95
3 years	88	88	89	90	85	87	78	84	61	79	80	86
5 years	78	79	83	84	78	81	68	77	45	72	70	79
Overall	(1573)		(2285)		(2469)		(2175)		(2098)		(10600)	
1 year	98	98	98	98	95	96	92	94	83	90	93	95
3 years	88	88	89	90	85	87	78	84	61	79	80	86
5 years	78	79	83	84	78	81	68	77	45	72	70	79

FRANCE

AREA	NUMBER OF CASES			PERIOD	MEAN AGE		
	Males	Females	All		Males	Females	All
Somme	11	1044	1055	1985-1989	68.0	58.0	58.1
Calvados	15	1373	1388	1985-1989	61.7	59.8	59.9
Côte d'Or	-	1104	1104	1985-1989	-	60.9	60.9
Doubs	4	977	981	1985-1989	64.5	60.0	60.0
Isere	-	1561	1561	1987-1989	-	59.2	59.2
French Registries	30	6059	6089		64.5	59.6	59.6

5-YR RELATIVE SURVIVAL (%)

Males — Somme, Calvad, Côte d, Doubs, Isere
Females — Somme, Calvad, Côte d, Doubs, Isere

OBSERVED AND RELATIVE SURVIVAL (%) BY AGE (number of cases in parentheses)

	AGE CLASS										ALL	
	15-44		45-54		55-64		65-74		75-99			
	obs	rel	obs	rel	obs	rel	obs	rel	obs	rel	obs	rel
Males	(1)		(6)		(8)		(7)		(8)		(30)	
1 year	100	100	67	67	100	100	86	89	59	64	79	82
3 years	100	100	67	69	100	100	86	96	0	0	65	73
5 years	100	100	50	53	88	97	86	100	0	0	57	70
Females	(1056)		(1257)		(1473)		(1144)		(1129)		(6059)	
1 year	98	98	98	98	95	96	94	95	85	92	94	96
3 years	89	89	89	90	84	86	82	86	67	85	83	87
5 years	80	81	83	84	76	78	73	80	51	78	73	81
Overall	(1057)		(1263)		(1481)		(1151)		(1137)		(6089)	
1 year	98	98	97	98	95	96	94	95	85	92	94	96
3 years	89	89	89	90	84	86	82	86	66	84	82	87
5 years	80	81	83	84	76	79	73	80	51	78	73	81

BREAST   (ICD-9 174-175)

GERMANY

AREA	NUMBER OF CASES			PERIOD	MEAN AGE		
	Males	Females	All		Males	Females	All
Saarland	11	2578	2589	1985-1989	61.0	61.8	61.8

OBSERVED AND RELATIVE SURVIVAL (%) BY AGE (number of cases in parentheses)

	AGE CLASS										ALL	
	15-44		45-54		55-64		65-74		75-99			
	obs	rel	obs	rel	obs	rel	obs	rel	obs	rel	obs	rel
Males	(0)		(3)		(5)		(1)		(2)		(11)	
1 year	-	-	100	100	80	81	100	100	100	100	91	94
3 years	-	-	100	100	60	63	100	100	100	100	82	90
5 years	-	-	100	100	60	66	100	100	-	-	82	96
Females	(278)		(548)		(617)		(575)		(560)		(2578)	
1 year	97	97	94	94	94	95	90	92	80	86	90	93
3 years	82	83	81	82	79	81	75	81	58	74	75	80
5 years	70	71	72	73	70	73	64	73	43	68	63	72
Overall	(278)		(551)		(622)		(576)		(562)		(2589)	
1 year	97	97	94	94	94	94	90	92	80	86	90	93
3 years	82	83	81	82	79	81	75	81	59	74	75	80
5 years	70	71	72	73	70	73	64	73	44	69	63	72

ICELAND

AREA	NUMBER OF CASES			PERIOD	MEAN AGE		
	Males	Females	All		Males	Females	All
Iceland	3	520	523	1985-1989	71.7	59.3	59.4

OBSERVED AND RELATIVE SURVIVAL (%) BY AGE (number of cases in parentheses)

	AGE CLASS										ALL	
	15-44		45-54		55-64		65-74		75-99			
	obs	rel	obs	rel	obs	rel	obs	rel	obs	rel	obs	rel
Males	(0)		(0)		(0)		(2)		(1)		(3)	
1 year	-	-	-	-	-	-	100	100	100	100	100	100
3 years	-	-	-	-	-	-	100	100	100	100	100	100
5 years	-	-	-	-	-	-	100	100	100	100	100	100
Females	(87)		(114)		(130)		(104)		(85)		(520)	
1 year	100	100	100	100	92	93	96	98	80	88	94	96
3 years	87	88	91	92	82	84	83	88	62	82	82	87
5 years	74	74	80	81	78	81	72	80	48	78	72	79
Overall	(87)		(114)		(130)		(106)		(86)		(523)	
1 year	100	100	100	100	92	93	96	98	80	88	94	96
3 years	87	88	91	92	82	84	83	88	63	83	82	87
5 years	74	74	80	81	78	81	73	81	49	79	72	79

BREAST   (ICD-9 174-175)

ITALY

AREA	NUMBER OF CASES			PERIOD	MEAN AGE			5-YR RELATIVE SURVIVAL (%)	
	Males	Females	All		Males	Females	All	Males	Females
Florence	32	3295	3327	1985-1989	64.6	61.2	61.3		
Genoa	6	1344	1350	1986-1988	53.5	61.8	61.8		
Latina	5	360	365	1985-1987	53.4	57.4	57.4		
Modena	3	640	643	1988-1989	60.0	60.9	60.9		
Parma	2	712	714	1985-1987	53.5	61.2	61.2		
Ragusa	5	467	472	1985-1989	72.2	59.2	59.3		
Romagna	8	725	733	1986-1988	65.1	60.7	60.8		
Turin	16	1624	1640	1985-1987	66.9	60.1	60.1		
Varese	9	2209	2218	1985-1989	73.0	60.8	60.9		
Italian Registries	86	11376	11462		64.6	60.8	60.8		

OBSERVED AND RELATIVE SURVIVAL (%) BY AGE (number of cases in parentheses)

	AGE CLASS										ALL	
	15-44		45-54		55-64		65-74		75-99			
	obs	rel	obs	rel	obs	rel	obs	rel	obs	rel	obs	rel
Males	(6)		(12)		(25)		(17)		(26)		(86)	
1 year	100	100	83	84	92	93	76	79	58	64	78	81
3 years	83	84	67	68	76	80	76	84	31	43	62	70
5 years	83	84	58	60	64	70	59	69	23	42	51	63
Females	(1459)		(2460)		(2822)		(2517)		(2118)		(11376)	
1 year	98	98	97	98	95	96	93	94	84	90	93	95
3 years	87	87	87	87	83	85	80	85	63	79	80	85
5 years	78	78	78	79	74	76	70	78	49	72	70	77
Overall	(1465)		(2472)		(2847)		(2534)		(2144)		(11462)	
1 year	98	98	97	98	95	96	93	94	83	89	93	95
3 years	87	87	86	87	83	85	80	85	63	78	80	85
5 years	78	78	78	79	74	76	70	78	48	72	70	77

NETHERLANDS

AREA	NUMBER OF CASES			PERIOD	MEAN AGE		
	Males	Females	All		Males	Females	All
Eindhoven	9	2119	2128	1985-1989	59.2	59.2	59.2

OBSERVED AND RELATIVE SURVIVAL (%) BY AGE (number of cases in parentheses)

	AGE CLASS										ALL	
	15-44		45-54		55-64		65-74		75-99			
	obs	rel	obs	rel	obs	rel	obs	rel	obs	rel	obs	rel
Males	(2)		(0)		(3)		(3)		(1)		(9)	
1 year	100	100	-	-	100	100	100	100	100	100	100	100
3 years	100	100	-	-	100	100	67	77	0	0	76	83
5 years	100	100	-	-	100	100	67	85	0	0	76	89
Females	(355)		(489)		(503)		(421)		(351)		(2119)	
1 year	97	97	97	97	92	93	92	94	85	91	93	95
3 years	87	87	87	88	79	81	76	81	61	78	79	83
5 years	76	76	79	80	69	71	65	73	47	73	68	75
Overall	(357)		(489)		(506)		(424)		(352)		(2128)	
1 year	97	97	97	97	92	93	92	94	85	91	93	95
3 years	87	87	87	88	79	81	76	81	61	77	79	83
5 years	76	76	79	80	69	71	65	73	47	73	68	75

BREAST   (ICD-9 174-175)

POLAND

AREA	NUMBER OF CASES			PERIOD	MEAN AGE			5-YR RELATIVE SURVIVAL (%)	
	Males	Females	All		Males	Females	All	Males	Females
Cracow	7	1068	1075	1985-1989	70.1	58.4	58.5		
Warsaw	9	982	991	1988-1989	59.7	58.4	58.4		
Polish Registries	16	2050	2066		64.4	58.4	58.5		

OBSERVED AND RELATIVE SURVIVAL (%) BY AGE (number of cases in parentheses)

	AGE CLASS										ALL	
	15-44		45-54		55-64		65-74		75-99			
	obs	rel	obs	rel	obs	rel	obs	rel	obs	rel	obs	rel
Males	(1)		(2)		(4)		(5)		(4)		(16)	
1 year	100	100	50	51	75	77	100	100	50	55	75	79
3 years	100	100	50	52	75	82	80	96	25	35	63	73
5 years	100	100	50	54	75	87	40	55	25	45	50	66
Females	(360)		(469)		(552)		(367)		(302)		(2050)	
1 year	91	91	90	91	89	90	80	83	70	76	85	87
3 years	73	74	76	77	67	69	60	65	49	64	66	71
5 years	62	63	64	65	55	59	47	56	32	51	54	60
Overall	(361)		(471)		(556)		(372)		(306)		(2066)	
1 year	91	92	90	91	89	90	81	83	69	76	85	87
3 years	73	74	76	77	67	70	60	66	49	64	66	71
5 years	62	63	64	65	55	59	47	56	32	51	54	60

SCOTLAND

AREA	NUMBER OF CASES			PERIOD	MEAN AGE		
	Males	Females	All		Males	Females	All
Scotland	57	12259	12316	1985-1989	69.8	62.4	62.4

OBSERVED AND RELATIVE SURVIVAL (%) BY AGE (number of cases in parentheses)

	AGE CLASS										ALL	
	15-44		45-54		55-64		65-74		75-99			
	obs	rel	obs	rel	obs	rel	obs	rel	obs	rel	obs	rel
Males	(1)		(4)		(11)		(22)		(19)		(57)	
1 year	100	100	75	75	73	74	82	86	68	78	75	81
3 years	100	100	50	51	64	68	64	75	42	64	56	69
5 years	100	100	50	52	64	73	50	67	26	54	46	65
Females	(1577)		(2312)		(2761)		(2718)		(2891)		(12259)	
1 year	96	96	94	94	90	91	86	88	71	78	86	89
3 years	80	81	78	79	74	76	68	74	47	63	68	74
5 years	70	70	68	70	63	67	56	66	31	54	56	66
Overall	(1578)		(2316)		(2772)		(2740)		(2910)		(12316)	
1 year	96	96	94	94	90	91	86	88	71	78	86	89
3 years	80	81	78	79	74	76	68	74	47	63	68	74
5 years	70	70	68	70	63	67	56	66	31	54	56	66

BREAST   (ICD-9 174-175)

SLOVAKIA

AREA	NUMBER OF CASES			PERIOD	MEAN AGE		
	Males	Females	All		Males	Females	All
Slovakia	66	5682	5748	1985-1989	59.3	58.4	58.4

OBSERVED AND RELATIVE SURVIVAL (%) BY AGE (number of cases in parentheses)

	AGE CLASS										ALL	
	15-44		45-54		55-64		65-74		75-99			
	obs	rel	obs	rel	obs	rel	obs	rel	obs	rel	obs	rel
Males	(11)		(12)		(18)		(14)		(11)		(66)	
1 year	82	82	75	76	72	74	64	68	55	60	70	72
3 years	73	74	42	43	50	54	43	50	27	38	47	53
5 years	50	52	19	21	38	45	27	36	27	49	32	39
Females	(983)		(1266)		(1549)		(1069)		(815)		(5682)	
1 year	93	94	90	91	85	86	83	85	66	72	84	86
3 years	71	72	71	72	65	67	63	69	42	57	64	69
5 years	57	57	59	60	54	58	50	59	32	56	52	59
Overall	(994)		(1278)		(1567)		(1083)		(826)		(5748)	
1 year	93	93	90	91	85	86	82	85	65	72	84	86
3 years	71	72	71	72	65	67	63	69	42	57	64	68
5 years	57	57	58	60	54	58	50	59	32	56	52	58

SLOVENIA

AREA	NUMBER OF CASES			PERIOD	MEAN AGE		
	Males	Females	All		Males	Females	All
Slovenia	20	3073	3093	1985-1989	67.3	58.6	58.6

OBSERVED AND RELATIVE SURVIVAL (%) BY AGE (number of cases in parentheses)

	AGE CLASS										ALL	
	15-44		45-54		55-64		65-74		75-99			
	obs	rel	obs	rel	obs	rel	obs	rel	obs	rel	obs	rel
Males	(0)		(2)		(8)		(3)		(7)		(20)	
1 year	-	-	50	51	75	77	33	35	57	66	60	64
3 years	-	-	0	0	63	67	33	38	29	46	40	49
5 years	-	-	0	0	63	70	33	42	29	68	40	56
Females	(506)		(707)		(842)		(579)		(439)		(3073)	
1 year	97	97	96	96	90	91	85	87	73	80	89	91
3 years	83	84	79	80	72	74	69	75	51	69	72	77
5 years	70	71	64	65	60	63	55	64	35	60	58	65
Overall	(506)		(709)		(850)		(582)		(446)		(3093)	
1 year	97	97	96	96	90	91	85	87	72	80	89	91
3 years	83	84	78	79	72	74	69	75	50	68	71	76
5 years	70	71	64	65	60	64	55	63	35	60	58	65

BREAST (ICD-9 174-175)

SPAIN

AREA	NUMBER OF CASES			PERIOD	MEAN AGE			5-YR RELATIVE SURVIVAL (%)	
	Males	Females	All		Males	Females	All	Males	Females
Basque Country	17	1872	1889	1986-1988	74.0	58.1	58.2		
Girona	0	730	730	1985-1989	-	61.6	61.6		
Granada	0	449	449	1985-1989	-	57.2	57.2		
Mallorca	2	400	402	1988-1989	83.5	60.2	60.4		
Navarra	6	824	830	1985-1989	65.5	59.8	59.9		
Tarragona	10	898	908	1985-1989	67.4	60.0	60.1		
Spanish Registries	35	5173	5208		71.3	59.3	59.4		

OBSERVED AND RELATIVE SURVIVAL (%) BY AGE (number of cases in parentheses)

	AGE CLASS										ALL	
	15-44		45-54		55-64		65-74		75-99			
	obs	rel	obs	rel	obs	rel	obs	rel	obs	rel	obs	rel
Males	(1)		(2)		(7)		(6)		(19)		(35)	
1 year	100	100	100	100	57	58	100	100	84	94	83	88
3 years	100	100	100	100	43	45	100	100	58	80	66	80
5 years	100	100	100	100	43	46	80	95	52	92	59	82
Females	(867)		(1092)		(1285)		(1138)		(791)		(5173)	
1 year	98	98	96	96	94	94	92	93	83	90	93	94
3 years	84	85	80	81	78	79	76	80	62	77	77	81
5 years	74	74	69	70	67	69	63	69	47	71	65	71
Overall	(868)		(1094)		(1292)		(1144)		(810)		(5208)	
1 year	98	98	96	96	93	94	92	93	84	90	93	94
3 years	84	85	80	81	78	79	76	80	61	77	77	81
5 years	74	74	69	70	67	69	63	70	47	71	65	71

SWEDEN

AREA	NUMBER OF CASES			PERIOD	MEAN AGE		
	Males	Females	All		Males	Females	All
South Sweden	32	3925	3957	1985-1989	65.8	63.6	63.6

OBSERVED AND RELATIVE SURVIVAL (%) BY AGE (number of cases in parentheses)

	AGE CLASS										ALL	
	15-44		45-54		55-64		65-74		75-99			
	obs	rel	obs	rel	obs	rel	obs	rel	obs	rel	obs	rel
Males	(1)		(5)		(11)		(6)		(9)		(32)	
1 year	100	100	100	100	100	100	100	100	67	75	91	95
3 years	100	100	40	41	100	100	100	100	22	32	69	78
5 years	100	100	20	21	100	100	83	100	22	41	63	78
Females	(437)		(708)		(815)		(951)		(1014)		(3925)	
1 year	97	97	97	98	98	98	94	95	84	91	93	95
3 years	84	85	86	87	89	91	84	88	65	83	80	87
5 years	77	78	79	80	80	84	75	83	49	77	70	81
Overall	(438)		(713)		(826)		(957)		(1023)		(3957)	
1 year	97	97	97	98	98	98	94	95	84	91	93	95
3 years	84	85	86	86	89	91	84	89	64	83	80	87
5 years	77	78	78	80	81	84	75	84	49	77	70	81

BREAST   (ICD-9 174-175)

SWITZERLAND

AREA	NUMBER OF CASES			PERIOD	MEAN AGE			5-YR RELATIVE SURVIVAL (%)	
	Males	Females	All		Males	Females	All	Males	Females
Basel	0	976	976	1985-1988	-	62.5	62.5		
Geneva	2	1075	1077	1985-1989	55.5	61.8	61.8		
Swiss Registries	2	2051	2053		56.0	62.2	62.1		

OBSERVED AND RELATIVE SURVIVAL (%) BY AGE (number of cases in parentheses)

	AGE CLASS										ALL	
	15-44		45-54		55-64		65-74		75-99			
	obs	rel	obs	rel	obs	rel	obs	rel	obs	rel	obs	rel
Males	(0)		(1)		(1)		(0)		(0)		(2)	
1 year	-	-	100	100	100	100	-	-	-	-	100	100
3 years	-	-	100	100	-	-	-	-	-	-	100	100
5 years	-	-	100	100	-	-	-	-	-	-	100	100
Females	(290)		(418)		(445)		(376)		(522)		(2051)	
1 year	100	100	99	99	95	96	94	95	87	94	94	97
3 years	92	93	86	87	86	87	82	87	67	86	81	88
5 years	81	82	77	78	78	80	72	79	50	79	70	80
Overall	(290)		(419)		(446)		(376)		(522)		(2053)	
1 year	100	100	99	99	95	96	94	95	87	94	94	97
3 years	92	93	86	87	86	87	82	87	67	86	81	88
5 years	81	82	77	78	78	80	72	79	50	79	70	80

BREAST (ICD-9 174-175)

EUROPE, 1985-89

Weighted analyses

COUNTRY	% COVERAGE WITH C.R.s	\ Males	YEARLY NO. OF CASES (Mean No. of cases recorded) Females	All
AUSTRIA	8	1	260	261
DENMARK	100	16	2782	2798
ENGLAND	50	96	12242	12338
ESTONIA	100	3	389	392
FINLAND	100	8	2112	2120
FRANCE	6	6	1420	1426
GERMANY	2	2	516	518
ICELAND	100	1	104	105
ITALY	10	23	3103	3126
NETHERLANDS	6	2	424	426
POLAND	6	6	705	711
SCOTLAND	100	11	2452	2463
SLOVAKIA	100	13	1136	1149
SLOVENIA	100	4	615	619
SPAIN	13	10	1464	1474
SWEDEN	17	6	785	791
SWITZERLAND	11	0	459	459

RELATIVE SURVIVAL (%) (Age-standardized)

□ 1 year ■ 5 years

OBSERVED AND RELATIVE SURVIVAL (%) BY AGE

	15-44 obs rel	45-54 obs rel	55-64 obs rel	65-74 obs rel	75-99 obs rel	ALL obs rel
Males						
1 year	100 100	83 83	86 87	89 91	70 76	82 85
3 years	90 90	72 73	76 79	81 88	42 53	66 76
5 years	85 86	65 67	68 74	67 78	25 46	57 72
Females						
1 year	96 97	95 96	93 94	90 92	80 87	91 93
3 years	84 84	83 84	79 81	76 81	59 75	76 81
5 years	74 74	74 75	70 73	65 73	44 68	65 73
Overall						
1 year	97 97	95 96	93 94	90 92	80 86	91 93
3 years	84 84	83 84	79 81	76 81	59 75	76 81
5 years	74 74	74 75	70 73	65 73	44 68	65 73

AGE STANDARDIZED RELATIVE SURVIVAL(%)

COUNTRY	MALES 1-year (95% C.I.)	5-years (95% C.I.)	FEMALES 1-year (95% C.I.)	5-years (95% C.I.)
AUSTRIA	-	-	86.5 (83.5 - 89.7)	63.2 (58.7 - 68.2)
DENMARK	95.9 (91.1 -101.0)	57.1 (43.8 - 74.4)	91.9 (91.4 - 92.4)	70.6 (69.7 - 71.6)
ENGLAND	88.1 (84.9 - 91.5)	68.4 (62.6 - 74.7)	89.5 (89.2 - 89.7)	66.7 (66.3 - 67.2)
ESTONIA	93.7 (83.7 -104.8)	52.3 (36.6 - 74.6)	86.8 (85.0 - 88.7)	59.5 (56.6 - 62.5)
FINLAND	92.7 (84.3 -101.9)	70.4 (55.7 - 88.8)	95.0 (94.5 - 95.6)	78.4 (77.4 - 79.5)
FRANCE	83.5 (71.7 - 97.2)	68.7 (57.5 - 82.2)	95.6 (95.0 - 96.3)	80.3 (78.9 - 81.8)
GERMANY	-	-	92.6 (91.4 - 93.7)	71.7 (69.5 - 74.1)
ICELAND	-	-	95.2 (92.8 - 97.6)	79.2 (74.4 - 84.4)
ITALY	83.0 (75.3 - 91.4)	63.7 (52.7 - 77.1)	94.9 (94.4 - 95.3)	76.7 (75.7 - 77.7)
NETHERLANDS	-	-	94.2 (93.0 - 95.4)	74.4 (71.9 - 77.0)
POLAND	75.5 (57.5 - 99.1)	66.4 (43.6 -101.1)	85.8 (84.0 - 87.6)	58.5 (55.9 - 61.3)
SCOTLAND	81.6 (70.2 - 94.7)	67.2 (52.7 - 85.8)	88.9 (88.3 - 89.6)	65.0 (64.0 - 66.0)
SLOVAKIA	71.2 (60.3 - 84.0)	40.0 (27.1 - 58.9)	84.8 (83.7 - 85.9)	58.3 (56.5 - 60.2)
SLOVENIA	-	-	89.6 (88.3 - 91.0)	64.2 (62.0 - 66.5)
SPAIN	88.9 (79.9 - 98.9)	84.7 (70.5 -101.9)	93.8 (92.9 - 94.6)	70.4 (68.8 - 72.1)
SWEDEN	94.6 (87.5 -102.2)	72.1 (58.2 - 89.2)	95.7 (95.0 - 96.5)	80.6 (79.0 - 82.2)
SWITZERLAND	-	-	96.6 (95.6 - 97.6)	79.6 (77.4 - 82.0)
EUROPE, 1985-89	86.4 (82.9 - 90.0)	69.3 (64.0 - 75.0)	92.7 (92.4 - 93.0)	72.5 (71.9 - 73.1)

CERVIX UTERI   (ICD-9 180)

AUSTRIA

AREA	NUMBER OF CASES Females	PERIOD	MEAN AGE Females
Tirol	164	1988-1989	51.2

OBSERVED AND RELATIVE SURVIVAL (%) BY AGE (number of cases in parentheses)

	15-44 obs rel	45-54 obs rel	55-64 obs rel	65-74 obs rel	75-99 obs rel	ALL obs rel
Females	(62)	(39)	(26)	(20)	(17)	(164)
1 year	94 94	85 85	81 81	60 61	59 63	82 83
3 years	92 92	79 80	58 59	45 48	35 44	72 74
5 years	90 91	72 73	58 59	40 44	29 43	68 72

DENMARK

AREA	NUMBER OF CASES Females	PERIOD	MEAN AGE Females
Denmark	2791	1985-1989	53.9

OBSERVED AND RELATIVE SURVIVAL (%) BY AGE (number of cases in parentheses)

	15-44 obs rel	45-54 obs rel	55-64 obs rel	65-74 obs rel	75-99 obs rel	ALL obs rel
Females	(958)	(464)	(510)	(519)	(340)	(2791)
1 year	95 95	88 88	81 82	76 78	55 59	83 84
3 years	86 87	71 72	60 62	55 60	30 38	66 70
5 years	83 83	66 67	52 56	46 52	19 29	60 65

CERVIX UTERI (ICD-9 180)

ENGLAND

AREA	NUMBER OF CASES Females	PERIOD	MEAN AGE Females	5-YR RELATIVE SURVIVAL (%) Females
East Anglia	766	1985-1989	53.3	
Mersey	1291	1985-1989	52.7	
Oxford	846	1985-1989	51.2	
South Thames	2101	1985-1989	53.0	
Wessex	1254	1985-1989	52.3	
West Midlands	2209	1985-1989	49.8	
Yorkshire	1845	1985-1989	50.9	
English Registries	10312		51.7	

OBSERVED AND RELATIVE SURVIVAL (%) BY AGE (number of cases in parentheses)

	AGE CLASS										ALL	
	15-44		45-54		55-64		65-74		75-99			
	obs	rel	obs	rel	obs	rel	obs	rel	obs	rel	obs	rel
Females	(4243)		(1589)		(1769)		(1644)		(1067)		(10312)	
1 year	93	93	87	87	83	84	72	74	51	55	83	84
3 years	82	82	71	71	65	67	52	56	28	36	67	70
5 years	78	78	65	66	56	59	43	48	20	31	61	65

ESTONIA

AREA	NUMBER OF CASES Females	PERIOD	MEAN AGE Females
Estonia	795	1985-1989	57.2

OBSERVED AND RELATIVE SURVIVAL (%) BY AGE (number of cases in parentheses)

	AGE CLASS										ALL	
	15-44		45-54		55-64		65-74		75-99			
	obs	rel	obs	rel	obs	rel	obs	rel	obs	rel	obs	rel
Females	(165)		(156)		(212)		(178)		(84)		(795)	
1 year	85	86	79	80	85	86	80	83	64	71	81	82
3 years	66	66	60	61	65	67	62	68	33	45	60	64
5 years	60	61	54	56	54	57	52	62	21	36	51	57

315

CERVIX UTERI (ICD-9 180)

FINLAND

AREA	NUMBER OF CASES Females	PERIOD	MEAN AGE Females
Finland	678	1985-1989	61.7

OBSERVED AND RELATIVE SURVIVAL (%) BY AGE (number of cases in parentheses)

Females	15-44 obs rel (121)	45-54 obs rel (92)	55-64 obs rel (123)	65-74 obs rel (170)	75-99 obs rel (172)	ALL obs rel (678)
1 year	93 93	89 89	82 83	79 81	62 67	79 81
3 years	77 77	76 77	67 69	55 58	34 43	59 63
5 years	72 72	63 64	58 60	41 47	23 36	48 55

FRANCE

AREA	NUMBER OF CASES Females	PERIOD	MEAN AGE Females
Somme	218	1985-1989	53.3
Calvados	246	1985-1989	56.4
Côte d'Or	154	1985-1989	57.3
Doubs	134	1985-1989	56.6
French Registries	752		55.7

5-YR RELATIVE SURVIVAL (%)

Females

OBSERVED AND RELATIVE SURVIVAL (%) BY AGE (number of cases in parentheses)

Females	15-44 obs rel (216)	45-54 obs rel (139)	55-64 obs rel (167)	65-74 obs rel (127)	75-99 obs rel (103)	ALL obs rel (752)
1 year	90 90	90 90	89 90	84 85	71 77	86 87
3 years	75 75	70 71	72 74	62 66	38 48	66 69
5 years	71 72	65 66	66 68	51 56	26 41	59 64

CERVIX UTERI   (ICD-9 180)

GERMANY

AREA	NUMBER OF CASES	PERIOD	MEAN AGE
	Females		Females
Saarland	429	1985-1989	56.4

OBSERVED AND RELATIVE SURVIVAL (%) BY AGE (number of cases in parentheses)

	15-44		45-54		55-64		65-74		75-99		ALL	
	obs	rel	obs	rel	obs	rel	obs	rel	obs	rel	obs	rel
Females	(114)		(78)		(92)		(86)		(59)		(429)	
1 year	92	92	81	81	86	87	87	89	59	64	83	85
3 years	79	79	55	56	65	67	64	69	32	41	62	66
5 years	77	78	54	55	58	61	55	63	26	42	57	63

ICELAND

AREA	NUMBER OF CASES	PERIOD	MEAN AGE
	Females		Females
Iceland	65	1985-1989	43.3

OBSERVED AND RELATIVE SURVIVAL (%) BY AGE (number of cases in parentheses)

	15-44		45-54		55-64		65-74		75-99		ALL	
	obs	rel	obs	rel	obs	rel	obs	rel	obs	rel	obs	rel
Females	(42)		(8)		(5)		(7)		(3)		(65)	
1 year	100	100	100	100	100	100	100	100	67	71	98	99
3 years	88	88	88	88	100	100	86	90	33	41	86	88
5 years	88	88	88	89	100	100	71	79	33	48	85	87

CERVIX UTERI   (ICD-9 180)

ITALY

AREA	NUMBER OF CASES	PERIOD	MEAN AGE	5-YR RELATIVE SURVIVAL (%)
	Females		Females	Females
Florence	317	1985-1989	59.7	
Genoa	168	1986-1988	58.4	
Latina	79	1985-1987	53.9	
Modena	59	1988-1989	57.7	
Parma	83	1985-1987	60.9	
Ragusa	100	1985-1989	57.1	
Romagna	105	1986-1988	56.5	
Turin	211	1985-1987	59.5	
Varese	196	1985-1989	57.2	
Italian Registries	1318		58.3	

OBSERVED AND RELATIVE SURVIVAL (%) BY AGE (number of cases in parentheses)

	AGE CLASS										ALL	
	15-44		45-54		55-64		65-74		75-99			
	obs	rel	obs	rel	obs	rel	obs	rel	obs	rel	obs	rel
Females	(274)		(270)		(267)		(299)		(208)		(1318)	
1 year	96	96	90	90	91	91	80	81	60	64	84	86
3 years	81	82	74	74	66	67	57	60	34	42	64	67
5 years	76	77	67	68	60	62	48	54	24	35	56	62

NETHERLANDS

AREA	NUMBER OF CASES	PERIOD	MEAN AGE
	Females		Females
Eindhoven	166	1985-1989	53.5

OBSERVED AND RELATIVE SURVIVAL (%) BY AGE (number of cases in parentheses)

	AGE CLASS										ALL	
	15-44		45-54		55-64		65-74		75-99			
	obs	rel	obs	rel	obs	rel	obs	rel	obs	rel	obs	rel
Females	(66)		(21)		(27)		(27)		(25)		(166)	
1 year	92	93	71	72	89	90	81	83	64	69	83	84
3 years	85	85	56	57	81	83	67	71	32	40	70	73
5 years	81	82	51	52	70	73	55	61	32	48	64	69

CERVIX UTERI   (ICD-9 180)

POLAND

AREA	NUMBER OF CASES Females	PERIOD	MEAN AGE Females	5-YR RELATIVE SURVIVAL (%) Females
Cracow	491	1985-1989	53.3	
Warsaw	353	1988-1989	53.4	
Polish Registries	844		53.4	

OBSERVED AND RELATIVE SURVIVAL (%) BY AGE (number of cases in parentheses)

	15-44		45-54		55-64		65-74		75-99		ALL	
	obs	rel	obs	rel	obs	rel	obs	rel	obs	rel	obs	rel
Females	(266)		(192)		(204)		(90)		(92)		(844)	
1 year	82	82	80	80	80	81	68	69	51	55	76	77
3 years	66	66	60	61	56	58	35	38	26	33	54	57
5 years	62	63	56	58	44	47	31	37	18	28	49	53

SCOTLAND

AREA	NUMBER OF CASES Females	PERIOD	MEAN AGE Females
Scotland	2093	1985-1989	52.0

OBSERVED AND RELATIVE SURVIVAL (%) BY AGE (number of cases in parentheses)

	15-44		45-54		55-64		65-74		75-99		ALL	
	obs	rel	obs	rel	obs	rel	obs	rel	obs	rel	obs	rel
Females	(805)		(350)		(402)		(333)		(203)		(2093)	
1 year	91	91	85	85	77	78	73	75	42	46	80	81
3 years	79	79	70	71	58	60	50	54	20	27	63	66
5 years	75	75	65	66	49	53	40	47	14	24	57	62

CERVIX UTERI   (ICD-9 180)

SLOVAKIA

AREA	NUMBER OF CASES Females	PERIOD	MEAN AGE Females
Slovakia	2390	1985-1989	49.8

OBSERVED AND RELATIVE SURVIVAL (%) BY AGE (number of cases in parentheses)

	AGE CLASS										ALL	
	15-44		45-54		55-64		65-74		75-99			
	obs	rel	obs	rel	obs	rel	obs	rel	obs	rel	obs	rel
Females	(1020)		(481)		(474)		(266)		(149)		(2390)	
1 year	90	90	87	87	82	83	73	75	50	55	83	84
3 years	75	75	70	71	65	67	53	58	28	38	67	69
5 years	70	71	64	66	58	62	44	52	25	42	61	65

SLOVENIA

AREA	NUMBER OF CASES Females	PERIOD	MEAN AGE Females
Slovenia	800	1985-1989	51.8

OBSERVED AND RELATIVE SURVIVAL (%) BY AGE (number of cases in parentheses)

	AGE CLASS										ALL	
	15-44		45-54		55-64		65-74		75-99			
	obs	rel	obs	rel	obs	rel	obs	rel	obs	rel	obs	rel
Females	(309)		(118)		(193)		(106)		(74)		(800)	
1 year	91	91	88	88	81	82	75	76	47	52	82	83
3 years	74	75	64	65	60	62	51	55	23	31	62	64
5 years	71	71	61	62	51	54	42	48	16	28	56	60

CERVIX UTERI   (ICD-9 180)

SPAIN

AREA	NUMBER OF CASES	PERIOD	MEAN AGE	5-YR RELATIVE SURVIVAL (%)
	Females		Females	Females
Basque Country	231	1986-1988	55.8	
Girona	99	1985-1989	56.1	
Mallorca	104	1988-1989	50.6	
Navarra	74	1985-1989	55.0	
Tarragona	148	1985-1989	56.6	
Spanish Registries	656		55.1	

OBSERVED AND RELATIVE SURVIVAL (%) BY AGE (number of cases in parentheses)

	AGE CLASS										ALL	
	15-44		45-54		55-64		65-74		75-99			
	obs	rel	obs	rel	obs	rel	obs	rel	obs	rel	obs	rel
Females	(178)		(147)		(143)		(116)		(72)		(656)	
1 year	88	88	92	92	84	84	71	72	60	64	82	83
3 years	77	77	71	72	68	69	50	52	29	37	64	66
5 years	74	74	65	66	63	65	43	48	21	31	58	62

SWEDEN

AREA	NUMBER OF CASES	PERIOD	MEAN AGE
	Females		Females
South Sweden	433	1985-1989	51.8

OBSERVED AND RELATIVE SURVIVAL (%) BY AGE (number of cases in parentheses)

	AGE CLASS										ALL	
	15-44		45-54		55-64		65-74		75-99			
	obs	rel	obs	rel	obs	rel	obs	rel	obs	rel	obs	rel
Females	(198)		(51)		(50)		(69)		(65)		(433)	
1 year	95	96	94	94	82	82	70	71	69	75	86	87
3 years	87	87	84	85	66	67	54	57	43	55	72	76
5 years	84	85	78	80	54	56	45	50	28	43	65	71

CERVIX UTERI   (ICD-9 180)

SWITZERLAND

AREA	NUMBER OF CASES	PERIOD	MEAN AGE	5-YR RELATIVE SURVIVAL (%)
	Females		Females	Females
Basel	74	1985-1988	55.6	
Geneva	107	1985-1989	56.8	
Swiss Registries	181		56.3	

OBSERVED AND RELATIVE SURVIVAL (%) BY AGE (number of cases in parentheses)

	AGE CLASS										ALL	
	15-44		45-54		55-64		65-74		75-99			
	obs	rel	obs	rel	obs	rel	obs	rel	obs	rel	obs	rel
Females	(53)		(31)		(40)		(27)		(30)		(181)	
1 year	94	94	94	94	90	90	85	87	73	78	88	90
3 years	77	77	80	81	71	73	52	55	47	56	67	70
5 years	75	75	77	78	55	57	52	57	40	56	61	66

CERVIX UTERI (ICD-9 180)

EUROPE, 1985-89
Weighted analyses

COUNTRY	% COVERAGE WITH C.R.s	YEARLY NO. OF CASES (Mean No. of cases recorded) Females	RELATIVE SURVIVAL (%) (Age-standardized) Females
AUSTRIA	8	82	A
DENMARK	100	558	DK
ENGLAND	50	2062	ENG
ESTONIA	100	159	EST
FINLAND	100	136	FIN
FRANCE	4	150	F
GERMANY	2	86	D
ICELAND	100	13	IS
ITALY	10	367	I
NETHERLANDS	6	33	NL
POLAND	6	275	PL
SCOTLAND	100	419	SCO
SLOVAKIA	100	478	SK
SLOVENIA	100	160	SLO
SPAIN	11	193	E
SWEDEN	17	87	S
SWITZERLAND	11	40	CH
			EUR

□ 1 year ■ 5 years

OBSERVED AND RELATIVE SURVIVAL (%) BY AGE

	AGE CLASS										ALL	
	15-44		45-54		55-64		65-74		75-99			
	obs	rel	obs	rel	obs	rel	obs	rel	obs	rel	obs	rel
Females												
1 year	91	91	85	86	85	86	77	78	58	63	82	84
3 years	78	78	67	67	65	66	54	57	32	40	63	66
5 years	74	75	62	63	57	60	46	52	23	36	57	62

AGE STANDARDIZED RELATIVE SURVIVAL(%) FEMALES

COUNTRY	1-year (95% C.I.)	5-years (95% C.I.)
AUSTRIA	81.0 (75.1 - 87.4)	68.7 (61.8 - 76.5)
DENMARK	84.5 (83.2 - 85.8)	64.2 (62.4 - 66.0)
ENGLAND	82.8 (82.1 - 83.6)	62.6 (61.6 - 63.6)
ESTONIA	82.5 (79.6 - 85.4)	56.8 (53.0 - 61.0)
FINLAND	85.7 (83.0 - 88.4)	60.4 (56.3 - 64.7)
FRANCE	87.7 (85.3 - 90.2)	64.1 (60.4 - 68.0)
GERMANY	85.6 (82.3 - 89.0)	64.1 (59.3 - 69.3)
ICELAND	96.8 (90.7 -103.3)	84.7 (73.6 - 97.3)
ITALY	88.1 (86.5 - 89.8)	64.0 (61.3 - 66.8)
NETHERLANDS	84.2 (78.7 - 90.1)	67.8 (60.5 - 76.0)
POLAND	76.4 (73.4 - 79.5)	51.0 (47.5 - 54.8)
SCOTLAND	79.9 (78.2 - 81.6)	59.0 (56.9 - 61.2)
SLOVAKIA	81.9 (80.2 - 83.6)	62.0 (59.6 - 64.4)
SLOVENIA	82.0 (79.3 - 84.8)	57.9 (54.3 - 61.7)
SPAIN	82.6 (79.6 - 85.6)	61.8 (58.0 - 66.0)
SWEDEN	86.5 (83.1 - 89.9)	68.0 (63.4 - 72.9)
SWITZERLAND	90.4 (86.1 - 94.8)	67.2 (60.2 - 75.1)
EUROPE, 1985-89	83.8 (82.9 - 84.8)	61.8 (60.4 - 63.1)

CORPUS UTERI (ICD-9 182)

AUSTRIA

AREA	NUMBER OF CASES	PERIOD	MEAN AGE
	Females		Females
Tirol	114	1988-1989	64.6

OBSERVED AND RELATIVE SURVIVAL (%) BY AGE (number of cases in parentheses)

	AGE CLASS										ALL	
	15-44		45-54		55-64		65-74		75-99			
	obs	rel	obs	rel	obs	rel	obs	rel	obs	rel	obs	rel
Females	(5)		(15)		(40)		(27)		(27)		(114)	
1 year	100	100	100	100	95	96	81	83	63	67	85	87
3 years	100	100	100	100	90	92	74	78	44	53	77	82
5 years	100	100	87	88	88	90	70	76	44	62	74	82

DENMARK

AREA	NUMBER OF CASES	PERIOD	MEAN AGE
	Females		Females
Denmark	3092	1985-1989	65.4

OBSERVED AND RELATIVE SURVIVAL (%) BY AGE (number of cases in parentheses)

	AGE CLASS										ALL	
	15-44		45-54		55-64		65-74		75-99			
	obs	rel	obs	rel	obs	rel	obs	rel	obs	rel	obs	rel
Females	(85)		(344)		(980)		(1100)		(583)		(3092)	
1 year	99	99	96	97	90	91	89	90	70	76	87	89
3 years	93	93	90	91	81	84	75	80	48	60	74	80
5 years	89	90	85	88	77	82	66	75	36	54	66	76

CORPUS UTERI (ICD-9 182)

ENGLAND

AREA	NUMBER OF CASES Females	PERIOD	MEAN AGE Females
East Anglia	861	1985-1989	65.6
Mersey	844	1985-1989	64.3
Oxford	1008	1985-1989	65.1
South Thames	2302	1985-1989	65.6
Wessex	1167	1985-1989	65.5
West Midlands	1799	1985-1989	65.2
Yorkshire	1151	1985-1989	65.7
English Registries	9132		65.3

5-YR RELATIVE SURVIVAL (%) Females

OBSERVED AND RELATIVE SURVIVAL (%) BY AGE (number of cases in parentheses)

	15-44 obs rel (364)	45-54 obs rel (1286)	55-64 obs rel (2685)	65-74 obs rel (2635)	75-99 obs rel (2162)	ALL obs rel (9132)
Females 1 year	94 94	94 95	90 91	82 83	66 71	83 85
3 years	87 88	88 89	81 83	68 73	44 56	70 76
5 years	85 85	86 87	76 80	60 68	35 54	64 73

ESTONIA

AREA	NUMBER OF CASES Females	PERIOD	MEAN AGE Females
Estonia	753	1985-1989	61.6

OBSERVED AND RELATIVE SURVIVAL (%) BY AGE (number of cases in parentheses)

	15-44 obs rel (43)	45-54 obs rel (154)	55-64 obs rel (263)	65-74 obs rel (176)	75-99 obs rel (117)	ALL obs rel (753)
Females 1 year	91 91	90 90	90 91	81 84	55 59	82 84
3 years	79 80	82 84	75 78	65 72	32 41	68 73
5 years	79 80	79 81	69 74	54 65	23 38	61 70

CORPUS UTERI (ICD-9 182)

FINLAND

AREA	NUMBER OF CASES	PERIOD	MEAN AGE
	Females		Females
Finland	2289	1985-1989	65.0

OBSERVED AND RELATIVE SURVIVAL (%) BY AGE (number of cases in parentheses)

	15-44		45-54		55-64		65-74		75-99		ALL	
	obs	rel	obs	rel	obs	rel	obs	rel	obs	rel	obs	rel
Females	(88)		(340)		(667)		(694)		(500)		(2289)	
1 year	97	97	97	97	94	95	88	90	67	73	87	89
3 years	97	97	90	91	84	86	75	80	40	52	73	79
5 years	95	96	87	89	80	83	68	76	31	50	67	77

FRANCE

AREA	NUMBER OF CASES	PERIOD	MEAN AGE
	Females		Females
Somme	194	1985-1989	64.6
Calvados	225	1985-1989	65.2
Côte d'Or	182	1985-1989	66.6
Doubs	147	1985-1989	65.8
French Registries	748		65.5

5-YR RELATIVE SURVIVAL (%)

Females

OBSERVED AND RELATIVE SURVIVAL (%) BY AGE (number of cases in parentheses)

	15-44		45-54		55-64		65-74		75-99		ALL	
	obs	rel	obs	rel	obs	rel	obs	rel	obs	rel	obs	rel
Females	(25)		(91)		(241)		(213)		(178)		(748)	
1 year	96	96	98	98	93	94	88	89	78	83	89	90
3 years	91	91	88	88	83	85	70	74	51	63	73	78
5 years	91	92	85	86	77	80	62	68	44	63	67	75

CORPUS UTERI (ICD-9 182)

GERMANY

AREA	NUMBER OF CASES Females	PERIOD	MEAN AGE Females
Saarland	646	1985-1989	66.1

OBSERVED AND RELATIVE SURVIVAL (%) BY AGE (number of cases in parentheses)

	AGE CLASS										ALL	
	15-44		45-54		55-64		65-74		75-99			
	obs	rel	obs	rel	obs	rel	obs	rel	obs	rel	obs	rel
Females	(18)		(70)		(191)		(209)		(158)		(646)	
1 year	89	89	93	93	88	89	83	85	76	81	84	86
3 years	89	89	87	88	79	81	69	74	51	63	70	76
5 years	83	83	84	85	73	77	59	67	42	64	62	73

ICELAND

AREA	NUMBER OF CASES Females	PERIOD	MEAN AGE Females
Iceland	78	1985-1989	62.5

OBSERVED AND RELATIVE SURVIVAL (%) BY AGE (number of cases in parentheses)

	AGE CLASS										ALL	
	15-44		45-54		55-64		65-74		75-99			
	obs	rel	obs	rel	obs	rel	obs	rel	obs	rel	obs	rel
Females	(6)		(16)		(26)		(12)		(18)		(78)	
1 year	100	100	100	100	85	85	92	93	72	78	87	89
3 years	67	67	94	95	77	79	83	88	39	50	72	77
5 years	67	67	88	89	77	80	83	92	28	43	68	77

CORPUS UTERI   (ICD-9 182)

ITALY

AREA	NUMBER OF CASES	PERIOD	MEAN AGE	5-YR RELATIVE SURVIVAL (%)
	Females		Females	Females
Florence	670	1985-1989	63.3	
Genoa	215	1986-1988	65.6	
Latina	86	1985-1987	61.7	
Modena	130	1988-1989	64.2	
Parma	152	1985-1987	64.5	
Ragusa	145	1985-1989	63.2	
Romagna	143	1986-1988	64.2	
Turin	297	1985-1987	63.1	
Varese	438	1985-1989	63.8	
Italian Registries	2276		63.7	

OBSERVED AND RELATIVE SURVIVAL (%) BY AGE (number of cases in parentheses)

	15-44		45-54		55-64		65-74		75-99		ALL	
	obs	rel	obs	rel	obs	rel	obs	rel	obs	rel	obs	rel
Females	(73)		(410)		(746)		(629)		(418)		(2276)	
1 year	97	97	93	93	91	91	89	90	72	76	87	89
3 years	93	93	85	86	80	81	74	78	43	53	73	77
5 years	92	92	82	84	75	78	67	74	35	51	68	75

NETHERLANDS

AREA	NUMBER OF CASES	PERIOD	MEAN AGE
	Females		Females
Eindhoven	300	1985-1989	62.7

OBSERVED AND RELATIVE SURVIVAL (%) BY AGE (number of cases in parentheses)

	15-44		45-54		55-64		65-74		75-99		ALL	
	obs	rel	obs	rel	obs	rel	obs	rel	obs	rel	obs	rel
Females	(10)		(66)		(103)		(73)		(48)		(300)	
1 year	100	100	98	99	94	95	92	93	81	88	93	94
3 years	100	100	94	95	86	88	75	80	56	72	81	86
5 years	100	100	94	96	82	85	73	81	48	74	77	86

CORPUS UTERI (ICD-9 182)

POLAND

AREA	NUMBER OF CASES	PERIOD	MEAN AGE	5-YR RELATIVE SURVIVAL (%)
	Females		Females	Females
Cracow	301	1985-1989	60.4	
Warsaw	307	1988-1989	61.9	
Polish Registries	608		61.2	

OBSERVED AND RELATIVE SURVIVAL (%) BY AGE (number of cases in parentheses)

	15-44		45-54		55-64		65-74		75-99		ALL	
	obs	rel	obs	rel	obs	rel	obs	rel	obs	rel	obs	rel
Females	(26)		(130)		(245)		(139)		(68)		(608)	
1 year	96	96	88	89	88	89	81	83	55	61	83	85
3 years	81	81	83	84	77	80	60	66	34	45	70	75
5 years	81	82	78	80	71	76	54	65	24	38	64	72

SCOTLAND

AREA	NUMBER OF CASES	PERIOD	MEAN AGE
	Females		Females
Scotland	1548	1985-1989	64.3

OBSERVED AND RELATIVE SURVIVAL (%) BY AGE (number of cases in parentheses)

	15-44		45-54		55-64		65-74		75-99		ALL	
	obs	rel	obs	rel	obs	rel	obs	rel	obs	rel	obs	rel
Females	(67)		(271)		(463)		(408)		(339)		(1548)	
1 year	94	94	94	95	91	92	82	84	60	66	83	85
3 years	88	88	89	90	80	83	64	70	39	51	69	75
5 years	81	81	87	89	74	79	56	66	27	45	62	72

CORPUS UTERI (ICD-9 182)

SLOVAKIA

AREA	NUMBER OF CASES	PERIOD	MEAN AGE
	Females		Females
Slovakia	2371	1985-1989	60.5

OBSERVED AND RELATIVE SURVIVAL (%) BY AGE (number of cases in parentheses)

	AGE CLASS										ALL	
	15-44		45-54		55-64		65-74		75-99			
	obs	rel	obs	rel	obs	rel	obs	rel	obs	rel	obs	rel
Females	(152)		(536)		(882)		(531)		(270)		(2371)	
1 year	93	93	94	94	89	90	80	83	64	70	86	88
3 years	91	91	87	88	76	79	63	69	38	51	72	77
5 years	87	88	85	87	70	74	54	64	30	51	66	75

SLOVENIA

AREA	NUMBER OF CASES	PERIOD	MEAN AGE
	Females		Females
Slovenia	917	1985-1989	62.5

OBSERVED AND RELATIVE SURVIVAL (%) BY AGE (number of cases in parentheses)

	AGE CLASS										ALL	
	15-44		45-54		55-64		65-74		75-99			
	obs	rel	obs	rel	obs	rel	obs	rel	obs	rel	obs	rel
Females	(28)		(179)		(351)		(223)		(136)		(917)	
1 year	96	97	94	94	93	94	85	87	63	68	87	89
3 years	93	93	90	91	83	86	65	70	43	57	74	80
5 years	93	94	85	88	79	83	55	63	32	54	68	77

CORPUS UTERI (ICD-9 182)

SPAIN

AREA	NUMBER OF CASES	PERIOD	MEAN AGE
	Females		Females
Basque Country	388	1986-1988	61.8
Girona	171	1985-1989	62.5
Mallorca	105	1988-1989	63.2
Navarra	202	1985-1989	62.3
Tarragona	231	1985-1989	61.8
Spanish Registries	1097		62.2

5-YR RELATIVE SURVIVAL (%)

Females

OBSERVED AND RELATIVE SURVIVAL (%) BY AGE (number of cases in parentheses)

	AGE CLASS										ALL	
	15-44		45-54		55-64		65-74		75-99			
	obs	rel	obs	rel	obs	rel	obs	rel	obs	rel	obs	rel
Females	(64)		(176)		(429)		(275)		(153)		(1097)	
1 year	98	99	94	94	92	92	84	86	73	77	88	89
3 years	97	97	88	89	80	81	69	73	46	57	75	78
5 years	97	97	86	87	76	78	63	69	37	55	70	76

SWEDEN

AREA	NUMBER OF CASES	PERIOD	MEAN AGE
	Females		Females
South Sweden	705	1985-1989	64.4

OBSERVED AND RELATIVE SURVIVAL (%) BY AGE (number of cases in parentheses)

	AGE CLASS										ALL	
	15-44		45-54		55-64		65-74		75-99			
	obs	rel	obs	rel	obs	rel	obs	rel	obs	rel	obs	rel
Females	(21)		(120)		(209)		(224)		(131)		(705)	
1 year	95	95	99	99	97	98	92	94	79	84	92	94
3 years	95	96	98	98	89	90	81	85	56	70	82	87
5 years	90	91	97	98	84	87	75	82	40	60	75	84

CORPUS UTERI   (ICD-9 182)

SWITZERLAND

AREA	NUMBER OF CASES Females	PERIOD	MEAN AGE Females	5-YR RELATIVE SURVIVAL (%) Females
Basel	219	1985-1988	67.2	
Geneva	217	1985-1989	66.3	
Swiss Registries	436		66.7	

OBSERVED AND RELATIVE SURVIVAL (%) BY AGE (number of cases in parentheses)

	AGE CLASS										ALL	
	15-44 obs rel		45-54 obs rel		55-64 obs rel		65-74 obs rel		75-99 obs rel		obs rel	
Females	(8)		(47)		(141)		(123)		(117)		(436)	
1 year	75	75	98	98	95	96	87	88	68	73	86	88
3 years	75	75	89	90	85	87	77	81	45	56	72	78
5 years	75	75	89	91	81	84	72	80	33	50	66	76

CORPUS UTERI   (ICD-9 182)

EUROPE, 1985-89
Weighted analyses

COUNTRY	% COVERAGE WITH C.R.s	YEARLY NO. OF CASES (Mean No. of cases recorded) Females
AUSTRIA	8	57
DENMARK	100	618
ENGLAND	50	1826
ESTONIA	100	151
FINLAND	100	458
FRANCE	4	150
GERMANY	2	129
ICELAND	100	16
ITALY	10	613
NETHERLANDS	6	60
POLAND	6	214
SCOTLAND	100	310
SLOVAKIA	100	474
SLOVENIA	100	183
SPAIN	11	303
SWEDEN	17	141
SWITZERLAND	11	98

RELATIVE SURVIVAL (%) (Age-standardized) Females

□ 1 year   ■ 5 years

OBSERVED AND RELATIVE SURVIVAL (%) BY AGE

	AGE CLASS										ALL	
	15-44 obs rel		45-54 obs rel		55-64 obs rel		65-74 obs rel		75-99 obs rel		obs	rel
Females												
1 year	94	94	94	94	91	91	85	87	71	76	86	88
3 years	90	90	88	88	80	82	70	75	46	57	72	77
5 years	88	88	84	86	76	79	62	70	37	56	66	75

AGE STANDARDIZED RELATIVE SURVIVAL(%) FEMALES

COUNTRY	1-year (95% C.I.)	5-years (95% C.I.)
AUSTRIA	86.9 (81.0 - 93.3)	80.7 (72.5 - 89.8)
DENMARK	89.0 (87.8 - 90.2)	75.6 (73.7 - 77.4)
ENGLAND	85.5 (84.8 - 86.3)	72.9 (71.8 - 74.0)
ESTONIA	82.3 (79.4 - 85.3)	65.4 (61.4 - 69.7)
FINLAND	89.4 (88.1 - 90.7)	75.9 (73.8 - 78.0)
FRANCE	90.9 (88.7 - 93.1)	74.7 (70.8 - 78.7)
GERMANY	87.0 (84.3 - 89.8)	73.0 (68.9 - 77.4)
ICELAND	88.9 (81.5 - 97.0)	76.9 (66.6 - 88.9)
ITALY	88.6 (87.2 - 90.0)	72.9 (70.8 - 75.0)
NETHERLANDS	93.8 (90.5 - 97.3)	83.7 (77.9 - 90.0)
POLAND	81.8 (78.3 - 85.5)	66.0 (61.3 - 71.1)
SCOTLAND	85.1 (83.3 - 87.0)	70.2 (67.5 - 73.0)
SLOVAKIA	84.8 (83.1 - 86.6)	69.3 (66.6 - 72.0)
SLOVENIA	87.0 (84.6 - 89.5)	72.7 (69.0 - 76.6)
SPAIN	87.9 (85.7 - 90.1)	73.0 (69.7 - 76.4)
SWEDEN	94.1 (92.1 - 96.1)	82.2 (78.7 - 85.9)
SWITZERLAND	88.6 (85.6 - 91.7)	76.6 (72.1 - 81.4)
EUROPE, 1985-89	87.6 (86.7 - 88.4)	73.2 (71.9 - 74.6)

OVARY (ICD-9 183)

AUSTRIA

AREA	NUMBER OF CASES Females	PERIOD	MEAN AGE Females
Tirol	119	1988-1989	64.0

OBSERVED AND RELATIVE SURVIVAL (%) BY AGE (number of cases in parentheses)

	AGE CLASS										ALL	
	15-44		45-54		55-64		65-74		75-99			
	obs	rel	obs	rel	obs	rel	obs	rel	obs	rel	obs	rel
Females	(11)		(16)		(25)		(40)		(27)		(119)	
1 year	100	100	81	81	76	76	43	43	56	59	63	64
3 years	91	91	50	50	44	45	30	32	37	45	43	46
5 years	82	82	44	44	44	45	18	19	37	52	37	41

DENMARK

AREA	NUMBER OF CASES Females	PERIOD	MEAN AGE Females
Denmark	2926	1985-1989	62.6

OBSERVED AND RELATIVE SURVIVAL (%) BY AGE (number of cases in parentheses)

	AGE CLASS										ALL	
	15-44		45-54		55-64		65-74		75-99			
	obs	rel	obs	rel	obs	rel	obs	rel	obs	rel	obs	rel
Females	(324)		(469)		(726)		(777)		(630)		(2926)	
1 year	90	90	81	81	71	71	54	55	33	36	62	63
3 years	71	71	47	48	36	37	27	29	17	21	35	38
5 years	65	65	37	38	28	30	20	23	10	16	28	32

OVARY   (ICD-9 183)

ENGLAND

AREA	NUMBER OF CASES Females	PERIOD	MEAN AGE Females
East Anglia	990	1985-1989	62.7
Mersey	1057	1985-1989	62.7
Oxford	1140	1985-1989	61.7
South Thames	2885	1985-1989	63.4
Wessex	1433	1985-1989	63.8
West Midlands	2465	1985-1989	62.5
Yorkshire	1503	1985-1989	62.3
English Registries	11473		62.8

5-YR RELATIVE SURVIVAL (%)
Females

OBSERVED AND RELATIVE SURVIVAL (%) BY AGE (number of cases in parentheses)

Females	15-44 obs rel (1241)		45-54 obs rel (1823)		55-64 obs rel (2836)		65-74 obs rel (3044)		75-99 obs rel (2529)		ALL obs rel (11473)	
1 year	84	84	75	75	60	60	46	47	29	32	54	56
3 years	67	67	47	48	35	36	24	26	15	20	33	36
5 years	61	62	39	40	29	30	19	21	11	16	27	31

ESTONIA

AREA	NUMBER OF CASES Females	PERIOD	MEAN AGE Females
Estonia	740	1985-1989	60.3

OBSERVED AND RELATIVE SURVIVAL (%) BY AGE (number of cases in parentheses)

Females	15-44 obs rel (97)		45-54 obs rel (141)		55-64 obs rel (213)		65-74 obs rel (168)		75-99 obs rel (121)		ALL obs rel (740)	
1 year	77	77	75	76	57	57	49	50	26	28	56	58
3 years	56	57	40	40	31	32	21	23	16	21	31	34
5 years	50	51	30	31	22	23	15	18	11	18	24	27

OVARY

(ICD-9 183)

FINLAND

AREA	NUMBER OF CASES	PERIOD	MEAN AGE
	Females		Females
Finland	1861	1985-1989	61.8

OBSERVED AND RELATIVE SURVIVAL (%) BY AGE (number of cases in parentheses)

	AGE CLASS						ALL
	15-44	45-54	55-64	65-74	75-99		
	obs rel	obs rel	obs rel	obs rel	obs rel		obs rel
Females	(240)	(292)	(496)	(452)	(381)		(1861)
1 year	87 87	83 83	73 74	61 62	38 41		66 68
3 years	72 73	60 61	42 43	32 34	19 24		42 45
5 years	69 70	48 49	33 34	23 26	12 19		33 38

FRANCE

AREA	NUMBER OF CASES	PERIOD	MEAN AGE
	Females		Females
Somme	190	1985-1989	62.6
Calvados	197	1985-1989	60.0
Côte d'Or	178	1985-1989	62.1
Doubs	142	1985-1989	60.3
French Registries	707		61.3

5-YR RELATIVE SURVIVAL (%)

Females

0 20 40 60 80 100

Somme
Calvad
Côte d
Doubs

OBSERVED AND RELATIVE SURVIVAL (%) BY AGE (number of cases in parentheses)

	AGE CLASS						ALL
	15-44	45-54	55-64	65-74	75-99		
	obs rel	obs rel	obs rel	obs rel	obs rel		obs rel
Females	(83)	(122)	(194)	(167)	(141)		(707)
1 year	82 82	86 86	83 84	63 64	53 56		73 74
3 years	70 71	50 50	46 47	32 34	26 32		43 45
5 years	65 65	42 43	39 40	21 23	20 29		35 38

OVARY (ICD-9 183)

GERMANY

AREA	NUMBER OF CASES Females	PERIOD	MEAN AGE Females
Saarland	408	1985-1989	62.9

OBSERVED AND RELATIVE SURVIVAL (%) BY AGE (number of cases in parentheses)

	AGE CLASS										ALL	
	15-44 obs rel		45-54 obs rel		55-64 obs rel		65-74 obs rel		75-99 obs rel		obs rel	
Females	(31)		(74)		(103)		(107)		(93)		(408)	
1 year	90	90	82	83	62	63	44	45	35	38	57	58
3 years	68	68	62	63	43	44	23	25	23	29	38	42
5 years	68	68	53	53	35	37	10	11	11	18	29	33

ICELAND

AREA	NUMBER OF CASES Females	PERIOD	MEAN AGE Females
Iceland	85	1985-1989	62.4

OBSERVED AND RELATIVE SURVIVAL (%) BY AGE (number of cases in parentheses)

	AGE CLASS										ALL	
	15-44 obs rel		45-54 obs rel		55-64 obs rel		65-74 obs rel		75-99 obs rel		obs rel	
Females	(12)		(8)		(25)		(21)		(19)		(85)	
1 year	92	92	75	75	68	68	57	58	47	51	65	66
3 years	92	92	50	51	24	25	33	36	32	40	40	43
5 years	92	92	38	38	20	21	19	22	21	32	32	36

<h1 style="text-align:center">OVARY</h1> (ICD-9 183)

ITALY

AREA	NUMBER OF CASES Females	PERIOD	MEAN AGE Females	5-YR RELATIVE SURVIVAL (%) Females
Florence	447	1985-1989	59.9	
Genoa	209	1986-1988	63.3	
Latina	50	1985-1987	59.5	
Modena	127	1988-1989	63.7	
Parma	130	1985-1987	62.1	
Ragusa	76	1985-1989	62.4	
Romagna	111	1986-1988	58.6	
Turin	236	1985-1987	62.6	
Varese	299	1985-1989	60.0	
Italian Registries	1685		61.2	

OBSERVED AND RELATIVE SURVIVAL (%) BY AGE (number of cases in parentheses)

	15-44		45-54		55-64		65-74		75-99		ALL	
	obs	rel	obs	rel	obs	rel	obs	rel	obs	rel	obs	rel
Females	(202)		(325)		(452)		(382)		(324)		(1685)	
1 year	81	81	79	79	74	74	56	56	32	34	63	65
3 years	65	65	54	55	41	42	26	28	15	19	38	40
5 years	59	60	44	45	33	34	18	20	9	14	30	34

NETHERLANDS

AREA	NUMBER OF CASES Females	PERIOD	MEAN AGE Females
Eindhoven	260	1985-1989	58.5

OBSERVED AND RELATIVE SURVIVAL (%) BY AGE (number of cases in parentheses)

	15-44		45-54		55-64		65-74		75-99		ALL	
	obs	rel	obs	rel	obs	rel	obs	rel	obs	rel	obs	rel
Females	(38)		(56)		(69)		(67)		(30)		(260)	
1 year	95	95	73	73	70	70	55	56	20	21	65	66
3 years	79	79	52	52	33	34	33	35	7	8	41	43
5 years	73	73	39	40	25	25	22	25	7	10	32	35

OVARY

(ICD-9 183)

POLAND

AREA	NUMBER OF CASES	PERIOD	MEAN AGE
	Females		Females
Cracow	317	1985-1989	57.1
Warsaw	293	1988-1989	59.1
Polish Registries	610		58.1

5-YR RELATIVE SURVIVAL (%)

Females

OBSERVED AND RELATIVE SURVIVAL (%) BY AGE (number of cases in parentheses)

	AGE CLASS									ALL	
	15-44		45-54		55-64		65-74		75-99			
	obs	rel	obs	rel	obs	rel	obs	rel	obs	rel	obs	rel
Females	(93)		(142)		(184)		(109)		(82)		(610)	
1 year	75	75	74	74	59	59	42	43	20	22	57	58
3 years	55	56	44	44	34	36	16	18	10	13	33	36
5 years	51	51	36	37	27	28	13	15	4	6	27	30

SCOTLAND

AREA	NUMBER OF CASES	PERIOD	MEAN AGE
	Females		Females
Scotland	2470	1985-1989	63.2

OBSERVED AND RELATIVE SURVIVAL (%) BY AGE (number of cases in parentheses)

	AGE CLASS									ALL	
	15-44		45-54		55-64		65-74		75-99			
	obs	rel	obs	rel	obs	rel	obs	rel	obs	rel	obs	rel
Females	(254)		(366)		(609)		(676)		(565)		(2470)	
1 year	88	88	72	73	60	61	45	47	21	23	52	53
3 years	69	70	47	48	34	36	23	26	9	12	31	34
5 years	63	64	38	39	28	30	18	21	7	11	25	30

OVARY

(ICD-9 183)

SLOVAKIA

AREA	NUMBER OF CASES	PERIOD	MEAN AGE
	Females		Females
Slovakia	1493	1985-1989	56.0

OBSERVED AND RELATIVE SURVIVAL (%) BY AGE (number of cases in parentheses)

	15-44		45-54		55-64		65-74		75-99		ALL	
	obs	rel	obs	rel	obs	rel	obs	rel	obs	rel	obs	rel
Females	(291)		(359)		(431)		(266)		(146)		(1493)	
1 year	82	82	71	71	54	55	43	44	27	30	59	60
3 years	63	63	43	44	30	31	22	24	15	20	37	39
5 years	57	58	36	37	24	26	19	22	11	18	31	34

SLOVENIA

AREA	NUMBER OF CASES	PERIOD	MEAN AGE
	Females		Females
Slovenia	685	1985-1989	59.9

OBSERVED AND RELATIVE SURVIVAL (%) BY AGE (number of cases in parentheses)

	15-44		45-54		55-64		65-74		75-99		ALL	
	obs	rel	obs	rel	obs	rel	obs	rel	obs	rel	obs	rel
Females	(77)		(152)		(212)		(144)		(100)		(685)	
1 year	82	82	80	80	65	66	48	50	22	24	60	62
3 years	66	67	53	54	29	30	21	23	9	11	34	36
5 years	56	56	41	42	22	24	15	17	4	7	26	29

OVARY

(ICD-9 183)

SPAIN

AREA	NUMBER OF CASES	PERIOD	MEAN AGE
	Females		Females
Basque Country	256	1986-1988	56.2
Girona	120	1985-1989	61.5
Mallorca	52	1988-1989	57.5
Navarra	150	1985-1989	59.3
Tarragona	139	1985-1989	61.0
Spanish Registries	717		58.8

5-YR RELATIVE SURVIVAL (%)

Females

OBSERVED AND RELATIVE SURVIVAL (%) BY AGE (number of cases in parentheses)

	15-44		45-54		55-64		65-74		75-99		ALL	
	obs	rel	obs	rel	obs	rel	obs	rel	obs	rel	obs	rel
Females	(121)		(124)		(195)		(172)		(105)		(717)	
1 year	90	90	77	77	72	72	59	60	42	45	68	69
3 years	82	82	54	54	44	45	35	37	28	34	48	50
5 years	76	77	47	48	35	36	30	33	20	28	41	44

SWEDEN

AREA	NUMBER OF CASES	PERIOD	MEAN AGE
	Females		Females
South Sweden	837	1985-1989	63.1

OBSERVED AND RELATIVE SURVIVAL (%) BY AGE (number of cases in parentheses)

	15-44		45-54		55-64		65-74		75-99		ALL	
	obs	rel	obs	rel	obs	rel	obs	rel	obs	rel	obs	rel
Females	(83)		(127)		(214)		(244)		(169)		(837)	
1 year	92	92	86	86	85	85	66	67	42	45	71	73
3 years	77	77	67	68	57	59	35	37	23	29	47	51
5 years	77	78	56	57	48	50	31	34	14	22	40	45

OVARY

(ICD-9 183)

SWITZERLAND

AREA	NUMBER OF CASES Females	PERIOD	MEAN AGE Females
Basel	169	1985-1988	63.0
Geneva	182	1985-1989	62.8
Swiss Registries	351		62.9

5-YR RELATIVE SURVIVAL (%)
Females

OBSERVED AND RELATIVE SURVIVAL (%) BY AGE (number of cases in parentheses)

Females	AGE CLASS 15-44 obs rel (37)		45-54 obs rel (59)		55-64 obs rel (88)		65-74 obs rel (81)		75-99 obs rel (86)		ALL obs rel (351)	
1 year	92	92	90	90	78	79	56	57	43	46	68	69
3 years	77	77	64	65	52	53	29	30	20	24	43	46
5 years	77	77	54	55	43	45	20	22	16	24	36	41

OVARY

EUROPE, 1985-89

Weighted analyses

COUNTRY	% COVERAGE WITH C.R.s	YEARLY NO. OF CASES (Mean No. of cases recorded) Females	RELATIVE SURVIVAL (%) (Age-standardized) Females
AUSTRIA	8	60	A
DENMARK	100	585	DK
ENGLAND	50	2295	ENG
ESTONIA	100	148	EST
FINLAND	100	372	FIN
FRANCE	4	141	F
GERMANY	2	82	D
ICELAND	100	17	IS
ITALY	10	473	I
NETHERLANDS	6	52	NL
POLAND	6	210	PL
SCOTLAND	100	494	SCO
SLOVAKIA	100	299	SK
SLOVENIA	100	137	SLO
SPAIN	11	193	E
SWEDEN	17	167	S
SWITZERLAND	11	79	CH
			EUR

□ 1 year   ■ 5 years

OBSERVED AND RELATIVE SURVIVAL (%) BY AGE

	AGE CLASS										ALL	
	15-44		45-54		55-64		65-74		75-99			
	obs	rel	obs	rel	obs	rel	obs	rel	obs	rel	obs	rel
Females												
1 year	85	85	79	80	69	69	51	52	35	37	62	63
3 years	68	69	53	53	41	42	26	28	19	23	38	41
5 years	64	65	44	45	33	35	18	20	12	18	31	35

AGE STANDARDIZED RELATIVE SURVIVAL(%) FEMALES

COUNTRY	1-year (95% C.I.)	5-years (95% C.I.)
AUSTRIA	68.1 (60.7 - 76.4)	44.3 (35.8 - 54.8)
DENMARK	63.8 (62.2 - 65.5)	30.8 (29.1 - 32.5)
ENGLAND	56.4 (55.5 - 57.3)	30.6 (29.7 - 31.4)
ESTONIA	55.1 (51.7 - 58.7)	25.6 (22.4 - 29.2)
FINLAND	67.2 (65.1 - 69.3)	35.8 (33.6 - 38.1)
FRANCE	73.5 (70.2 - 76.9)	37.0 (33.2 - 41.4)
GERMANY	59.8 (55.5 - 64.5)	33.0 (28.7 - 38.1)
ICELAND	66.2 (56.7 - 77.3)	34.5 (25.5 - 46.7)
ITALY	63.2 (61.0 - 65.5)	31.2 (29.0 - 33.5)
NETHERLANDS	60.2 (54.9 - 66.1)	30.1 (25.1 - 36.1)
POLAND	52.0 (48.2 - 56.1)	24.5 (21.3 - 28.2)
SCOTLAND	54.7 (52.9 - 56.6)	29.4 (27.6 - 31.3)
SLOVAKIA	53.1 (50.4 - 55.8)	29.0 (26.4 - 31.9)
SLOVENIA	57.5 (54.0 - 61.2)	25.6 (22.5 - 29.1)
SPAIN	66.6 (63.2 - 70.2)	40.6 (36.9 - 44.8)
SWEDEN	73.3 (70.5 - 76.2)	44.5 (41.2 - 48.1)
SWITZERLAND	70.1 (65.7 - 74.8)	40.1 (35.3 - 45.7)
EUROPE, 1985-89	62.1 (60.9 - 63.2)	32.9 (31.7 - 34.1)

VAGINA & VULVA (ICD-9 184)

AUSTRIA

AREA	NUMBER OF CASES	PERIOD	MEAN AGE
	Females		Females
Tirol	24	1988-1989	69.2

OBSERVED AND RELATIVE SURVIVAL (%) BY AGE (number of cases in parentheses)

	AGE CLASS						ALL	
	15-44		45-54		55-64		65-74		75-99			
	obs rel		obs rel		obs rel		obs rel		obs rel		obs rel	
Females	(3)		(2)		(2)		(5)		(12)		(24)	
1 year	100	100	50	50	50	50	80	81	50	54	63	65
3 years	100	100	50	50	50	51	80	84	25	31	50	56
5 years	100	100	50	51	50	52	60	66	8	12	38	46

DENMARK

AREA	NUMBER OF CASES	PERIOD	MEAN AGE
	Females		Females
Denmark	546	1985-1989	70.8

OBSERVED AND RELATIVE SURVIVAL (%) BY AGE (number of cases in parentheses)

	AGE CLASS						ALL	
	15-44		45-54		55-64		65-74		75-99			
	obs rel		obs rel		obs rel		obs rel		obs rel		obs rel	
Females	(37)		(35)		(85)		(139)		(250)		(546)	
1 year	84	84	94	95	86	87	81	83	60	66	73	77
3 years	68	68	86	87	65	67	63	68	39	53	54	63
5 years	59	60	77	79	62	66	53	61	29	51	45	60

VAGINA & VULVA (ICD-9 184)

ENGLAND

AREA	NUMBER OF CASES Females	PERIOD	MEAN AGE Females
East Anglia	205	1985-1989	73.8
Mersey	232	1985-1989	73.3
Oxford	219	1985-1989	72.0
South Thames	527	1985-1989	72.4
Wessex	318	1985-1989	71.9
West Midlands	486	1985-1989	71.3
Yorkshire	382	1985-1989	72.8
English Registries	2369		72.4

5-YR RELATIVE SURVIVAL (%)
Females

OBSERVED AND RELATIVE SURVIVAL (%) BY AGE (number of cases in parentheses)

	15-44 obs rel	45-54 obs rel	55-64 obs rel	65-74 obs rel	75-99 obs rel	ALL obs rel
Females	(112)	(139)	(283)	(637)	(1198)	(2369)
1 year	91 91	92 92	84 85	73 75	59 65	69 73
3 years	83 83	74 75	66 68	56 61	36 49	49 59
5 years	79 80	68 70	60 63	48 56	27 45	41 55

ESTONIA

AREA	NUMBER OF CASES Females	PERIOD	MEAN AGE Females
Estonia	137	1985-1989	70.8

OBSERVED AND RELATIVE SURVIVAL (%) BY AGE (number of cases in parentheses)

	15-44 obs rel	45-54 obs rel	55-64 obs rel	65-74 obs rel	75-99 obs rel	ALL obs rel
Females	(2)	(7)	(28)	(43)	(57)	(137)
1 year	50 50	71 72	71 72	67 70	58 64	64 68
3 years	50 50	57 58	54 56	58 65	28 39	45 53
5 years	50 50	57 59	46 50	51 62	18 32	36 49

VAGINA & VULVA   (ICD-9 184)

FINLAND

AREA	NUMBER OF CASES	PERIOD	MEAN AGE
	Females		Females
Finland	340	1985-1989	70.8

OBSERVED AND RELATIVE SURVIVAL (%) BY AGE (number of cases in parentheses)

	AGE CLASS						ALL
	15-44	45-54	55-64	65-74	75-99		
	obs rel	obs rel	obs rel	obs rel	obs rel		obs rel
Females	(14)	(31)	(52)	(84)	(159)		(340)
1 year	100 100	81 81	83 83	89 91	57 62		73 76
3 years	100 100	55 55	58 59	63 68	31 42		48 56
5 years	100 100	52 52	52 54	55 62	19 34		39 51

FRANCE

AREA	NUMBER OF CASES	PERIOD	MEAN AGE
	Females		Females
Somme	47	1985-1989	68.3
Calvados	44	1985-1989	74.0
Côte d'Or	14	1985-1989	76.1
Doubs	40	1985-1989	74.0
French Registries	145		72.4

5-YR RELATIVE SURVIVAL (%)
Females
0 20 40 60 80 100
Somme
Calvad
Côte d
Doubs

OBSERVED AND RELATIVE SURVIVAL (%) BY AGE (number of cases in parentheses)

	AGE CLASS						ALL
	15-44	45-54	55-64	65-74	75-99		
	obs rel	obs rel	obs rel	obs rel	obs rel		obs rel
Females	(7)	(11)	(15)	(33)	(79)		(145)
1 year	100 100	91 91	100 100	70 71	71 77		77 81
3 years	100 100	58 58	64 66	48 51	31 40		45 52
5 years	100 100	43 44	64 67	44 49	17 27		36 46

VAGINA & VULVA (ICD-9 184)

GERMANY

AREA	NUMBER OF CASES Females	PERIOD	MEAN AGE Females
Saarland	117	1985-1989	71.8

OBSERVED AND RELATIVE SURVIVAL (%) BY AGE (number of cases in parentheses)

	AGE CLASS										ALL	
	15-44		45-54		55-64		65-74		75-99			
	obs	rel	obs	rel	obs	rel	obs	rel	obs	rel	obs	rel
Females	(4)		(8)		(16)		(33)		(56)		(117)	
1 year	100	100	75	75	88	88	79	81	50	55	67	70
3 years	75	75	63	63	75	77	61	66	29	38	48	56
5 years	75	75	31	32	69	72	54	63	27	45	43	57

ICELAND

AREA	NUMBER OF CASES Females	PERIOD	MEAN AGE Females
Iceland	9	1985-1989	71.7

OBSERVED AND RELATIVE SURVIVAL (%) BY AGE (number of cases in parentheses)

	AGE CLASS										ALL	
	15-44		45-54		55-64		65-74		75-99			
	obs	rel	obs	rel	obs	rel	obs	rel	obs	rel	obs	rel
Females	(0)		(1)		(2)		(2)		(4)		(9)	
1 year	-	-	100	100	100	100	100	100	50	58	78	83
3 years	-	-	0	0	100	100	100	100	50	78	67	81
5 years	-	-	0	0	100	100	100	100	25	51	56	74

VAGINA & VULVA   (ICD-9 184)

ITALY

AREA	NUMBER OF CASES	PERIOD	MEAN AGE	5-YR RELATIVE SURVIVAL (%)
	Females		Females	Females
Florence	133	1985-1989	73.0	
Genoa	48	1986-1988	74.5	
Latina	20	1985-1987	66.8	
Modena	34	1988-1989	72.7	
Parma	28	1985-1987	73.5	
Ragusa	15	1985-1989	70.6	
Romagna	36	1986-1988	74.9	
Turin	44	1985-1987	68.8	
Varese	59	1985-1989	72.8	
Italian Registries	417		72.5	

OBSERVED AND RELATIVE SURVIVAL (%) BY AGE (number of cases in parentheses)

	15-44		45-54		55-64		65-74		75-99		ALL	
	obs	rel	obs	rel	obs	rel	obs	rel	obs	rel	obs	rel
Females	(15)		(23)		(57)		(104)		(218)		(417)	
1 year	87	87	65	65	84	85	76	77	65	70	71	74
3 years	73	74	65	66	63	64	56	59	35	45	47	54
5 years	67	67	61	62	54	56	45	50	26	41	38	49

NETHERLANDS

AREA	NUMBER OF CASES	PERIOD	MEAN AGE
	Females		Females
Eindhoven	43	1985-1989	70.6

OBSERVED AND RELATIVE SURVIVAL (%) BY AGE (number of cases in parentheses)

	15-44		45-54		55-64		65-74		75-99		ALL	
	obs	rel	obs	rel	obs	rel	obs	rel	obs	rel	obs	rel
Females	(2)		(1)		(8)		(13)		(19)		(43)	
1 year	100	100	100	100	75	75	92	94	95	100	91	94
3 years	100	100	100	100	63	64	62	65	51	63	60	67
5 years	100	100	100	100	63	65	54	61	39	58	53	65

VAGINA & VULVA (ICD-9 184)

POLAND

AREA	NUMBER OF CASES Females	PERIOD	MEAN AGE Females
Cracow	55	1985-1989	69.7
Warsaw	57	1988-1989	65.6
Polish Registries	112		67.6

5-YR RELATIVE SURVIVAL (%)

Females

OBSERVED AND RELATIVE SURVIVAL (%) BY AGE (number of cases in parentheses)

	15-44		45-54		55-64		65-74		75-99		ALL	
	obs	rel	obs	rel	obs	rel	obs	rel	obs	rel	obs	rel
Females	(6)		(13)		(21)		(27)		(45)		(112)	
1 year	83	83	76	76	76	77	77	80	18	19	53	55
3 years	83	84	50	51	57	59	58	64	7	9	37	43
5 years	83	84	50	52	52	56	50	60	4	7	34	42

SCOTLAND

AREA	NUMBER OF CASES Females	PERIOD	MEAN AGE Females
Scotland	459	1985-1989	70.4

OBSERVED AND RELATIVE SURVIVAL (%) BY AGE (number of cases in parentheses)

	15-44		45-54		55-64		65-74		75-99		ALL	
	obs	rel	obs	rel	obs	rel	obs	rel	obs	rel	obs	rel
Females	(34)		(32)		(62)		(122)		(209)		(459)	
1 year	94	94	84	85	79	80	71	73	60	67	70	74
3 years	71	71	66	66	61	64	52	58	36	50	48	57
5 years	71	71	59	61	55	59	43	52	28	49	41	55

VAGINA & VULVA (ICD-9 184)

SLOVAKIA

AREA	NUMBER OF CASES Females	PERIOD	MEAN AGE Females
Slovakia	336	1985-1989	67.6

OBSERVED AND RELATIVE SURVIVAL (%) BY AGE (number of cases in parentheses)

	15-44 obs rel	45-54 obs rel	55-64 obs rel	65-74 obs rel	75-99 obs rel	ALL obs rel
Females	(20)	(24)	(81)	(92)	(119)	(336)
1 year	80 80	71 71	73 74	61 63	41 45	59 61
3 years	50 50	58 59	47 49	41 46	23 31	38 43
5 years	44 45	58 60	44 47	37 44	21 36	35 44

SLOVENIA

AREA	NUMBER OF CASES Females	PERIOD	MEAN AGE Females
Slovenia	157	1985-1989	68.4

OBSERVED AND RELATIVE SURVIVAL (%) BY AGE (number of cases in parentheses)

	15-44 obs rel	45-54 obs rel	55-64 obs rel	65-74 obs rel	75-99 obs rel	ALL obs rel
Females	(8)	(14)	(25)	(49)	(61)	(157)
1 year	100 100	86 86	76 77	53 54	62 68	66 69
3 years	88 88	64 65	56 58	37 40	28 38	41 48
5 years	63 63	64 66	56 59	27 31	23 40	35 45

VAGINA & VULVA   (ICD-9 184)

SPAIN

AREA	NUMBER OF CASES	PERIOD	MEAN AGE
	Females		Females
Basque Country	101	1986-1988	67.7
Girona	28	1985-1989	72.1
Mallorca	31	1988-1989	71.6
Navarra	45	1985-1989	71.7
Tarragona	49	1985-1989	72.8
Spanish Registries	254		70.3

5-YR RELATIVE SURVIVAL (%)

Females

OBSERVED AND RELATIVE SURVIVAL (%) BY AGE (number of cases in parentheses)

	AGE CLASS										ALL	
	15-44		45-54		55-64		65-74		75-99			
	obs	rel	obs	rel	obs	rel	obs	rel	obs	rel	obs	rel
Females	(10)		(21)		(40)		(75)		(108)		(254)	
1 year	90	90	76	76	63	63	66	67	54	59	62	65
3 years	90	90	67	67	52	53	49	52	35	45	46	53
5 years	80	80	67	68	50	52	46	51	31	50	43	54

SWEDEN

AREA	NUMBER OF CASES	PERIOD	MEAN AGE
	Females		Females
South Sweden	132	1985-1989	69.8

OBSERVED AND RELATIVE SURVIVAL (%) BY AGE (number of cases in parentheses)

	AGE CLASS										ALL	
	15-44		45-54		55-64		65-74		75-99			
	obs	rel	obs	rel	obs	rel	obs	rel	obs	rel	obs	rel
Females	(6)		(16)		(16)		(39)		(55)		(132)	
1 year	100	100	88	88	94	94	92	94	55	59	77	80
3 years	83	84	75	76	69	70	64	68	38	49	56	63
5 years	83	84	63	63	69	72	64	72	29	46	51	63

VAGINA & VULVA (ICD-9 184)

SWITZERLAND

AREA	NUMBER OF CASES Females	PERIOD	MEAN AGE Females
Geneva	28·	1985-1989	68.7

OBSERVED AND RELATIVE SURVIVAL (%) BY AGE (number of cases in parentheses)

	15-44 obs rel	45-54 obs rel	55-64 obs rel	65-74 obs rel	75-99 obs rel	ALL obs rel
Females	(4)	(4)	(3)	(1)	(16)	(28)
1 year	100 100	75 75	100 100	0 0	44 48	61 64
3 years	75 75	75 76	100 100	0 0	25 33	46 55
5 years	75 75	75 76	100 100	0 0	25 42	46 62

VAGINA & VULVA

(ICD-9 184)

EUROPE, 1985-89

Weighted analyses

COUNTRY	% COVERAGE WITH C.R.s	YEARLY NO. OF CASES (Mean No. of cases recorded) Females	RELATIVE SURVIVAL (%) (Age-standardized) Females
AUSTRIA	8	12	
DENMARK	100	109	
ENGLAND	50	474	
ESTONIA	100	27	
FINLAND	100	68	
FRANCE	4	29	
GERMANY	2	23	
ICELAND	100	2	
ITALY	10	118	
NETHERLANDS	6	9	
POLAND	6	40	
SCOTLAND	100	92	
SLOVAKIA	100	67	
SLOVENIA	100	31	
SPAIN	11	74	
SWEDEN	17	26	
SWITZERLAND	6	6	

□ 1 year ■ 5 years

OBSERVED AND RELATIVE SURVIVAL (%) BY AGE

	AGE CLASS										ALL	
	15-44 obs rel		45-54 obs rel		55-64 obs rel		65-74 obs rel		75-99 obs rel		obs rel	
Females												
1 year	93	93	79	79	83	83	74	76	55	60	68	71
3 years	82	82	65	65	65	66	55	60	30	40	47	54
5 years	79	80	54	55	60	63	48	55	23	38	40	52

AGE STANDARDIZED RELATIVE SURVIVAL(%) FEMALES

COUNTRY	1-year (95% C.I.)	5-years (95% C.I.)
AUSTRIA	62.6 (45.2 - 86.7)	39.4 (23.6 - 65.8)
DENMARK	76.5 (72.7 - 80.5)	58.3 (52.9 - 64.3)
ENGLAND	73.6 (71.7 - 75.5)	53.9 (51.4 - 56.5)
ESTONIA	66.6 (58.1 - 76.4)	45.2 (35.4 - 57.6)
FINLAND	76.1 (71.5 - 81.0)	48.8 (42.8 - 55.7)
FRANCE	80.9 (74.0 - 88.4)	43.2 (34.0 - 54.9)
GERMANY	70.1 (62.2 - 78.9)	54.2 (43.5 - 67.4)
ICELAND	-	-
ITALY	74.7 (70.3 - 79.3)	48.4 (42.9 - 54.6)
NETHERLANDS	94.9 (87.5 -103.0)	64.9 (48.7 - 86.5)
POLAND	50.6 (43.2 - 59.3)	35.0 (27.3 - 44.8)
SCOTLAND	73.0 (68.7 - 77.7)	53.1 (47.1 - 59.7)
SLOVAKIA	57.4 (51.9 - 63.4)	41.8 (35.2 - 49.6)
SLOVENIA	68.6 (61.2 - 76.9)	43.0 (33.9 - 54.5)
SPAIN	64.4 (58.5 - 71.0)	52.9 (45.4 - 61.7)
SWEDEN	77.4 (70.3 - 85.2)	59.5 (49.6 - 71.3)
SWITZERLAND	47.0 (35.7 - 61.9)	43.2 (28.9 - 64.6)
EUROPE, 1985-89	70.5 (68.1 - 72.9)	49.5 (46.3 - 52.9)

PROSTATE (ICD-9 185)

AUSTRIA

AREA	NUMBER OF CASES	PERIOD	MEAN AGE
	Males		Males
Tirol	364	1988-1989	73.1

OBSERVED AND RELATIVE SURVIVAL (%) BY AGE (number of cases in parentheses)

	15-54		55-64		65-74		75-84		85-99		ALL	
	obs	rel	obs	rel	obs	rel	obs	rel	obs	rel	obs	rel
Males	(3)		(49)		(130)		(163)		(19)		(364)	
1 year	33	33	88	89	92	95	73	78	47	56	80	84
3 years	33	34	71	74	68	74	49	61	5	9	56	66
5 years	33	34	67	72	55	64	33	48	5	15	44	58

DENMARK

AREA	NUMBER OF CASES	PERIOD	MEAN AGE
	Males		Males
Denmark	6939	1985-1989	73.9

OBSERVED AND RELATIVE SURVIVAL (%) BY AGE (number of cases in parentheses)

	15-54		55-64		65-74		75-84		85-99		ALL	
	obs	rel	obs	rel	obs	rel	obs	rel	obs	rel	obs	rel
Males	(102)		(817)		(2597)		(2773)		(650)		(6939)	
1 year	81	82	85	87	84	87	73	80	55	67	77	83
3 years	44	45	54	58	53	61	40	54	25	47	45	57
5 years	27	29	36	40	35	45	23	39	11	34	28	42

PROSTATE   (ICD-9 185)

ENGLAND

AREA	NUMBER OF CASES Males	PERIOD	MEAN AGE Males	5-YR RELATIVE SURVIVAL (%) Males
East Anglia	2906	1985-1989	74.6	
Mersey	2366	1985-1989	73.4	
Oxford	2779	1985-1989	74.0	
South Thames	6341	1985-1989	73.7	
Wessex	4097	1985-1989	75.0	
West Midlands	5278	1985-1989	73.5	
Yorkshire	3844	1985-1989	73.8	
English Registries	27611		74.0	

100 80 60 40 20 0

E.Angl
Mersey
Oxford
S.Tham
Wessex
W.Midl
Yorksh

OBSERVED AND RELATIVE SURVIVAL (%) BY AGE (number of cases in parentheses)

	AGE CLASS										ALL	
	15-54		55-64		65-74		75-84		85-99			
	obs	rel	obs	rel	obs	rel	obs	rel	obs	rel	obs	rel
Males	(375)		(3213)		(10202)		(11423)		(2398)		(27611)	
1 year	84	84	84	86	79	83	69	76	51	62	73	79
3 years	52	53	57	61	51	59	40	55	24	45	45	57
5 years	39	40	43	48	36	46	25	44	11	36	30	45

ESTONIA

AREA	NUMBER OF CASES Males	PERIOD	MEAN AGE Males
Estonia	703	1985-1989	71.2

OBSERVED AND RELATIVE SURVIVAL (%) BY AGE (number of cases in parentheses)

	AGE CLASS										ALL	
	15-54		55-64		65-74		75-84		85-99			
	obs	rel	obs	rel	obs	rel	obs	rel	obs	rel	obs	rel
Males	(23)		(121)		(295)		(243)		(21)		(703)	
1 year	70	71	73	75	70	74	61	68	38	48	66	72
3 years	39	40	42	46	42	50	36	51	14	30	39	49
5 years	24	26	28	33	28	40	21	41	5	18	25	38

PROSTATE (ICD-9 185)

FINLAND

AREA	NUMBER OF CASES	PERIOD	MEAN AGE
	Males		Males
Finland	5566	1985-1989	72.8

OBSERVED AND RELATIVE SURVIVAL (%) BY AGE (number of cases in parentheses)

	AGE CLASS										ALL	
	15-54		55-64		65-74		75-84		85-99			
	obs	rel	obs	rel	obs	rel	obs	rel	obs	rel	obs	rel
Males	(94)		(853)		(2101)		(2138)		(380)		(5566)	
1 year	90	91	90	92	88	93	81	89	67	82	84	91
3 years	51	52	66	70	66	76	54	73	33	64	59	73
5 years	43	44	52	58	50	64	36	63	16	52	42	62

FRANCE

AREA	NUMBER OF CASES	PERIOD	MEAN AGE
	Males		Males
Somme	757	1985-1989	73.3
Calvados	838	1985-1989	72.7
Doubs	558	1985-1989	73.8
French Registries	2153		73.2

5-YR RELATIVE SURVIVAL (%)
Males

OBSERVED AND RELATIVE SURVIVAL (%) BY AGE (number of cases in parentheses)

	AGE CLASS										ALL	
	15-54		55-64		65-74		75-84		85-99			
	obs	rel	obs	rel	obs	rel	obs	rel	obs	rel	obs	rel
Males	(34)		(332)		(755)		(869)		(163)		(2153)	
1 year	91	92	89	90	88	92	77	85	68	85	83	88
3 years	67	69	65	69	68	77	48	64	32	66	57	70
5 years	48	51	53	58	54	68	33	56	19	70	43	62

PROSTATE   (ICD-9 185)

GERMANY

AREA	NUMBER OF CASES Males	PERIOD	MEAN AGE Males
Saarland	1035	1985-1989	71.8

OBSERVED AND RELATIVE SURVIVAL (%) BY AGE (number of cases in parentheses)

	AGE CLASS					ALL
	15-54 obs rel	55-64 obs rel	65-74 obs rel	75-84 obs rel	85-99 obs rel	obs rel
Males	(32)	(190)	(373)	(386)	(54)	(1035)
1 year	100 100	92 94	87 91	78 87	61 75	84 90
3 years	72 74	74 78	65 76	49 70	31 65	59 74
5 years	72 75	64 71	55 73	30 58	21 82	46 69

ICELAND

AREA	NUMBER OF CASES Males	PERIOD	MEAN AGE Males
Iceland	438	1985-1989	73.6

OBSERVED AND RELATIVE SURVIVAL (%) BY AGE (number of cases in parentheses)

	AGE CLASS					ALL
	15-54 obs rel	55-64 obs rel	65-74 obs rel	75-84 obs rel	85-99 obs rel	obs rel
Males	(6)	(73)	(147)	(165)	(47)	(438)
1 year	100 100	97 98	90 93	83 90	72 87	87 92
3 years	83 85	85 88	71 78	53 68	40 72	63 76
5 years	50 51	71 77	59 70	38 60	23 64	49 68

PROSTATE (ICD-9 185)

ITALY

AREA	NUMBER OF CASES Males	PERIOD	MEAN AGE Males	5-YR RELATIVE SURVIVAL (%) Males
Florence	1297	1985-1989	74.1	
Genoa	424	1986-1988	73.6	
Latina	109	1985-1987	70.4	
Modena	278	1988-1989	72.2	
Parma	234	1985-1987	74.2	
Ragusa	176	1985-1989	74.7	
Romagna	280	1986-1988	73.5	
Turin	478	1985-1987	72.8	
Varese	716	1985-1989	72.0	
Italian Registries	3992		73.3	

OBSERVED AND RELATIVE SURVIVAL (%) BY AGE (number of cases in parentheses)

	AGE CLASS									ALL	
	15-54 obs rel		55-64 obs rel		65-74 obs rel		75-84 obs rel		85-99 obs rel		obs rel
Males	(72)		(531)		(1496)		(1619)		(274)		(3992)
1 year	85	85	87	88	84	87	72	78	52	63	77	82
3 years	58	59	63	66	57	65	41	54	22	41	49	60
5 years	44	46	50	55	43	53	27	43	10	30	35	49

NETHERLANDS

AREA	NUMBER OF CASES Males	PERIOD	MEAN AGE Males
Eindhoven	819	1985-1989	72.7

OBSERVED AND RELATIVE SURVIVAL (%) BY AGE (number of cases in parentheses)

	AGE CLASS									ALL	
	15-54 obs rel		55-64 obs rel		65-74 obs rel		75-84 obs rel		85-99 obs rel		obs rel
Males	(22)		(130)		(312)		(285)		(70)		(819)
1 year	82	82	85	86	89	93	78	86	68	84	82	88
3 years	64	65	68	71	66	76	46	63	31	62	56	70
5 years	48	50	53	58	51	66	26	46	13	45	39	58

PROSTATE   (ICD-9 185)

POLAND

AREA	NUMBER OF CASES Males	PERIOD	MEAN AGE Males
Cracow	212	1985-1989	70.6
Warsaw	225	1988-1989	70.2
Polish Registries	437		70.4

5-YR RELATIVE SURVIVAL (%)
Males

OBSERVED AND RELATIVE SURVIVAL (%) BY AGE (number of cases in parentheses)

	15-54 obs rel (13)		55-64 obs rel (105)		65-74 obs rel (167)		75-84 obs rel (127)		85-99 obs rel (25)		ALL obs rel (437)	
Males												
1 year	69	70	72	74	67	71	54	60	32	39	62	67
3 years	31	32	42	46	47	57	25	35	20	36	38	47
5 years	15	17	36	43	30	42	13	25	16	44	25	37

SCOTLAND

AREA	NUMBER OF CASES Males	PERIOD	MEAN AGE Males
Scotland	5476	1985-1989	73.6

OBSERVED AND RELATIVE SURVIVAL (%) BY AGE (number of cases in parentheses)

	15-54 obs rel (85)		55-64 obs rel (638)		65-74 obs rel (2137)		75-84 obs rel (2159)		85-99 obs rel (457)		ALL obs rel (5476)	
Males												
1 year	75	76	86	88	79	83	69	77	46	58	73	79
3 years	46	47	62	66	53	63	40	57	21	42	46	60
5 years	36	38	48	54	37	50	24	45	9	32	31	48

PROSTATE (ICD-9 185)

SLOVAKIA

AREA	NUMBER OF CASES Males	PERIOD	MEAN AGE Males
Slovakia	2725	1985-1989	71.6

OBSERVED AND RELATIVE SURVIVAL (%) BY AGE (number of cases in parentheses)

	15-54 obs rel	55-64 obs rel	65-74 obs rel	75-84 obs rel	85-99 obs rel	ALL obs rel
Males	(70)	(508)	(1004)	(1031)	(112)	(2725)
1 year	77 78	81 84	75 80	67 75	46 59	72 78
3 years	50 52	57 63	51 62	44 64	29 63	49 63
5 years	45 49	44 52	40 55	33 64	19 76	37 57

SLOVENIA

AREA	NUMBER OF CASES Males	PERIOD	MEAN AGE Males
Slovenia	1012	1985-1989	72.8

OBSERVED AND RELATIVE SURVIVAL (%) BY AGE (number of cases in parentheses)

	15-54 obs rel	55-64 obs rel	65-74 obs rel	75-84 obs rel	85-99 obs rel	ALL obs rel
Males	(23)	(142)	(359)	(446)	(42)	(1012)
1 year	70 70	80 81	71 75	67 74	40 51	69 75
3 years	35 36	51 55	48 56	36 51	12 26	41 53
5 years	26 28	37 43	31 41	22 41	2 11	26 40

PROSTATE   (ICD-9 185)

SPAIN

AREA	NUMBER OF CASES	PERIOD	MEAN AGE	5-YR RELATIVE SURVIVAL (%)
	Males		Males	Males
Basque Country	648	1986-1988	73.2	
Mallorca	222	1988-1989	74.3	
Navarra	527	1985-1989	72.8	
Tarragona	409	1985-1989	74.3	
Spanish Registries	1806		73.5	

5-YR RELATIVE SURVIVAL (%) Males: scale 100 80 60 40 20 0 — Basque, Mallor, Navarr, Tarrag

OBSERVED AND RELATIVE SURVIVAL (%) BY AGE (number of cases in parentheses)

	AGE CLASS										ALL	
	15-54		55-64		65-74		75-84		85-99			
	obs	rel	obs	rel	obs	rel	obs	rel	obs	rel	obs	rel
Males	(31)		(234)		(670)		(738)		(133)		(1806)	
1 year	71	71	85	86	84	87	75	81	54	66	78	83
3 years	52	53	62	64	57	64	48	63	29	54	52	63
5 years	45	47	50	54	43	53	34	56	19	56	39	54

SWEDEN

AREA	NUMBER OF CASES	PERIOD	MEAN AGE
	Males		Males
South Sweden	3580	1985-1989	73.8

OBSERVED AND RELATIVE SURVIVAL (%) BY AGE (number of cases in parentheses)

	AGE CLASS										ALL	
	15-54		55-64		65-74		75-84		85-99			
	obs	rel	obs	rel	obs	rel	obs	rel	obs	rel	obs	rel
Males	(41)		(436)		(1338)		(1473)		(292)		(3580)	
1 year	90	91	94	95	91	94	84	91	68	83	86	92
3 years	66	67	75	79	70	79	58	76	38	73	63	77
5 years	49	50	61	66	55	68	38	64	18	58	46	65

PROSTATE   (ICD-9 185)

SWITZERLAND

AREA	NUMBER OF CASES Males	PERIOD	MEAN AGE Males	5-YR RELATIVE SURVIVAL (%) Males
Basel	565	1985-1988	73.6	
Geneva	507	1985-1989	74.4	
Swiss Registries	1072		74.0	

100 80 60 40 20 0

Basel
Geneva

OBSERVED AND RELATIVE SURVIVAL (%) BY AGE (number of cases in parentheses)

	15-54 obs rel	55-64 obs rel	65-74 obs rel	75-84 obs rel	85-99 obs rel	ALL obs rel
Males	(16)	(129)	(391)	(433)	(103)	(1072)
1 year	100 100	94 95	91 94	85 92	66 79	87 92
3 years	80 82	71 75	73 82	64 84	31 56	65 80
5 years	58 61	59 64	59 73	46 77	17 52	50 72

PROSTATE   (ICD-9 185)

EUROPE, 1985-89

Weighted analyses

COUNTRY	% COVERAGE WITH C.R.s	YEARLY NO. OF CASES (Mean No. of cases recorded) Males	RELATIVE SURVIVAL (%) (Age-standardized) Males
AUSTRIA	8	182	A
DENMARK	100	1388	DK
ENGLAND	50	5522	ENG
ESTONIA	100	141	EST
FINLAND	100	1113	FIN
FRANCE	3	431	F
GERMANY	2	207	D
ICELAND	100	88	IS
ITALY	10	1085	I
NETHERLANDS	6	164	NL
POLAND	6	155	PL
SCOTLAND	100	1095	SCO
SLOVAKIA	100	545	SK
SLOVENIA	100	202	SLO
SPAIN	10	514	E
SWEDEN	17	716	S
SWITZERLAND	11	243	CH
			EUR

□ 1 year ■ 5 years

OBSERVED AND RELATIVE SURVIVAL (%) BY AGE

	AGE CLASS										ALL	
	15-54 obs rel		55-64 obs rel		65-74 obs rel		75-84 obs rel		85-99 obs rel		obs rel	
Males												
1 year	86	86	87	89	85	88	75	82	58	71	79	85
3 years	60	61	65	68	61	70	46	62	28	54	53	66
5 years	48	50	52	58	47	60	30	52	15	53	39	56

AGE STANDARDIZED RELATIVE SURVIVAL(%) MALES

COUNTRY	1-year (95% C.I.)	5-years (95% C.I.)
AUSTRIA	83.2 (79.1 - 87.6)	54.4 (48.3 - 61.2)
DENMARK	82.7 (81.7 - 83.8)	41.0 (39.4 - 42.7)
ENGLAND	78.9 (78.4 - 79.5)	44.3 (43.5 - 45.1)
ESTONIA	69.7 (65.6 - 74.0)	37.4 (32.1 - 43.5)
FINLAND	90.3 (89.3 - 91.4)	61.6 (59.6 - 63.8)
FRANCE	88.0 (86.2 - 89.8)	61.7 (58.0 - 65.6)
GERMANY	88.7 (86.1 - 91.4)	67.6 (62.0 - 73.7)
ICELAND	92.0 (88.7 - 95.5)	66.2 (59.9 - 73.2)
ITALY	81.6 (80.3 - 83.0)	47.4 (45.3 - 49.5)
NETHERLANDS	88.4 (85.5 - 91.3)	55.3 (50.2 - 60.8)
POLAND	64.1 (59.1 - 69.6)	34.7 (28.7 - 42.1)
SCOTLAND	79.2 (78.0 - 80.5)	47.2 (45.3 - 49.2)
SLOVAKIA	76.6 (74.7 - 78.6)	59.9 (56.2 - 64.0)
SLOVENIA	73.6 (70.5 - 76.9)	38.6 (34.5 - 43.1)
SPAIN	82.6 (80.5 - 84.6)	54.5 (51.1 - 58.1)
SWEDEN	92.3 (91.1 - 93.5)	64.7 (62.3 - 67.2)
SWITZERLAND	92.5 (90.4 - 94.7)	71.4 (67.1 - 76.0)
EUROPE, 1985-89	84.5 (83.8 - 85.2)	55.7 (54.3 - 57.1)

TESTIS (ICD-9 186)

AUSTRIA

AREA	NUMBER OF CASES	PERIOD	MEAN AGE
	Males		Males
Tirol	38	1988-1989	34.2

OBSERVED AND RELATIVE SURVIVAL (%) BY AGE (number of cases in parentheses)

	AGE CLASS					ALL
	15-44	45-54	55-64	65-74	75-99	
	obs rel	obs rel	obs rel	obs rel	obs rel	obs rel
Males	(31)	(4)	(2)	(1)	(0)	(38)
1 year	94 94	100 100	100 100	100 100	- -	95 95
3 years	94 94	100 100	100 100	100 100	- -	95 95
5 years	94 94	100 100	100 100	100 100	- -	95 96

DENMARK

AREA	NUMBER OF CASES	PERIOD	MEAN AGE
	Males		Males
Denmark	1252	1985-1989	36.2

OBSERVED AND RELATIVE SURVIVAL (%) BY AGE (number of cases in parentheses)

	AGE CLASS					ALL
	15-44	45-54	55-64	65-74	75-99	
	obs rel	obs rel	obs rel	obs rel	obs rel	obs rel
Males	(987)	(154)	(61)	(33)	(17)	(1252)
1 year	97 97	92 93	90 92	82 85	65 74	95 96
3 years	94 95	86 88	84 88	61 69	35 54	91 93
5 years	93 94	84 87	77 85	55 70	18 38	89 92

TESTIS (ICD-9 186)

ENGLAND

AREA	NUMBER OF CASES Males	PERIOD	MEAN AGE Males	5-YR RELATIVE SURVIVAL (%)
East Anglia	270	1985-1989	35.8	
Mersey	312	1985-1989	35.9	
Oxford	351	1985-1989	35.6	
South Thames	787	1985-1989	34.4	
Wessex	407	1985-1989	36.3	
West Midlands	431	1985-1989	35.7	
Yorkshire	397	1985-1989	36.7	
English Registries	2955		35.6	

OBSERVED AND RELATIVE SURVIVAL (%) BY AGE (number of cases in parentheses)

	AGE CLASS									ALL	
	15-44		45-54		55-64		65-74		75-99			
	obs	rel	obs	rel	obs	rel	obs	rel	obs	rel	obs	rel
Males	(2409)		(291)		(136)		(64)		(55)		(2955)	
1 year	96	96	96	96	91	93	80	83	58	65	94	95
3 years	92	92	90	91	85	89	64	73	45	65	90	91
5 years	91	91	89	91	81	88	55	68	34	64	88	90

ESTONIA

AREA	NUMBER OF CASES Males	PERIOD	MEAN AGE Males
Estonia	54	1985-1989	40.1

OBSERVED AND RELATIVE SURVIVAL (%) BY AGE (number of cases in parentheses)

	AGE CLASS									ALL	
	15-44		45-54		55-64		65-74		75-99			
	obs	rel	obs	rel	obs	rel	obs	rel	obs	rel	obs	rel
Males	(36)		(10)		(1)		(4)		(3)		(54)	
1 year	67	67	80	81	100	100	0	0	33	38	63	64
3 years	53	53	58	60	100	100	0	0	33	50	50	52
5 years	50	51	46	50	0	0	0	0	33	69	44	48

TESTIS (ICD-9 186)

FINLAND

AREA	NUMBER OF CASES	PERIOD	MEAN AGE
	Males		Males
Finland	292	1985-1989	36.5

OBSERVED AND RELATIVE SURVIVAL (%) BY AGE (number of cases in parentheses)

	15-44		45-54		55-64		65-74		75-99		ALL	
	obs	rel	obs	rel	obs	rel	obs	rel	obs	rel	obs	rel
Males	(227)		(36)		(14)		(5)		(10)		(292)	
1 year	96	96	94	95	93	94	60	63	70	77	94	95
3 years	92	93	89	91	79	83	40	47	40	54	88	90
5 years	91	92	89	92	71	78	40	53	10	17	86	90

FRANCE

AREA	NUMBER OF CASES	PERIOD	MEAN AGE
	Males		Males
Somme	53	1985-1989	33.6
Calvados	57	1985-1989	36.6
Doubs	49	1985-1989	31.8
French Registries	159		34.2

5-YR RELATIVE SURVIVAL (%)

Males

OBSERVED AND RELATIVE SURVIVAL (%) BY AGE (number of cases in parentheses)

	15-44		45-54		55-64		65-74		75-99		ALL	
	obs	rel	obs	rel	obs	rel	obs	rel	obs	rel	obs	rel
Males	(137)		(14)		(7)		(1)		(0)		(159)	
1 year	96	96	100	100	100	100	100	100	-	-	97	97
3 years	89	89	77	79	100	100	100	100	-	-	88	89
5 years	86	87	77	81	100	100	0	0	-	-	84	86

TESTIS (ICD-9 186)

GERMANY

AREA	NUMBER OF CASES Males	PERIOD	MEAN AGE Males
Saarland	172	1985-1989	34.8

OBSERVED AND RELATIVE SURVIVAL (%) BY AGE (number of cases in parentheses)

	AGE CLASS										ALL	
	15-44 obs rel		45-54 obs rel		55-64 obs rel		65-74 obs rel		75-99 obs rel			obs rel
Males	(134)		(23)		(11)		(2)		(2)			(172)
1 year	98	98	96	96	100	100	100	100	50	57	97	98
3 years	94	94	96	97	91	95	50	59	50	81	93	94
5 years	92	93	96	99	80	87	50	68	50	100	91	93

ICELAND

AREA	NUMBER OF CASES Males	PERIOD	MEAN AGE Males
Iceland	36	1985-1989	30.8

OBSERVED AND RELATIVE SURVIVAL (%) BY AGE (number of cases in parentheses)

	AGE CLASS										ALL	
	15-44 obs rel		45-54 obs rel		55-64 obs rel		65-74 obs rel		75-99 obs rel			obs rel
Males	(36)		(0)		(0)		(0)		(0)			(36)
1 year	100	100	-	-	-	-	-	-	-	-	100	100
3 years	97	98	-	-	-	-	-	-	-	-	97	98
5 years	94	95	-	-	-	-	-	-	-	-	94	95

TESTIS (ICD-9 186)

ITALY

AREA	NUMBER OF CASES Males	PERIOD	MEAN AGE Males	5-YR RELATIVE SURVIVAL (%) Males
Florence	114	1985-1989	40.9	
Genoa	33	1986-1988	34.9	
Latina	11	1985-1987	34.2	
Modena	19	1988-1989	40.3	
Parma	15	1985-1987	42.0	
Ragusa	10	1985-1989	44.9	
Romagna	26	1986-1988	40.0	
Turin	45	1985-1987	38.7	
Varese	94	1985-1989	34.6	
Italian Registries	367		38.4	

OBSERVED AND RELATIVE SURVIVAL (%) BY AGE (number of cases in parentheses)

	AGE CLASS										ALL	
	15-44		45-54		55-64		65-74		75-99			
	obs	rel	obs	rel	obs	rel	obs	rel	obs	rel	obs	rel
Males	(264)		(50)		(29)		(14)		(10)		(367)	
1 year	98	98	96	96	83	84	79	82	50	55	94	95
3 years	93	94	92	93	83	86	64	72	40	53	90	91
5 years	92	93	90	92	79	85	57	71	30	49	88	91

NETHERLANDS

AREA	NUMBER OF CASES Males	PERIOD	MEAN AGE Males
Eindhoven	86	1985-1989	33.4

OBSERVED AND RELATIVE SURVIVAL (%) BY AGE (number of cases in parentheses)

	AGE CLASS										ALL	
	15-44		45-54		55-64		65-74		75-99			
	obs	rel	obs	rel	obs	rel	obs	rel	obs	rel	obs	rel
Males	(70)		(6)		(5)		(5)		(0)		(86)	
1 year	99	99	100	100	100	100	80	83	-	-	98	98
3 years	94	94	100	100	100	100	80	91	-	-	94	95
5 years	94	95	100	100	100	100	80	99	-	-	94	96

TESTIS (ICD-9 186)

POLAND

AREA	NUMBER OF CASES Males	PERIOD	MEAN AGE Males	5-YR RELATIVE SURVIVAL (%) Males
Cracow	49	1985-1989	33.0	
Warsaw	75	1988-1989	35.1	
Polish Registries	124		34.3	

100 80 60 40 20 0

Cracow
Warsaw

OBSERVED AND RELATIVE SURVIVAL (%) BY AGE (number of cases in parentheses)

	15-44 obs rel	45-54 obs rel	55-64 obs rel	65-74 obs rel	75-99 obs rel	ALL obs rel
Males	(110)	(5)	(4)	(3)	(2)	(124)
1 year	95 95	80 81	100 100	0 0	0 0	90 91
3 years	82 82	80 83	75 82	0 0	0 0	78 80
5 years	82 83	80 86	50 59	0 0	0 0	77 80

SCOTLAND

AREA	NUMBER OF CASES Males	PERIOD	MEAN AGE Males
Scotland	692	1985-1989	35.7

OBSERVED AND RELATIVE SURVIVAL (%) BY AGE (number of cases in parentheses)

	15-44 obs rel	45-54 obs rel	55-64 obs rel	65-74 obs rel	75-99 obs rel	ALL obs rel
Males	(567)	(75)	(30)	(11)	(9)	(692)
1 year	97 97	93 94	83 85	91 95	33 39	95 95
3 years	93 93	89 91	80 85	73 85	33 53	91 92
5 years	92 93	88 91	73 81	73 97	22 49	90 92

TESTIS (ICD-9 186)

SLOVAKIA

AREA	NUMBER OF CASES	PERIOD	MEAN AGE
	Males		Males
Slovakia	564	1985-1989	32.5

OBSERVED AND RELATIVE SURVIVAL (%) BY AGE (number of cases in parentheses)

	15-44		45-54		55-64		65-74		75-99		ALL	
	obs	rel	obs	rel	obs	rel	obs	rel	obs	rel	obs	rel
Males	(509)		(20)		(13)		(14)		(8)		(564)	
1 year	90	90	100	100	77	79	50	52	63	73	89	89
3 years	82	83	90	93	62	67	50	58	50	81	81	82
5 years	81	82	85	90	53	62	40	53	50	100	79	82

SLOVENIA

AREA	NUMBER OF CASES	PERIOD	MEAN AGE
	Males		Males
Slovenia	197	1985-1989	32.7

OBSERVED AND RELATIVE SURVIVAL (%) BY AGE (number of cases in parentheses)

	15-44		45-54		55-64		65-74		75-99		ALL	
	obs	rel	obs	rel	obs	rel	obs	rel	obs	rel	obs	rel
Males	(174)		(15)		(6)		(1)		(1)		(197)	
1 year	94	94	93	94	100	100	100	100	0	0	93	94
3 years	88	89	87	89	100	100	0	0	0	0	88	89
5 years	87	88	87	90	67	76	0	0	0	0	85	87

TESTIS $\qquad$ (ICD-9 186)

SPAIN

AREA	NUMBER OF CASES	PERIOD	MEAN AGE	5-YR RELATIVE SURVIVAL (%)
	Males		Males	Males
Basque Country	56	1986-1988	37.3	
Mallorca	4	1988-1989	29.0	
Navarra	20	1985-1989	37.0	
Tarragona	25	1985-1989	35.5	
Spanish Registries	105		36.5	

OBSERVED AND RELATIVE SURVIVAL (%) BY AGE (number of cases in parentheses)

	AGE CLASS										ALL	
	15-44		45-54		55-64		65-74		75-99			
	obs	rel	obs	rel	obs	rel	obs	rel	obs	rel	obs	rel
Males	(81)		(11)		(4)		(7)		(2)		(105)	
1 year	100	100	82	82	75	76	57	59	0	0	92	93
3 years	96	97	82	83	75	78	43	48	0	0	89	90
5 years	96	97	82	84	75	81	43	52	0	0	89	92

SWEDEN

AREA	NUMBER OF CASES	PERIOD	MEAN AGE
	Males		Males
South Sweden	176	1985-1989	35.6

OBSERVED AND RELATIVE SURVIVAL (%) BY AGE (number of cases in parentheses)

	AGE CLASS										ALL	
	15-44		45-54		55-64		65-74		75-99			
	obs	rel	obs	rel	obs	rel	obs	rel	obs	rel	obs	rel
Males	(140)		(20)		(12)		(2)		(2)		(176)	
1 year	96	97	95	95	92	93	100	100	100	100	96	96
3 years	94	94	90	91	83	86	100	100	0	0	91	93
5 years	94	94	85	87	75	80	100	100	0	0	90	92

TESTIS (ICD-9 186)

SWITZERLAND

AREA	NUMBER OF CASES	PERIOD	MEAN AGE	5-YR RELATIVE SURVIVAL (%)
	Males		Males	Males
Basel	85	1985-1988	33.4	
Geneva	72	1985-1989	34.0	
Swiss Registries	157		33.7	

OBSERVED AND RELATIVE SURVIVAL (%) BY AGE (number of cases in parentheses)

	AGE CLASS									ALL	
	15-44		45-54		55-64		65-74		75-99		
	obs	rel	obs	rel	obs	rel	obs	rel	obs	rel	obs	rel
Males	(133)		(12)		(8)		(2)		(2)		(157)	
1 year	98	98	92	92	100	100	50	52	50	54	96	96
3 years	96	97	92	93	100	100	50	55	50	64	95	96
5 years	96	97	92	94	88	94	50	59	-	-	94	96

TESTIS (ICD-9 186)

EUROPE, 1985-89
Weighted analyses

COUNTRY	% COVERAGE WITH C.R.s	YEARLY NO. OF CASES (Mean No. of cases recorded) Males	
AUSTRIA	8	19	A
DENMARK	100	250	DK
ENGLAND	50	591	ENG
ESTONIA	100	11	EST
FINLAND	100	58	FIN
FRANCE	3	32	F
GERMANY	2	34	D
ICELAND	100	7	IS
ITALY	10	97	I
NETHERLANDS	6	17	NL
POLAND	6	47	PL
SCOTLAND	100	138	SCO
SLOVAKIA	100	113	SK
SLOVENIA	100	39	SLO
SPAIN	10	30	E
SWEDEN	17	35	S
SWITZERLAND	11	36	CH

RELATIVE SURVIVAL (%)
(Age-standardized)
Males

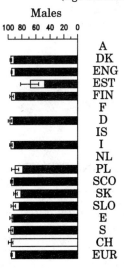

□ 1 year ■ 5 years

OBSERVED AND RELATIVE SURVIVAL (%) BY AGE

	AGE CLASS										ALL	
	15-44		45-54		55-64		65-74		75-99			
	obs	rel	obs	rel	obs	rel	obs	rel	obs	rel	obs	rel
Males												
1 year	97	97	94	95	94	95	79	80	45	50	95	96
3 years	92	92	89	91	88	91	60	66	36	55	90	91
5 years	90	91	88	92	80	86	44	55	31	59	88	90

AGE STANDARDIZED RELATIVE SURVIVAL(%)

COUNTRY	MALES	
	1-year (95% C.I.)	5-years (95% C.I.)
AUSTRIA	-	-
DENMARK	95.9 (94.8 - 97.1)	91.4 (89.7 - 93.1)
ENGLAND	94.9 (94.1 - 95.7)	90.0 (88.8 - 91.2)
ESTONIA	67.8 (56.1 - 82.0)	47.6 (35.3 - 64.1)
FINLAND	95.0 (92.4 - 97.6)	89.4 (85.8 - 93.2)
FRANCE	-	-
GERMANY	97.2 (94.7 - 99.8)	92.7 (87.3 - 98.5)
ICELAND	-	-
ITALY	96.0 (94.1 - 97.8)	91.1 (88.0 - 94.2)
NETHERLANDS	-	-
POLAND	89.9 (85.0 - 95.0)	78.8 (71.6 - 86.8)
SCOTLAND	95.1 (93.5 - 96.7)	91.5 (89.1 - 94.1)
SLOVAKIA	89.5 (87.0 - 92.1)	81.6 (77.7 - 85.6)
SLOVENIA	92.7 (89.5 - 96.0)	83.9 (79.0 - 89.0)
SPAIN	94.5 (91.4 - 97.7)	92.5 (87.9 - 97.4)
SWEDEN	96.4 (93.6 - 99.2)	91.4 (87.6 - 95.4)
SWITZERLAND	95.6 (92.3 - 98.9)	-
EUROPE, 1985-89	95.3 (94.3 - 96.4)	89.5 (87.4 - 91.7)

PENIS (ICD-9 187)

AUSTRIA

AREA	NUMBER OF CASES	PERIOD	MEAN AGE
	Males		Males
Tirol	5	1988-1989	64.0

OBSERVED AND RELATIVE SURVIVAL (%) BY AGE (number of cases in parentheses)

	AGE CLASS										ALL	
	15-44		45-54		55-64		65-74		75-99			
	obs	rel	obs	rel	obs	rel	obs	rel	obs	rel	obs	rel
Males	(1)		(0)		(1)		(1)		(2)		(5)	
1 year	100	100	-	-	100	100	100	100	50	59	80	86
3 years	100	100	-	-	100	100	100	100	0	0	60	75
5 years	100	100	-	-	100	100	100	100	0	0	60	86

DENMARK

AREA	NUMBER OF CASES	PERIOD	MEAN AGE
	Males		Males
Denmark	214	1985-1989	68.0

OBSERVED AND RELATIVE SURVIVAL (%) BY AGE (number of cases in parentheses)

	AGE CLASS										ALL	
	15-44		45-54		55-64		65-74		75-99			
	obs	rel	obs	rel	obs	rel	obs	rel	obs	rel	obs	rel
Males	(12)		(20)		(46)		(63)		(73)		(214)	
1 year	83	84	95	96	80	82	92	96	63	72	79	84
3 years	67	67	90	92	72	76	70	80	37	56	61	73
5 years	50	51	90	94	63	70	57	73	32	65	52	71

PENIS (ICD-9 187)

ENGLAND

AREA	NUMBER OF CASES Males	PERIOD	MEAN AGE Males	5-YR RELATIVE SURVIVAL (%) Males
East Anglia	67	1985-1989	66.6	
Mersey	101	1985-1989	65.6	
Oxford	90	1985-1989	64.1	
South Thames	179	1985-1989	66.3	
Wessex	110	1985-1989	67.9	
West Midlands	184	1985-1989	64.0	
Yorkshire	131	1985-1989	68.1	
English Registries	862		66.0	

OBSERVED AND RELATIVE SURVIVAL (%) BY AGE (number of cases in parentheses)

	AGE CLASS										ALL	
	15-44 obs rel		45-54 obs rel		55-64 obs rel		65-74 obs rel		75-99 obs rel		obs rel	
Males	(73)		(93)		(172)		(254)		(270)		(862)	
1 year	90	91	92	93	87	89	79	82	74	83	82	86
3 years	78	78	81	82	70	74	61	70	51	74	63	74
5 years	77	77	77	80	66	73	51	65	36	67	54	71

ESTONIA

AREA	NUMBER OF CASES Males	PERIOD	MEAN AGE Males
Estonia	35	1985-1989	63.8

OBSERVED AND RELATIVE SURVIVAL (%) BY AGE (number of cases in parentheses)

	AGE CLASS										ALL	
	15-44 obs rel		45-54 obs rel		55-64 obs rel		65-74 obs rel		75-99 obs rel		obs rel	
Males	(2)		(9)		(8)		(9)		(7)		(35)	
1 year	100	100	78	79	75	77	89	94	29	33	71	76
3 years	0	0	56	58	50	54	78	94	14	24	49	58
5 years	0	0	56	61	38	44	67	95	14	35	43	58

PENIS (ICD-9 187)

FINLAND

AREA	NUMBER OF CASES	PERIOD	MEAN AGE
	Males		Males
Finland	66	1985-1989	59.2

OBSERVED AND RELATIVE SURVIVAL (%) BY AGE (number of cases in parentheses)

	AGE CLASS										ALL	
	15-44		45-54		55-64		65-74		75-99			
	obs	rel	obs	rel	obs	rel	obs	rel	obs	rel	obs	rel
Males	(13)		(15)		(11)		(13)		(14)		(66)	
1 year	92	93	87	87	82	83	85	88	79	87	85	88
3 years	85	85	73	75	64	68	62	71	43	59	65	73
5 years	85	86	67	69	55	61	38	50	43	76	58	69

FRANCE

AREA	NUMBER OF CASES	PERIOD	MEAN AGE
	Males		Males
Somme	13	1985-1989	63.9
Calvados	17	1985-1989	69.2
Doubs	15	1985-1989	60.2
French Registries	45		64.8

5-YR RELATIVE SURVIVAL (%)

Males

OBSERVED AND RELATIVE SURVIVAL (%) BY AGE (number of cases in parentheses)

	AGE CLASS										ALL	
	15-44		45-54		55-64		65-74		75-99			
	obs	rel	obs	rel	obs	rel	obs	rel	obs	rel	obs	rel
Males	(4)		(4)		(14)		(8)		(15)		(45)	
1 year	100	100	100	100	78	79	100	100	86	95	89	92
3 years	100	100	100	100	60	64	83	93	63	86	72	82
5 years	-	-	100	100	60	66	63	77	54	97	62	80

PENIS (ICD-9 187)

GERMANY

AREA	NUMBER OF CASES	PERIOD	MEAN AGE
	Males		Males
Saarland	24	1985-1989	65.7

OBSERVED AND RELATIVE SURVIVAL (%) BY AGE (number of cases in parentheses)

	15-44		45-54		55-64		65-74		75-99		ALL	
	obs	rel	obs	rel	obs	rel	obs	rel	obs	rel	obs	rel
Males	(0)		(4)		(6)		(9)		(5)		(24)	
1 year	-	-	100	100	83	85	78	81	40	46	75	79
3 years	-	-	75	76	67	71	78	87	20	31	63	72
5 years	-	-	50	52	67	75	56	68	-	-	52	66

ICELAND

AREA	NUMBER OF CASES	PERIOD	MEAN AGE
	Males		Males
Iceland	6	1985-1989	73.7

OBSERVED AND RELATIVE SURVIVAL (%) BY AGE (number of cases in parentheses)

	15-44		45-54		55-64		65-74		75-99		ALL	
	obs	rel	obs	rel	obs	rel	obs	rel	obs	rel	obs	rel
Males	(0)		(0)		(2)		(0)		(4)		(6)	
1 year	-	-	-	-	100	100	-	-	50	55	67	71
3 years	-	-	-	-	100	100	-	-	50	67	67	81
5 years	-	-	-	-	100	100	-	-	50	83	67	93

PENIS (ICD-9 187)

ITALY

AREA	NUMBER OF CASES Males	PERIOD	MEAN AGE Males	5-YR RELATIVE SURVIVAL (%) Males
Florence	41	1985-1989	68.1	
Genoa	15	1986-1988	62.3	
Latina	6	1985-1987	64.8	
Modena	4	1988-1989	62.3	
Parma	3	1985-1987	80.0	
Ragusa	2	1985-1989	36.5	
Romagna	11	1986-1988	65.2	
Turin	21	1985-1987	64.5	
Varese	23	1985-1989	60.4	
Italian Registries	126		64.7	

OBSERVED AND RELATIVE SURVIVAL (%) BY AGE (number of cases in parentheses)

	AGE CLASS										ALL	
	15-44		45-54		55-64		65-74		75-99			
	obs	rel	obs	rel	obs	rel	obs	rel	obs	rel	obs	rel
Males	(14)		(17)		(26)		(35)		(34)		(126)	
1 year	100	100	100	100	81	82	89	92	74	83	86	90
3 years	86	86	94	96	65	69	66	74	53	78	68	78
5 years	86	86	94	97	62	67	48	59	41	81	59	75

NETHERLANDS

AREA	NUMBER OF CASES Males	PERIOD	MEAN AGE Males
Eindhoven	26	1985-1989	64.9

OBSERVED AND RELATIVE SURVIVAL (%) BY AGE (number of cases in parentheses)

	AGE CLASS										ALL	
	15-44		45-54		55-64		65-74		75-99			
	obs	rel	obs	rel	obs	rel	obs	rel	obs	rel	obs	rel
Males	(4)		(5)		(3)		(5)		(9)		(26)	
1 year	100	100	100	100	100	100	80	84	56	63	81	85
3 years	100	100	80	82	67	70	80	95	33	51	64	77
5 years	100	100	80	83	67	73	60	80	11	24	51	70

PENIS (ICD-9 187)

POLAND

AREA	NUMBER OF CASES Males	PERIOD	MEAN AGE Males	5-YR RELATIVE SURVIVAL (%) Males
Cracow	9	1985-1989	63.0	
Warsaw	10	1988-1989	63.7	
Polish Registries	19		63.5	

5-YR RELATIVE SURVIVAL (%) Males

100 80 60 40 20 0

Cracow
Warsaw

OBSERVED AND RELATIVE SURVIVAL (%) BY AGE (number of cases in parentheses)

	15-44 obs rel (1)		45-54 obs rel (4)		55-64 obs rel (2)		65-74 obs rel (9)		75-99 obs rel (3)		ALL obs rel (19)	
Males												
1 year	100	100	50	51	50	51	78	82	67	74	68	72
3 years	100	100	25	26	50	53	44	52	67	92	47	55
5 years	100	100	25	27	50	56	44	60	67	100	47	61

SCOTLAND

AREA	NUMBER OF CASES Males	PERIOD	MEAN AGE Males
Scotland	189	1985-1989	64.8

OBSERVED AND RELATIVE SURVIVAL (%) BY AGE (number of cases in parentheses)

	15-44 obs rel (15)		45-54 obs rel (26)		55-64 obs rel (45)		65-74 obs rel (55)		75-99 obs rel (48)		ALL obs rel (189)	
Males												
1 year	100	100	88	89	82	84	84	88	73	83	83	87
3 years	93	94	69	71	53	57	55	64	50	75	58	68
5 years	93	94	69	72	51	58	45	60	31	64	50	66

PENIS (ICD-9 187)

SLOVAKIA

AREA	NUMBER OF CASES	PERIOD	MEAN AGE
	Males		Males
Slovakia	136	1985-1989	61.8

OBSERVED AND RELATIVE SURVIVAL (%) BY AGE (number of cases in parentheses)

	AGE CLASS									ALL	
	15-44		45-54		55-64		65-74		75-99			
	obs	rel	obs	rel	obs	rel	obs	rel	obs	rel	obs	rel
Males	(17)		(19)		(37)		(31)		(32)		(136)	
1 year	82	83	79	80	84	86	77	81	66	74	77	81
3 years	65	66	63	66	62	68	48	57	56	83	58	68
5 years	54	55	50	54	59	70	41	54	44	87	50	64

SLOVENIA

AREA	NUMBER OF CASES	PERIOD	MEAN AGE
	Males		Males
Slovenia	40	1985-1989	61.6

OBSERVED AND RELATIVE SURVIVAL (%) BY AGE (number of cases in parentheses)

	AGE CLASS									ALL	
	15-44		45-54		55-64		65-74		75-99			
	obs	rel	obs	rel	obs	rel	obs	rel	obs	rel	obs	rel
Males	(7)		(5)		(9)		(10)		(9)		(40)	
1 year	86	86	100	100	78	79	80	84	67	75	80	84
3 years	57	58	80	82	44	47	40	47	22	33	45	52
5 years	57	58	80	84	44	50	40	53	22	46	45	57

PENIS
(ICD-9 187)

SPAIN

AREA	NUMBER OF CASES	PERIOD	MEAN AGE
	Males		Males
Basque Country	55	1986-1988	64.9
Mallorca	10	1988-1989	68.1
Navarra	17	1985-1989	59.9
Tarragona	16	1985-1989	66.4
Spanish Registries	98		64.7

5-YR RELATIVE SURVIVAL (%)

Males

OBSERVED AND RELATIVE SURVIVAL (%) BY AGE (number of cases in parentheses)

	AGE CLASS										ALL	
	15-44		45-54		55-64		65-74		75-99			
	obs	rel	obs	rel	obs	rel	obs	rel	obs	rel	obs	rel
Males	(8)		(11)		(34)		(23)		(22)		(98)	
1 year	100	100	100	100	94	95	96	99	77	88	92	96
3 years	100	100	100	100	79	83	70	79	41	60	72	82
5 years	100	100	89	93	59	64	59	74	41	79	62	77

SWEDEN

AREA	NUMBER OF CASES	PERIOD	MEAN AGE
	Males		Males
South Sweden	53	1985-1989	67.5

OBSERVED AND RELATIVE SURVIVAL (%) BY AGE (number of cases in parentheses)

	AGE CLASS										ALL	
	15-44		45-54		55-64		65-74		75-99			
	obs	rel	obs	rel	obs	rel	obs	rel	obs	rel	obs	rel
Males	(8)		(2)		(10)		(14)		(19)		(53)	
1 year	88	88	100	100	90	91	71	74	74	85	79	84
3 years	88	88	100	100	90	94	57	64	58	90	70	84
5 years	88	88	50	52	80	87	43	53	37	80	55	74

PENIS (ICD-9 187)

SWITZERLAND

AREA	NUMBER OF CASES	PERIOD	MEAN AGE
	Males		Males
Geneva	11	1985-1989	54.5

OBSERVED AND RELATIVE SURVIVAL (%) BY AGE (number of cases in parentheses)

	AGE CLASS										ALL	
	15-44		45-54		55-64		65-74		75-99			
	obs	rel	obs	rel	obs	rel	obs	rel	obs	rel	obs	rel
Males	(3)		(3)		(2)		(1)		(2)		(11)	
1 year	100	100	100	100	50	51	100	100	100	100	91	93
3 years	67	67	67	68	50	53	100	100	100	100	73	78
5 years	67	67	67	68	0	0	100	100	100	100	64	72

PENIS   (ICD-9 187)

EUROPE, 1985-89

Weighted analyses

COUNTRY	% COVERAGE WITH C.R.s	YEARLY NO. OF CASES (Mean No. of cases recorded) Males	RELATIVE SURVIVAL (%) (Age-standardized) Males
AUSTRIA	8	3	A
DENMARK	100	43	DK
ENGLAND	50	172	ENG
ESTONIA	100	7	EST
FINLAND	100	13	FIN
FRANCE	3	9	F
GERMANY	2	5	D
ICELAND	100	1	IS
ITALY	10	35	I
NETHERLANDS	6	5	NL
POLAND	6	12	PL
SCOTLAND	100	38	SCO
SLOVAKIA	100	27	SK
SLOVENIA	100	8	SLO
SPAIN	10	30	E
SWEDEN	17	11	S
SWITZERLAND	6	2	CH
			EUR

□ 1 year   ■ 5 years

OBSERVED AND RELATIVE SURVIVAL (%) BY AGE

	AGE CLASS										ALL	
	15-44		45-54		55-64		65-74		75-99			
	obs	rel	obs	rel	obs	rel	obs	rel	obs	rel	obs	rel
Males												
1 year	97	97	93	94	82	83	86	89	70	78	83	87
3 years	90	90	83	84	67	71	69	78	48	68	65	75
5 years	87	87	75	78	61	67	55	68	43	78	56	72

COUNTRY	AGE STANDARDIZED RELATIVE SURVIVAL(%) MALES	
	1-year (95% C.I.)	5-years (95% C.I.)
AUSTRIA	-	-
DENMARK	84.6 (79.4 - 90.2)	70.3 (61.9 - 79.8)
ENGLAND	86.0 (83.4 - 88.7)	70.2 (66.0 - 74.8)
ESTONIA	71.5 (58.1 - 88.1)	53.5 (34.0 - 84.0)
FINLAND	87.2 (77.2 - 98.4)	65.4 (49.6 - 86.4)
FRANCE	93.9 (86.7 -101.7)	-
GERMANY	-	-
ICELAND	-	-
ITALY	88.9 (82.5 - 95.8)	74.2 (63.1 - 87.3)
NETHERLANDS	85.1 (71.5 -101.3)	64.4 (44.1 - 94.1)
POLAND	70.7 (49.6 -100.9)	70.5 (43.2 -115.3)
SCOTLAND	86.9 (81.3 - 92.9)	65.4 (56.0 - 76.4)
SLOVAKIA	80.2 (72.7 - 88.5)	67.3 (55.0 - 82.4)
SLOVENIA	82.6 (69.7 - 97.9)	54.5 (36.3 - 81.6)
SPAIN	95.3 (89.0 -102.1)	77.9 (64.5 - 94.1)
SWEDEN	85.3 (75.4 - 96.5)	71.4 (54.3 - 93.8)
SWITZERLAND	89.2 (75.1 -106.1)	71.2 (63.4 - 80.1)
EUROPE, 1985-89	86.0 (82.3 - 89.9)	73.7 (67.6 - 80.4)

BLADDER (ICD-9 188)

AUSTRIA

AREA	NUMBER OF CASES			PERIOD	MEAN AGE		
	Males	Females	All		Males	Females	All
Tirol	206	70	276	1988-1989	70.4	69.4	70.2

OBSERVED AND RELATIVE SURVIVAL (%) BY AGE (number of cases in parentheses)

	AGE CLASS										ALL	
	15-44		45-54		55-64		65-74		75-99			
	obs	rel	obs	rel	obs	rel	obs	rel	obs	rel	obs	rel
Males	(8)		(12)		(30)		(67)		(89)		(206)	
1 year	100	100	92	92	93	94	84	86	71	77	81	85
3 years	100	100	75	76	83	87	69	75	48	63	64	74
5 years	100	100	75	77	77	82	51	60	36	59	51	67
Females	(4)		(4)		(11)		(22)		(29)		(70)	
1 year	75	75	75	75	100	100	86	88	62	66	77	79
3 years	75	75	50	50	91	92	68	72	38	46	59	64
5 years	75	75	50	51	91	94	55	60	34	48	53	62
Overall	(12)		(16)		(41)		(89)		(118)		(276)	
1 year	92	92	88	88	95	96	84	86	69	74	80	83
3 years	92	92	69	70	85	88	69	74	46	59	62	71
5 years	92	92	69	70	80	85	52	60	36	56	52	66

DENMARK

AREA	NUMBER OF CASES			PERIOD	MEAN AGE		
	Males	Females	All		Males	Females	All
Denmark	3522	1196	4718	1985-1989	69.9	71.6	70.3

OBSERVED AND RELATIVE SURVIVAL (%) BY AGE (number of cases in parentheses)

	AGE CLASS										ALL	
	15-44		45-54		55-64		65-74		75-99			
	obs	rel	obs	rel	obs	rel	obs	rel	obs	rel	obs	rel
Males	(64)		(192)		(695)		(1329)		(1242)		(3522)	
1 year	97	97	81	81	79	80	75	78	60	67	71	75
3 years	89	90	67	68	59	62	50	58	34	48	48	57
5 years	88	89	59	62	51	56	40	51	21	40	37	51
Females	(18)		(70)		(208)		(354)		(546)		(1196)	
1 year	78	78	76	76	71	72	67	68	50	54	61	63
3 years	67	67	60	61	51	53	52	56	27	35	41	47
5 years	67	67	57	59	46	49	42	49	20	31	34	44
Overall	(82)		(262)		(903)		(1683)		(1788)		(4718)	
1 year	93	93	79	80	77	78	73	76	57	63	68	72
3 years	84	85	65	66	57	60	51	57	32	44	46	55
5 years	83	84	59	61	50	54	40	51	21	37	37	49

BLADDER (ICD-9 188)

ENGLAND

AREA	Males	Females	All	PERIOD	Males	Females	All
East Anglia	1391	509	1900	1985-1989	70.1	73.2	70.9
Mersey	1819	815	2634	1985-1989	68.7	70.4	69.2
Oxford	1815	646	2461	1985-1989	68.6	71.5	69.3
South Thames	4634	1771	6405	1985-1989	69.6	72.4	70.4
Wessex	2696	990	3686	1985-1989	69.6	71.6	70.2
West Midlands	3569	1283	4852	1985-1989	68.2	71.1	68.9
Yorkshire	2634	1103	3737	1985-1989	69.0	71.6	69.8
English Registries	18558	7117	25675		69.1	71.7	69.8

(NUMBER OF CASES / MEAN AGE / 5-YR RELATIVE SURVIVAL chart for Males and Females: E.Angl, Mersey, Oxford, S.Tham, Wessex, W.Midl, Yorksh)

OBSERVED AND RELATIVE SURVIVAL (%) BY AGE (number of cases in parentheses)

	15-44 obs rel	45-54 obs rel	55-64 obs rel	65-74 obs rel	75-99 obs rel	ALL obs rel
Males	(486)	(1302)	(3895)	(6607)	(6268)	(18558)
1 year	94 95	91 92	85 87	79 82	66 74	77 81
3 years	90 91	81 83	73 77	61 70	44 62	60 71
5 years	89 90	76 79	66 73	51 64	31 58	50 67
Females	(167)	(374)	(1231)	(2165)	(3180)	(7117)
1 year	85 85	86 87	81 82	73 75	56 61	68 71
3 years	77 78	78 78	71 73	59 64	40 52	54 62
5 years	76 77	75 76	65 68	52 59	30 49	46 59
Overall	(653)	(1676)	(5126)	(8772)	(9448)	(25675)
1 year	92 92	90 90	85 86	77 80	62 69	75 79
3 years	87 87	80 82	72 76	61 68	42 59	58 69
5 years	86 86	76 78	65 71	51 63	31 55	49 65

ESTONIA

AREA	Males	Females	All	PERIOD	Males	Females	All
Estonia	381	164	545	1985-1989	65.6	72.2	67.6

OBSERVED AND RELATIVE SURVIVAL (%) BY AGE (number of cases in parentheses)

	15-44 obs rel	45-54 obs rel	55-64 obs rel	65-74 obs rel	75-99 obs rel	ALL obs rel
Males	(8)	(55)	(108)	(118)	(92)	(381)
1 year	100 100	71 72	72 74	55 58	42 48	60 64
3 years	100 100	47 49	46 51	34 40	22 32	38 45
5 years	75 78	36 39	43 50	22 30	11 22	28 38
Females	(0)	(4)	(26)	(57)	(77)	(164)
1 year	- -	100 100	73 74	65 67	36 40	54 57
3 years	- -	75 76	58 60	37 41	19 26	33 39
5 years	- -	75 77	42 45	26 32	16 26	25 34
Overall	(8)	(59)	(134)	(175)	(169)	(545)
1 year	100 100	73 74	72 74	58 61	40 44	58 61
3 years	100 100	49 51	49 52	35 40	21 29	36 43
5 years	75 78	39 42	43 49	23 31	13 24	27 37

385

BLADDER

(ICD-9 188)

FINLAND

AREA	NUMBER OF CASES			PERIOD	MEAN AGE		
	Males	Females	All		Males	Females	All
Finland	2011	601	2612	1985-1989	68.2	71.1	68.9

OBSERVED AND RELATIVE SURVIVAL (%) BY AGE (number of cases in parentheses)

	15-44		45-54		55-64		65-74		75-99		ALL	
	obs	rel	obs	rel	obs	rel	obs	rel	obs	rel	obs	rel
Males	(79)		(145)		(446)		(684)		(657)		(2011)	
1 year	97	98	93	94	89	90	83	87	74	83	83	87
3 years	95	96	83	85	73	77	66	76	48	68	64	76
5 years	94	95	76	79	66	73	53	68	33	61	53	70
Females	(15)		(32)		(113)		(176)		(265)		(601)	
1 year	100	100	91	91	90	91	82	84	64	70	77	80
3 years	100	100	84	85	78	80	72	77	43	57	62	71
5 years	87	87	75	76	70	73	61	70	31	52	51	65
Overall	(94)		(177)		(559)		(860)		(922)		(2612)	
1 year	98	98	93	93	89	90	83	86	71	79	81	86
3 years	96	97	83	85	74	78	67	76	46	65	63	75
5 years	93	94	76	79	67	73	55	69	32	58	52	69

FRANCE

AREA	NUMBER OF CASES			PERIOD	MEAN AGE		
	Males	Females	All		Males	Females	All
Somme	244	55	299	1985-1989	68.5	71.4	69.0
Calvados	296	84	380	1985-1989	66.3	72.5	67.7
Doubs	187	46	233	1985-1989	66.3	70.6	67.1
French Registries	727	185	912		67.0	71.7	68.0

5-YR RELATIVE SURVIVAL (%)

OBSERVED AND RELATIVE SURVIVAL (%) BY AGE (number of cases in parentheses)

	15-44		45-54		55-64		65-74		75-99		ALL	
	obs	rel	obs	rel	obs	rel	obs	rel	obs	rel	obs	rel
Males	(18)		(67)		(216)		(223)		(203)		(727)	
1 year	94	95	88	89	86	88	79	82	69	76	80	83
3 years	94	95	78	80	69	73	59	67	37	53	59	68
5 years	94	96	67	70	58	65	50	61	26	48	49	62
Females	(5)		(15)		(33)		(38)		(94)		(185)	
1 year	100	100	72	72	81	82	81	83	61	67	71	75
3 years	78	78	57	58	71	72	54	57	28	37	45	52
5 years	78	78	57	59	67	69	48	53	27	44	43	55
Overall	(23)		(82)		(249)		(261)		(297)		(912)	
1 year	96	96	85	86	86	87	80	82	66	73	78	82
3 years	91	92	74	76	69	73	59	65	35	48	56	65
5 years	91	92	65	68	60	65	49	60	26	47	47	61

BLADDER (ICD-9 188)

GERMANY

AREA	NUMBER OF CASES			PERIOD	MEAN AGE		
	Males	Females	All		Males	Females	All
Saarland	763	263	1026	1985-1989	67.0	71.2	68.1

OBSERVED AND RELATIVE SURVIVAL (%) BY AGE (number of cases in parentheses)

	AGE CLASS										ALL	
	15-44		45-54		55-64		65-74		75-99			
	obs	rel	obs	rel	obs	rel	obs	rel	obs	rel	obs	rel
Males	(23)		(58)		(215)		(267)		(200)		(763)	
1 year	96	96	93	94	90	91	84	88	71	79	83	87
3 years	87	88	86	88	81	86	66	77	49	70	68	80
5 years	81	82	84	88	72	80	54	71	36	72	57	76
Females	(4)		(13)		(52)		(75)		(119)		(263)	
1 year	100	100	85	85	79	80	80	82	59	64	71	74
3 years	100	100	85	85	67	69	59	63	42	55	55	63
5 years	100	100	75	77	63	66	51	59	36	59	48	62
Overall	(27)		(71)		(267)		(342)		(319)		(1026)	
1 year	96	97	92	92	88	89	83	87	66	73	80	84
3 years	89	90	86	88	79	83	65	73	46	64	65	75
5 years	83	84	83	86	70	77	54	68	36	66	55	73

ICELAND

AREA	NUMBER OF CASES			PERIOD	MEAN AGE		
	Males	Females	All		Males	Females	All
Iceland	128	47	175	1985-1989	66.1	65.4	65.9

OBSERVED AND RELATIVE SURVIVAL (%) BY AGE (number of cases in parentheses)

	AGE CLASS										ALL	
	15-44		45-54		55-64		65-74		75-99			
	obs	rel	obs	rel	obs	rel	obs	rel	obs	rel	obs	rel
Males	(8)		(13)		(40)		(30)		(37)		(128)	
1 year	100	100	100	100	95	96	83	86	54	60	81	85
3 years	100	100	92	94	88	91	63	70	41	55	70	78
5 years	100	100	92	95	80	86	53	63	30	50	62	75
Females	(5)		(6)		(9)		(12)		(15)		(47)	
1 year	100	100	100	100	89	90	83	85	67	74	83	86
3 years	100	100	67	67	89	91	75	80	53	72	72	81
5 years	100	100	50	51	78	81	58	66	47	77	62	74
Overall	(13)		(19)		(49)		(42)		(52)		(175)	
1 year	100	100	100	100	94	95	83	86	58	64	82	85
3 years	100	100	84	85	88	91	67	73	44	60	70	79
5 years	100	100	79	81	80	85	55	64	35	58	62	75

BLADDER

(ICD-9 188)

ITALY

AREA	NUMBER OF CASES			PERIOD	MEAN AGE			5-YR RELATIVE SURVIVAL (%)	
	Males	Females	All		Males	Females	All	Males	Females
Florence	1701	412	2113	1985-1989	67.3	70.8	68.0		
Genoa	530	133	663	1986-1988	68.0	70.7	68.5		
Latina	169	24	193	1985-1987	67.5	66.8	67.5		
Modena	315	66	381	1988-1989	65.3	69.9	66.1		
Parma	244	51	295	1985-1987	66.7	69.2	67.1		
Ragusa	155	17	172	1985-1989	70.0	71.5	70.1		
Romagna	362	54	416	1986-1988	67.8	70.7	68.2		
Turin	692	175	867	1985-1987	66.0	70.7	67.0		
Varese	588	139	727	1985-1989	66.6	71.3	67.5		
Italian Registries	4756	1071	5827		67.1	70.6	67.7		

OBSERVED AND RELATIVE SURVIVAL (%) BY AGE (number of cases in parentheses)

	AGE CLASS										ALL	
	15-44		45-54		55-64		65-74		75-99			
	obs	rel	obs	rel	obs	rel	obs	rel	obs	rel	obs	rel
Males	(138)		(433)		(1288)		(1619)		(1278)		(4756)	
1 year	98	98	94	95	89	91	84	87	68	75	82	86
3 years	89	89	88	89	76	79	65	73	44	60	65	74
5 years	85	85	83	86	68	74	53	64	31	54	55	69
Females	(34)		(59)		(207)		(313)		(458)		(1071)	
1 year	97	97	88	88	84	85	81	83	66	71	76	79
3 years	94	94	81	82	74	76	68	72	46	59	61	69
5 years	94	95	76	77	67	70	58	64	35	54	52	64
Overall	(172)		(492)		(1495)		(1932)		(1736)		(5827)	
1 year	98	98	93	94	89	90	83	86	68	74	81	85
3 years	90	90	87	89	76	79	66	73	45	60	64	73
5 years	86	87	82	85	68	74	53	64	32	54	54	68

NETHERLANDS

AREA	NUMBER OF CASES			PERIOD	MEAN AGE		
	Males	Females	All		Males	Females	All
Eindhoven	421	128	549	1985-1989	67.3	70.3	68.0

OBSERVED AND RELATIVE SURVIVAL (%) BY AGE (number of cases in parentheses)

	AGE CLASS										ALL	
	15-44		45-54		55-64		65-74		75-99			
	obs	rel	obs	rel	obs	rel	obs	rel	obs	rel	obs	rel
Males	(15)		(43)		(97)		(155)		(111)		(421)	
1 year	100	100	93	93	87	88	82	85	68	76	81	85
3 years	100	100	81	82	68	72	60	69	49	71	63	73
5 years	100	100	79	81	58	64	49	63	32	62	51	67
Females	(7)		(5)		(26)		(34)		(56)		(128)	
1 year	100	100	60	60	88	89	65	66	61	66	70	73
3 years	86	86	60	61	81	82	44	47	32	43	49	56
5 years	86	86	60	61	77	80	35	39	16	27	39	49
Overall	(22)		(48)		(123)		(189)		(167)		(549)	
1 year	100	100	89	90	87	88	79	82	65	73	78	82
3 years	95	96	79	80	71	74	57	65	43	61	59	69
5 years	95	96	77	79	62	68	46	58	27	49	48	63

BLADDER (ICD-9 188)

POLAND

AREA	NUMBER OF CASES			PERIOD	MEAN AGE			5-YR RELATIVE SURVIVAL (%)	
	Males	Females	All		Males	Females	All	Males	Females
Cracow	213	39	252	1985-1989	65.3	70.2	66.1		
Warsaw	225	82	307	1988-1989	66.4	69.3	67.2		
Polish Registries	438	121	559		65.9	69.6	66.7		

OBSERVED AND RELATIVE SURVIVAL (%) BY AGE (number of cases in parentheses)

	AGE CLASS										ALL	
	15-44		45-54		55-64		65-74		75-99			
	obs	rel	obs	rel	obs	rel	obs	rel	obs	rel	obs	rel
Males	(16)		(34)		(148)		(146)		(94)		(438)	
1 year	88	88	74	74	64	66	56	59	50	56	60	63
3 years	75	76	47	49	37	41	40	48	29	42	39	46
5 years	75	77	44	47	28	33	25	35	18	34	28	37
Females	(2)		(9)		(27)		(34)		(49)		(121)	
1 year	50	50	89	89	48	49	73	75	39	42	54	57
3 years	50	50	56	56	41	42	52	57	22	29	38	43
5 years	50	50	44	46	33	36	46	55	16	25	31	39
Overall	(18)		(43)		(175)		(180)		(143)		(559)	
1 year	83	84	77	78	62	63	59	62	46	51	59	62
3 years	72	73	49	51	38	41	42	49	27	37	38	45
5 years	72	74	44	47	29	33	29	39	18	31	29	38

SCOTLAND

AREA	NUMBER OF CASES			PERIOD	MEAN AGE		
	Males	Females	All		Males	Females	All
Scotland	3937	1777	5714	1985-1989	68.2	70.2	68.8

OBSERVED AND RELATIVE SURVIVAL (%) BY AGE (number of cases in parentheses)

	AGE CLASS										ALL	
	15-44		45-54		55-64		65-74		75-99			
	obs	rel	obs	rel	obs	rel	obs	rel	obs	rel	obs	rel
Males	(119)		(300)		(923)		(1390)		(1205)		(3937)	
1 year	95	95	95	96	85	87	77	81	64	72	77	81
3 years	89	90	80	82	72	76	57	67	38	57	58	69
5 years	87	89	73	76	63	71	46	61	26	51	47	65
Females	(42)		(133)		(345)		(555)		(702)		(1777)	
1 year	83	83	90	91	85	86	74	76	53	58	69	73
3 years	76	77	80	81	72	74	59	65	34	45	54	62
5 years	74	74	77	79	66	70	50	59	25	42	46	59
Overall	(161)		(433)		(1268)		(1945)		(1907)		(5714)	
1 year	92	92	94	94	85	87	76	79	60	67	74	79
3 years	86	86	80	82	72	76	58	67	37	52	56	67
5 years	84	85	74	77	64	71	47	61	25	48	47	63

BLADDER (ICD-9 188)

SLOVAKIA

AREA	NUMBER OF CASES			PERIOD	MEAN AGE		
	Males	Females	All		Males	Females	All
Slovakia	2021	515	2536	1985-1989	66.4	67.9	66.7

OBSERVED AND RELATIVE SURVIVAL (%) BY AGE (number of cases in parentheses)

	AGE CLASS										ALL	
	15-44		45-54		55-64		65-74		75-99			
	obs	rel	obs	rel	obs	rel	obs	rel	obs	rel	obs	rel
Males	(77)		(211)		(566)		(619)		(548)		(2021)	
1 year	90	90	90	91	77	79	67	71	57	65	70	75
3 years	82	83	75	78	61	67	48	57	36	55	52	63
5 years	77	79	65	70	54	63	39	54	28	59	45	62
Females	(23)		(46)		(123)		(128)		(195)		(515)	
1 year	87	87	80	81	73	74	71	73	50	55	65	68
3 years	83	83	72	73	63	65	51	56	34	47	50	58
5 years	76	76	64	65	60	65	48	57	27	47	45	59
Overall	(100)		(257)		(689)		(747)		(743)		(2536)	
1 year	89	89	88	89	76	78	68	72	55	62	69	74
3 years	82	83	74	77	61	66	48	56	36	53	52	62
5 years	77	78	65	69	55	64	41	54	28	56	45	61

SLOVENIA

AREA	NUMBER OF CASES			PERIOD	MEAN AGE		
	Males	Females	All		Males	Females	All
Slovenia	554	171	725	1985-1989	67.3	69.5	67.8

OBSERVED AND RELATIVE SURVIVAL (%) BY AGE (number of cases in parentheses)

	AGE CLASS										ALL	
	15-44		45-54		55-64		65-74		75-99			
	obs	rel	obs	rel	obs	rel	obs	rel	obs	rel	obs	rel
Males	(15)		(49)		(163)		(153)		(174)		(554)	
1 year	100	100	78	78	72	74	72	75	50	57	66	70
3 years	100	100	63	65	53	57	46	53	26	39	45	54
5 years	80	82	49	52	42	47	33	43	16	31	33	44
Females	(6)		(8)		(36)		(49)		(72)		(171)	
1 year	100	100	63	63	58	59	63	65	49	53	57	60
3 years	100	100	38	38	38	39	37	40	26	35	35	40
5 years	100	100	38	38	29	31	31	36	18	30	28	36
Overall	(21)		(57)		(199)		(202)		(246)		(725)	
1 year	100	100	75	76	70	71	70	73	50	55	64	68
3 years	100	100	60	61	51	54	44	50	26	38	43	51
5 years	86	87	47	50	39	44	32	41	16	31	32	42

BLADDER (ICD-9 188)

SPAIN

AREA	NUMBER OF CASES			PERIOD	MEAN AGE			5-YR RELATIVE SURVIVAL (%)	
	Males	Females	All		Males	Females	All	Males	Females
Basque Country	1031	145	1176	1986-1988	65.3	69.4	65.8		
Mallorca	217	34	251	1988-1989	68.4	74.8	69.3		
Navarra	442	64	506	1985-1989	66.2	71.3	66.8		
Tarragona	462	95	557	1985-1989	68.0	71.1	68.5		
Spanish Registries	2152	338	2490		66.4	70.8	67.0		

OBSERVED AND RELATIVE SURVIVAL (%) BY AGE (number of cases in parentheses)

	AGE CLASS										ALL	
	15-44		45-54		55-64		65-74		75-99			
	obs	rel	obs	rel	obs	rel	obs	rel	obs	rel	obs	rel
Males	(94)		(198)		(586)		(731)		(543)		(2152)	
1 year	97	97	93	93	89	90	84	87	69	75	83	86
3 years	94	94	83	85	75	79	65	73	47	64	66	75
5 years	93	94	78	80	68	74	56	68	36	63	58	72
Females	(10)		(21)		(47)		(118)		(142)		(338)	
1 year	100	100	95	95	87	88	83	84	68	74	79	82
3 years	90	90	90	91	85	87	69	73	50	63	65	73
5 years	90	90	80	81	83	86	57	63	42	65	57	70
Overall	(104)		(219)		(633)		(849)		(685)		(2490)	
1 year	97	97	93	94	88	90	84	86	68	75	82	85
3 years	93	94	84	85	76	79	66	73	48	64	66	75
5 years	92	93	78	80	69	75	56	67	38	64	58	71

SWEDEN

AREA	NUMBER OF CASES			PERIOD	MEAN AGE		
	Males	Females	All		Males	Females	All
South Sweden	1185	330	1515	1985-1989	69.4	70.8	69.7

OBSERVED AND RELATIVE SURVIVAL (%) BY AGE (number of cases in parentheses)

	AGE CLASS										ALL	
	15-44		45-54		55-64		65-74		75-99			
	obs	rel	obs	rel	obs	rel	obs	rel	obs	rel	obs	rel
Males	(32)		(78)		(232)		(426)		(417)		(1185)	
1 year	97	97	91	91	93	94	87	90	67	74	82	86
3 years	97	97	86	87	80	83	72	81	43	59	65	76
5 years	97	98	82	84	71	76	66	80	32	58	57	75
Females	(14)		(12)		(63)		(100)		(141)		(330)	
1 year	93	93	92	92	86	86	84	85	67	72	78	81
3 years	79	79	92	92	78	80	68	72	50	65	64	72
5 years	71	72	92	93	73	76	62	69	40	63	56	70
Overall	(46)		(90)		(295)		(526)		(558)		(1515)	
1 year	96	96	91	92	91	92	87	89	67	74	81	85
3 years	91	92	87	88	79	82	71	79	45	61	65	75
5 years	89	90	83	86	71	76	65	78	34	59	57	74

BLADDER

(ICD-9 188)

SWITZERLAND

AREA	NUMBER OF CASES			PERIOD	MEAN AGE			5-YR RELATIVE SURVIVAL (%)	
	Males	Females	All		Males	Females	All	Males	Females
Basel	136	57	193	1985-1988	69.3	69.7	69.4		
Geneva	196	46	242	1985-1989	68.4	74.2	69.5		
Swiss Registries	332	103	435		68.8	71.7	69.5		

OBSERVED AND RELATIVE SURVIVAL (%) BY AGE (number of cases in parentheses)

	AGE CLASS										ALL	
	15-44		45-54		55-64		65-74		75-99			
	obs	rel	obs	rel	obs	rel	obs	rel	obs	rel	obs	rel
Males	(7)		(39)		(68)		(101)		(117)		(332)	
1 year	100	100	95	95	87	88	80	83	61	68	77	81
3 years	100	100	79	81	71	75	53	60	34	48	54	64
5 years	67	67	69	71	67	72	40	50	24	45	44	58
Females	(4)		(5)		(16)		(33)		(45)		(103)	
1 year	50	50	100	100	88	88	55	55	56	60	62	65
3 years	50	50	78	78	63	64	42	45	38	48	45	51
5 years	25	25	52	53	50	52	30	34	30	48	34	43
Overall	(11)		(44)		(84)		(134)		(162)		(435)	
1 year	82	82	95	96	87	88	74	76	59	65	73	77
3 years	82	82	79	81	70	72	51	56	35	48	52	61
5 years	51	52	67	69	63	68	38	46	26	46	42	54

BLADDER   (ICD-9 188)

EUROPE, 1985-89
Weighted analyses

COUNTRY	% COVERAGE WITH C.R.s	YEARLY NO. OF CASES (Mean No. of cases recorded)			RELATIVE SURVIVAL (%) (Age-standardized)
		Males	Females	All	
AUSTRIA	8	103	35	138	A
DENMARK	100	704	239	943	DK
ENGLAND	50	3712	1423	5135	ENG
ESTONIA	100	76	33	109	EST
FINLAND	100	402	120	522	FIN
FRANCE	3	145	37	182	F
GERMANY	2	153	53	206	D
ICELAND	100	26	9	35	IS
ITALY	10	1312	292	1604	I
NETHERLANDS	6	84	26	110	NL
POLAND	6	155	49	204	PL
SCOTLAND	100	787	355	1142	SCO
SLOVAKIA	100	404	103	507	SK
SLOVENIA	100	111	34	145	SLO
SPAIN	10	633	97	730	E
SWEDEN	17	237	66	303	S
SWITZERLAND	11	73	24	97	CH
					EUR

□ 1 year   ■ 5 years

OBSERVED AND RELATIVE SURVIVAL (%) BY AGE

	AGE CLASS										ALL	
	15-44		45-54		55-64		65-74		75-99			
	obs	rel	obs	rel	obs	rel	obs	rel	obs	rel	obs	rel
Males												
1 year	96	96	91	92	87	88	81	84	67	75	80	84
3 years	90	91	82	83	73	77	62	71	44	61	62	72
5 years	87	88	77	80	65	71	51	64	31	58	52	68
Females												
1 year	91	91	85	85	81	82	78	79	59	64	71	74
3 years	85	85	76	77	71	72	60	64	40	52	55	62
5 years	84	84	71	72	65	68	52	59	32	51	47	60
Overall												
1 year	95	95	90	90	86	87	80	83	65	72	78	82
3 years	89	90	81	82	73	76	62	69	43	59	61	70
5 years	86	87	75	78	65	71	51	63	32	56	51	66

AGE STANDARDIZED RELATIVE SURVIVAL(%)

COUNTRY	MALES		FEMALES	
	1-year (95% C.I.)	5-years (95% C.I.)	1-year (95% C.I.)	5-years (95% C.I.)
AUSTRIA	85.6 (80.5 - 91.0)	66.7 (58.8 - 75.6)	81.5 (73.2 - 90.7)	63.0 (51.6 - 76.8)
DENMARK	75.2 (73.7 - 76.8)	50.3 (48.2 - 52.5)	65.1 (62.3 - 68.0)	44.1 (40.9 - 47.5)
ENGLAND	81.2 (80.6 - 81.9)	65.6 (64.7 - 66.6)	72.9 (71.8 - 73.9)	59.4 (58.0 - 60.8)
ESTONIA	60.3 (55.1 - 66.1)	33.7 (28.0 - 40.6)	-	-
FINLAND	87.0 (85.3 - 88.8)	68.6 (65.6 - 71.8)	81.5 (78.3 - 84.8)	65.2 (60.6 - 70.2)
FRANCE	82.2 (78.9 - 85.7)	59.2 (53.8 - 65.0)	76.7 (70.3 - 83.8)	54.5 (46.0 - 64.7)
GERMANY	86.2 (83.2 - 89.3)	74.8 (69.3 - 80.8)	75.8 (70.6 - 81.3)	62.6 (55.4 - 70.8)
ICELAND	80.6 (73.1 - 88.9)	66.9 (56.3 - 79.6)	83.7 (72.1 - 97.2)	73.3 (56.3 - 95.3)
ITALY	84.5 (83.2 - 85.7)	65.1 (63.2 - 67.1)	80.0 (77.6 - 82.6)	63.7 (60.3 - 67.4)
NETHERLANDS	83.8 (79.6 - 88.3)	65.3 (58.4 - 72.9)	71.6 (63.7 - 80.5)	46.5 (37.9 - 57.1)
POLAND	61.5 (56.4 - 67.0)	36.5 (30.5 - 43.6)	58.3 (50.1 - 67.7)	39.6 (30.6 - 51.3)
SCOTLAND	80.5 (79.1 - 81.9)	61.8 (59.6 - 64.1)	73.3 (71.2 - 75.4)	57.5 (54.7 - 60.4)
SLOVAKIA	72.7 (70.5 - 75.0)	59.7 (56.2 - 63.4)	68.2 (64.0 - 72.6)	56.5 (51.0 - 62.6)
SLOVENIA	69.5 (65.4 - 73.8)	41.6 (36.5 - 47.5)	60.3 (53.1 - 68.5)	34.8 (27.3 - 44.3)
SPAIN	84.2 (82.4 - 86.1)	69.2 (66.1 - 72.4)	82.6 (78.4 - 86.9)	70.5 (64.5 - 77.1)
SWEDEN	85.8 (83.6 - 88.1)	72.6 (69.0 - 76.4)	81.7 (77.4 - 86.2)	70.3 (64.2 - 76.9)
SWITZERLAND	80.1 (75.5 - 85.0)	55.1 (48.4 - 62.6)	67.1 (58.9 - 76.5)	43.7 (33.6 - 57.0)
EUROPE, 1985-89	82.6 (81.8 - 83.4)	65.2 (63.8 - 66.6)	75.4 (73.9 - 77.0)	59.7 (57.5 - 61.9)

KIDNEY (ICD-9 189)

AUSTRIA

AREA	NUMBER OF CASES			PERIOD	MEAN AGE		
	Males	Females	All		Males	Females	All
Tirol	107	77	184	1988-1989	62.4	70.0	65.6

OBSERVED AND RELATIVE SURVIVAL (%) BY AGE (number of cases in parentheses)

	AGE CLASS										ALL	
	15-44		45-54		55-64		65-74		75-99			
	obs	rel	obs	rel	obs	rel	obs	rel	obs	rel	obs	rel
Males	(10)		(19)		(27)		(35)		(16)		(107)	
1 year	90	90	79	79	78	79	60	62	63	67	71	73
3 years	70	70	79	80	63	65	43	47	38	47	56	60
5 years	70	71	79	81	56	60	37	44	31	47	51	59
Females	(3)		(6)		(9)		(26)		(33)		(77)	
1 year	100	100	100	100	100	100	73	74	61	64	74	76
3 years	100	100	100	100	89	90	62	65	58	69	68	74
5 years	67	67	100	100	89	91	54	59	48	68	60	71
Overall	(13)		(25)		(36)		(61)		(49)		(184)	
1 year	92	92	84	84	83	84	66	67	61	65	72	74
3 years	77	77	84	85	69	72	51	55	51	62	61	66
5 years	69	70	84	86	64	68	44	50	43	62	55	64

DENMARK

AREA	NUMBER OF CASES			PERIOD	MEAN AGE		
	Males	Females	All		Males	Females	All
Denmark	1550	1297	2847	1985-1989	65.6	67.9	66.7

OBSERVED AND RELATIVE SURVIVAL (%) BY AGE (number of cases in parentheses)

	AGE CLASS										ALL	
	15-44		45-54		55-64		65-74		75-99			
	obs	rel	obs	rel	obs	rel	obs	rel	obs	rel	obs	rel
Males	(93)		(172)		(378)		(524)		(383)		(1550)	
1 year	82	82	60	61	59	60	56	58	40	44	55	57
3 years	67	67	45	46	40	43	36	41	23	32	37	42
5 years	60	61	39	40	32	35	27	35	15	27	29	36
Females	(51)		(121)		(290)		(435)		(400)		(1297)	
1 year	67	67	66	66	53	54	49	50	41	44	50	51
3 years	51	51	50	51	36	37	31	33	25	31	33	36
5 years	49	49	44	45	31	33	25	29	19	29	27	33
Overall	(144)		(293)		(668)		(959)		(783)		(2847)	
1 year	76	77	63	63	57	57	53	54	40	44	52	54
3 years	61	62	47	48	38	40	34	38	24	32	35	39
5 years	56	57	41	42	32	34	26	32	17	28	28	35

KIDNEY (ICD-9 189)

ENGLAND

AREA	NUMBER OF CASES			PERIOD	MEAN AGE			5-YR RELATIVE SURVIVAL (%)	
	Males	Females	All		Males	Females	All	Males	Females
East Anglia	453	207	660	1985-1989	66.0	68.7	66.8		
Mersey	469	261	730	1985-1989	64.8	67.6	65.8		
Oxford	498	302	800	1985-1989	63.9	65.3	64.4		
South Thames	1069	614	1683	1985-1989	64.8	67.2	65.7		
Wessex	698	383	1081	1985-1989	64.4	68.2	65.8		
West Midlands	990	591	1581	1985-1989	64.0	67.1	65.2		
Yorkshire	714	447	1161	1985-1989	64.7	66.2	65.3		
English Registries	4891	2805	7696		64.6	67.1	65.5		

OBSERVED AND RELATIVE SURVIVAL (%) BY AGE (number of cases in parentheses)

	AGE CLASS										ALL	
	15-44		45-54		55-64		65-74		75-99			
	obs	rel	obs	rel	obs	rel	obs	rel	obs	rel	obs	rel
Males	(299)		(648)		(1311)		(1550)		(1083)		(4891)	
1 year	74	74	69	69	57	58	53	55	42	46	55	57
3 years	60	60	53	54	42	44	36	41	27	37	39	44
5 years	55	56	46	48	36	40	29	37	19	33	33	40
Females	(163)		(276)		(618)		(869)		(879)		(2805)	
1 year	71	71	65	65	56	56	53	54	38	41	51	53
3 years	55	55	49	49	43	44	38	41	24	31	37	41
5 years	50	51	45	45	36	38	31	36	19	29	31	37
Overall	(462)		(924)		(1929)		(2419)		(1962)		(7696)	
1 year	73	73	68	68	57	58	53	55	40	44	54	56
3 years	58	59	52	52	42	44	37	41	26	34	38	43
5 years	54	54	46	47	36	39	30	36	19	31	32	39

ESTONIA

AREA	NUMBER OF CASES			PERIOD	MEAN AGE		
	Males	Females	All		Males	Females	All
Estonia	330	250	580	1985-1989	60.0	63.4	61.5

OBSERVED AND RELATIVE SURVIVAL (%) BY AGE (number of cases in parentheses)

	AGE CLASS										ALL	
	15-44		45-54		55-64		65-74		75-99			
	obs	rel	obs	rel	obs	rel	obs	rel	obs	rel	obs	rel
Males	(18)		(78)		(127)		(83)		(24)		(330)	
1 year	39	39	53	53	48	49	45	47	46	51	48	49
3 years	28	28	35	36	30	33	28	33	25	36	30	34
5 years	22	23	32	35	23	27	22	30	21	39	25	30
Females	(15)		(43)		(75)		(67)		(50)		(250)	
1 year	60	60	76	77	60	61	37	38	38	42	52	54
3 years	40	40	55	56	46	48	19	21	16	22	34	37
5 years	40	40	48	49	37	39	13	16	10	17	27	32
Overall	(33)		(121)		(202)		(150)		(74)		(580)	
1 year	48	49	61	62	52	53	41	43	41	45	50	51
3 years	33	34	42	43	36	38	24	28	19	26	32	35
5 years	30	31	38	40	28	32	18	23	14	24	26	31

KIDNEY (ICD-9 189)

FINLAND

AREA	NUMBER OF CASES			PERIOD	MEAN AGE		
	Males	Females	All		Males	Females	All
Finland	1446	1159	2605	1985-1989	62.7	67.1	64.7

OBSERVED AND RELATIVE SURVIVAL (%) BY AGE (number of cases in parentheses)

	AGE CLASS										ALL	
	15-44		45-54		55-64		65-74		75-99			
	obs	rel	obs	rel	obs	rel	obs	rel	obs	rel	obs	rel
Males	(99)		(240)		(452)		(411)		(244)		(1446)	
1 year	83	83	75	76	67	68	62	65	48	53	65	67
3 years	71	71	61	63	51	54	44	50	32	44	49	54
5 years	65	66	54	56	42	46	34	44	19	35	39	48
Females	(58)		(100)		(255)		(417)		(329)		(1159)	
1 year	83	83	88	88	70	70	70	71	53	58	67	69
3 years	78	78	76	77	52	54	53	56	36	46	51	56
5 years	72	73	73	74	48	50	44	50	25	39	43	51
Overall	(157)		(340)		(707)		(828)		(573)		(2605)	
1 year	83	83	79	80	68	69	66	68	51	56	66	68
3 years	73	74	66	67	51	54	48	53	34	45	50	55
5 years	68	68	59	61	44	48	39	47	22	37	41	49

FRANCE

AREA	NUMBER OF CASES			PERIOD	MEAN AGE		
	Males	Females	All		Males	Females	All
Somme	134	58	192	1985-1989	61.2	65.4	62.5
Calvados	151	84	235	1985-1989	63.5	64.3	63.8
Doubs	102	68	170	1985-1989	66.0	65.4	65.8
French Registries	387	210	597		63.4	65.0	64.0

5-YR RELATIVE SURVIVAL (%)

Males — Females

Somme / Calvad / Doubs

OBSERVED AND RELATIVE SURVIVAL (%) BY AGE (number of cases in parentheses)

	AGE CLASS										ALL	
	15-44		45-54		55-64		65-74		75-99			
	obs	rel	obs	rel	obs	rel	obs	rel	obs	rel	obs	rel
Males	(21)		(55)		(132)		(116)		(63)		(387)	
1 year	85	85	75	76	73	74	72	74	62	68	72	74
3 years	74	75	59	61	59	62	53	59	43	58	56	61
5 years	54	55	54	58	53	59	46	57	34	58	49	58
Females	(15)		(20)		(59)		(61)		(55)		(210)	
1 year	100	100	90	90	78	78	68	69	47	51	70	71
3 years	91	91	74	75	65	67	57	60	29	36	56	60
5 years	58	58	74	76	65	68	49	54	23	35	50	58
Overall	(36)		(75)		(191)		(177)		(118)		(597)	
1 year	91	91	79	80	74	75	70	72	55	59	71	73
3 years	81	82	63	65	61	64	54	59	36	46	56	61
5 years	56	57	60	63	57	62	47	55	28	45	49	58

KIDNEY

(ICD-9 189)

GERMANY

AREA	NUMBER OF CASES			PERIOD	MEAN AGE		
	Males	Females	All		Males	Females	All
Saarland	324	231	555	1985-1989	62.3	66.8	64.2

OBSERVED AND RELATIVE SURVIVAL (%) BY AGE (number of cases in parentheses)

	AGE CLASS										ALL	
	15-44		45-54		55-64		65-74		75-99			
	obs	rel	obs	rel	obs	rel	obs	rel	obs	rel	obs	rel
Males	(14)		(67)		(101)		(86)		(56)		(324)	
1 year	86	86	78	78	76	78	65	68	46	52	69	71
3 years	71	72	64	66	56	60	52	59	21	31	52	58
5 years	61	62	53	55	46	51	39	49	16	33	41	50
Females	(7)		(30)		(54)		(84)		(56)		(231)	
1 year	100	100	80	80	83	84	68	69	55	60	71	73
3 years	71	72	70	71	67	68	52	56	27	35	52	58
5 years	71	72	67	68	63	66	44	51	21	34	46	55
Overall	(21)		(97)		(155)		(170)		(112)		(555)	
1 year	90	91	78	79	79	80	66	69	51	56	70	72
3 years	71	72	66	67	60	63	52	58	24	33	52	58
5 years	65	66	57	59	52	56	41	50	19	34	44	52

ICELAND

AREA	NUMBER OF CASES			PERIOD	MEAN AGE		
	Males	Females	All		Males	Females	All
Iceland	74	63	137	1985-1989	64.5	67.3	65.8

OBSERVED AND RELATIVE SURVIVAL (%) BY AGE (number of cases in parentheses)

	AGE CLASS										ALL	
	15-44		45-54		55-64		65-74		75-99			
	obs	rel	obs	rel	obs	rel	obs	rel	obs	rel	obs	rel
Males	(6)		(10)		(16)		(29)		(13)		(74)	
1 year	67	67	90	90	63	63	69	71	69	76	70	72
3 years	50	50	70	71	50	52	52	57	23	31	49	54
5 years	33	34	60	61	44	47	41	50	15	25	39	46
Females	(2)		(5)		(17)		(22)		(17)		(63)	
1 year	50	50	80	80	71	71	59	60	24	25	54	55
3 years	50	50	60	61	59	60	36	39	24	29	41	45
5 years	50	50	60	61	47	49	32	36	12	17	33	39
Overall	(8)		(15)		(33)		(51)		(30)		(137)	
1 year	63	63	87	87	67	67	65	66	43	47	63	65
3 years	50	50	67	67	55	56	45	49	23	30	45	50
5 years	38	38	60	61	45	48	37	44	13	21	36	43

KIDNEY (ICD-9 189)

ITALY

AREA	NUMBER OF CASES			PERIOD	MEAN AGE			5-YR RELATIVE SURVIVAL (%)	
	Males	Females	All		Males	Females	All	Males	Females
Florence	481	249	730	1985-1989	65.2	66.2	65.5		
Genoa	147	87	234	1986-1988	65.0	66.3	65.5		
Latina	37	23	60	1985-1987	60.9	65.9	62.8		
Modena	96	70	166	1988-1989	64.6	67.9	66.0		
Parma	107	47	154	1985-1987	65.8	66.1	65.9		
Ragusa	38	17	55	1985-1989	59.5	64.8	61.2		
Romagna	140	60	200	1986-1988	65.0	68.2	66.0		
Turin	180	113	293	1985-1987	63.7	68.2	65.4		
Varese	277	155	432	1985-1989	64.2	65.1	64.5		
Italian Registries	1503	821	2324		64.6	66.5	65.3		

OBSERVED AND RELATIVE SURVIVAL (%) BY AGE (number of cases in parentheses)

	15-44		45-54		55-64		65-74		75-99		ALL	
	obs	rel	obs	rel	obs	rel	obs	rel	obs	rel	obs	rel
Males	(74)		(180)		(471)		(472)		(306)		(1503)	
1 year	85	85	86	87	73	74	65	68	56	61	69	72
3 years	78	79	71	72	57	60	50	56	31	41	52	58
5 years	73	74	64	66	52	57	38	47	24	40	45	54
Females	(47)		(85)		(204)		(247)		(238)		(821)	
1 year	85	85	80	80	82	83	68	69	50	54	69	71
3 years	74	75	69	70	67	68	53	56	34	43	54	59
5 years	72	73	67	68	62	64	44	48	26	40	47	55
Overall	(121)		(265)		(675)		(719)		(544)		(2324)	
1 year	85	85	84	84	76	77	66	68	54	58	69	71
3 years	77	77	70	71	60	63	51	56	33	42	53	58
5 years	73	73	65	67	55	59	40	48	25	40	46	54

NETHERLANDS

AREA	NUMBER OF CASES			PERIOD	MEAN AGE		
	Males	Females	All		Males	Females	All
Eindhoven	201	135	336	1985-1989	62.8	64.7	63.6

OBSERVED AND RELATIVE SURVIVAL (%) BY AGE (number of cases in parentheses)

	15-44		45-54		55-64		65-74		75-99		ALL	
	obs	rel	obs	rel	obs	rel	obs	rel	obs	rel	obs	rel
Males	(13)		(35)		(61)		(54)		(38)		(201)	
1 year	69	69	86	86	80	81	74	77	55	61	74	77
3 years	69	70	63	64	65	69	57	64	32	43	56	63
5 years	69	70	56	58	58	64	39	49	24	41	47	56
Females	(9)		(17)		(33)		(47)		(29)		(135)	
1 year	89	89	88	89	70	70	64	65	59	63	69	70
3 years	76	76	76	77	51	52	53	57	24	30	51	54
5 years	61	61	71	72	45	46	41	47	14	20	41	47
Overall	(22)		(52)		(94)		(101)		(67)		(336)	
1 year	77	77	87	87	77	77	69	71	57	62	72	74
3 years	72	73	67	68	60	63	55	60	28	37	54	59
5 years	66	67	61	63	53	57	40	48	19	31	45	52

KIDNEY (ICD-9 189)

POLAND

AREA	NUMBER OF CASES			PERIOD	MEAN AGE			5-YR RELATIVE SURVIVAL (%)	
	Males	Females	All		Males	Females	All	Males	Females
Cracow	177	97	274	1985-1989	58.9	59.5	59.1		
Warsaw	208	152	360	1988-1989	61.2	64.9	62.8		
Polish Registries	385	249	634		60.2	62.8	61.2		

OBSERVED AND RELATIVE SURVIVAL (%) BY AGE (number of cases in parentheses)

	AGE CLASS										ALL	
	15-44		45-54		55-64		65-74		75-99			
	obs	rel	obs	rel	obs	rel	obs	rel	obs	rel	obs	rel
Males	(33)		(83)		(144)		(74)		(51)		(385)	
1 year	70	70	58	58	61	62	60	64	25	28	56	58
3 years	58	58	37	39	40	43	29	34	18	25	36	40
5 years	45	47	31	34	31	36	25	34	14	25	29	35
Females	(12)		(49)		(78)		(71)		(39)		(249)	
1 year	58	58	73	74	55	56	47	48	36	39	54	55
3 years	50	50	57	58	41	43	30	33	16	21	38	41
5 years	50	51	53	54	36	38	22	27	11	17	32	37
Overall	(45)		(132)		(222)		(145)		(90)		(634)	
1 year	67	67	64	64	59	60	54	56	30	33	55	57
3 years	56	56	45	46	40	43	29	34	17	23	37	40
5 years	47	48	39	42	33	37	24	30	13	21	30	36

SCOTLAND

AREA	NUMBER OF CASES			PERIOD	MEAN AGE		
	Males	Females	All		Males	Females	All
Scotland	1162	840	2002	1985-1989	64.7	67.3	65.8

OBSERVED AND RELATIVE SURVIVAL (%) BY AGE (number of cases in parentheses)

	AGE CLASS										ALL	
	15-44		45-54		55-64		65-74		75-99			
	obs	rel	obs	rel	obs	rel	obs	rel	obs	rel	obs	rel
Males	(53)		(153)		(354)		(368)		(234)		(1162)	
1 year	77	78	65	65	59	60	54	56	34	38	54	56
3 years	62	63	53	54	41	44	35	41	15	22	36	42
5 years	55	56	48	50	35	39	26	34	11	21	30	38
Females	(37)		(79)		(197)		(278)		(249)		(840)	
1 year	57	57	65	65	62	63	48	49	38	42	50	52
3 years	46	46	52	53	44	45	33	36	23	30	35	39
5 years	46	46	48	49	37	39	26	31	16	25	28	35
Overall	(90)		(232)		(551)		(646)		(483)		(2002)	
1 year	69	69	65	65	60	61	51	53	36	40	52	55
3 years	56	56	53	54	42	45	34	39	19	26	36	41
5 years	51	52	48	50	36	39	26	33	13	23	29	37

KIDNEY (ICD-9 189)

SLOVAKIA

AREA	NUMBER OF CASES			PERIOD	MEAN AGE		
	Males	Females	All		Males	Females	All
Slovakia	1020	686	1706	1985-1989	60.4	62.1	61.1

OBSERVED AND RELATIVE SURVIVAL (%) BY AGE (number of cases in parentheses)

	AGE CLASS										ALL	
	15-44		45-54		55-64		65-74		75-99			
	obs	rel	obs	rel	obs	rel	obs	rel	obs	rel	obs	rel
Males	(95)		(189)		(359)		(253)		(124)		(1020)	
1 year	72	72	64	65	59	61	56	59	40	44	58	60
3 years	61	62	49	51	42	45	37	44	26	37	42	47
5 years	58	59	40	43	36	42	30	41	22	43	36	44
Females	(46)		(116)		(240)		(176)		(108)		(686)	
1 year	70	70	72	72	69	70	53	54	44	49	61	63
3 years	65	66	57	58	52	54	40	44	29	39	47	51
5 years	61	62	54	55	48	52	31	36	22	38	42	48
Overall	(141)		(305)		(599)		(429)		(232)		(1706)	
1 year	71	71	67	68	63	64	55	57	42	46	59	61
3 years	62	63	52	54	46	49	38	44	27	38	44	49
5 years	59	60	45	48	41	46	31	39	22	40	38	46

SLOVENIA

AREA	NUMBER OF CASES			PERIOD	MEAN AGE		
	Males	Females	All		Males	Females	All
Slovenia	310	197	507	1985-1989	61.4	63.4	62.2

OBSERVED AND RELATIVE SURVIVAL (%) BY AGE (number of cases in parentheses)

	AGE CLASS										ALL	
	15-44		45-54		55-64		65-74		75-99			
	obs	rel	obs	rel	obs	rel	obs	rel	obs	rel	obs	rel
Males	(23)		(58)		(102)		(84)		(43)		(310)	
1 year	70	70	74	75	56	57	59	62	49	55	60	62
3 years	70	70	60	62	35	38	37	43	30	44	42	48
5 years	65	67	48	51	28	32	29	38	19	36	34	41
Females	(14)		(27)		(62)		(57)		(37)		(197)	
1 year	93	93	89	89	66	67	65	67	41	44	66	68
3 years	93	93	73	74	55	56	53	57	24	33	54	58
5 years	93	94	73	75	48	51	40	47	22	37	48	55
Overall	(37)		(85)		(164)		(141)		(80)		(507)	
1 year	78	79	79	79	60	61	62	64	45	50	62	65
3 years	78	79	64	66	43	45	44	49	28	38	47	52
5 years	76	77	56	59	36	40	34	42	20	36	39	47

KIDNEY (ICD-9 189)

SPAIN

AREA	NUMBER OF CASES			PERIOD	MEAN AGE			5-YR RELATIVE SURVIVAL (%)	
	Males	Females	All		Males	Females	All	Males	Females
Basque Country	292	119	411	1986-1988	61.7	64.8	62.6		
Mallorca	46	19	65	1988-1989	63.5	70.4	65.5		
Navarra	108	70	178	1985-1989	64.7	66.3	65.3		
Tarragona	74	37	111	1985-1989	66.0	68.1	66.7		
Spanish Registries	520	245	765		63.1	66.2	64.1		

OBSERVED AND RELATIVE SURVIVAL (%) BY AGE (number of cases in parentheses)

	15-44		45-54		55-64		65-74		75-99		ALL	
	obs	rel	obs	rel	obs	rel	obs	rel	obs	rel	obs	rel
Males	(47)		(69)		(141)		(157)		(106)		(520)	
1 year	72	72	74	74	70	70	64	66	55	60	66	68
3 years	57	58	65	66	57	60	48	54	33	44	51	56
5 years	57	58	60	62	53	58	41	49	24	39	44	53
Females	(19)		(24)		(53)		(80)		(69)		(245)	
1 year	95	95	83	84	72	72	65	66	51	54	67	68
3 years	89	90	71	71	55	56	51	54	35	43	52	56
5 years	84	84	71	72	48	50	48	52	23	33	46	52
Overall	(66)		(93)		(194)		(237)		(175)		(765)	
1 year	79	79	76	77	70	71	65	66	53	57	66	68
3 years	67	67	67	68	57	59	49	54	34	43	51	56
5 years	65	66	63	64	52	55	43	50	24	37	45	53

SWEDEN

AREA	NUMBER OF CASES			PERIOD	MEAN AGE		
	Males	Females	All		Males	Females	All
South Sweden	489	346	835	1985-1989	66.4	67.5	66.9

OBSERVED AND RELATIVE SURVIVAL (%) BY AGE (number of cases in parentheses)

	15-44		45-54		55-64		65-74		75-99		ALL	
	obs	rel	obs	rel	obs	rel	obs	rel	obs	rel	obs	rel
Males	(18)		(56)		(119)		(177)		(119)		(489)	
1 year	83	83	73	74	74	75	61	63	50	55	64	66
3 years	67	67	59	60	59	61	45	50	29	38	47	53
5 years	56	56	54	55	52	56	36	44	24	40	40	49
Females	(15)		(26)		(81)		(122)		(102)		(346)	
1 year	87	87	77	77	74	75	64	65	48	51	64	65
3 years	87	87	58	58	54	55	50	53	28	35	47	51
5 years	80	80	58	59	48	50	42	46	23	34	40	47
Overall	(33)		(82)		(200)		(299)		(221)		(835)	
1 year	85	85	74	75	74	75	62	64	49	53	64	66
3 years	76	76	59	59	57	59	47	51	29	37	47	52
5 years	67	67	55	56	51	54	38	45	23	37	40	48

KIDNEY (ICD-9 189)

SWITZERLAND

AREA	NUMBER OF CASES			PERIOD	MEAN AGE			5-YR RELATIVE SURVIVAL (%)	
	Males	Females	All		Males	Females	All	Males	Females
Basel	100	80	180	1985-1988	64.0	67.8	65.7		
Geneva	106	76	182	1985-1989	63.5	67.7	65.2		
Swiss Registries	206	156	362		63.7	67.8	65.5		

OBSERVED AND RELATIVE SURVIVAL (%) BY AGE (number of cases in parentheses)

	AGE CLASS										ALL	
	15-44		45-54		55-64		65-74		75-99			
	obs	rel	obs	rel	obs	rel	obs	rel	obs	rel	obs	rel
Males	(13)		(29)		(59)		(64)		(41)		(206)	
1 year	85	85	93	93	85	86	59	61	41	46	69	72
3 years	85	85	68	69	72	75	44	49	27	36	54	60
5 years	76	77	61	63	59	63	38	45	22	38	46	55
Females	(6)		(18)		(37)		(45)		(50)		(156)	
1 year	83	83	83	84	84	84	64	66	40	43	64	66
3 years	83	84	56	56	62	63	38	40	24	30	43	47
5 years	83	84	50	51	57	59	33	37	18	27	38	44
Overall	(19)		(47)		(96)		(109)		(91)		(362)	
1 year	84	84	89	90	84	85	61	63	41	44	67	69
3 years	84	85	63	64	68	70	41	45	25	33	49	54
5 years	79	79	56	58	58	61	36	42	20	32	42	51

KIDNEY

(ICD-9 189)

EUROPE, 1985-89

Weighted analyses

COUNTRY	% COVERAGE WITH C.R.s	YEARLY NO. OF CASES (Mean No. of cases recorded)			RELATIVE SURVIVAL (%) (Age-standardized)
		Males	Females	All	
AUSTRIA	8	54	39	93	
DENMARK	100	310	259	569	
ENGLAND	50	978	561	1539	
ESTONIA	100	66	50	116	
FINLAND	100	289	232	521	
FRANCE	3	77	42	119	
GERMANY	2	65	46	111	
ICELAND	100	15	13	28	
ITALY	10	411	229	640	
NETHERLANDS	6	40	27	67	
POLAND	6	139	95	234	
SCOTLAND	100	232	168	400	
SLOVAKIA	100	204	137	341	
SLOVENIA	100	62	39	101	
SPAIN	10	157	71	228	
SWEDEN	17	98	69	167	
SWITZERLAND	11	46	35	81	

□ 1 year ■ 5 years

OBSERVED AND RELATIVE SURVIVAL (%) BY AGE

	15-44 obs rel	45-54 obs rel	55-64 obs rel	65-74 obs rel	75-99 obs rel	ALL obs rel
Males						
1 year	80 81	75 76	70 71	64 66	49 54	66 68
3 years	69 70	60 62	54 57	46 52	29 39	49 54
5 years	61 61	54 56	47 51	37 46	22 38	41 49
Females						
1 year	86 86	80 80	74 75	63 64	48 52	65 67
3 years	72 73	67 67	59 60	48 51	28 36	49 54
5 years	65 66	64 65	55 57	40 45	22 33	43 50
Overall						
1 year	82 83	77 78	72 73	63 65	49 53	65 67
3 years	70 71	63 64	56 58	47 52	29 38	49 54
5 years	62 63	58 59	50 54	38 45	22 36	42 50

AGE STANDARDIZED RELATIVE SURVIVAL(%)

COUNTRY	MALES 1-year (95% C.I.)	MALES 5-years (95% C.I.)	FEMALES 1-year (95% C.I.)	FEMALES 5-years (95% C.I.)
AUSTRIA	71.5 (62.8 - 81.5)	55.2 (44.8 - 68.2)	83.8 (77.3 - 90.8)	75.6 (65.6 - 87.1)
DENMARK	57.2 (54.7 - 59.8)	35.5 (32.8 - 38.4)	52.6 (49.9 - 55.5)	33.3 (30.6 - 36.4)
ENGLAND	56.9 (55.5 - 58.3)	39.4 (37.8 - 41.1)	54.3 (52.4 - 56.2)	36.9 (34.9 - 38.9)
ESTONIA	49.0 (42.5 - 56.4)	31.5 (24.0 - 41.3)	51.4 (45.5 - 58.1)	28.3 (22.9 - 35.0)
FINLAND	65.4 (62.8 - 68.1)	45.1 (42.0 - 48.5)	70.7 (68.1 - 73.4)	51.9 (48.8 - 55.2)
FRANCE	73.6 (68.7 - 78.9)	57.4 (50.2 - 65.7)	71.9 (66.0 - 78.3)	56.3 (48.8 - 65.0)
GERMANY	69.1 (63.9 - 74.8)	47.3 (40.4 - 55.5)	74.4 (69.0 - 80.2)	54.6 (47.7 - 62.5)
ICELAND	72.3 (62.0 - 84.3)	43.8 (32.5 - 59.0)	57.1 (46.4 - 70.2)	39.3 (28.3 - 54.6)
ITALY	71.4 (69.1 - 73.9)	52.0 (49.1 - 55.1)	71.7 (68.7 - 74.9)	54.6 (51.0 - 58.5)
NETHERLANDS	75.3 (69.1 - 82.1)	53.4 (45.3 - 62.8)	70.3 (62.9 - 78.7)	44.5 (36.4 - 54.3)
POLAND	54.8 (49.6 - 60.7)	33.3 (27.3 - 40.4)	51.8 (45.6 - 58.9)	32.6 (26.7 - 39.8)
SCOTLAND	55.6 (52.8 - 58.7)	35.8 (32.7 - 39.2)	53.6 (50.2 - 57.1)	35.2 (31.7 - 39.0)
SLOVAKIA	57.5 (54.1 - 61.1)	43.0 (38.6 - 47.9)	60.3 (56.5 - 64.4)	44.9 (40.3 - 50.0)
SLOVENIA	61.1 (55.3 - 67.5)	39.3 (32.5 - 47.4)	65.9 (59.6 - 73.0)	52.1 (44.5 - 60.9)
SPAIN	67.3 (63.2 - 71.7)	51.2 (46.1 - 56.8)	68.8 (63.2 - 74.9)	51.7 (45.2 - 59.0)
SWEDEN	67.1 (62.9 - 71.5)	48.7 (43.7 - 54.2)	67.3 (62.5 - 72.5)	48.0 (42.5 - 54.2)
SWITZERLAND	69.9 (63.9 - 76.4)	52.7 (45.0 - 61.6)	68.8 (62.1 - 76.2)	45.3 (37.7 - 54.4)
EUROPE, 1985-89	66.9 (65.3 - 68.5)	47.7 (45.6 - 49.9)	67.4 (65.6 - 69.3)	49.3 (47.1 - 51.6)

CHOROID (MELANOMA) (ICD-9 190.6)

AUSTRIA

AREA	NUMBER OF CASES			PERIOD	MEAN AGE		
	Males	Females	All		Males	Females	All
Tirol	4	1	5	1988-1989	46.5	73.0	52.0

OBSERVED AND RELATIVE SURVIVAL (%) BY AGE (number of cases in parentheses)

	AGE CLASS										ALL	
	15-44		45-54		55-64		65-74		75-99			
	obs	rel	obs	rel	obs	rel	obs	rel	obs	rel	obs	rel
Males	(1)		(2)		(1)		(0)		(0)		(4)	
1 year	100	100	100	100	100	100	-	-	-	-	100	100
3 years	100	100	50	50	0	0	-	-	-	-	50	51
5 years	100	100	50	51	0	0	-	-	-	-	50	51
Females	(0)		(0)		(0)		(1)		(0)		(1)	
1 year	-	-	-	-	-	-	100	100	-	-	100	100
3 years	-	-	-	-	-	-	100	100	-	-	100	100
5 years	-	-	-	-	-	-	0	0	-	-	0	0
Overall	(1)		(2)		(1)		(1)		(0)		(5)	
1 year	100	100	100	100	100	100	100	100	-	-	100	100
3 years	100	100	50	50	0	0	100	100	-	-	60	62
5 years	100	100	50	51	0	0	0	0	-	-	40	42

DENMARK

AREA	NUMBER OF CASES			PERIOD	MEAN AGE		
	Males	Females	All		Males	Females	All
Denmark	104	99	203	1985-1989	61.6	63.8	62.6

OBSERVED AND RELATIVE SURVIVAL (%) BY AGE (number of cases in parentheses)

	AGE CLASS										ALL	
	15-44		45-54		55-64		65-74		75-99			
	obs	rel	obs	rel	obs	rel	obs	rel	obs	rel	obs	rel
Males	(16)		(16)		(22)		(32)		(18)		(104)	
1 year	94	94	100	100	95	97	97	100	83	93	94	98
3 years	94	95	75	77	73	77	72	82	50	71	72	81
5 years	88	89	63	65	64	71	41	52	33	63	55	67
Females	(10)		(13)		(21)		(34)		(21)		(99)	
1 year	100	100	100	100	95	96	94	96	95	100	96	98
3 years	100	100	92	94	81	84	74	79	52	66	76	82
5 years	100	100	77	79	62	66	53	61	24	37	57	65
Overall	(26)		(29)		(43)		(66)		(39)		(203)	
1 year	96	96	100	100	95	97	95	98	90	98	95	98
3 years	96	97	83	84	77	80	73	80	51	68	74	81
5 years	92	93	69	71	63	68	47	56	28	48	56	66

CHOROID (MELANOMA) (ICD-9 190.6)

ENGLAND

AREA	NUMBER OF CASES			PERIOD	MEAN AGE			5-YR RELATIVE SURVIVAL (%)	
	Males	Females	All		Males	Females	All	Males	Females
East Anglia	13	7	20	1985-1989	64.2	60.6	63.0		
Mersey	18	8	26	1985-1989	64.3	66.0	64.8		
Oxford	11	15	26	1985-1989	56.8	54.7	55.7		
South Thames	53	46	99	1985-1989	54.1	58.2	56.0		
Wessex	23	21	44	1985-1989	57.9	64.3	61.0		
West Midlands	49	37	86	1985-1989	59.5	63.0	61.0		
Yorkshire	36	41	77	1985-1989	63.3	59.9	61.5		
English Registries	203	175	378		59.2	60.5	59.8		

OBSERVED AND RELATIVE SURVIVAL (%) BY AGE (number of cases in parentheses)

	AGE CLASS										ALL	
	15-44		45-54		55-64		65-74		75-99			
	obs	rel	obs	rel	obs	rel	obs	rel	obs	rel	obs	rel
Males	(32)		(30)		(57)		(55)		(29)		(203)	
1 year	100	100	97	97	96	98	91	94	90	98	95	97
3 years	94	94	83	85	79	83	75	84	69	91	79	87
5 years	88	88	80	83	63	70	71	88	51	85	70	81
Females	(25)		(35)		(45)		(34)		(36)		(175)	
1 year	96	96	100	100	93	94	94	96	81	87	93	95
3 years	88	88	97	98	80	82	79	85	47	60	78	83
5 years	80	80	83	84	58	61	59	67	39	60	62	70
Overall	(57)		(65)		(102)		(89)		(65)		(378)	
1 year	98	98	98	99	95	96	92	95	85	92	94	96
3 years	91	92	91	92	79	83	76	85	57	74	79	85
5 years	84	85	82	84	61	66	66	79	44	70	66	76

ESTONIA

AREA	NUMBER OF CASES			PERIOD	MEAN AGE		
	Males	Females	All		Males	Females	All
Estonia	13	27	40	1985-1989	54.6	62.4	59.9

OBSERVED AND RELATIVE SURVIVAL (%) BY AGE (number of cases in parentheses)

	AGE CLASS										ALL	
	15-44		45-54		55-64		65-74		75-99			
	obs	rel	obs	rel	obs	rel	obs	rel	obs	rel	obs	rel
Males	(1)		(6)		(4)		(2)		(0)		(13)	
1 year	100	100	83	84	100	100	100	100	-	-	92	95
3 years	0	0	83	87	50	55	100	100	-	-	69	75
5 years	0	0	83	90	50	59	0	0	-	-	54	62
Females	(3)		(4)		(6)		(10)		(4)		(27)	
1 year	100	100	100	100	100	100	100	100	50	57	93	96
3 years	67	67	100	100	100	100	60	66	25	38	70	78
5 years	67	67	50	51	83	89	60	72	25	53	59	70
Overall	(4)		(10)		(10)		(12)		(4)		(40)	
1 year	100	100	90	91	100	100	100	100	50	57	93	95
3 years	50	50	90	93	80	85	67	75	25	38	70	77
5 years	50	51	70	74	70	78	50	62	25	53	58	68

CHOROID (MELANOMA)   (ICD-9 190.6)

FINLAND

AREA	NUMBER OF CASES			PERIOD	MEAN AGE		
	Males	Females	All		Males	Females	All
Finland	60	80	140	1985-1989	59.0	60.8	60.0

OBSERVED AND RELATIVE SURVIVAL (%) BY AGE (number of cases in parentheses)

	AGE CLASS										ALL	
	15-44		45-54		55-64		65-74		75-99			
	obs	rel	obs	rel	obs	rel	obs	rel	obs	rel	obs	rel
Males	(7)		(16)		(15)		(8)		(14)		(60)	
1 year	100	100	100	100	100	100	100	100	86	95	97	100
3 years	100	100	94	96	73	77	50	57	50	69	73	81
5 years	100	100	81	85	60	65	50	63	21	39	60	72
Females	(8)		(16)		(24)		(19)		(13)		(80)	
1 year	100	100	100	100	96	96	100	100	85	90	96	98
3 years	100	100	81	82	63	64	84	90	46	57	73	77
5 years	88	88	75	76	42	43	68	78	23	34	56	62
Overall	(15)		(32)		(39)		(27)		(27)		(140)	
1 year	100	100	100	100	97	98	100	100	85	93	96	99
3 years	100	100	88	89	67	69	74	81	48	63	73	79
5 years	93	94	78	80	49	52	63	73	22	36	58	66

FRANCE

AREA	NUMBER OF CASES			PERIOD	MEAN AGE			5-YR RELATIVE SURVIVAL (%)	
	Males	Females	All		Males	Females	All	Males	Females
Somme	10	3	13	1985-1989	68.1	57.0	65.6		
Calvados	7	3	10	1985-1989	58.1	44.0	54.0		
Doubs	2	3	5	1985-1989	46.0	59.7	54.4		
French Registries	19	9	28		62.3	53.9	59.6		

OBSERVED AND RELATIVE SURVIVAL (%) BY AGE (number of cases in parentheses)

	AGE CLASS										ALL	
	15-44		45-54		55-64		65-74		75-99			
	obs	rel	obs	rel	obs	rel	obs	rel	obs	rel	obs	rel
Males	(1)		(2)		(10)		(3)		(3)		(19)	
1 year	100	100	100	100	90	92	100	100	67	76	89	93
3 years	0	0	100	100	70	74	67	75	33	51	63	70
5 years	0	0	100	100	70	77	67	82	0	0	58	70
Females	(1)		(4)		(2)		(2)		(0)		(9)	
1 year	100	100	75	75	100	100	100	100	-	-	89	89
3 years	100	100	75	76	100	100	100	100	-	-	89	90
5 years	100	100	75	77	100	100	100	100	-	-	89	92
Overall	(2)		(6)		(12)		(5)		(3)		(28)	
1 year	100	100	83	84	92	93	100	100	67	76	89	92
3 years	50	50	83	85	74	77	80	87	33	51	71	77
5 years	50	50	83	86	74	80	80	93	0	0	67	77

CHOROID (MELANOMA) (ICD-9 190.6)

GERMANY

AREA	NUMBER OF CASES			PERIOD	MEAN AGE		
	Males	Females	All		Males	Females	All
Saarland	2	4	6	1985-1989	57.5	62.5	61.0

OBSERVED AND RELATIVE SURVIVAL (%) BY AGE (number of cases in parentheses)

	AGE CLASS										ALL	
	15-44		45-54		55-64		65-74		75-99			
	obs	rel	obs	rel	obs	rel	obs	rel	obs	rel	obs	rel
Males	(1)		(0)		(0)		(0)		(1)		(2)	
1 year	100	100	-	-	-	-	-	-	100	100	100	100
3 years	100	100	-	-	-	-	-	-	0	0	50	62
5 years	-	-	-	-	-	-	-	-	0	0	-	-
Females	(0)		(1)		(1)		(1)		(1)		(4)	
1 year	-	-	100	100	100	100	100	100	100	100	100	100
3 years	-	-	100	100	0	0	100	100	100	100	75	80
5 years	-	-	-	-	0	0	100	100	100	100	75	86
Overall	(1)		(1)		(1)		(1)		(2)		(6)	
1 year	100	100	100	100	100	100	100	100	100	100	100	100
3 years	100	100	100	100	0	0	100	100	50	68	67	74
5 years	-	-	-	-	0	0	100	100	50	86	67	83

ICELAND

AREA	NUMBER OF CASES			PERIOD	MEAN AGE		
	Males	Females	All		Males	Females	All
Iceland	2	0	2	1985-1989	77.0	-	77.0

OBSERVED AND RELATIVE SURVIVAL (%) BY AGE (number of cases in parentheses)

	AGE CLASS										ALL	
	15-44		45-54		55-64		65-74		75-99			
	obs	rel	obs	rel	obs	rel	obs	rel	obs	rel	obs	rel
Males	(0)		(0)		(0)		(1)		(1)		(2)	
1 year	-	-	-	-	-	-	100	100	100	100	100	100
3 years	-	-	-	-	-	-	100	100	100	100	100	100
5 years	-	-	-	-	-	-	0	0	100	100	50	76
Females	(0)		(0)		(0)		(0)		(0)		(0)	
1 year	-	-	-	-	-	-	-	-	-	-	-	-
3 years	-	-	-	-	-	-	-	-	-	-	-	-
5 years	-	-	-	-	-	-	-	-	-	-	-	-
Overall	(0)		(0)		(0)		(1)		(1)		(2)	
1 year	-	-	-	-	-	-	100	100	100	100	100	100
3 years	-	-	-	-	-	-	100	100	100	100	100	100
5 years	-	-	-	-	-	-	0	0	100	100	50	76

CHOROID (MELANOMA) (ICD-9 190.6)

ITALY

AREA	NUMBER OF CASES			PERIOD	MEAN AGE			5-YR RELATIVE SURVIVAL (%)
	Males	Females	All		Males	Females	All	Males / Females
Florence	8	7	15	1985-1989	61.0	65.3	63.1	
Genoa	0	1	1	1986-1988	-	76.0	76.0	
Latina	2	1	3	1985-1987	63.5	34.0	54.0	
Modena	2	2	4	1988-1989	53.0	59.5	56.5	
Parma	3	3	6	1985-1987	53.3	60.0	56.8	
Ragusa	1	0	1	1985-1989	77.0	-	77.0	
Romagna	1	5	6	1986-1988	59.0	67.2	66.0	
Turin	3	9	12	1985-1987	69.0	52.4	56.7	
Varese	3	5	8	1985-1989	64.7	70.4	68.4	
Italian Registries	23	33	56		62.0	61.6	61.8	

OBSERVED AND RELATIVE SURVIVAL (%) BY AGE (number of cases in parentheses)

	AGE CLASS										ALL	
	15-44		45-54		55-64		65-74		75-99			
	obs	rel	obs	rel	obs	rel	obs	rel	obs	rel	obs	rel
Males	(2)		(5)		(6)		(4)		(6)		(23)	
1 year	100	100	100	100	83	85	100	100	67	73	87	90
3 years	50	50	75	76	67	70	75	83	50	66	64	71
5 years	50	50	75	77	50	54	75	89	33	55	55	66
Females	(5)		(5)		(7)		(8)		(8)		(33)	
1 year	100	100	100	100	100	100	100	100	100	100	100	100
3 years	80	80	100	100	86	87	88	94	88	100	88	93
5 years	80	80	100	100	43	44	50	57	38	51	56	63
Overall	(7)		(10)		(13)		(12)		(14)		(56)	
1 year	100	100	100	100	92	93	100	100	86	91	95	97
3 years	71	72	88	89	77	79	83	90	71	88	78	84
5 years	71	72	88	89	46	49	58	67	36	52	56	64

NETHERLANDS

AREA	NUMBER OF CASES			PERIOD	MEAN AGE		
	Males	Females	All		Males	Females	All
Eindhoven	3	3	6	1985-1989	58.3	62.3	60.5

OBSERVED AND RELATIVE SURVIVAL (%) BY AGE (number of cases in parentheses)

	AGE CLASS										ALL	
	15-44		45-54		55-64		65-74		75-99			
	obs	rel	obs	rel	obs	rel	obs	rel	obs	rel	obs	rel
Males	(0)		(0)		(3)		(0)		(0)		(3)	
1 year	-	-	-	-	67	68	-	-	-	-	67	68
3 years	-	-	-	-	67	70	-	-	-	-	67	70
5 years	-	-	-	-	67	72	-	-	-	-	67	72
Females	(0)		(1)		(1)		(0)		(1)		(3)	
1 year	-	-	100	100	100	100	-	-	100	100	100	100
3 years	-	-	100	100	0	0	-	-	100	100	67	73
5 years	-	-	100	100	0	0	-	-	100	100	67	78
Overall	(0)		(1)		(4)		(0)		(1)		(6)	
1 year	-	-	100	100	75	76	-	-	100	100	83	85
3 years	-	-	100	100	50	52	-	-	100	100	67	71
5 years	-	-	100	100	50	53	-	-	100	100	67	75

CHOROID (MELANOMA) (ICD-9 190.6)

POLAND

AREA	NUMBER OF CASES			PERIOD	MEAN AGE			5-YR RELATIVE SURVIVAL (%)	
	Males	Females	All		Males	Females	All	Males	Females
Cracow	1	0	1	1985-1989	48.0	-	48.0		
Warsaw	3	1	4	1988-1989	63.0	46.0	59.0		
Polish Registries	4	1	5		59.8	47.0	57.2		

OBSERVED AND RELATIVE SURVIVAL (%) BY AGE (number of cases in parentheses)

	AGE CLASS										ALL	
	15-44		45-54		55-64		65-74		75-99			
	obs	rel	obs	rel	obs	rel	obs	rel	obs	rel	obs	rel
Males	(0)		(2)		(1)		(0)		(1)		(4)	
1 year	-	-	100	100	100	100	-	-	100	100	100	100
3 years	-	-	100	100	100	100	-	-	100	100	100	100
5 years	-	-	100	100	100	100	-	-	100	100	100	100
Females	(0)		(1)		(0)		(0)		(0)		(1)	
1 year	-	-	100	100	-	-	-	-	-	-	100	100
3 years	-	-	100	100	-	-	-	-	-	-	100	100
5 years	-	-	100	100	-	-	-	-	-	-	100	100
Overall	(0)		(3)		(1)		(0)		(1)		(5)	
1 year	-	-	100	100	100	100	-	-	100	100	100	100
3 years	-	-	100	100	100	100	-	-	100	100	100	100
5 years	-	-	100	100	100	100	-	-	100	100	100	100

SCOTLAND

AREA	NUMBER OF CASES			PERIOD	MEAN AGE		
	Males	Females	All		Males	Females	All
Scotland	75	67	142	1985-1989	57.1	61.9	59.4

OBSERVED AND RELATIVE SURVIVAL (%) BY AGE (number of cases in parentheses)

	AGE CLASS										ALL	
	15-44		45-54		55-64		65-74		75-99			
	obs	rel	obs	rel	obs	rel	obs	rel	obs	rel	obs	rel
Males	(13)		(19)		(24)		(11)		(8)		(75)	
1 year	100	100	100	100	96	98	91	96	100	100	97	100
3 years	100	100	95	97	83	90	73	85	100	100	89	97
5 years	100	100	84	88	67	76	64	85	75	100	77	89
Females	(11)		(9)		(16)		(11)		(20)		(67)	
1 year	100	100	100	100	88	88	91	94	90	96	93	95
3 years	100	100	100	100	75	78	82	90	65	80	81	88
5 years	100	100	100	100	63	67	82	97	40	59	70	82
Overall	(24)		(28)		(40)		(22)		(28)		(142)	
1 year	100	100	100	100	93	94	91	95	93	100	95	98
3 years	100	100	96	98	80	85	77	88	75	95	85	93
5 years	100	100	89	93	65	72	73	92	50	77	74	86

CHOROID (MELANOMA) (ICD-9 190.6)

SLOVAKIA

AREA	NUMBER OF CASES			PERIOD	MEAN AGE		
	Males	Females	All		Males	Females	All
Slovakia	28	43	71	1985-1989	57.7	58.9	58.5

OBSERVED AND RELATIVE SURVIVAL (%) BY AGE (number of cases in parentheses)

	AGE CLASS										ALL	
	15-44		45-54		55-64		65-74		75-99			
	obs	rel	obs	rel	obs	rel	obs	rel	obs	rel	obs	rel
Males	(6)		(5)		(11)		(1)		(5)		(28)	
1 year	83	84	80	81	91	93	100	100	40	45	79	81
3 years	67	68	60	62	82	90	0	0	40	58	64	72
5 years	67	69	60	65	70	83	0	0	20	39	56	68
Females	(6)		(9)		(12)		(12)		(4)		(43)	
1 year	100	100	89	89	100	100	100	100	50	54	93	95
3 years	83	84	78	79	92	95	75	83	50	63	79	84
5 years	83	84	78	80	66	71	75	90	-	-	71	79
Overall	(12)		(14)		(23)		(13)		(9)		(71)	
1 year	92	92	86	86	96	97	100	100	44	49	87	90
3 years	75	76	71	73	87	93	69	77	44	60	73	79
5 years	75	76	71	75	68	76	69	84	32	55	65	75

SPAIN

AREA	NUMBER OF CASES			PERIOD	MEAN AGE			5-YR RELATIVE SURVIVAL (%)	
	Males	Females	All		Males	Females	All	Males	Females
Basque Country	6	10	16	1986-1988	61.8	56.6	58.6		
Mallorca	0	2	2	1988-1989	-	70.0	70.0		
Navarra	3	3	6	1985-1989	65.0	68.3	66.8		
Spanish Registries	9	15	24		63.1	60.9	61.8		

OBSERVED AND RELATIVE SURVIVAL (%) BY AGE (number of cases in parentheses)

	AGE CLASS										ALL	
	15-44		45-54		55-64		65-74		75-99			
	obs	rel	obs	rel	obs	rel	obs	rel	obs	rel	obs	rel
Males	(0)		(0)		(5)		(4)		(0)		(9)	
1 year	-	-	-	-	100	100	100	100	-	-	100	100
3 years	-	-	-	-	40	41	75	84	-	-	56	60
5 years	-	-	-	-	40	43	45	56	-	-	43	49
Females	(1)		(3)		(4)		(6)		(1)		(15)	
1 year	100	100	100	100	100	100	100	100	0	0	93	94
3 years	100	100	100	100	75	76	100	100	0	0	87	90
5 years	100	100	100	100	75	77	80	88	0	0	79	84
Overall	(1)		(3)		(9)		(10)		(1)		(24)	
1 year	100	100	100	100	100	100	100	100	0	0	96	97
3 years	100	100	100	100	56	57	90	97	0	0	75	79
5 years	100	100	100	100	56	58	66	75	0	0	66	71

CHOROID (MELANOMA) (ICD-9 190.6)

SWEDEN

AREA	NUMBER OF CASES			PERIOD	MEAN AGE		
	Males	Females	All		Males	Females	All
South Sweden	6	5	11	1985-1989	58.0	57.2	57.7

OBSERVED AND RELATIVE SURVIVAL (%) BY AGE (number of cases in parentheses)

	AGE CLASS										ALL	
	15-44		45-54		55-64		65-74		75-99			
	obs	rel	obs	rel	obs	rel	obs	rel	obs	rel	obs	rel
Males	(1)		(1)		(2)		(2)		(0)		(6)	
1 year	100	100	100	100	100	100	100	100	-	-	100	100
3 years	100	100	100	100	100	100	100	100	-	-	100	100
5 years	100	100	100	100	50	55	50	63	-	-	67	75
Females	(2)		(0)		(1)		(0)		(2)		(5)	
1 year	100	100	-	-	100	100	-	-	100	100	100	100
3 years	100	100	-	-	100	100	-	-	50	66	80	89
5 years	100	100	-	-	100	100	-	-	50	84	80	96
Overall	(3)		(1)		(3)		(2)		(2)		(11)	
1 year	100	100	100	100	100	100	100	100	100	100	100	100
3 years	100	100	100	100	100	100	100	100	50	66	91	99
5 years	100	100	100	100	67	72	50	63	50	84	73	84

CHOROID (MELANOMA) (ICD-9 190.6)

EUROPE, 1985-89

Weighted analyses

COUNTRY	% COVERAGE WITH C.R.s	YEARLY NO. OF CASES (Mean No. of cases recorded) Males	Females	All
AUSTRIA	8	2	1	3
DENMARK	100	21	20	41
ENGLAND	50	41	35	76
ESTONIA	100	3	5	8
FINLAND	100	12	16	28
FRANCE	3	4	2	6
GERMANY	2	0	1	1
ICELAND	100	1	0	1
ITALY	10	8	11	19
NETHERLANDS	6	1	1	2
POLAND	6	4	1	5
SCOTLAND	100	15	13	28
SLOVAKIA	100	6	9	15
SPAIN	10	3	5	8
SWEDEN	17	2	2	4

RELATIVE SURVIVAL (%) (Age-standardized) Males / Females

□ 1 year ■ 5 years

OBSERVED AND RELATIVE SURVIVAL (%) BY AGE

	AGE CLASS 15-44 obs rel	45-54 obs rel	55-64 obs rel	65-74 obs rel	75-99 obs rel	ALL obs rel
Males						
1 year	99 99	99 99	93 94	98 99	80 86	93 95
3 years	54 54	88 89	71 74	71 79	54 69	71 77
5 years	50 50	86 88	63 68	63 78	35 48	64 73
Females						
1 year	99 99	96 96	98 98	98 99	78 80	96 96
3 years	91 91	94 95	73 74	90 93	61 70	83 88
5 years	89 89	89 90	56 58	71 77	41 53	69 76
Overall						
1 year	99 99	98 98	95 96	98 99	79 83	94 96
3 years	71 71	91 92	72 74	80 86	58 69	77 82
5 years	68 68	88 89	60 63	67 77	38 50	66 74

AGE STANDARDIZED RELATIVE SURVIVAL(%)

COUNTRY	MALES 1-year (95% C.I.)	5-years (95% C.I.)	FEMALES 1-year (95% C.I.)	5-years (95% C.I.)
AUSTRIA	-	-	-	-
DENMARK	97.2 (92.6 -102.0)	66.4 (55.5 - 79.3)	98.1 (94.6 -101.7)	66.6 (57.3 - 77.3)
ENGLAND	97.3 (94.0 -100.7)	81.6 (74.0 - 90.1)	94.7 (90.9 - 98.6)	69.0 (61.4 - 77.5)
ESTONIA	-	-	92.3 (83.1 -102.7)	68.7 (49.1 - 96.3)
FINLAND	99.1 (95.6 -102.7)	68.3 (55.1 - 84.7)	97.4 (93.2 -101.7)	61.9 (51.8 - 74.1)
FRANCE	93.5 (82.3 -106.1)	58.2 (43.1 - 78.6)	-	-
GERMANY	-	-	-	-
ICELAND	-	-	-	-
ITALY	91.0 (80.7 -102.6)	66.2 (46.4 - 94.4)	100.0 (100.0 -100.0)	63.5 (48.9 - 82.4)
NETHERLANDS	-	-	-	-
POLAND	-	-	-	-
SCOTLAND	98.4 (93.8 -103.3)	87.8 (74.5 -103.5)	94.7 (88.4 -101.4)	83.2 (73.0 - 94.8)
SLOVAKIA	82.8 (71.3 - 96.2)	50.3 (35.2 - 72.1)	89.8 (80.4 -100.4)	-
SPAIN	-	-	82.4 (82.2 - 82.5)	73.3 (59.9 - 89.7)
SWEDEN	-	-	-	-
EUROPE, 1985-89	95.4 (91.3 - 99.7)	67.9 (59.8 - 77.1)	95.0 (93.5 - 96.5)	71.5 (65.9 - 77.6)

413

BRAIN (ICD-9 191)

AUSTRIA

AREA	NUMBER OF CASES			PERIOD	MEAN AGE		
	Males	Females	All		Males	Females	All
Tirol	32	22	54	1988-1989	48.7	55.2	51.4

OBSERVED AND RELATIVE SURVIVAL (%) BY AGE (number of cases in parentheses)

	AGE CLASS										ALL	
	15-44		45-54		55-64		65-74		75-99			
	obs	rel	obs	rel	obs	rel	obs	rel	obs	rel	obs	rel
Males	(11)		(7)		(7)		(6)		(1)		(32)	
1 year	91	91	57	57	57	58	17	17	100	100	63	63
3 years	64	64	29	29	14	15	0	0	0	0	31	32
5 years	45	46	14	15	14	15	0	0	0	0	22	23
Females	(5)		(7)		(5)		(4)		(1)		(22)	
1 year	60	60	43	43	60	60	50	51	0	0	50	50
3 years	40	40	0	0	0	0	25	26	0	0	14	14
5 years	40	40	0	0	0	0	25	27	0	0	14	14
Overall	(16)		(14)		(12)		(10)		(2)		(54)	
1 year	81	81	50	50	58	59	30	31	50	53	57	58
3 years	56	56	14	14	8	9	10	11	0	0	24	25
5 years	44	44	7	7	8	9	10	11	0	0	19	20

DENMARK

AREA	NUMBER OF CASES			PERIOD	MEAN AGE		
	Males	Females	All		Males	Females	All
Denmark	1083	894	1977	1985-1989	54.5	56.9	55.6

OBSERVED AND RELATIVE SURVIVAL (%) BY AGE (number of cases in parentheses)

	AGE CLASS										ALL	
	15-44		45-54		55-64		65-74		75-99			
	obs	rel	obs	rel	obs	rel	obs	rel	obs	rel	obs	rel
Males	(298)		(182)		(253)		(250)		(100)		(1083)	
1 year	73	73	35	35	25	25	10	11	5	5	35	35
3 years	52	53	20	20	10	11	4	5	1	1	21	23
5 years	47	47	18	19	8	9	1	2	0	0	18	20
Females	(211)		(137)		(181)		(251)		(114)		(894)	
1 year	74	74	39	40	22	22	15	15	7	7	33	34
3 years	57	58	27	27	15	16	9	9	4	5	24	25
5 years	52	52	24	25	12	13	7	8	4	5	21	23
Overall	(509)		(319)		(434)		(501)		(214)		(1977)	
1 year	73	73	37	37	24	24	13	13	6	7	34	35
3 years	54	55	23	23	12	13	6	7	3	4	22	24
5 years	49	49	21	21	10	11	4	5	2	3	19	22

BRAIN (ICD-9 191)

ENGLAND

AREA	NUMBER OF CASES			PERIOD	MEAN AGE			5-YR RELATIVE SURVIVAL (%)	
	Males	Females	All		Males	Females	All	Males	Females
East Anglia	368	259	627	1985-1989	59.2	60.5	59.8		
Mersey	342	273	615	1985-1989	55.1	55.9	55.4		
Oxford	445	356	801	1985-1989	56.6	56.7	56.7		
South Thames	928	664	1592	1985-1989	54.2	56.9	55.4		
Wessex	542	395	937	1985-1989	57.0	57.7	57.3		
West Midlands	724	471	1195	1985-1989	54.3	54.4	54.4		
Yorkshire	530	384	914	1985-1989	55.6	57.6	56.4		
English Registries	3879	2802	6681		55.7	56.9	56.2		

OBSERVED AND RELATIVE SURVIVAL (%) BY AGE (number of cases in parentheses)

	AGE CLASS										ALL	
	15-44		45-54		55-64		65-74		75-99			
	obs	rel	obs	rel	obs	rel	obs	rel	obs	rel	obs	rel
Males	(902)		(680)		(1047)		(928)		(322)		(3879)	
1 year	72	72	37	37	18	19	11	12	5	5	31	32
3 years	50	50	18	18	6	6	4	5	3	4	18	19
5 years	40	41	13	14	4	5	4	5	3	5	14	16
Females	(622)		(415)		(712)		(719)		(334)		(2802)	
1 year	73	73	39	39	21	22	10	10	5	5	31	31
3 years	55	56	23	23	10	10	5	5	3	4	20	21
5 years	46	46	18	18	8	8	4	4	3	4	16	18
Overall	(1524)		(1095)		(1759)		(1647)		(656)		(6681)	
1 year	72	72	38	38	20	20	11	11	5	5	31	32
3 years	52	53	20	20	7	8	5	5	3	4	19	20
5 years	43	43	15	16	6	6	4	4	3	4	15	17

ESTONIA

AREA	NUMBER OF CASES			PERIOD	MEAN AGE		
	Males	Females	All		Males	Females	All
Estonia	147	123	270	1985-1989	48.7	48.8	48.8

OBSERVED AND RELATIVE SURVIVAL (%) BY AGE (number of cases in parentheses)

	AGE CLASS										ALL	
	15-44		45-54		55-64		65-74		75-99			
	obs	rel	obs	rel	obs	rel	obs	rel	obs	rel	obs	rel
Males	(47)		(40)		(40)		(18)		(2)		(147)	
1 year	60	60	35	35	23	23	11	12	0	0	36	37
3 years	43	43	5	5	5	5	6	6	0	0	17	18
5 years	28	28	3	3	3	3	0	0	0	0	10	11
Females	(42)		(27)		(38)		(11)		(5)		(123)	
1 year	69	69	36	36	26	27	27	28	0	0	42	43
3 years	52	53	16	16	11	11	9	10	0	0	26	26
5 years	42	43	12	12	8	8	9	10	0	0	21	22
Overall	(89)		(67)		(78)		(29)		(7)		(270)	
1 year	64	64	36	36	24	25	17	18	0	0	39	39
3 years	47	48	9	10	8	8	7	8	0	0	21	22
5 years	35	35	6	7	5	6	3	4	0	0	15	16

BRAIN (ICD-9 191)

FINLAND

AREA	NUMBER OF CASES			PERIOD	MEAN AGE		
	Males	Females	All		Males	Females	All
Finland	610	555	1165	1985-1989	49.1	52.6	50.8

OBSERVED AND RELATIVE SURVIVAL (%) BY AGE (number of cases in parentheses)

	AGE CLASS										ALL	
	15-44		45-54		55-64		65-74		75-99			
	obs	rel	obs	rel	obs	rel	obs	rel	obs	rel	obs	rel
Males	(248)		(113)		(113)		(96)		(40)		(610)	
1 year	79	80	53	54	37	38	16	16	3	3	52	53
3 years	63	63	31	32	19	20	3	4	0	0	35	37
5 years	55	56	20	21	10	11	3	4	0	0	28	31
Females	(194)		(80)		(117)		(108)		(56)		(555)	
1 year	82	83	64	64	38	38	19	19	9	10	50	51
3 years	61	61	31	32	14	14	5	5	4	5	30	31
5 years	54	54	25	25	12	12	4	4	0	0	26	28
Overall	(442)		(193)		(230)		(204)		(96)		(1165)	
1 year	81	81	58	58	37	38	17	18	6	7	51	52
3 years	62	62	31	32	16	17	4	4	2	3	33	34
5 years	55	55	22	23	11	12	3	4	0	0	27	29

FRANCE

AREA	NUMBER OF CASES			PERIOD	MEAN AGE			5-YR RELATIVE SURVIVAL (%)	
	Males	Females	All		Males	Females	All	Males	Females
Somme	69	49	118	1985-1989	52.5	55.3	53.7		
Calvados	58	39	97	1985-1989	50.2	50.2	50.2		
Doubs	53	34	87	1985-1989	52.4	60.1	55.4		
French Registries	180	122	302		51.7	55.0	53.1		

OBSERVED AND RELATIVE SURVIVAL (%) BY AGE (number of cases in parentheses)

	AGE CLASS										ALL	
	15-44		45-54		55-64		65-74		75-99			
	obs	rel	obs	rel	obs	rel	obs	rel	obs	rel	obs	rel
Males	(53)		(38)		(46)		(30)		(13)		(180)	
1 year	87	87	38	39	43	44	24	24	17	19	51	51
3 years	67	67	14	15	4	5	5	5	17	22	26	28
5 years	46	47	14	15	-	-	-	-	17	26	20	22
Females	(33)		(14)		(36)		(25)		(14)		(122)	
1 year	75	76	45	45	47	47	20	20	9	9	45	45
3 years	56	57	18	18	16	16	5	5	0	0	24	25
5 years	44	45	18	18	16	16	0	0	0	0	19	20
Overall	(86)		(52)		(82)		(55)		(27)		(302)	
1 year	82	82	40	40	45	45	22	22	13	14	48	49
3 years	63	63	15	15	9	9	5	5	9	10	25	26
5 years	46	46	15	15	9	10	0	0	9	12	19	21

BRAIN
(ICD-9 191)

GERMANY

AREA	NUMBER OF CASES			PERIOD	MEAN AGE		
	Males	Females	All		Males	Females	All
Saarland	132	121	253	1985-1989	54.0	54.2	54.1

OBSERVED AND RELATIVE SURVIVAL (%) BY AGE (number of cases in parentheses)

	AGE CLASS										ALL	
	15-44		45-54		55-64		65-74		75-99			
	obs	rel	obs	rel	obs	rel	obs	rel	obs	rel	obs	rel
Males	(31)		(25)		(45)		(18)		(13)		(132)	
1 year	81	81	52	52	22	23	28	29	8	9	41	42
3 years	55	55	32	33	9	9	0	0	8	11	23	25
5 years	46	46	32	33	3	3	0	0	8	15	19	22
Females	(36)		(17)		(31)		(26)		(11)		(121)	
1 year	83	83	41	41	23	23	19	20	0	0	40	41
3 years	72	72	35	36	16	17	12	12	0	0	33	34
5 years	60	60	26	27	16	17	8	9	0	0	27	29
Overall	(67)		(42)		(76)		(44)		(24)		(253)	
1 year	82	82	48	48	22	23	23	23	4	5	41	41
3 years	64	64	33	34	12	12	7	8	4	6	28	29
5 years	53	54	30	31	9	10	5	5	4	7	23	26

ICELAND

AREA	NUMBER OF CASES			PERIOD	MEAN AGE		
	Males	Females	All		Males	Females	All
Iceland	47	34	81	1985-1989	52.0	58.7	54.8

OBSERVED AND RELATIVE SURVIVAL (%) BY AGE (number of cases in parentheses)

	AGE CLASS										ALL	
	15-44		45-54		55-64		65-74		75-99			
	obs	rel	obs	rel	obs	rel	obs	rel	obs	rel	obs	rel
Males	(18)		(8)		(6)		(10)		(5)		(47)	
1 year	72	72	50	50	50	51	0	0	40	47	47	48
3 years	44	45	0	0	17	17	0	0	0	0	19	21
5 years	33	34	0	0	17	18	0	0	0	0	15	17
Females	(7)		(6)		(6)		(12)		(3)		(34)	
1 year	86	86	17	17	50	50	8	8	0	0	32	33
3 years	71	72	17	17	0	0	0	0	0	0	18	19
5 years	57	57	17	17	0	0	0	0	0	0	15	16
Overall	(25)		(14)		(12)		(22)		(8)		(81)	
1 year	76	76	36	36	50	50	5	5	25	28	41	42
3 years	52	52	7	7	8	9	0	0	0	0	19	20
5 years	40	40	7	7	8	9	0	0	0	0	15	16

BRAIN (ICD-9 191)

ITALY

AREA	NUMBER OF CASES			PERIOD	MEAN AGE			5-YR RELATIVE SURVIVAL (%)	
	Males	Females	All		Males	Females	All	Males	Females
Florence	249	176	425	1985-1989	58.8	59.9	59.2		
Genoa	75	70	145	1986-1988	59.6	64.3	61.9		
Latina	32	29	61	1985-1987	52.7	55.1	53.9		
Modena	35	32	67	1988-1989	59.5	59.7	59.6		
Parma	36	24	60	1985-1987	60.0	65.1	62.1		
Ragusa	43	27	70	1985-1989	56.4	54.7	55.8		
Romagna	57	50	107	1986-1988	54.5	55.3	54.9		
Turin	110	75	185	1985-1987	54.6	60.8	57.1		
Varese	122	103	225	1985-1989	54.2	59.7	56.7		
Italian Registries	759	586	1345		56.9	59.9	58.2		

5-YR RELATIVE SURVIVAL (%) chart scale: Males 100 80 60 40 20 0 ; Females 0 20 40 60 80 100. Bars for: Floren, Genoa, Latina, Modena, Parma, Ragusa, Romagn, Turin, Varese.

OBSERVED AND RELATIVE SURVIVAL (%) BY AGE (number of cases in parentheses)

	AGE CLASS										ALL	
	15-44		45-54		55-64		65-74		75-99			
	obs	rel	obs	rel	obs	rel	obs	rel	obs	rel	obs	rel
Males	(155)		(127)		(209)		(178)		(90)		(759)	
1 year	73	74	38	38	31	32	19	20	11	12	36	36
3 years	50	50	16	16	11	11	5	6	4	6	17	19
5 years	43	44	15	15	9	9	4	5	2	4	15	17
Females	(95)		(86)		(154)		(144)		(107)		(586)	
1 year	75	75	59	59	32	32	13	14	14	15	35	36
3 years	57	57	22	23	15	15	6	6	7	8	19	20
5 years	49	50	19	19	13	14	5	5	2	3	16	17
Overall	(250)		(213)		(363)		(322)		(197)		(1345)	
1 year	74	74	46	46	32	32	17	17	13	14	35	36
3 years	53	53	18	19	12	13	5	6	6	7	18	19
5 years	46	46	16	17	11	11	5	5	2	3	15	17

NETHERLANDS

AREA	NUMBER OF CASES			PERIOD	MEAN AGE		
	Males	Females	All		Males	Females	All
Eindhoven	74	69	143	1985-1989	49.1	51.7	50.4

OBSERVED AND RELATIVE SURVIVAL (%) BY AGE (number of cases in parentheses)

	AGE CLASS										ALL	
	15-44		45-54		55-64		65-74		75-99			
	obs	rel	obs	rel	obs	rel	obs	rel	obs	rel	obs	rel
Males	(24)		(20)		(14)		(16)		(0)		(74)	
1 year	79	79	45	45	36	36	6	7	-	-	46	46
3 years	57	57	15	15	0	0	0	0	-	-	22	23
5 years	20	20	15	15	0	0	0	0	-	-	11	11
Females	(27)		(10)		(9)		(14)		(9)		(69)	
1 year	67	67	50	50	22	22	43	44	11	12	46	47
3 years	52	52	30	30	11	11	21	23	11	13	32	33
5 years	44	44	30	31	0	0	21	24	11	15	27	29
Overall	(51)		(30)		(23)		(30)		(9)		(143)	
1 year	72	73	47	47	30	31	23	24	11	12	46	47
3 years	54	54	20	20	4	4	10	11	11	13	27	28
5 years	33	34	20	20	0	0	10	12	11	15	19	20

BRAIN (ICD-9 191)

POLAND

AREA	NUMBER OF CASES			PERIOD	MEAN AGE			5-YR RELATIVE SURVIVAL (%)	
	Males	Females	All		Males	Females	All	Males	Females
Cracow	73	46	119	1985-1989	51.0	56.4	53.1		
Warsaw	56	94	150	1988-1989	54.0	57.8	56.4		
Polish Registries	129	140	269		52.3	57.3	54.9		

OBSERVED AND RELATIVE SURVIVAL (%) BY AGE (number of cases in parentheses)

	15-44 obs rel		45-54 obs rel		55-64 obs rel		65-74 obs rel		75-99 obs rel		ALL obs rel	
Males	(39)		(30)		(35)		(17)		(8)		(129)	
1 year	53	53	42	42	17	17	0	0	0	0	30	31
3 years	29	29	24	25	0	0	0	0	0	0	15	16
5 years	26	27	17	19	0	0	0	0	0	0	12	14
Females	(22)		(23)		(54)		(28)		(13)		(140)	
1 year	64	64	39	39	26	26	7	7	15	17	29	30
3 years	27	27	9	9	17	17	4	4	15	19	14	15
5 years	27	27	9	9	15	16	4	4	15	23	14	15
Overall	(61)		(53)		(89)		(45)		(21)		(269)	
1 year	57	57	41	41	22	23	5	5	10	10	30	30
3 years	28	29	17	18	11	11	2	3	10	12	15	15
5 years	27	27	14	14	9	10	2	3	10	15	13	15

SCOTLAND

AREA	NUMBER OF CASES			PERIOD	MEAN AGE		
	Males	Females	All		Males	Females	All
Scotland	702	568	1270	1985-1989	55.1	57.0	56.0

OBSERVED AND RELATIVE SURVIVAL (%) BY AGE (number of cases in parentheses)

	15-44 obs rel		45-54 obs rel		55-64 obs rel		65-74 obs rel		75-99 obs rel		ALL obs rel	
Males	(163)		(115)		(212)		(145)		(67)		(702)	
1 year	64	64	35	35	17	17	5	5	1	2	27	28
3 years	49	49	13	13	5	6	2	2	1	2	16	17
5 years	38	38	8	8	2	2	1	1	1	3	11	13
Females	(127)		(85)		(145)		(138)		(73)		(568)	
1 year	69	69	29	30	17	17	8	8	4	4	27	27
3 years	49	49	11	11	5	5	5	6	0	0	15	16
5 years	37	37	8	8	3	3	4	5	0	0	11	13
Overall	(290)		(200)		(357)		(283)		(140)		(1270)	
1 year	66	66	33	33	17	17	6	7	3	3	27	27
3 years	49	49	12	12	5	5	4	4	1	1	15	17
5 years	38	38	8	8	2	2	2	3	1	1	11	13

BRAIN (ICD-9 191)

SLOVAKIA

AREA	NUMBER OF CASES			PERIOD	MEAN AGE		
	Males	Females	All		Males	Females	All
Slovakia	436	375	811	1985-1989	49.7	50.3	50.0

OBSERVED AND RELATIVE SURVIVAL (%) BY AGE (number of cases in parentheses)

	AGE CLASS										ALL	
	15-44		45-54		55-64		65-74		75-99			
	obs	rel	obs	rel	obs	rel	obs	rel	obs	rel	obs	rel
Males	(148)		(89)		(115)		(76)		(8)		(436)	
1 year	70	70	30	31	19	20	9	10	13	14	37	37
3 years	52	52	17	18	7	8	5	6	13	18	24	26
5 years	41	41	17	18	7	8	-	-	-	-	20	22
Females	(125)		(64)		(120)		(54)		(12)		(375)	
1 year	67	67	38	38	15	15	6	6	8	9	35	35
3 years	46	47	19	19	6	6	4	4	0	0	21	22
5 years	38	38	16	16	6	6	-	-	0	0	18	19
Overall	(273)		(153)		(235)		(130)		(20)		(811)	
1 year	68	69	33	34	17	17	8	8	10	11	36	36
3 years	49	50	18	18	6	7	5	5	5	7	23	24
5 years	39	40	17	18	6	7	-	-	-	-	19	21

SLOVENIA

AREA	NUMBER OF CASES			PERIOD	MEAN AGE		
	Males	Females	All		Males	Females	All
Slovenia	172	131	303	1985-1989	48.9	51.7	50.1

OBSERVED AND RELATIVE SURVIVAL (%) BY AGE (number of cases in parentheses)

	AGE CLASS										ALL	
	15-44		45-54		55-64		65-74		75-99			
	obs	rel	obs	rel	obs	rel	obs	rel	obs	rel	obs	rel
Males	(59)		(40)		(46)		(23)		(4)		(172)	
1 year	68	68	38	38	17	18	9	9	0	0	38	38
3 years	46	46	15	15	7	7	4	5	0	0	22	23
5 years	36	36	10	11	7	7	0	0	0	0	16	18
Females	(37)		(33)		(39)		(18)		(4)		(131)	
1 year	76	76	42	43	21	22	6	6	25	27	40	40
3 years	49	49	15	15	13	14	6	6	0	0	22	23
5 years	43	44	12	12	11	11	0	0	0	0	19	20
Overall	(96)		(73)		(85)		(41)		(8)		(303)	
1 year	71	71	40	40	19	20	7	8	13	13	39	39
3 years	47	47	15	15	10	10	5	5	0	0	22	23
5 years	39	39	11	11	8	9	0	0	0	0	17	19

BRAIN
(ICD-9 191)

SPAIN

AREA	NUMBER OF CASES			PERIOD	MEAN AGE			5-YR RELATIVE SURVIVAL (%)	
	Males	Females	All		Males	Females	All	Males	Females
Basque Country	177	129	306	1986-1988	57.0	58.3	57.5		
Mallorca	45	32	77	1988-1989	60.3	54.5	57.9		
Navarra	102	72	174	1985-1989	59.1	61.1	59.9		
Tarragona	70	56	126	1985-1989	56.4	51.9	54.4		
Spanish Registries	394	289	683		57.8	57.4	57.6		

OBSERVED AND RELATIVE SURVIVAL (%) BY AGE (number of cases in parentheses)

	AGE CLASS										ALL	
	15-44		45-54		55-64		65-74		75-99			
	obs	rel	obs	rel	obs	rel	obs	rel	obs	rel	obs	rel
Males	(76)		(51)		(115)		(112)		(40)		(394)	
1 year	74	74	37	37	24	25	13	13	8	8	31	31
3 years	55	56	16	16	7	7	5	6	5	6	17	18
5 years	48	49	9	10	7	7	2	3	5	8	14	16
Females	(53)		(50)		(78)		(70)		(38)		(289)	
1 year	55	55	48	48	27	27	17	17	5	6	30	31
3 years	47	47	14	14	17	17	7	7	3	3	18	18
5 years	40	41	9	9	14	14	7	8	3	4	15	16
Overall	(129)		(101)		(193)		(182)		(78)		(683)	
1 year	66	66	43	43	25	26	14	15	6	7	31	31
3 years	52	52	15	15	11	11	6	6	4	5	17	18
5 years	45	45	9	9	10	10	4	5	4	6	14	16

SWEDEN

AREA	NUMBER OF CASES			PERIOD	MEAN AGE		
	Males	Females	All		Males	Females	All
South Sweden	242	210	452	1985-1989	57.1	55.7	56.5

OBSERVED AND RELATIVE SURVIVAL (%) BY AGE (number of cases in parentheses)

	AGE CLASS										ALL	
	15-44		45-54		55-64		65-74		75-99			
	obs	rel	obs	rel	obs	rel	obs	rel	obs	rel	obs	rel
Males	(49)		(38)		(69)		(69)		(17)		(242)	
1 year	90	90	55	55	32	32	20	21	6	6	42	43
3 years	51	51	18	19	10	11	3	3	0	0	17	18
5 years	47	47	8	8	4	5	1	2	0	0	12	14
Females	(57)		(37)		(39)		(55)		(22)		(210)	
1 year	81	81	59	60	41	41	9	9	5	5	43	43
3 years	68	69	35	35	13	13	2	2	5	6	28	29
5 years	61	62	30	30	8	8	2	2	5	7	24	26
Overall	(106)		(75)		(108)		(124)		(39)		(452)	
1 year	85	85	57	58	35	36	15	16	5	6	42	43
3 years	60	61	27	27	11	12	2	3	3	3	22	23
5 years	55	55	19	19	6	6	2	2	3	4	18	20

BRAIN (ICD-9 191)

SWITZERLAND

AREA	NUMBER OF CASES			PERIOD	MEAN AGE			5-YR RELATIVE SURVIVAL (%)	
	Males	Females	All		Males	Females	All	Males	Females
Basel	57	46	103	1985-1988	56.8	58.7	57.6		
Geneva	67	39	106	1985-1989	53.4	58.7	55.4		
Swiss Registries	124	85	209		55.0	58.8	56.5		

100 80 60 40 20 0   0 20 40 60 80 100   Basel   Geneva

OBSERVED AND RELATIVE SURVIVAL (%) BY AGE (number of cases in parentheses)

	AGE CLASS										ALL	
	15-44		45-54		55-64		65-74		75-99			
	obs	rel	obs	rel	obs	rel	obs	rel	obs	rel	obs	rel
Males	(31)		(24)		(32)		(27)		(10)		(124)	
1 year	74	74	61	62	38	38	22	23	0	0	45	45
3 years	49	49	44	44	7	7	0	0	0	0	22	24
5 years	42	42	35	36	7	8	0	0	0	0	19	21
Females	(20)		(10)		(20)		(19)		(16)		(85)	
1 year	90	90	60	60	30	30	0	0	6	7	37	38
3 years	55	55	20	20	20	20	0	0	0	0	20	21
5 years	45	45	10	10	13	14	0	0	0	0	15	17
Overall	(51)		(34)		(52)		(46)		(26)		(209)	
1 year	80	80	61	61	35	35	14	14	4	4	42	42
3 years	51	52	37	37	12	13	0	0	0	0	21	23
5 years	43	44	27	28	10	10	0	0	0	0	17	19

BRAIN (ICD-9 191)

EUROPE, 1985-89
Weighted analyses

COUNTRY	% COVERAGE WITH C.R.s	Males	Females	All
AUSTRIA	8	16	11	27
DENMARK	100	217	179	396
ENGLAND	50	776	560	1336
ESTONIA	100	29	25	54
FINLAND	100	122	111	233
FRANCE	3	36	24	60
GERMANY	2	26	24	50
ICELAND	100	9	7	16
ITALY	10	204	160	364
NETHERLANDS	6	15	14	29
POLAND	6	43	56	99
SCOTLAND	100	140	114	254
SLOVAKIA	100	87	75	162
SLOVENIA	100	34	26	60
SPAIN	10	116	85	201
SWEDEN	17	48	42	90
SWITZERLAND	11	28	19	47

YEARLY NO. OF CASES (Mean No. of cases recorded)

RELATIVE SURVIVAL (%) (Age-standardized)

□ 1 year ■ 5 years

OBSERVED AND RELATIVE SURVIVAL (%) BY AGE

	15-44 obs rel	45-54 obs rel	55-64 obs rel	65-74 obs rel	75-99 obs rel	ALL obs rel
Males						
1 year	75 76	42 42	28 28	17 17	10 11	38 39
3 years	53 53	20 21	7 8	3 4	6 7	20 21
5 years	43 43	17 18	5 6	2 3	5 8	16 18
Females						
1 year	73 73	47 47	29 29	15 16	8 8	36 37
3 years	55 55	22 22	14 15	7 7	4 5	22 23
5 years	47 47	18 18	12 13	5 6	3 5	19 20
Overall						
1 year	74 74	44 44	28 29	16 17	9 10	37 38
3 years	54 54	21 21	10 11	5 5	5 6	21 22
5 years	44 45	17 18	9 9	4 4	4 7	17 19

AGE STANDARDIZED RELATIVE SURVIVAL(%)

COUNTRY	MALES 1-year (95% C.I.)	MALES 5-years (95% C.I.)	FEMALES 1-year (95% C.I.)	FEMALES 5-years (95% C.I.)
AUSTRIA	60.8 (48.3 - 76.5)	17.8 (9.5 - 33.3)	49.3 (32.8 - 74.2)	16.2 (6.4 - 41.1)
DENMARK	33.6 (31.2 - 36.1)	17.5 (15.6 - 19.7)	35.1 (32.4 - 38.1)	22.8 (20.3 - 25.6)
ENGLAND	32.2 (30.9 - 33.5)	15.3 (14.2 - 16.4)	33.3 (31.8 - 34.8)	18.0 (16.7 - 19.4)
ESTONIA	29.5 (23.6 - 36.8)	8.3 (5.3 - 12.9)	36.6 (29.0 - 46.2)	17.3 (11.8 - 25.4)
FINLAND	42.6 (39.2 - 46.3)	21.1 (18.5 - 24.0)	46.3 (42.8 - 50.2)	22.0 (19.2 - 25.2)
FRANCE	46.9 (40.6 - 54.2)	-	44.0 (36.4 - 53.3)	18.5 (12.8 - 26.7)
GERMANY	42.2 (35.2 - 50.7)	19.5 (13.8 - 27.5)	38.1 (31.6 - 46.0)	25.9 (19.6 - 34.1)
ICELAND	44.1 (32.1 - 60.4)	13.0 (6.1 - 27.8)	39.1 (27.6 - 55.5)	17.2 (9.3 - 31.7)
ITALY	38.5 (35.5 - 41.8)	17.5 (15.1 - 20.4)	41.4 (37.9 - 45.3)	20.6 (17.4 - 24.2)
NETHERLANDS	-	-	41.9 (31.7 - 55.4)	23.2 (15.6 - 34.4)
POLAND	24.8 (19.4 - 31.6)	9.9 (6.4 - 15.4)	32.5 (25.9 - 40.8)	15.6 (10.2 - 23.8)
SCOTLAND	27.6 (24.9 - 30.6)	12.0 (9.9 - 14.4)	28.9 (25.8 - 32.3)	12.6 (10.3 - 15.5)
SLOVAKIA	31.2 (27.2 - 35.8)	-	29.2 (25.5 - 33.4)	-
SLOVENIA	30.0 (24.9 - 36.1)	12.7 (9.2 - 17.5)	35.5 (28.7 - 43.9)	15.9 (11.4 - 22.0)
SPAIN	34.9 (30.8 - 39.4)	17.1 (13.7 - 21.2)	33.2 (28.3 - 38.9)	17.5 (13.5 - 22.7)
SWEDEN	45.5 (40.7 - 50.9)	14.8 (11.2 - 19.5)	43.4 (38.0 - 49.6)	23.6 (19.2 - 29.0)
SWITZERLAND	43.8 (36.7 - 52.2)	18.6 (13.3 - 26.0)	41.0 (33.7 - 50.0)	16.6 (10.5 - 26.2)
EUROPE, 1985-89	38.2 (36.4 - 40.2)	16.7 (15.1 - 18.4)	37.9 (35.9 - 40.1)	19.9 (18.1 - 22.0)

THYROID GLAND (ICD-9 193)

AUSTRIA

AREA	NUMBER OF CASES			PERIOD	MEAN AGE		
	Males	Females	All		Males	Females	All
Tirol	16	57	73	1988-1989	53.4	54.6	54.4

OBSERVED AND RELATIVE SURVIVAL (%) BY AGE (number of cases in parentheses)

	15-44		45-54		55-64		65-74		75-99		ALL	
	obs	rel	obs	rel	obs	rel	obs	rel	obs	rel	obs	rel
Males	(4)		(4)		(3)		(3)		(2)		(16)	
1 year	100	100	100	100	100	100	100	100	100	100	100	100
3 years	100	100	100	100	100	100	100	100	100	100	100	100
5 years	100	100	100	100	100	100	100	100	100	100	100	100
Females	(19)		(11)		(6)		(12)		(9)		(57)	
1 year	100	100	100	100	83	84	92	93	44	47	88	89
3 years	100	100	100	100	83	85	92	96	33	40	86	89
5 years	100	100	100	100	83	86	92	100	22	31	84	90
Overall	(23)		(15)		(9)		(15)		(11)		(73)	
1 year	100	100	100	100	89	89	93	95	55	58	90	92
3 years	100	100	100	100	89	91	93	98	45	54	89	93
5 years	100	100	100	100	89	92	93	100	36	51	88	94

DENMARK

AREA	NUMBER OF CASES			PERIOD	MEAN AGE		
	Males	Females	All		Males	Females	All
Denmark	141	341	482	1985-1989	57.3	56.2	56.5

OBSERVED AND RELATIVE SURVIVAL (%) BY AGE (number of cases in parentheses)

	15-44		45-54		55-64		65-74		75-99		ALL	
	obs	rel	obs	rel	obs	rel	obs	rel	obs	rel	obs	rel
Males	(33)		(25)		(23)		(35)		(25)		(141)	
1 year	88	88	68	68	65	66	63	65	36	40	65	67
3 years	85	85	56	57	52	55	49	55	36	50	57	63
5 years	85	86	44	46	43	48	34	44	36	66	50	59
Females	(111)		(48)		(44)		(63)		(75)		(341)	
1 year	98	98	88	88	77	78	62	63	31	34	72	74
3 years	97	98	83	85	75	78	52	56	20	27	67	73
5 years	95	96	83	85	68	72	46	53	12	20	63	72
Overall	(144)		(73)		(67)		(98)		(100)		(482)	
1 year	96	96	81	81	73	74	62	64	32	35	70	72
3 years	94	95	74	75	67	70	51	56	24	33	64	70
5 years	93	94	70	72	60	64	42	50	18	31	59	68

THYROID GLAND (ICD-9 193)

ENGLAND

AREA	NUMBER OF CASES			PERIOD	MEAN AGE			5-YR RELATIVE SURVIVAL (%)	
	Males	Females	All		Males	Females	All	Males	Females
East Anglia	50	112	162	1985-1989	60.2	51.6	54.2		
Mersey	49	98	147	1985-1989	55.8	57.1	56.7		
Oxford	58	177	235	1985-1989	51.1	51.9	51.7		
South Thames	138	324	462	1985-1989	55.4	56.5	56.2		
Wessex	74	178	252	1985-1989	60.8	54.8	56.5		
West Midlands	125	284	409	1985-1989	56.1	57.4	57.0		
Yorkshire	70	196	266	1985-1989	56.4	52.7	53.7		
English Registries	564	1369	1933		56.4	55.0	55.4		

OBSERVED AND RELATIVE SURVIVAL (%) BY AGE (number of cases in parentheses)

	AGE CLASS										ALL	
	15-44		45-54		55-64		65-74		75-99			
	obs	rel	obs	rel	obs	rel	obs	rel	obs	rel	obs	rel
Males	(144)		(82)		(128)		(132)		(78)		(564)	
1 year	92	92	87	87	72	73	56	58	36	40	71	73
3 years	92	92	76	77	61	64	34	39	22	32	59	65
5 years	91	92	63	66	57	63	29	37	17	32	55	64
Females	(462)		(195)		(205)		(232)		(275)		(1369)	
1 year	98	99	96	96	76	77	59	60	35	38	75	77
3 years	98	98	92	93	70	72	48	51	24	32	70	75
5 years	98	98	91	93	67	70	44	50	20	32	67	75
Overall	(606)		(277)		(333)		(364)		(353)		(1933)	
1 year	97	97	93	94	74	75	58	59	35	38	74	76
3 years	97	97	87	88	67	69	43	47	24	32	67	72
5 years	96	96	83	85	63	67	39	46	19	32	64	72

ESTONIA

AREA	NUMBER OF CASES			PERIOD	MEAN AGE		
	Males	Females	All		Males	Females	All
Estonia	25	159	184	1985-1989	54.9	56.9	56.6

OBSERVED AND RELATIVE SURVIVAL (%) BY AGE (number of cases in parentheses)

	AGE CLASS										ALL	
	15-44		45-54		55-64		65-74		75-99			
	obs	rel	obs	rel	obs	rel	obs	rel	obs	rel	obs	rel
Males	(6)		(6)		(6)		(4)		(3)		(25)	
1 year	100	100	67	67	67	68	75	79	33	38	72	74
3 years	100	100	33	35	67	72	25	30	0	0	52	58
5 years	100	100	17	18	67	77	25	35	0	0	48	57
Females	(47)		(23)		(27)		(30)		(32)		(159)	
1 year	100	100	91	92	74	75	63	65	50	55	77	79
3 years	94	94	87	88	70	73	50	55	28	37	67	73
5 years	94	94	87	89	67	71	50	61	25	42	66	76
Overall	(53)		(29)		(33)		(34)		(35)		(184)	
1 year	100	100	86	87	73	74	65	67	49	53	77	79
3 years	94	95	76	77	70	73	47	53	26	34	65	71
5 years	94	95	72	75	67	72	47	58	23	39	64	74

THYROID GLAND (ICD-9 193)

FINLAND

AREA	NUMBER OF CASES			PERIOD	MEAN AGE		
	Males	Females	All		Males	Females	All
Finland	233	923	1156	1985-1989	52.2	50.3	50.7

OBSERVED AND RELATIVE SURVIVAL (%) BY AGE (number of cases in parentheses)

	AGE CLASS										ALL	
	15-44		45-54		55-64		65-74		75-99			
	obs	rel	obs	rel	obs	rel	obs	rel	obs	rel	obs	rel
Males	(85)		(43)		(42)		(42)		(21)		(233)	
1 year	96	97	95	96	79	80	69	72	38	43	83	85
3 years	95	96	93	95	64	68	57	65	24	36	76	82
5 years	95	97	91	94	64	71	52	66	14	29	74	83
Females	(404)		(164)		(123)		(119)		(113)		(923)	
1 year	100	100	98	98	93	93	76	78	49	53	89	91
3 years	99	99	96	97	89	91	65	69	38	49	85	89
5 years	98	99	95	97	83	86	58	66	27	43	82	88
Overall	(489)		(207)		(165)		(161)		(134)		(1156)	
1 year	99	99	98	98	89	90	75	77	47	51	88	89
3 years	98	99	96	97	83	86	63	68	36	48	83	88
5 years	98	98	94	96	78	83	57	66	25	41	80	87

FRANCE

AREA	NUMBER OF CASES			PERIOD	MEAN AGE			5-YR RELATIVE SURVIVAL (%)	
	Males	Females	All		Males	Females	All	Males	Females
Somme	15	53	68	1985-1989	48.8	52.9	52.0		
Calvados	21	75	96	1985-1989	49.0	48.1	48.3		
Doubs	19	47	66	1985-1989	47.4	51.2	50.1		
French Registries	55	175	230		48.5	50.4	49.9		

OBSERVED AND RELATIVE SURVIVAL (%) BY AGE (number of cases in parentheses)

	AGE CLASS										ALL	
	15-44		45-54		55-64		65-74		75-99			
	obs	rel	obs	rel	obs	rel	obs	rel	obs	rel	obs	rel
Males	(23)		(13)		(10)		(8)		(1)		(55)	
1 year	95	95	68	68	88	90	45	46	0	0	78	79
3 years	90	91	39	40	74	77	45	50	0	0	67	69
5 years	90	91	39	41	74	80	45	55	0	0	67	72
Females	(78)		(26)		(26)		(25)		(20)		(175)	
1 year	100	100	96	96	96	97	66	67	57	61	89	90
3 years	98	99	92	92	92	93	61	64	51	65	86	89
5 years	97	97	80	81	88	91	50	56	38	61	79	85
Overall	(101)		(39)		(36)		(33)		(21)		(230)	
1 year	99	99	86	87	94	95	61	62	54	58	87	88
3 years	97	97	74	75	88	90	57	61	49	62	81	85
5 years	95	96	67	69	84	88	49	56	37	58	76	82

THYROID GLAND (ICD-9 193)

GERMANY

AREA	NUMBER OF CASES			PERIOD	MEAN AGE		
	Males	Females	All		Males	Females	All
Saarland	54	135	189	1985-1989	52.8	56.4	55.3

OBSERVED AND RELATIVE SURVIVAL (%) BY AGE (number of cases in parentheses)

	AGE CLASS										ALL	
	15-44		45-54		55-64		65-74		75-99			
	obs	rel	obs	rel	obs	rel	obs	rel	obs	rel	obs	rel
Males	(17)		(12)		(10)		(11)		(4)		(54)	
1 year	94	94	83	84	60	61	73	76	25	28	76	78
3 years	94	95	83	85	50	53	55	62	0	0	69	73
5 years	94	95	75	78	50	55	32	41	0	0	62	70
Females	(37)		(22)		(24)		(33)		(19)		(135)	
1 year	100	100	91	91	71	71	76	77	37	41	79	80
3 years	97	98	82	83	63	64	73	78	32	43	73	78
5 years	97	98	82	83	63	66	52	59	32	55	68	75
Overall	(54)		(34)		(34)		(44)		(23)		(189)	
1 year	98	98	88	89	68	68	75	77	35	38	78	79
3 years	96	97	82	83	59	61	68	74	26	35	72	77
5 years	96	97	79	81	59	63	47	55	26	46	66	74

ICELAND

AREA	NUMBER OF CASES			PERIOD	MEAN AGE		
	Males	Females	All		Males	Females	All
Iceland	31	50	81	1985-1989	54.0	50.8	52.0

OBSERVED AND RELATIVE SURVIVAL (%) BY AGE (number of cases in parentheses)

	AGE CLASS										ALL	
	15-44		45-54		55-64		65-74		75-99			
	obs	rel	obs	rel	obs	rel	obs	rel	obs	rel	obs	rel
Males	(8)		(6)		(9)		(4)		(4)		(31)	
1 year	100	100	100	100	100	100	75	77	75	83	94	95
3 years	100	100	100	100	100	100	75	80	75	100	94	99
5 years	100	100	100	100	89	95	75	85	25	44	84	93
Females	(23)		(6)		(6)		(6)		(9)		(50)	
1 year	100	100	100	100	83	84	100	100	67	72	92	94
3 years	100	100	100	100	83	85	100	100	56	71	90	95
5 years	100	100	83	85	83	86	100	100	44	68	86	94
Overall	(31)		(12)		(15)		(10)		(13)		(81)	
1 year	100	100	100	100	93	94	90	92	69	75	93	94
3 years	100	100	100	100	93	96	90	96	62	81	91	97
5 years	100	100	92	93	87	91	90	100	38	61	85	93

THYROID GLAND (ICD-9 193)

ITALY

AREA	NUMBER OF CASES			PERIOD	MEAN AGE			5-YR RELATIVE SURVIVAL (%)	
	Males	Females	All		Males	Females	All	Males	Females
Florence	75	189	264	1985-1989	51.5	50.6	50.9		
Genoa	27	79	106	1986-1988	59.6	57.3	57.9		
Latina	3	17	20	1985-1987	52.3	40.0	41.9		
Modena	12	44	56	1988-1989	49.1	48.6	48.7		
Parma	18	54	72	1985-1987	55.8	49.2	50.9		
Ragusa	10	18	28	1985-1989	50.1	50.2	50.2		
Romagna	19	70	89	1986-1988	50.5	48.7	49.1		
Turin	26	78	104	1985-1987	44.1	49.5	48.1		
Varese	54	144	198	1985-1989	50.9	49.3	49.8		
Italian Registries	244	693	937		51.6	50.3	50.6		

OBSERVED AND RELATIVE SURVIVAL (%) BY AGE (number of cases in parentheses)

	AGE CLASS										ALL	
	15-44		45-54		55-64		65-74		75-99			
	obs	rel	obs	rel	obs	rel	obs	rel	obs	rel	obs	rel
Males	(88)		(40)		(60)		(36)		(20)		(244)	
1 year	95	96	95	95	71	72	47	49	40	44	78	79
3 years	93	94	87	89	56	59	36	41	10	14	68	72
5 years	92	93	82	84	52	57	36	44	10	17	66	72
Females	(279)		(133)		(111)		(98)		(72)		(693)	
1 year	99	99	97	97	89	90	61	62	49	53	87	87
3 years	99	99	95	95	80	82	50	53	31	38	81	84
5 years	99	99	93	94	77	80	45	50	24	35	79	83
Overall	(367)		(173)		(171)		(134)		(92)		(937)	
1 year	98	98	96	97	83	84	57	59	47	51	84	85
3 years	98	98	93	94	72	74	46	50	26	33	78	81
5 years	97	97	91	92	69	72	43	48	21	32	75	81

NETHERLANDS

AREA	NUMBER OF CASES			PERIOD	MEAN AGE		
	Males	Females	All		Males	Females	All
Eindhoven	23	73	96	1985-1989	51.7	52.9	52.6

OBSERVED AND RELATIVE SURVIVAL (%) BY AGE (number of cases in parentheses)

	AGE CLASS										ALL	
	15-44		45-54		55-64		65-74		75-99			
	obs	rel	obs	rel	obs	rel	obs	rel	obs	rel	obs	rel
Males	(6)		(7)		(6)		(3)		(1)		(23)	
1 year	83	83	100	100	83	85	67	70	100	100	87	88
3 years	67	67	100	100	67	70	67	76	100	100	78	82
5 years	67	67	71	73	67	73	67	85	100	100	69	75
Females	(29)		(8)		(10)		(13)		(13)		(73)	
1 year	100	100	100	100	70	70	92	94	77	83	90	92
3 years	100	100	100	100	60	61	69	74	62	77	82	87
5 years	100	100	100	100	60	62	62	70	46	70	78	85
Overall	(35)		(15)		(16)		(16)		(14)		(96)	
1 year	97	97	100	100	75	76	88	90	79	84	90	91
3 years	94	94	100	100	63	65	69	74	64	81	81	85
5 years	94	95	87	88	63	66	63	72	50	76	75	83

THYROID GLAND (ICD-9 193)

POLAND

AREA	NUMBER OF CASES			PERIOD	MEAN AGE			5-YR RELATIVE SURVIVAL (%)	
	Males	Females	All		Males	Females	All	Males	Females
Cracow	15	56	71	1985-1989	57.4	58.3	58.1		
Warsaw	7	54	61	1988-1989	54.0	54.1	54.1		
Polish Registries	22	110	132		56.4	56.3	56.3		

100 80 60 40 20 0   0 20 40 60 80 100

Cracow
Warsaw

OBSERVED AND RELATIVE SURVIVAL (%) BY AGE (number of cases in parentheses)

	AGE CLASS										ALL	
	15-44		45-54		55-64		65-74		75-99			
	obs	rel	obs	rel	obs	rel	obs	rel	obs	rel	obs	rel
Males	(4)		(1)		(12)		(3)		(2)		(22)	
1 year	100	100	100	100	42	43	33	35	0	0	50	52
3 years	100	100	100	100	33	36	33	40	0	0	45	51
5 years	100	100	100	100	25	30	33	47	0	0	40	49
Females	(32)		(18)		(20)		(20)		(20)		(110)	
1 year	100	100	83	84	65	66	30	31	35	38	66	68
3 years	97	97	72	73	50	52	30	33	25	32	59	63
5 years	97	98	72	74	50	53	25	30	25	39	58	66
Overall	(36)		(19)		(32)		(23)		(22)		(132)	
1 year	100	100	84	85	56	57	30	31	32	35	64	65
3 years	97	98	74	75	44	46	30	34	23	30	57	61
5 years	97	98	74	76	41	45	26	32	23	36	55	63

SCOTLAND

AREA	NUMBER OF CASES			PERIOD	MEAN AGE		
	Males	Females	All		Males	Females	All
Scotland	122	351	473	1985-1989	53.4	55.1	54.6

OBSERVED AND RELATIVE SURVIVAL (%) BY AGE (number of cases in parentheses)

	AGE CLASS										ALL	
	15-44		45-54		55-64		65-74		75-99			
	obs	rel	obs	rel	obs	rel	obs	rel	obs	rel	obs	rel
Males	(40)		(22)		(23)		(20)		(17)		(122)	
1 year	98	98	91	92	70	71	45	47	41	46	75	77
3 years	98	98	86	88	57	60	40	46	12	17	66	72
5 years	98	99	86	90	48	54	25	33	12	23	62	72
Females	(116)		(54)		(49)		(63)		(69)		(351)	
1 year	98	98	94	95	73	74	59	61	33	36	74	76
3 years	97	98	89	90	67	70	46	51	20	27	68	73
5 years	97	98	85	87	65	70	44	53	13	22	65	74
Overall	(156)		(76)		(72)		(83)		(86)		(473)	
1 year	98	98	93	94	72	73	55	57	35	38	74	76
3 years	97	98	88	90	64	67	45	50	19	25	67	73
5 years	97	98	86	88	60	65	40	49	13	22	64	74

THYROID GLAND (ICD-9 193)

SLOVAKIA

AREA	NUMBER OF CASES			PERIOD	MEAN AGE		
	Males	Females	All		Males	Females	All
Slovakia	99	366	465	1985-1989	53.8	53.9	53.9

OBSERVED AND RELATIVE SURVIVAL (%) BY AGE (number of cases in parentheses)

	AGE CLASS										ALL	
	15-44		45-54		55-64		65-74		75-99			
	obs	rel	obs	rel	obs	rel	obs	rel	obs	rel	obs	rel
Males	(31)		(16)		(21)		(18)		(13)		(99)	
1 year	94	94	81	82	57	59	28	29	15	18	62	64
3 years	90	91	75	78	57	62	28	33	15	24	60	66
5 years	87	88	68	73	57	66	28	38	8	17	56	67
Females	(124)		(64)		(60)		(61)		(57)		(366)	
1 year	97	97	94	94	68	69	57	59	35	38	75	77
3 years	95	95	88	89	63	66	48	52	25	32	70	74
5 years	95	96	88	90	63	68	36	43	17	29	67	75
Overall	(155)		(80)		(81)		(79)		(70)		(465)	
1 year	96	96	91	92	65	66	51	52	31	35	72	74
3 years	94	95	85	87	62	65	43	48	23	31	68	73
5 years	94	94	83	86	62	68	34	41	15	26	64	73

SLOVENIA

AREA	NUMBER OF CASES			PERIOD	MEAN AGE		
	Males	Females	All		Males	Females	All
Slovenia	65	172	237	1985-1989	53.7	54.5	54.3

OBSERVED AND RELATIVE SURVIVAL (%) BY AGE (number of cases in parentheses)

	AGE CLASS										ALL	
	15-44		45-54		55-64		65-74		75-99			
	obs	rel	obs	rel	obs	rel	obs	rel	obs	rel	obs	rel
Males	(22)		(10)		(10)		(14)		(9)		(65)	
1 year	95	96	90	91	30	31	43	45	33	37	65	67
3 years	91	92	70	72	20	21	21	25	11	16	51	56
5 years	91	92	70	74	20	23	21	28	11	20	51	59
Females	(50)		(29)		(44)		(29)		(20)		(172)	
1 year	98	98	86	87	70	71	45	46	55	60	75	76
3 years	98	98	83	84	66	68	38	41	50	66	72	75
5 years	94	95	83	85	61	65	31	36	25	42	65	72
Overall	(72)		(39)		(54)		(43)		(29)		(237)	
1 year	97	97	87	88	63	64	44	46	48	53	72	74
3 years	96	96	79	81	57	60	33	36	38	51	66	70
5 years	93	94	79	82	54	57	28	34	21	36	61	68

THYROID GLAND (ICD-9 193)

SPAIN

AREA	NUMBER OF CASES			PERIOD	MEAN AGE			5-YR RELATIVE SURVIVAL (%)	
	Males	Females	All		Males	Females	All	Males	Females
Basque Country	30	80	110	1986-1988	52.9	51.2	51.6		
Mallorca	2	22	24	1988-1989	62.0	45.5	46.9		
Navarra	26	113	139	1985-1989	48.2	49.8	49.5		
Tarragona	17	52	69	1985-1989	52.6	49.1	50.0		
Spanish Registries	75	267	342		51.5	49.7	50.1		

OBSERVED AND RELATIVE SURVIVAL (%) BY AGE (number of cases in parentheses)

	AGE CLASS										ALL	
	15-44		45-54		55-64		65-74		75-99			
	obs	rel	obs	rel	obs	rel	obs	rel	obs	rel	obs	rel
Males	(30)		(9)		(13)		(11)		(12)		(75)	
1 year	100	100	100	100	77	78	82	84	50	54	85	87
3 years	93	94	100	100	69	72	45	50	50	64	76	81
5 years	93	94	100	100	60	65	27	33	22	33	68	76
Females	(110)		(46)		(46)		(44)		(21)		(267)	
1 year	100	100	91	91	93	94	75	76	43	45	89	90
3 years	99	99	87	88	91	93	61	64	24	29	84	86
5 years	99	99	87	88	89	92	61	67	19	27	83	87
Overall	(140)		(55)		(59)		(55)		(33)		(342)	
1 year	100	100	93	93	90	90	76	78	45	49	88	89
3 years	98	98	89	90	86	88	58	62	33	41	82	85
5 years	98	98	89	90	83	86	56	62	20	30	80	85

SWEDEN

AREA	NUMBER OF CASES			PERIOD	MEAN AGE		
	Males	Females	All		Males	Females	All
South Sweden	140	287	427	1985-1989	53.6	55.3	54.7

OBSERVED AND RELATIVE SURVIVAL (%) BY AGE (number of cases in parentheses)

	AGE CLASS										ALL	
	15-44		45-54		55-64		65-74		75-99			
	obs	rel	obs	rel	obs	rel	obs	rel	obs	rel	obs	rel
Males	(42)		(25)		(23)		(30)		(20)		(140)	
1 year	98	98	96	96	91	92	83	86	10	11	81	83
3 years	90	91	92	93	78	81	73	82	10	13	74	79
5 years	86	86	92	95	78	84	57	69	10	17	69	78
Females	(87)		(41)		(46)		(66)		(47)		(287)	
1 year	98	98	98	98	91	92	73	74	62	66	85	86
3 years	97	97	95	96	87	89	65	69	47	59	79	84
5 years	97	97	95	96	83	86	64	71	34	51	76	84
Overall	(129)		(66)		(69)		(96)		(67)		(427)	
1 year	98	98	97	97	91	92	76	78	46	50	84	85
3 years	95	95	94	95	84	86	68	73	36	46	78	82
5 years	93	93	94	96	81	85	61	70	27	42	74	82

THYROID GLAND (ICD-9 193)

SWITZERLAND

AREA	NUMBER OF CASES			PERIOD	MEAN AGE		
	Males	Females	All		Males	Females	All
Geneva	13	51	64	1985-1989	53.6	50.6	51.2

OBSERVED AND RELATIVE SURVIVAL (%) BY AGE (number of cases in parentheses)

	AGE CLASS										ALL	
	15-44		45-54		55-64		65-74		75-99			
	obs	rel	obs	rel	obs	rel	obs	rel	obs	rel	obs	rel
Males	(2)		(4)		(4)		(3)		(0)		(13)	
1 year	100	100	75	75	75	76	67	69	-	-	77	78
3 years	100	100	75	76	50	52	67	74	-	-	68	71
5 years	100	100	75	77	50	54	33	40	-	-	60	65
Females	(26)		(4)		(6)		(7)		(8)		(51)	
1 year	100	100	75	75	83	84	86	87	13	14	80	81
3 years	100	100	75	76	83	85	86	90	0	0	78	82
5 years	100	100	75	76	83	86	86	95	0	0	78	85
Overall	(28)		(8)		(10)		(10)		(8)		(64)	
1 year	100	100	75	75	80	81	80	82	13	14	79	81
3 years	100	100	75	76	70	72	80	86	0	0	76	80
5 years	100	100	75	76	70	74	70	80	0	0	75	81

THYROID GLAND (ICD-9 193)

EUROPE, 1985-89
Weighted analyses

COUNTRY	% COVERAGE WITH C.R.s	YEARLY NO. OF CASES (Mean No. of cases recorded)			RELATIVE SURVIVAL (%) (Age-standardized)
		Males	Females	All	
AUSTRIA	8	8	29	37	
DENMARK	100	28	68	96	
ENGLAND	50	113	274	387	
ESTONIA	100	5	32	37	
FINLAND	100	47	185	232	
FRANCE	3	11	35	46	
GERMANY	2	11	27	38	
ICELAND	100	6	10	16	
ITALY	10	65	192	257	
NETHERLANDS	6	5	15	20	
POLAND	6	7	38	45	
SCOTLAND	100	24	70	94	
SLOVAKIA	100	20	73	93	
SLOVENIA	100	13	34	47	
SPAIN	10	20	71	91	
SWEDEN	17	28	57	85	
SWITZERLAND	6	3	10	13	

□ 1 year ■ 5 years

OBSERVED AND RELATIVE SURVIVAL (%) BY AGE

	AGE CLASS										ALL	
	15-44		45-54		55-64		65-74		75-99			
	obs	rel	obs	rel	obs	rel	obs	rel	obs	rel	obs	rel
Males												
1 year	95	95	88	88	73	74	61	63	32	34	77	79
3 years	93	93	81	82	61	64	49	54	17	20	69	73
5 years	92	93	76	78	58	64	40	49	14	19	65	72
Females												
1 year	99	100	94	94	83	83	67	68	45	49	83	84
3 years	98	99	89	90	76	78	60	63	34	43	78	82
5 years	98	98	87	88	74	77	51	57	27	43	74	81
Overall												
1 year	98	98	92	93	80	81	66	67	42	45	81	83
3 years	97	97	87	88	72	74	57	61	29	37	76	79
5 years	96	97	84	86	70	74	49	55	24	37	72	78

AGE STANDARDIZED RELATIVE SURVIVAL(%)

COUNTRY	MALES		FEMALES	
	1-year (95% C.I.)	5-years (95% C.I.)	1-year (95% C.I.)	5-years (95% C.I.)
AUSTRIA	100.0 (100.0 -100.0)	100.0 (100.0 -100.0)	88.2 (80.9 - 96.2)	87.3 (79.6 - 95.8)
DENMARK	70.2 (63.3 - 77.9)	62.6 (54.2 - 72.3)	77.6 (73.8 - 81.5)	71.7 (67.3 - 76.3)
ENGLAND	74.7 (71.5 - 78.1)	64.3 (60.3 - 68.5)	78.9 (77.0 - 80.7)	74.4 (72.3 - 76.6)
ESTONIA	76.6 (63.1 - 93.0)	56.7 (44.6 - 72.2)	81.7 (76.5 - 87.3)	76.1 (69.4 - 83.5)
FINLAND	81.6 (76.7 - 86.9)	76.8 (70.4 - 83.7)	87.8 (85.6 - 90.0)	82.3 (79.4 - 85.3)
FRANCE	67.4 (58.8 - 77.3)	61.4 (50.7 - 74.5)	87.3 (82.2 - 92.7)	81.0 (73.4 - 89.3)
GERMANY	74.0 (63.6 - 86.0)	62.3 (52.7 - 73.8)	81.1 (75.6 - 87.0)	77.0 (69.4 - 85.4)
ICELAND	93.5 (83.8 -104.3)	88.3 (75.1 -103.8)	93.1 (86.3 -100.4)	90.4 (80.7 -101.3)
ITALY	76.0 (70.9 - 81.5)	65.9 (60.2 - 72.2)	83.9 (81.2 - 86.7)	77.0 (73.8 - 80.4)
NETHERLANDS	86.4 (72.6 -102.9)	77.0 (59.6 - 99.6)	91.4 (85.1 - 98.2)	84.0 (74.9 - 94.1)
POLAND	64.4 (54.4 - 76.3)	64.1 (51.7 - 79.5)	70.5 (64.1 - 77.5)	66.0 (58.3 - 74.7)
SCOTLAND	75.9 (69.2 - 83.1)	67.0 (59.6 - 75.3)	78.0 (74.4 - 81.9)	72.5 (68.2 - 77.1)
SLOVAKIA	63.6 (56.4 - 71.7)	63.0 (53.8 - 73.7)	76.6 (72.8 - 80.5)	71.1 (66.5 - 75.9)
SLOVENIA	66.5 (57.7 - 76.7)	55.9 (46.0 - 67.8)	77.0 (71.4 - 83.1)	70.1 (63.3 - 77.7)
SPAIN	86.8 (79.9 - 94.3)	70.6 (60.7 - 82.1)	85.4 (81.1 - 89.9)	79.9 (75.1 - 85.1)
SWEDEN	81.8 (77.6 - 86.2)	74.0 (67.2 - 81.5)	88.0 (84.6 - 91.5)	83.7 (79.3 - 88.4)
SWITZERLAND	-	-	78.2 (68.5 - 89.3)	78.0 (68.7 - 88.7)
EUROPE, 1985-89	76.1 (72.7 - 79.8)	66.9 (63.2 - 70.7)	83.0 (81.3 - 84.7)	77.8 (75.5 - 80.1)

NON-HODGKIN'S LYMPHOMAS   (ICD-9 200,202)

AUSTRIA

AREA	NUMBER OF CASES			PERIOD	MEAN AGE		
	Males	Females	All		Males	Females	All
Tirol	44	86	130	1988-1989	64.9	68.0	67.0

OBSERVED AND RELATIVE SURVIVAL (%) BY AGE (number of cases in parentheses)

	AGE CLASS										ALL	
	15-44		45-54		55-64		65-74		75-99			
	obs	rel	obs	rel	obs	rel	obs	rel	obs	rel	obs	rel
Males	(5)		(2)		(13)		(13)		(11)		(44)	
1 year	100	100	50	50	85	86	77	79	45	50	73	75
3 years	100	100	50	51	77	80	69	75	27	37	64	71
5 years	100	100	50	51	69	75	54	63	18	31	55	66
Females	(6)		(5)		(14)		(33)		(28)		(86)	
1 year	100	100	40	40	100	100	67	68	54	57	69	70
3 years	100	100	40	40	86	87	55	57	46	56	59	64
5 years	100	100	40	41	86	89	55	60	29	41	53	62
Overall	(11)		(7)		(27)		(46)		(39)		(130)	
1 year	100	100	43	43	93	93	70	71	51	55	70	72
3 years	100	100	43	43	81	84	59	62	41	51	61	67
5 years	100	100	43	44	78	82	54	61	26	38	54	63

DENMARK

AREA	NUMBER OF CASES			PERIOD	MEAN AGE		
	Males	Females	All		Males	Females	All
Denmark	1514	1354	2868	1985-1989	61.2	65.6	63.3

OBSERVED AND RELATIVE SURVIVAL (%) BY AGE (number of cases in parentheses)

	AGE CLASS										ALL	
	15-44		45-54		55-64		65-74		75-99			
	obs	rel	obs	rel	obs	rel	obs	rel	obs	rel	obs	rel
Males	(273)		(192)		(285)		(423)		(341)		(1514)	
1 year	79	79	76	76	74	75	58	61	46	51	64	67
3 years	64	64	61	63	50	53	40	46	27	38	46	52
5 years	56	57	54	56	43	47	29	37	17	32	37	46
Females	(153)		(146)		(219)		(406)		(430)		(1354)	
1 year	90	90	88	88	74	74	66	68	41	44	64	67
3 years	80	81	76	77	63	65	48	51	24	31	49	55
5 years	73	74	70	72	52	55	39	44	17	26	41	49
Overall	(426)		(338)		(504)		(829)		(771)		(2868)	
1 year	83	83	81	81	74	75	62	64	43	47	64	67
3 years	70	70	68	69	56	58	44	49	25	34	48	53
5 years	62	63	61	63	47	51	34	41	17	28	39	47

NON-HODGKIN'S LYMPHOMAS   (ICD-9 200,202)

ENGLAND

AREA	NUMBER OF CASES			PERIOD	MEAN AGE			5-YR RELATIVE SURVIVAL (%)	
	Males	Females	All		Males	Females	All	Males	Females
East Anglia	685	558	1243	1985-1989	62.3	66.1	64.0		
Mersey	572	595	1167	1985-1989	61.6	65.5	63.6		
Oxford	672	553	1225	1985-1989	60.7	66.5	63.4		
South Thames	1698	1601	3299	1985-1989	60.1	65.5	62.7		
Wessex	1060	978	2038	1985-1989	63.2	66.8	64.9		
West Midlands	1134	1007	2141	1985-1989	60.8	64.0	62.3		
Yorkshire	919	822	1741	1985-1989	61.5	66.1	63.7		
English Registries	6740	6114	12854		61.3	65.7	63.4		

OBSERVED AND RELATIVE SURVIVAL (%) BY AGE (number of cases in parentheses)

	AGE CLASS										ALL	
	15-44		45-54		55-64		65-74		75-99			
	obs	rel	obs	rel	obs	rel	obs	rel	obs	rel	obs	rel
Males	(1043)		(933)		(1472)		(1863)		(1429)		(6740)	
1 year	80	80	75	76	70	71	59	61	44	49	64	66
3 years	69	69	61	62	53	56	39	44	22	31	46	52
5 years	64	65	53	55	44	49	29	37	15	26	38	46
Females	(674)		(633)		(1098)		(1696)		(2013)		(6114)	
1 year	84	84	81	81	74	74	62	64	43	47	62	65
3 years	72	72	68	69	59	60	46	49	28	36	47	52
5 years	67	67	61	62	49	52	37	42	19	29	39	47
Overall	(1717)		(1566)		(2570)		(3559)		(3442)		(12854)	
1 year	81	82	78	78	72	73	61	63	43	47	63	65
3 years	70	70	64	65	56	58	42	46	25	34	47	52
5 years	65	66	56	58	47	50	33	39	17	28	39	46

ESTONIA

AREA	NUMBER OF CASES			PERIOD	MEAN AGE		
	Males	Females	All		Males	Females	All
Estonia	156	111	267	1985-1989	56.7	59.9	58.0

OBSERVED AND RELATIVE SURVIVAL (%) BY AGE (number of cases in parentheses)

	AGE CLASS										ALL	
	15-44		45-54		55-64		65-74		75-99			
	obs	rel	obs	rel	obs	rel	obs	rel	obs	rel	obs	rel
Males	(27)		(29)		(46)		(34)		(20)		(156)	
1 year	44	45	62	63	54	56	53	56	35	39	51	53
3 years	33	34	37	39	26	28	26	31	15	22	28	31
5 years	33	34	30	32	17	20	21	28	0	0	21	25
Females	(18)		(15)		(27)		(32)		(19)		(111)	
1 year	56	56	80	80	70	71	59	61	42	46	61	63
3 years	28	28	47	47	56	58	44	48	16	21	40	43
5 years	17	17	40	41	48	52	34	41	5	9	31	36
Overall	(45)		(44)		(73)		(66)		(39)		(267)	
1 year	49	49	68	69	60	61	56	58	38	43	55	57
3 years	31	31	40	42	37	39	35	40	15	22	33	36
5 years	27	27	33	35	29	32	27	35	3	5	25	30

NON-HODGKIN'S LYMPHOMAS (ICD-9 200,202)

FINLAND

AREA	NUMBER OF CASES			PERIOD	MEAN AGE		
	Males	Females	All		Males	Females	All
Finland	1114	1234	2348	1985-1989	59.4	64.8	62.2

OBSERVED AND RELATIVE SURVIVAL (%) BY AGE (number of cases in parentheses)

	AGE CLASS										ALL	
	15-44		45-54		55-64		65-74		75-99			
	obs	rel	obs	rel	obs	rel	obs	rel	obs	rel	obs	rel
Males	(204)		(172)		(280)		(260)		(198)		(1114)	
1 year	82	82	76	77	74	75	55	58	43	49	66	68
3 years	69	70	60	62	54	57	36	41	20	28	47	53
5 years	62	63	52	54	43	47	28	35	9	17	38	46
Females	(165)		(113)		(230)		(353)		(373)		(1234)	
1 year	87	87	86	86	78	78	65	67	42	46	65	68
3 years	78	78	71	71	62	64	49	53	25	33	50	55
5 years	71	71	61	62	49	51	37	42	17	28	40	47
Overall	(369)		(285)		(510)		(613)		(571)		(2348)	
1 year	84	84	80	80	75	76	61	63	43	47	66	68
3 years	73	73	65	66	57	60	44	48	23	31	49	54
5 years	66	67	55	57	45	49	33	39	15	24	39	47

FRANCE

AREA	NUMBER OF CASES			PERIOD	MEAN AGE		
	Males	Females	All		Males	Females	All
Somme	121	115	236	1985-1989	58.2	67.9	62.9
Calvados	141	149	290	1985-1989	59.6	66.9	63.3
Côte d'Or	127	111	238	1985-1989	61.7	67.2	64.2
Doubs	125	93	218	1985-1989	61.9	60.5	61.3
French Registries	514	468	982		60.3	65.9	63.0

5-YR RELATIVE SURVIVAL (%)

OBSERVED AND RELATIVE SURVIVAL (%) BY AGE (number of cases in parentheses)

	AGE CLASS										ALL	
	15-44		45-54		55-64		65-74		75-99			
	obs	rel	obs	rel	obs	rel	obs	rel	obs	rel	obs	rel
Males	(94)		(61)		(128)		(129)		(102)		(514)	
1 year	79	79	87	88	74	75	67	70	60	67	72	75
3 years	69	69	70	72	55	58	47	52	36	51	53	60
5 years	62	63	70	74	44	48	37	45	29	53	45	55
Females	(44)		(55)		(96)		(107)		(166)		(468)	
1 year	90	90	84	85	82	82	79	80	52	56	72	74
3 years	73	73	70	70	69	70	58	62	31	39	54	59
5 years	66	66	67	69	62	65	44	48	22	33	45	53
Overall	(138)		(116)		(224)		(236)		(268)		(982)	
1 year	83	83	86	86	77	78	73	75	55	60	72	74
3 years	70	71	70	71	61	63	52	57	33	43	54	59
5 years	63	64	69	71	52	56	40	47	24	40	45	54

NON-HODGKIN'S LYMPHOMAS   (ICD-9 200,202)

GERMANY

AREA	NUMBER OF CASES			PERIOD	MEAN AGE		
	Males	Females	All		Males	Females	All
Saarland	217	171	388	1985-1989	58.5	66.0	61.8

OBSERVED AND RELATIVE SURVIVAL (%) BY AGE (number of cases in parentheses)

	15-44		45-54		55-64		65-74		75-99		ALL	
	obs	rel	obs	rel	obs	rel	obs	rel	obs	rel	obs	rel
Males	(37)		(32)		(72)		(42)		(34)		(217)	
1 year	73	73	94	94	69	71	60	62	47	53	68	70
3 years	62	63	81	83	57	60	52	61	24	34	55	61
5 years	59	60	61	63	44	49	26	34	17	34	42	51
Females	(15)		(18)		(37)		(42)		(59)		(171)	
1 year	87	87	83	84	76	76	71	73	46	49	66	68
3 years	67	67	67	67	65	67	60	64	31	39	52	58
5 years	58	59	60	61	55	57	54	62	15	23	42	51
Overall	(52)		(50)		(109)		(84)		(93)		(388)	
1 year	77	77	90	90	72	73	65	68	46	50	67	69
3 years	63	64	76	77	60	62	56	62	28	37	54	60
5 years	59	60	61	63	48	52	42	50	16	27	42	51

ICELAND

AREA	NUMBER OF CASES			PERIOD	MEAN AGE		
	Males	Females	All		Males	Females	All
Iceland	51	27	78	1985-1989	62.6	63.3	62.9

OBSERVED AND RELATIVE SURVIVAL (%) BY AGE (number of cases in parentheses)

	15-44		45-54		55-64		65-74		75-99		ALL	
	obs	rel	obs	rel	obs	rel	obs	rel	obs	rel	obs	rel
Males	(7)		(7)		(14)		(12)		(11)		(51)	
1 year	71	72	86	86	79	80	50	51	55	60	67	69
3 years	71	72	71	72	64	67	17	18	27	37	47	52
5 years	57	58	71	73	64	69	17	20	18	31	43	51
Females	(6)		(2)		(5)		(4)		(10)		(27)	
1 year	100	100	100	100	80	81	75	76	50	55	74	77
3 years	83	83	100	100	60	61	75	79	50	67	67	75
5 years	67	67	100	100	60	62	50	56	50	86	59	72
Overall	(13)		(9)		(19)		(16)		(21)		(78)	
1 year	85	85	89	89	79	80	56	58	52	58	69	72
3 years	77	77	78	79	63	65	31	34	38	52	54	60
5 years	62	62	78	79	63	67	25	29	33	57	49	58

NON-HODGKIN'S LYMPHOMAS (ICD-9 200,202)

ITALY

AREA	NUMBER OF CASES			PERIOD	MEAN AGE			5-YR RELATIVE SURVIVAL (%)
	Males	Females	All		Males	Females	All	Males / Females
Florence	327	304	631	1985-1989	61.1	64.9	62.9	
Genoa	136	134	270	1986-1988	60.3	63.7	62.0	
Latina	55	41	96	1985-1987	61.5	57.7	59.9	
Modena	138	103	241	1988-1989	64.0	63.0	63.6	
Parma	66	74	140	1985-1987	63.2	65.2	64.3	
Ragusa	47	32	79	1985-1989	60.4	65.3	62.4	
Romagna	124	123	247	1986-1988	59.8	64.2	62.0	
Turin	149	129	278	1985-1987	57.3	60.8	58.9	
Varese	296	284	580	1985-1989	60.4	65.8	63.0	
Italian Registries	1338	1224	2562		60.7	64.1	62.3	

OBSERVED AND RELATIVE SURVIVAL (%) BY AGE (number of cases in parentheses)

	AGE CLASS									ALL	
	15-44		45-54		55-64		65-74		75-99			
	obs	rel	obs	rel	obs	rel	obs	rel	obs	rel	obs	rel
Males	(203)		(212)		(310)		(344)		(269)		(1338)	
1 year	74	74	74	74	76	77	65	68	52	57	68	70
3 years	58	59	58	58	54	57	44	50	31	42	48	53
5 years	53	54	51	52	46	50	33	41	20	34	39	47
Females	(152)		(139)		(260)		(321)		(352)		(1224)	
1 year	81	81	83	84	75	76	64	66	46	49	66	67
3 years	70	70	70	70	63	64	48	51	27	33	50	54
5 years	64	65	65	66	56	58	40	44	17	25	43	49
Overall	(355)		(351)		(570)		(665)		(621)		(2562)	
1 year	77	77	78	78	76	77	65	67	49	53	67	69
3 years	63	63	62	63	58	60	46	50	29	37	49	54
5 years	58	59	56	58	51	54	36	43	18	28	41	48

NETHERLANDS

AREA	NUMBER OF CASES			PERIOD	MEAN AGE		
	Males	Females	All		Males	Females	All
Eindhoven	221	167	388	1985-1989	59.5	63.0	61.0

OBSERVED AND RELATIVE SURVIVAL (%) BY AGE (number of cases in parentheses)

	AGE CLASS									ALL	
	15-44		45-54		55-64		65-74		75-99			
	obs	rel	obs	rel	obs	rel	obs	rel	obs	rel	obs	rel
Males	(45)		(30)		(44)		(58)		(44)		(221)	
1 year	86	87	73	73	75	76	62	65	50	56	69	71
3 years	74	75	55	56	55	57	41	48	25	35	49	55
5 years	72	73	39	40	38	42	31	40	11	21	37	45
Females	(23)		(31)		(25)		(37)		(51)		(167)	
1 year	87	87	81	81	92	93	70	71	45	49	70	72
3 years	63	63	65	65	76	77	41	43	20	25	47	51
5 years	63	63	48	49	67	70	35	39	15	23	40	46
Overall	(68)		(61)		(69)		(95)		(95)		(388)	
1 year	87	87	77	77	81	82	65	67	47	52	69	72
3 years	71	71	60	61	62	65	41	46	22	29	48	53
5 years	69	69	44	45	49	52	32	39	13	22	38	46

NON-HODGKIN'S LYMPHOMAS (ICD-9 200,202)

POLAND

AREA	NUMBER OF CASES			PERIOD	MEAN AGE			5-YR RELATIVE SURVIVAL (%)	
	Males	Females	All		Males	Females	All	Males	Females
Cracow	85	66	151	1985-1989	56.5	61.3	58.6		
Warsaw	107	83	190	1988-1989	57.4	63.7	60.1		
Polish Registries	192	149	341		57.0	62.7	59.5		

OBSERVED AND RELATIVE SURVIVAL (%) BY AGE (number of cases in parentheses)

	AGE CLASS										ALL	
	15-44		45-54		55-64		65-74		75-99			
	obs	rel	obs	rel	obs	rel	obs	rel	obs	rel	obs	rel
Males	(38)		(34)		(64)		(37)		(19)		(192)	
1 year	74	74	65	65	55	56	37	40	21	24	54	55
3 years	61	61	53	55	36	39	14	17	21	30	38	43
5 years	53	54	32	35	28	33	14	20	16	30	30	36
Females	(19)		(23)		(30)		(36)		(41)		(149)	
1 year	74	74	70	70	70	71	64	66	37	40	60	62
3 years	47	48	35	35	52	54	32	35	20	25	35	39
5 years	31	31	35	36	42	44	26	31	12	19	27	33
Overall	(57)		(57)		(94)		(73)		(60)		(341)	
1 year	74	74	67	67	60	61	51	53	32	35	56	58
3 years	56	57	46	47	41	44	23	27	20	27	37	41
5 years	46	46	33	35	32	37	20	26	13	22	29	34

SCOTLAND

AREA	NUMBER OF CASES			PERIOD	MEAN AGE		
	Males	Females	All		Males	Females	All
Scotland	1397	1505	2902	1985-1989	61.1	66.8	64.1

OBSERVED AND RELATIVE SURVIVAL (%) BY AGE (number of cases in parentheses)

	AGE CLASS										ALL	
	15-44		45-54		55-64		65-74		75-99			
	obs	rel	obs	rel	obs	rel	obs	rel	obs	rel	obs	rel
Males	(229)		(188)		(292)		(404)		(284)		(1397)	
1 year	79	79	75	76	67	68	50	52	32	36	58	60
3 years	68	69	54	56	52	56	32	38	18	26	42	48
5 years	63	64	50	52	43	49	25	33	11	22	36	45
Females	(147)		(134)		(253)		(456)		(515)		(1505)	
1 year	81	81	78	78	68	69	61	62	38	42	58	60
3 years	73	73	67	68	53	55	41	45	21	28	42	47
5 years	67	67	60	62	43	46	33	39	14	24	34	42
Overall	(376)		(322)		(545)		(860)		(799)		(2902)	
1 year	80	80	76	77	68	69	55	58	36	40	58	60
3 years	70	70	60	61	52	55	37	42	20	28	42	48
5 years	65	65	54	56	43	48	29	36	13	23	35	44

NON-HODGKIN'S LYMPHOMAS   (ICD-9 200,202)

SLOVAKIA

AREA	NUMBER OF CASES			PERIOD	MEAN AGE		
	Males	Females	All		Males	Females	All
Slovakia	622	447	1069	1985-1989	56.9	60.7	58.5

OBSERVED AND RELATIVE SURVIVAL (%) BY AGE (number of cases in parentheses)

	AGE CLASS										ALL	
	15-44		45-54		55-64		65-74		75-99			
	obs	rel	obs	rel	obs	rel	obs	rel	obs	rel	obs	rel
Males	(137)		(100)		(156)		(142)		(87)		(622)	
1 year	75	75	65	66	58	60	51	54	44	49	59	62
3 years	63	63	51	53	43	47	29	34	25	37	43	48
5 years	59	60	43	47	32	37	22	31	9	17	34	42
Females	(74)		(60)		(108)		(108)		(97)		(447)	
1 year	78	78	82	82	69	70	57	59	42	46	64	66
3 years	61	61	65	66	47	49	31	35	21	27	42	46
5 years	61	61	59	60	39	42	31	37	17	28	38	45
Overall	(211)		(160)		(264)		(250)		(184)		(1069)	
1 year	76	76	71	72	63	64	54	56	43	48	61	63
3 years	62	63	56	58	45	48	30	35	23	32	43	47
5 years	60	60	49	52	35	39	26	33	14	24	36	43

SLOVENIA

AREA	NUMBER OF CASES			PERIOD	MEAN AGE		
	Males	Females	All		Males	Females	All
Slovenia	273	268	541	1985-1989	57.4	60.7	59.0

OBSERVED AND RELATIVE SURVIVAL (%) BY AGE (number of cases in parentheses)

	AGE CLASS										ALL	
	15-44		45-54		55-64		65-74		75-99			
	obs	rel	obs	rel	obs	rel	obs	rel	obs	rel	obs	rel
Males	(53)		(48)		(75)		(55)		(42)		(273)	
1 year	77	78	60	61	72	74	65	68	50	56	66	69
3 years	68	69	52	54	43	46	44	50	12	17	45	49
5 years	62	63	44	46	25	29	29	38	12	22	34	41
Females	(47)		(41)		(49)		(68)		(63)		(268)	
1 year	91	92	78	78	86	86	56	57	44	48	68	70
3 years	77	77	66	67	71	73	43	46	25	34	53	58
5 years	68	69	61	62	59	61	34	40	19	32	45	53
Overall	(100)		(89)		(124)		(123)		(105)		(541)	
1 year	84	84	69	69	77	79	60	62	47	51	67	69
3 years	72	72	58	60	54	57	43	48	20	27	49	54
5 years	65	66	52	54	38	42	32	39	16	28	40	47

NON-HODGKIN'S LYMPHOMAS (ICD-9 200,202)

SPAIN

AREA	NUMBER OF CASES			PERIOD	MEAN AGE			5-YR RELATIVE SURVIVAL (%)	
	Males	Females	All		Males	Females	All	Males	Females
Basque Country	226	177	403	1986-1988	56.5	60.5	58.3		
Mallorca	63	46	109	1988-1989	58.8	66.1	61.9		
Navarra	107	88	195	1985-1989	59.5	65.5	62.2		
Tarragona	78	77	155	1985-1989	59.3	65.0	62.1		
Spanish Registries	474	388	862		58.0	63.2	60.3		

OBSERVED AND RELATIVE SURVIVAL (%) BY AGE (number of cases in parentheses)

	AGE CLASS										ALL	
	15-44		45-54		55-64		65-74		75-99			
	obs	rel	obs	rel	obs	rel	obs	rel	obs	rel	obs	rel
Males	(108)		(66)		(100)		(111)		(89)		(474)	
1 year	72	72	76	76	76	77	62	64	49	54	67	69
3 years	64	64	68	69	58	61	50	55	26	35	53	58
5 years	62	62	62	64	51	55	42	51	21	37	47	55
Females	(52)		(44)		(79)		(106)		(107)		(388)	
1 year	90	90	80	80	77	78	54	55	56	60	67	69
3 years	75	75	66	66	63	64	39	41	36	44	51	55
5 years	73	73	59	59	51	53	28	31	28	41	42	48
Overall	(160)		(110)		(179)		(217)		(196)		(862)	
1 year	78	78	77	78	77	77	58	60	53	58	67	69
3 years	68	68	67	68	60	62	44	48	31	40	52	56
5 years	65	66	61	62	51	54	36	41	25	39	45	52

SWEDEN

AREA	NUMBER OF CASES			PERIOD	MEAN AGE		
	Males	Females	All		Males	Females	All
South Sweden	496	400	896	1985-1989	65.8	67.8	66.7

OBSERVED AND RELATIVE SURVIVAL (%) BY AGE (number of cases in parentheses)

	AGE CLASS										ALL	
	15-44		45-54		55-64		65-74		75-99			
	obs	rel	obs	rel	obs	rel	obs	rel	obs	rel	obs	rel
Males	(36)		(57)		(92)		(179)		(132)		(496)	
1 year	94	95	82	83	74	75	69	71	49	54	68	71
3 years	75	75	70	71	57	59	49	54	30	41	50	56
5 years	61	62	63	65	48	52	34	41	18	32	38	47
Females	(31)		(30)		(75)		(121)		(143)		(400)	
1 year	94	94	97	97	80	81	74	75	43	47	67	70
3 years	81	81	67	67	63	64	56	59	30	39	51	56
5 years	71	71	67	68	53	55	49	54	17	28	42	50
Overall	(67)		(87)		(167)		(300)		(275)		(896)	
1 year	94	94	87	88	77	77	71	73	46	50	68	70
3 years	78	78	69	70	59	61	52	56	30	40	50	56
5 years	66	66	64	66	50	53	40	47	18	29	39	48

NON-HODGKIN'S LYMPHOMAS   (ICD-9 200,202)

SWITZERLAND

AREA	NUMBER OF CASES			PERIOD	MEAN AGE			5-YR RELATIVE SURVIVAL (%)	
	Males	Females	All		Males	Females	All	Males	Females
Basel	116	106	222	1985-1988	63.9	67.9	65.8		
Geneva	126	124	250	1985-1989	60.4	67.5	63.9		
Swiss Registries	242	230	472		62.1	67.7	64.8		

5-YR RELATIVE SURVIVAL (%) chart: Males scale 100 80 60 40 20 0; Females scale 0 20 40 60 80 100. Bars for Basel and Geneva.

OBSERVED AND RELATIVE SURVIVAL (%) BY AGE (number of cases in parentheses)

	AGE CLASS										ALL	
	15-44		45-54		55-64		65-74		75-99			
	obs	rel	obs	rel	obs	rel	obs	rel	obs	rel	obs	rel
Males	(34)		(32)		(59)		(61)		(56)		(242)	
1 year	76	77	78	78	81	82	77	80	59	65	74	77
3 years	49	50	65	66	68	71	51	57	39	54	54	60
5 years	46	47	56	57	49	53	34	42	28	50	41	49
Females	(22)		(25)		(33)		(52)		(98)		(230)	
1 year	82	82	96	96	79	79	71	72	42	46	64	66
3 years	77	78	74	75	67	68	52	55	23	29	47	52
5 years	77	78	66	67	55	56	46	51	18	27	40	49
Overall	(56)		(57)		(92)		(113)		(154)		(472)	
1 year	79	79	86	86	80	81	74	76	48	53	69	71
3 years	61	61	69	70	67	70	51	56	29	37	50	56
5 years	59	59	60	61	51	54	40	47	21	35	40	49

NON-HODGKIN'S LYMPHOMAS (ICD-9 200,202)

EUROPE, 1985-89

Weighted analyses

COUNTRY	% COVERAGE WITH C.R.s	YEARLY NO. OF CASES (Mean No. of cases recorded)			RELATIVE SURVIVAL (%) (Age-standardized)
		Males	Females	All	
AUSTRIA	8	22	43	65	A
DENMARK	100	303	271	574	DK
ENGLAND	50	1348	1223	2571	ENG
ESTONIA	100	31	22	53	EST
FINLAND	100	223	247	470	FIN
FRANCE	4	103	94	197	F
GERMANY	2	43	34	77	D
ICELAND	100	10	5	15	IS
ITALY	10	380	343	723	I
NETHERLANDS	6	44	33	77	NL
POLAND	6	71	55	126	PL
SCOTLAND	100	279	301	580	SCO
SLOVAKIA	100	124	89	213	SK
SLOVENIA	100	55	54	109	SLO
SPAIN	10	133	107	240	E
SWEDEN	17	99	80	179	S
SWITZERLAND	11	54	51	105	CH
					EUR

□ 1 year ■ 5 years

OBSERVED AND RELATIVE SURVIVAL (%) BY AGE

	AGE CLASS										ALL	
	15-44		45-54		55-64		65-74		75-99			
	obs	rel	obs	rel	obs	rel	obs	rel	obs	rel	obs	rel
Males												
1 year	77	78	79	79	72	73	62	64	48	54	67	69
3 years	65	65	64	66	54	57	44	49	28	38	50	55
5 years	60	60	55	57	44	49	31	39	19	35	40	49
Females												
1 year	85	85	81	81	78	78	67	69	46	50	66	68
3 years	71	71	66	66	64	65	49	52	29	36	50	54
5 years	65	65	60	61	55	58	41	46	18	28	41	49
Overall												
1 year	81	81	80	80	75	76	64	66	47	52	66	69
3 years	68	68	65	66	59	61	46	51	28	37	50	55
5 years	62	63	58	59	50	53	36	42	19	32	41	49

AGE STANDARDIZED RELATIVE SURVIVAL(%)

COUNTRY	MALES		FEMALES	
	1-year (95% C.I.)	5-years (95% C.I.)	1-year (95% C.I.)	5-years (95% C.I.)
AUSTRIA	72.3 (59.4 - 88.0)	60.8 (46.1 - 80.2)	72.7 (64.6 - 81.8)	64.0 (54.4 - 75.2)
DENMARK	65.8 (63.3 - 68.3)	43.0 (40.1 - 46.2)	68.6 (66.3 - 71.1)	49.4 (46.6 - 52.4)
ENGLAND	64.5 (63.3 - 65.7)	42.8 (41.4 - 44.2)	66.5 (65.4 - 67.7)	46.7 (45.4 - 48.1)
ESTONIA	50.9 (42.6 - 60.7)	20.6 (14.9 - 28.4)	60.9 (52.1 - 71.3)	31.5 (23.7 - 42.0)
FINLAND	64.7 (61.7 - 67.8)	39.2 (36.1 - 42.7)	68.9 (66.4 - 71.5)	46.7 (43.7 - 49.8)
FRANCE	73.9 (69.7 - 78.3)	53.8 (47.9 - 60.3)	76.3 (72.5 - 80.3)	52.8 (47.7 - 58.5)
GERMANY	67.0 (60.2 - 74.5)	44.2 (35.3 - 55.4)	70.7 (64.3 - 77.8)	50.3 (42.3 - 59.8)
ICELAND	66.7 (54.3 - 81.8)	44.8 (32.0 - 62.6)	77.9 (63.2 - 96.1)	71.8 (52.3 - 98.6)
ITALY	68.7 (66.0 - 71.4)	44.1 (41.0 - 47.4)	67.9 (65.3 - 70.5)	47.6 (44.7 - 50.6)
NETHERLANDS	68.9 (62.6 - 75.9)	40.0 (33.1 - 48.3)	73.2 (67.0 - 80.1)	45.8 (38.3 - 54.7)
POLAND	46.9 (39.6 - 55.5)	31.8 (23.2 - 43.5)	61.7 (54.3 - 70.0)	31.4 (24.1 - 41.0)
SCOTLAND	58.0 (55.4 - 60.7)	40.1 (37.2 - 43.3)	63.0 (60.6 - 65.5)	43.3 (40.6 - 46.2)
SLOVAKIA	58.4 (54.1 - 63.0)	34.6 (29.5 - 40.5)	63.6 (59.2 - 68.3)	41.8 (36.8 - 47.5)
SLOVENIA	66.6 (60.4 - 73.3)	36.5 (29.9 - 44.5)	68.4 (63.1 - 74.2)	49.0 (42.6 - 56.3)
SPAIN	66.9 (62.5 - 71.7)	51.3 (45.9 - 57.4)	68.9 (64.5 - 73.6)	47.5 (42.3 - 53.4)
SWEDEN	72.3 (68.4 - 76.4)	46.7 (41.8 - 52.2)	74.2 (70.3 - 78.2)	51.6 (46.5 - 57.3)
SWITZERLAND	75.9 (70.3 - 82.0)	48.9 (41.4 - 57.7)	71.1 (65.6 - 77.2)	51.8 (45.1 - 59.4)
EUROPE, 1985-89	67.0 (65.5 - 68.6)	45.2 (43.1 - 47.4)	69.7 (68.2 - 71.1)	48.4 (46.6 - 50.2)

HODGKIN'S DISEASE (ICD-9 201)

AUSTRIA

AREA	NUMBER OF CASES			PERIOD	MEAN AGE		
	Males	Females	All		Males	Females	All
Tirol	14	11	25	1988-1989	44.2	35.3	40.3

OBSERVED AND RELATIVE SURVIVAL (%) BY AGE (number of cases in parentheses)

	15-44		45-54		55-64		65-74		75-99		ALL	
	obs	rel	obs	rel	obs	rel	obs	rel	obs	rel	obs	rel
Males	(8)		(3)		(1)		(1)		(1)		(14)	
1 year	100	100	100	100	100	100	100	100	100	100	100	100
3 years	88	88	100	100	100	100	100	100	0	0	86	88
5 years	88	88	100	100	100	100	100	100	0	0	86	91
Females	(8)		(1)		(1)		(0)		(1)		(11)	
1 year	100	100	100	100	100	100	-	-	0	0	91	91
3 years	100	100	100	100	100	100	-	-	0	0	91	92
5 years	100	100	100	100	100	100	-	-	0	0	91	93
Overall	(16)		(4)		(2)		(1)		(2)		(25)	
1 year	100	100	100	100	100	100	100	100	50	53	96	97
3 years	94	94	100	100	100	100	100	100	0	0	88	90
5 years	94	94	100	100	100	100	100	100	0	0	88	92

DENMARK

AREA	NUMBER OF CASES			PERIOD	MEAN AGE		
	Males	Females	All		Males	Females	All
Denmark	382	220	602	1985-1989	44.1	44.6	44.3

OBSERVED AND RELATIVE SURVIVAL (%) BY AGE (number of cases in parentheses)

	15-44		45-54		55-64		65-74		75-99		ALL	
	obs	rel	obs	rel	obs	rel	obs	rel	obs	rel	obs	rel
Males	(218)		(53)		(44)		(39)		(28)		(382)	
1 year	95	96	87	87	89	90	67	69	36	39	86	87
3 years	87	87	74	75	75	79	49	56	14	19	74	78
5 years	81	81	64	67	68	75	28	36	4	6	66	71
Females	(130)		(16)		(28)		(22)		(24)		(220)	
1 year	97	97	75	75	82	83	59	60	42	45	84	85
3 years	92	92	69	70	82	85	41	44	29	39	77	80
5 years	87	87	56	58	57	61	32	36	17	28	68	73
Overall	(348)		(69)		(72)		(61)		(52)		(602)	
1 year	96	96	84	85	86	87	64	66	38	42	85	86
3 years	89	89	72	74	78	82	46	51	21	28	75	79
5 years	83	84	62	65	64	70	30	36	10	16	67	72

HODGKIN'S DISEASE (ICD-9 201)

ENGLAND

AREA	NUMBER OF CASES			PERIOD	MEAN AGE			5-YR RELATIVE SURVIVAL (%)	
	Males	Females	All		Males	Females	All	Males	Females
East Anglia	143	132	275	1985-1989	42.1	42.8	42.4		
Mersey	150	107	257	1985-1989	39.5	43.6	41.2		
Oxford	175	146	321	1985-1989	40.7	41.0	40.8		
South Thames	436	307	743	1985-1989	39.6	37.8	38.9		
Wessex	208	155	363	1985-1989	40.4	39.4	40.0		
West Midlands	329	215	544	1985-1989	42.1	39.9	41.2		
Yorkshire	245	181	426	1985-1989	41.4	40.1	40.9		
English Registries	1686	1243	2929		40.8	40.1	40.5		

OBSERVED AND RELATIVE SURVIVAL (%) BY AGE (number of cases in parentheses)

	AGE CLASS										ALL	
	15-44		45-54		55-64		65-74		75-99			
	obs	rel	obs	rel	obs	rel	obs	rel	obs	rel	obs	rel
Males	(1045)		(214)		(187)		(167)		(73)		(1686)	
1 year	97	97	88	88	80	81	57	59	34	38	87	88
3 years	89	89	76	77	67	70	40	45	15	21	77	79
5 years	83	84	67	69	53	58	30	38	12	22	69	74
Females	(826)		(85)		(90)		(120)		(122)		(1243)	
1 year	96	96	91	91	78	78	64	66	51	54	87	88
3 years	89	89	82	83	68	70	48	51	27	34	77	79
5 years	86	86	75	77	63	67	39	44	22	34	73	77
Overall	(1871)		(299)		(277)		(287)		(195)		(2929)	
1 year	97	97	89	89	79	80	60	62	44	48	87	88
3 years	89	89	78	79	67	70	43	48	23	30	77	79
5 years	84	85	69	71	56	61	34	41	19	30	71	75

ESTONIA

AREA	NUMBER OF CASES			PERIOD	MEAN AGE		
	Males	Females	All		Males	Females	All
Estonia	102	72	174	1985-1989	41.4	44.3	42.6

OBSERVED AND RELATIVE SURVIVAL (%) BY AGE (number of cases in parentheses)

	AGE CLASS										ALL	
	15-44		45-54		55-64		65-74		75-99			
	obs	rel	obs	rel	obs	rel	obs	rel	obs	rel	obs	rel
Males	(60)		(13)		(16)		(9)		(4)		(102)	
1 year	87	87	69	70	75	77	11	12	0	0	72	74
3 years	68	69	31	32	47	52	0	0	0	0	52	54
5 years	57	58	23	25	27	32	0	0	0	0	41	44
Females	(43)		(3)		(6)		(12)		(8)		(72)	
1 year	91	91	67	67	83	84	58	60	25	28	76	78
3 years	77	77	33	34	33	34	33	37	0	0	56	59
5 years	67	68	33	34	33	35	25	31	0	0	48	54
Overall	(103)		(16)		(22)		(21)		(12)		(174)	
1 year	88	89	69	69	77	79	38	40	17	19	74	75
3 years	72	72	31	32	43	47	19	22	0	0	53	56
5 years	61	62	25	27	29	33	14	18	0	0	44	48

HODGKIN'S DISEASE (ICD-9 201)

FINLAND

AREA	NUMBER OF CASES			PERIOD	MEAN AGE		
	Males	Females	All		Males	Females	All
Finland	283	245	528	1985-1989	45.1	47.5	46.2

OBSERVED AND RELATIVE SURVIVAL (%) BY AGE (number of cases in parentheses)

	AGE CLASS										ALL	
	15-44		45-54		55-64		65-74		75-99			
	obs	rel	obs	rel	obs	rel	obs	rel	obs	rel	obs	rel
Males	(161)		(36)		(39)		(25)		(22)		(283)	
1 year	94	94	92	92	87	89	64	67	18	21	84	86
3 years	88	89	81	82	72	76	32	37	5	7	73	78
5 years	83	84	75	78	62	68	32	42	5	10	68	75
Females	(125)		(21)		(29)		(28)		(42)		(245)	
1 year	98	98	86	86	86	87	71	73	52	56	84	86
3 years	94	94	86	86	76	77	50	53	31	39	75	79
5 years	90	90	81	82	59	61	43	48	19	30	68	74
Overall	(286)		(57)		(68)		(53)		(64)		(528)	
1 year	95	96	89	90	87	88	68	70	41	45	84	86
3 years	91	91	82	84	74	77	42	46	22	30	74	78
5 years	86	86	77	80	60	65	38	45	14	24	68	74

FRANCE

AREA	NUMBER OF CASES			PERIOD	MEAN AGE			5-YR RELATIVE SURVIVAL (%)	
	Males	Females	All		Males	Females	All	Males	Females
Somme	39	23	62	1985-1989	47.4	37.8	43.8		
Calvados	45	30	75	1985-1989	39.4	37.3	38.6		
Côte d'Or	37	22	59	1985-1989	50.1	44.1	47.9		
Doubs	32	21	53	1985-1989	36.2	34.6	35.6		
French Registries	153	96	249		43.4	38.4	41.5		

OBSERVED AND RELATIVE SURVIVAL (%) BY AGE (number of cases in parentheses)

	AGE CLASS										ALL	
	15-44		45-54		55-64		65-74		75-99			
	obs	rel	obs	rel	obs	rel	obs	rel	obs	rel	obs	rel
Males	(93)		(13)		(18)		(15)		(14)		(153)	
1 year	98	98	100	100	78	79	60	62	79	86	90	91
3 years	94	95	92	94	78	82	18	21	20	27	77	81
5 years	84	85	92	96	43	48	18	23	10	17	66	72
Females	(66)		(12)		(4)		(9)		(5)		(96)	
1 year	98	99	100	100	100	100	89	90	80	84	97	97
3 years	97	97	90	91	100	100	77	81	40	46	91	93
5 years	93	93	90	91	100	100	39	42	40	53	84	86
Overall	(159)		(25)		(22)		(24)		(19)		(249)	
1 year	98	98	100	100	82	83	71	73	79	85	93	94
3 years	95	96	91	93	82	86	42	46	26	33	83	86
5 years	88	88	91	94	51	56	26	31	19	30	73	78

HODGKIN'S DISEASE (ICD-9 201)

GERMANY

AREA	NUMBER OF CASES			PERIOD	MEAN AGE		
	Males	Females	All		Males	Females	All
Saarland	70	52	122	1985-1989	43.1	44.8	43.8

OBSERVED AND RELATIVE SURVIVAL (%) BY AGE (number of cases in parentheses)

	AGE CLASS										ALL	
	15-44		45-54		55-64		65-74		75-99			
	obs	rel	obs	rel	obs	rel	obs	rel	obs	rel	obs	rel
Males	(42)		(8)		(9)		(7)		(4)		(70)	
1 year	100	100	100	100	78	79	71	75	50	54	91	93
3 years	90	91	88	89	67	70	43	51	50	65	80	83
5 years	80	81	75	78	55	60	43	59	50	82	71	76
Females	(29)		(6)		(6)		(9)		(2)		(52)	
1 year	97	97	100	100	50	50	56	57	50	53	83	83
3 years	93	93	83	84	50	51	33	36	0	0	73	75
5 years	85	85	83	85	33	35	17	19	0	0	63	67
Overall	(71)		(14)		(15)		(16)		(6)		(122)	
1 year	99	99	100	100	67	67	63	65	50	54	88	89
3 years	92	92	86	87	60	63	38	42	33	43	77	80
5 years	82	83	78	80	44	48	28	35	33	54	68	72

ICELAND

AREA	NUMBER OF CASES			PERIOD	MEAN AGE		
	Males	Females	All		Males	Females	All
Iceland	11	3	14	1985-1989	36.9	39.0	37.4

OBSERVED AND RELATIVE SURVIVAL (%) BY AGE (number of cases in parentheses)

	AGE CLASS										ALL	
	15-44		45-54		55-64		65-74		75-99			
	obs	rel	obs	rel	obs	rel	obs	rel	obs	rel	obs	rel
Males	(7)		(2)		(2)		(0)		(0)		(11)	
1 year	100	100	100	100	100	100	-	-	-	-	100	100
3 years	100	100	100	100	100	100	-	-	-	-	100	100
5 years	86	86	100	100	100	100	-	-	-	-	91	92
Females	(2)		(0)		(0)		(1)		(0)		(3)	
1 year	100	100	-	-	-	-	100	100	-	-	100	100
3 years	100	100	-	-	-	-	100	100	-	-	100	100
5 years	100	100	-	-	-	-	100	100	-	-	100	100
Overall	(9)		(2)		(2)		(1)		(0)		(14)	
1 year	100	100	100	100	100	100	100	100	-	-	100	100
3 years	100	100	100	100	100	100	100	100	-	-	100	100
5 years	89	89	100	100	100	100	100	100	-	-	93	94

HODGKIN'S DISEASE (ICD-9 201)

ITALY

AREA	NUMBER OF CASES			PERIOD	MEAN AGE			5-YR RELATIVE SURVIVAL (%)	
	Males	Females	All		Males	Females	All	Males	Females
Florence	108	104	212	1985-1989	50.2	43.4	46.9		
Genoa	43	33	76	1986-1988	44.0	44.6	44.3		
Latina	22	17	39	1985-1987	48.6	33.2	41.9		
Modena	17	12	29	1988-1989	45.5	41.5	43.9		
Parma	33	20	53	1985-1987	47.9	61.9	53.2		
Ragusa	10	12	22	1985-1989	40.8	37.3	38.9		
Romagna	20	22	42	1986-1988	44.0	44.7	44.4		
Turin	50	45	95	1985-1987	48.9	44.2	46.7		
Varese	74	70	144	1985-1989	41.5	42.6	42.0		
Italian Registries	377	335	712		46.5	43.9	45.3		

OBSERVED AND RELATIVE SURVIVAL (%) BY AGE (number of cases in parentheses)

	AGE CLASS										ALL	
	15-44		45-54		55-64		65-74		75-99			
	obs	rel	obs	rel	obs	rel	obs	rel	obs	rel	obs	rel
Males	(190)		(47)		(56)		(49)		(35)		(377)	
1 year	96	96	87	88	75	76	63	65	46	50	83	84
3 years	90	90	66	67	63	65	53	59	26	35	72	76
5 years	82	83	64	66	54	58	40	49	13	23	64	69
Females	(194)		(25)		(43)		(42)		(31)		(335)	
1 year	95	95	88	88	81	82	67	68	45	48	85	86
3 years	91	91	76	77	60	62	48	50	13	16	73	75
5 years	84	85	76	77	56	58	45	50	6	10	68	71
Overall	(384)		(72)		(99)		(91)		(66)		(712)	
1 year	96	96	88	88	78	79	65	67	45	49	84	85
3 years	90	91	69	70	62	64	50	55	20	26	73	75
5 years	83	84	68	70	55	58	42	49	10	16	66	70

NETHERLANDS

AREA	NUMBER OF CASES			PERIOD	MEAN AGE		
	Males	Females	All		Males	Females	All
Eindhoven	50	37	87	1985-1989	40.4	40.9	40.6

OBSERVED AND RELATIVE SURVIVAL (%) BY AGE (number of cases in parentheses)

	AGE CLASS										ALL	
	15-44		45-54		55-64		65-74		75-99			
	obs	rel	obs	rel	obs	rel	obs	rel	obs	rel	obs	rel
Males	(32)		(6)		(6)		(3)		(3)		(50)	
1 year	97	97	100	100	83	84	100	100	67	72	94	95
3 years	93	94	100	100	83	87	67	74	0	0	85	88
5 years	85	86	80	82	63	67	67	80	0	0	75	79
Females	(28)		(1)		(0)		(3)		(5)		(37)	
1 year	100	100	100	100	-	-	100	100	60	68	94	96
3 years	96	97	100	100	-	-	67	71	40	60	86	91
5 years	96	97	100	100	-	-	67	75	20	41	83	91
Overall	(60)		(7)		(6)		(6)		(8)		(87)	
1 year	98	98	100	100	83	84	100	100	63	69	94	95
3 years	95	95	100	100	83	87	67	72	25	35	86	89
5 years	91	91	83	85	63	67	67	77	13	23	79	84

HODGKIN'S DISEASE (ICD-9 201)

POLAND

AREA	NUMBER OF CASES			PERIOD	MEAN AGE			5-YR RELATIVE SURVIVAL (%)	
	Males	Females	All		Males	Females	All	Males	Females
Cracow	49	42	91	1985-1989	42.4	43.8	43.1		
Warsaw	38	27	65	1988-1989	45.2	35.4	41.2		
Polish Registries	87	69	156		43.7	40.6	42.3		

OBSERVED AND RELATIVE SURVIVAL (%) BY AGE (number of cases in parentheses)

	AGE CLASS										ALL	
	15-44		45-54		55-64		65-74		75-99			
	obs	rel	obs	rel	obs	rel	obs	rel	obs	rel	obs	rel
Males	(51)		(11)		(14)		(9)		(2)		(87)	
1 year	92	92	73	74	71	73	56	59	100	100	83	84
3 years	78	79	45	47	50	54	33	39	100	100	65	68
5 years	68	69	45	49	36	41	22	30	100	100	56	60
Females	(43)		(9)		(10)		(4)		(3)		(69)	
1 year	95	95	100	100	80	81	25	26	67	73	88	89
3 years	83	84	100	100	60	62	0	0	33	44	75	77
5 years	81	81	100	100	49	52	0	0	33	55	72	75
Overall	(94)		(20)		(24)		(13)		(5)		(156)	
1 year	94	94	85	86	75	76	46	48	80	88	85	86
3 years	81	81	70	72	54	58	23	27	60	80	70	72
5 years	74	75	70	74	41	46	15	20	60	99	63	67

SCOTLAND

AREA	NUMBER OF CASES			PERIOD	MEAN AGE		
	Males	Females	All		Males	Females	All
Scotland	336	289	625	1985-1989	42.3	43.9	43.0

OBSERVED AND RELATIVE SURVIVAL (%) BY AGE (number of cases in parentheses)

	AGE CLASS										ALL	
	15-44		45-54		55-64		65-74		75-99			
	obs	rel	obs	rel	obs	rel	obs	rel	obs	rel	obs	rel
Males	(200)		(38)		(37)		(32)		(29)		(336)	
1 year	93	93	92	93	49	50	56	59	31	35	79	81
3 years	86	86	74	75	38	40	44	51	7	10	68	72
5 years	81	81	68	71	30	33	31	41	3	6	62	68
Females	(165)		(21)		(37)		(41)		(25)		(289)	
1 year	95	95	81	81	76	77	51	53	40	44	80	81
3 years	88	89	76	77	59	62	24	27	24	32	69	72
5 years	82	82	67	68	57	61	15	17	16	26	62	67
Overall	(365)		(59)		(74)		(73)		(54)		(625)	
1 year	94	94	88	89	62	63	53	55	35	39	80	81
3 years	87	87	75	76	49	51	33	37	15	20	69	72
5 years	81	82	68	70	43	47	22	27	9	16	62	67

HODGKIN'S DISEASE (ICD-9 201)

SLOVAKIA

AREA	NUMBER OF CASES			PERIOD	MEAN AGE		
	Males	Females	All		Males	Females	All
Slovakia	248	200	448	1985-1989	42.8	39.8	41.4

OBSERVED AND RELATIVE SURVIVAL (%) BY AGE (number of cases in parentheses)

	AGE CLASS										ALL	
	15-44		45-54		55-64		65-74		75-99			
	obs	rel	obs	rel	obs	rel	obs	rel	obs	rel	obs	rel
Males	(143)		(30)		(38)		(23)		(14)		(248)	
1 year	92	93	80	81	63	65	43	46	29	32	78	80
3 years	82	82	57	59	42	46	30	36	14	20	64	68
5 years	73	74	49	53	37	43	6	9	14	27	56	61
Females	(132)		(21)		(16)		(11)		(20)		(200)	
1 year	93	93	86	86	75	76	36	38	35	38	82	83
3 years	86	87	76	77	44	45	27	31	25	32	73	75
5 years	79	80	76	78	31	33	27	34	25	39	67	71
Overall	(275)		(51)		(54)		(34)		(34)		(448)	
1 year	93	93	82	83	67	68	41	43	32	35	80	81
3 years	84	84	65	66	43	46	29	34	21	28	68	71
5 years	76	77	60	63	34	39	13	18	21	35	61	66

SLOVENIA

AREA	NUMBER OF CASES			PERIOD	MEAN AGE		
	Males	Females	All		Males	Females	All
Slovenia	80	62	142	1985-1989	40.0	44.6	42.0

OBSERVED AND RELATIVE SURVIVAL (%) BY AGE (number of cases in parentheses)

	AGE CLASS										ALL	
	15-44		45-54		55-64		65-74		75-99			
	obs	rel	obs	rel	obs	rel	obs	rel	obs	rel	obs	rel
Males	(53)		(9)		(8)		(7)		(3)		(80)	
1 year	94	95	78	79	100	100	71	75	33	37	89	90
3 years	83	84	67	69	88	93	71	82	0	0	77	80
5 years	79	80	56	59	75	83	43	55	0	0	70	74
Females	(32)		(6)		(8)		(11)		(5)		(62)	
1 year	97	97	100	100	75	76	73	74	80	86	89	90
3 years	91	91	83	85	63	64	73	79	40	51	79	82
5 years	91	91	67	68	63	66	52	60	40	63	74	79
Overall	(85)		(15)		(16)		(18)		(8)		(142)	
1 year	95	95	87	87	88	89	72	74	63	68	89	90
3 years	86	86	73	75	75	78	72	80	25	33	78	81
5 years	83	84	60	63	69	74	48	58	25	41	72	76

HODGKIN'S DISEASE (ICD-9 201)

SPAIN

AREA	NUMBER OF CASES			PERIOD	MEAN AGE			5-YR RELATIVE SURVIVAL (%)	
	Males	Females	All		Males	Females	All	Males	Females
Basque Country	92	59	151	1986-1988	44.1	46.3	44.9		
Mallorca	9	15	24	1988-1989	44.9	36.7	39.8		
Navarra	43	25	68	1985-1989	46.0	42.7	44.8		
Tarragona	33	16	49	1985-1989	47.6	48.8	48.0		
Spanish Registries	177	115	292		45.3	44.6	45.0		

OBSERVED AND RELATIVE SURVIVAL (%) BY AGE (number of cases in parentheses)

	AGE CLASS										ALL	
	15-44		45-54		55-64		65-74		75-99			
	obs	rel	obs	rel	obs	rel	obs	rel	obs	rel	obs	rel
Males	(91)		(28)		(27)		(19)		(12)		(177)	
1 year	93	94	86	86	85	86	63	65	33	37	84	85
3 years	86	86	71	73	74	77	42	47	17	23	72	75
5 years	83	84	71	74	57	61	25	31	-	-	66	71
Females	(63)		(11)		(9)		(18)		(14)		(115)	
1 year	97	97	100	100	78	78	61	62	36	38	83	84
3 years	87	87	82	82	78	79	39	41	21	27	70	73
5 years	83	84	82	83	39	40	33	36	7	11	62	66
Overall	(154)		(39)		(36)		(37)		(26)		(292)	
1 year	95	95	90	90	83	84	62	64	35	38	83	84
3 years	86	87	74	75	75	77	41	44	19	25	72	74
5 years	83	84	74	76	52	55	29	33	6	10	64	69

SWEDEN

AREA	NUMBER OF CASES			PERIOD	MEAN AGE		
	Males	Females	All		Males	Females	All
South Sweden	80	71	151	1985-1989	44.9	41.1	43.1

OBSERVED AND RELATIVE SURVIVAL (%) BY AGE (number of cases in parentheses)

	AGE CLASS										ALL	
	15-44		45-54		55-64		65-74		75-99			
	obs	rel	obs	rel	obs	rel	obs	rel	obs	rel	obs	rel
Males	(46)		(4)		(11)		(11)		(8)		(80)	
1 year	96	96	100	100	64	64	73	75	38	41	83	84
3 years	91	92	100	100	55	57	45	51	13	17	73	76
5 years	87	88	100	100	45	49	27	33	13	21	66	72
Females	(50)		(3)		(4)		(9)		(5)		(71)	
1 year	98	98	67	67	100	100	67	68	60	64	90	91
3 years	94	94	33	34	100	100	44	47	40	51	82	84
5 years	92	92	0	0	75	77	33	37	20	31	75	78
Overall	(96)		(7)		(15)		(20)		(13)		(151)	
1 year	97	97	86	86	73	74	70	72	46	50	86	87
3 years	93	93	71	72	67	69	45	49	23	30	77	80
5 years	90	90	57	58	53	57	30	35	15	25	70	75

HODGKIN'S DISEASE (ICD-9 201)

SWITZERLAND

AREA	NUMBER OF CASES			PERIOD	MEAN AGE			5-YR RELATIVE SURVIVAL (%)	
	Males	Females	All		Males	Females	All	Males	Females
Basel	26	24	50	1985-1988	46.9	38.4	42.8		
Geneva	36	21	57	1985-1989	49.5	41.7	46.6		
Swiss Registries	62	45	107		48.4	40.0	44.9		

OBSERVED AND RELATIVE SURVIVAL (%) BY AGE (number of cases in parentheses)

	AGE CLASS										ALL	
	15-44		45-54		55-64		65-74		75-99			
	obs	rel	obs	rel	obs	rel	obs	rel	obs	rel	obs	rel
Males	(31)		(6)		(10)		(6)		(9)		(62)	
1 year	100	100	100	100	90	91	83	87	44	49	89	90
3 years	97	97	100	100	80	84	67	76	22	30	80	86
5 years	93	94	80	83	70	76	17	21	0	0	66	74
Females	(32)		(1)		(3)		(4)		(5)		(45)	
1 year	100	100	100	100	100	100	75	77	40	43	91	92
3 years	90	90	100	100	100	100	25	27	40	50	79	82
5 years	83	83	100	100	100	100	0	0	40	61	72	77
Overall	(63)		(7)		(13)		(10)		(14)		(107)	
1 year	100	100	100	100	92	93	80	83	43	47	90	91
3 years	93	94	100	100	85	88	50	56	29	38	80	84
5 years	88	88	83	86	77	83	10	12	14	24	68	75

HODGKIN'S DISEASE (ICD-9 201)

EUROPE, 1985-89

Weighted analyses

COUNTRY	% COVERAGE WITH C.R.s	Males	Females	All
		\multicolumn{3}{c}{YEARLY NO. OF CASES (Mean No. of cases recorded)}	
AUSTRIA	8	7	6	13
DENMARK	100	76	44	120
ENGLAND	50	337	249	586
ESTONIA	100	20	14	34
FINLAND	100	57	49	106
FRANCE	4	31	19	50
GERMANY	2	14	10	24
ICELAND	100	2	1	3
ITALY	10	103	89	192
NETHERLANDS	6	10	7	17
POLAND	6	29	22	51
SCOTLAND	100	67	58	125
SLOVAKIA	100	50	40	90
SLOVENIA	100	16	12	28
SPAIN	10	50	35	85
SWEDEN	17	16	14	30
SWITZERLAND	11	14	10	24

RELATIVE SURVIVAL (%) (Age-standardized) — Males / Females

□ 1 year ■ 5 years

OBSERVED AND RELATIVE SURVIVAL (%) BY AGE

	15-44 obs	15-44 rel	45-54 obs	45-54 rel	55-64 obs	55-64 rel	65-74 obs	65-74 rel	75-99 obs	75-99 rel	ALL obs	ALL rel
Males												
1 year	97	97	91	91	78	79	65	67	54	58	87	88
3 years	89	89	77	78	68	71	42	47	31	38	75	78
5 years	81	82	72	74	52	57	33	41	26	37	66	72
Females												
1 year	97	97	94	94	79	79	64	65	52	56	87	88
3 years	91	91	83	84	70	71	43	46	22	27	77	79
5 years	86	87	81	82	59	61	32	35	17	25	71	74
Overall												
1 year	97	97	92	93	78	79	64	66	53	57	87	88
3 years	90	90	80	81	68	71	42	47	27	33	76	79
5 years	83	84	76	78	55	58	32	39	22	32	68	73

AGE STANDARDIZED RELATIVE SURVIVAL(%)

COUNTRY	MALES 1-year (95% C.I.)	MALES 5-years (95% C.I.)	FEMALES 1-year (95% C.I.)	FEMALES 5-years (95% C.I.)
AUSTRIA	100.0 (100.0 -100.0)	85.0 (72.1 -100.1)	-	-
DENMARK	87.0 (83.9 - 90.2)	68.6 (64.4 - 73.2)	85.3 (81.2 - 89.7)	71.4 (65.8 - 77.3)
ENGLAND	85.8 (84.2 - 87.4)	69.7 (67.4 - 71.9)	87.3 (85.4 - 89.1)	74.4 (72.0 - 77.0)
ESTONIA	69.4 (63.0 - 76.4)	40.9 (33.1 - 50.5)	79.5 (70.8 - 89.3)	51.4 (41.0 - 64.5)
FINLAND	84.7 (81.1 - 88.5)	71.2 (66.1 - 76.5)	89.4 (86.1 - 92.9)	76.8 (72.0 - 81.9)
FRANCE	91.4 (87.2 - 95.8)	70.2 (63.3 - 77.8)	96.8 (92.9 -100.9)	85.3 (78.2 - 93.1)
GERMANY	91.5 (85.4 - 98.1)	76.1 (64.4 - 89.9)	84.3 (75.7 - 93.9)	66.2 (56.6 - 77.4)
ICELAND	-	-	-	-
ITALY	86.4 (83.4 - 89.5)	70.0 (65.5 - 74.7)	86.6 (83.3 - 90.0)	71.4 (67.1 - 76.0)
NETHERLANDS	94.3 (87.8 -101.3)	75.9 (64.6 - 89.2)	-	-
POLAND	85.4 (78.8 - 92.6)	62.2 (52.9 - 73.0)	85.3 (77.6 - 93.6)	69.6 (59.7 - 81.0)
SCOTLAND	80.1 (76.4 - 84.0)	64.7 (60.1 - 69.6)	82.9 (79.1 - 86.9)	67.1 (62.2 - 72.4)
SLOVAKIA	78.6 (74.1 - 83.4)	57.9 (51.8 - 64.7)	80.4 (75.4 - 85.8)	66.3 (59.7 - 73.7)
SLOVENIA	86.9 (79.7 - 94.8)	69.3 (60.2 - 79.8)	91.7 (85.5 - 98.3)	80.4 (70.6 - 91.7)
SPAIN	84.6 (79.8 - 89.7)	-	86.9 (81.9 - 92.1)	68.0 (60.4 - 76.5)
SWEDEN	86.3 (80.3 - 92.8)	73.7 (65.9 - 82.4)	89.3 (81.8 - 97.3)	70.6 (62.4 - 79.8)
SWITZERLAND	93.6 (89.0 - 98.5)	75.6 (67.4 - 84.7)	93.1 (87.5 - 99.1)	76.4 (67.2 - 86.8)
EUROPE, 1985-89	88.1 (86.5 - 89.8)	70.7 (67.8 - 73.7)	88.0 (86.0 - 90.0)	73.1 (70.4 - 75.9)

MULTIPLE MYELOMA (ICD-9 203)

AUSTRIA

AREA	NUMBER OF CASES			PERIOD	MEAN AGE		
	Males	Females	All		Males	Females	All
Tirol	19	22	41	1988-1989	61.6	66.2	64.1

OBSERVED AND RELATIVE SURVIVAL (%) BY AGE (number of cases in parentheses)

	AGE CLASS										ALL	
	15-44		45-54		55-64		65-74		75-99			
	obs	rel	obs	rel	obs	rel	obs	rel	obs	rel	obs	rel
Males	(1)		(2)		(8)		(7)		(1)		(19)	
1 year	100	100	100	100	75	76	100	100	0	0	84	86
3 years	0	0	100	100	75	78	57	62	0	0	63	67
5 years	0	0	100	100	50	53	43	50	0	0	47	52
Females	(1)		(3)		(6)		(6)		(6)		(22)	
1 year	0	0	67	67	100	100	67	68	67	71	73	74
3 years	0	0	67	67	83	85	33	35	50	60	55	58
5 years	0	0	33	34	67	69	33	36	0	0	32	36
Overall	(2)		(5)		(14)		(13)		(7)		(41)	
1 year	50	50	80	80	86	87	85	86	57	60	78	80
3 years	0	0	80	81	79	81	46	49	43	52	59	62
5 years	0	0	60	61	57	60	38	43	0	0	39	44

DENMARK

AREA	NUMBER OF CASES			PERIOD	MEAN AGE		
	Males	Females	All		Males	Females	All
Denmark	655	584	1239	1985-1989	69.0	70.0	69.5

OBSERVED AND RELATIVE SURVIVAL (%) BY AGE (number of cases in parentheses)

	AGE CLASS										ALL	
	15-44		45-54		55-64		65-74		75-99			
	obs	rel	obs	rel	obs	rel	obs	rel	obs	rel	obs	rel
Males	(20)		(44)		(119)		(259)		(213)		(655)	
1 year	70	70	82	82	71	72	56	58	44	48	57	60
3 years	45	45	48	49	39	41	31	35	16	23	29	34
5 years	30	30	32	33	21	23	19	24	10	18	17	23
Females	(10)		(45)		(107)		(208)		(214)		(584)	
1 year	100	100	73	74	78	78	64	65	41	44	59	62
3 years	70	70	51	52	47	48	27	29	18	23	30	34
5 years	40	40	40	41	32	34	15	17	9	14	18	23
Overall	(30)		(89)		(226)		(467)		(427)		(1239)	
1 year	80	80	78	78	74	75	60	62	42	46	58	61
3 years	53	54	49	50	42	45	29	32	17	23	29	34
5 years	33	34	36	37	26	28	17	21	9	16	18	23

MULTIPLE MYELOMA (ICD-9 203)

ENGLAND

AREA	NUMBER OF CASES			PERIOD	MEAN AGE			5-YR RELATIVE SURVIVAL (%)	
	Males	Females	All		Males	Females	All	Males	Females
East Anglia	273	258	531	1985-1989	69.6	72.7	71.1		
Mersey	234	226	460	1985-1989	68.6	71.4	70.0		
Oxford	299	280	579	1985-1989	68.8	72.2	70.5		
South Thames	662	590	1252	1985-1989	68.7	71.0	69.8		
Wessex	438	451	889	1985-1989	69.1	71.7	70.4		
West Midlands	582	531	1113	1985-1989	68.4	70.8	69.6		
Yorkshire	478	418	896	1985-1989	68.1	71.9	69.9		
English Registries	2966	2754	5720		68.7	71.5	70.1		

5-YR RELATIVE SURVIVAL (%)
100 80 60 40 20 0 — E.Angl — 0 20 40 60 80 100
Mersey / Oxford / S.Tham / Wessex / W.Midl / Yorksh

OBSERVED AND RELATIVE SURVIVAL (%) BY AGE (number of cases in parentheses)

	AGE CLASS										ALL	
	15-44		45-54		55-64		65-74		75-99			
	obs	rel	obs	rel	obs	rel	obs	rel	obs	rel	obs	rel
Males	(80)		(233)		(678)		(997)		(978)		(2966)	
1 year	84	84	72	73	63	65	54	57	36	40	53	55
3 years	61	62	50	51	37	39	27	31	15	22	28	34
5 years	46	47	30	31	22	24	13	17	8	14	16	21
Females	(43)		(182)		(453)		(870)		(1206)		(2754)	
1 year	88	88	72	72	68	68	58	59	41	44	53	56
3 years	70	70	46	47	41	42	30	33	19	25	29	33
5 years	60	61	34	35	26	28	17	19	9	15	17	21
Overall	(123)		(415)		(1131)		(1867)		(2184)		(5720)	
1 year	85	85	72	72	65	66	56	58	39	43	53	56
3 years	64	65	48	49	39	40	29	32	17	23	29	33
5 years	51	52	32	33	24	26	15	18	9	15	16	21

ESTONIA

AREA	NUMBER OF CASES			PERIOD	MEAN AGE		
	Males	Females	All		Males	Females	All
Estonia	62	81	143	1985-1989	61.8	63.6	62.8

OBSERVED AND RELATIVE SURVIVAL (%) BY AGE (number of cases in parentheses)

	AGE CLASS										ALL	
	15-44		45-54		55-64		65-74		75-99			
	obs	rel	obs	rel	obs	rel	obs	rel	obs	rel	obs	rel
Males	(2)		(13)		(21)		(22)		(4)		(62)	
1 year	50	50	54	55	62	64	55	57	0	0	53	55
3 years	50	51	23	24	33	36	18	22	0	0	24	27
5 years	50	51	8	8	33	39	9	12	0	0	18	22
Females	(4)		(13)		(26)		(24)		(14)		(81)	
1 year	100	100	77	77	58	58	67	69	36	39	62	64
3 years	100	100	61	62	31	32	42	46	7	9	38	42
5 years	100	100	52	54	15	16	17	20	7	12	24	28
Overall	(6)		(26)		(47)		(46)		(18)		(143)	
1 year	83	84	65	66	60	61	61	63	28	31	58	60
3 years	83	84	42	43	32	34	30	35	6	8	32	36
5 years	83	85	29	31	23	26	13	17	6	10	21	26

MULTIPLE MYELOMA   (ICD-9 203)

FINLAND

AREA	NUMBER OF CASES			PERIOD	MEAN AGE		
	Males	Females	All		Males	Females	All
Finland	544	624	1168	1985-1989	66.9	70.2	68.6

OBSERVED AND RELATIVE SURVIVAL (%) BY AGE (number of cases in parentheses)

	AGE CLASS										ALL	
	15-44		45-54		55-64		65-74		75-99			
	obs	rel	obs	rel	obs	rel	obs	rel	obs	rel	obs	rel
Males	(23)		(54)		(135)		(176)		(156)		(544)	
1 year	87	87	85	86	81	82	65	68	47	53	67	70
3 years	70	70	57	59	56	60	39	44	21	30	41	48
5 years	52	53	48	50	36	39	21	27	9	17	25	33
Females	(14)		(38)		(118)		(213)		(241)		(624)	
1 year	93	93	79	79	82	83	74	75	52	56	68	70
3 years	86	86	63	64	57	58	44	47	26	33	42	47
5 years	57	58	50	51	38	40	28	32	11	18	25	32
Overall	(37)		(92)		(253)		(389)		(397)		(1168)	
1 year	89	89	83	83	81	82	70	72	50	55	67	70
3 years	76	76	60	61	57	59	42	46	24	32	41	47
5 years	54	55	49	50	37	40	25	30	10	18	25	32

FRANCE

AREA	NUMBER OF CASES			PERIOD	MEAN AGE			5-YR RELATIVE SURVIVAL (%)	
	Males	Females	All		Males	Females	All	Males	Females
Somme	38	52	90	1985-1989	66.5	69.4	68.2		
Calvados	37	53	90	1985-1989	66.1	66.2	66.2		
Côte d'Or	44	45	89	1985-1989	72.7	73.8	73.3		
Doubs	35	42	77	1985-1989	65.7	68.3	67.1		
French Registries	154	192	346		68.0	69.3	68.8		

OBSERVED AND RELATIVE SURVIVAL (%) BY AGE (number of cases in parentheses)

	AGE CLASS										ALL	
	15-44		45-54		55-64		65-74		75-99			
	obs	rel	obs	rel	obs	rel	obs	rel	obs	rel	obs	rel
Males	(4)		(16)		(40)		(42)		(52)		(154)	
1 year	75	75	88	88	70	71	73	75	47	53	65	69
3 years	50	50	61	62	47	50	40	45	10	14	34	39
5 years	-	-	53	55	36	40	31	38	8	15	27	36
Females	(7)		(14)		(43)		(57)		(71)		(192)	
1 year	71	71	56	56	91	91	64	65	58	63	68	70
3 years	57	57	56	56	59	60	38	40	25	32	40	44
5 years	57	57	35	36	38	40	31	34	10	16	26	32
Overall	(11)		(30)		(83)		(99)		(123)		(346)	
1 year	73	73	73	73	81	82	68	69	54	59	66	69
3 years	55	55	58	59	53	55	39	42	18	25	37	42
5 years	55	55	43	45	37	40	31	36	9	16	26	33

MULTIPLE MYELOMA (ICD-9 203)

GERMANY

AREA	NUMBER OF CASES			PERIOD	MEAN AGE		
	Males	Females	All		Males	Females	All
Saarland	72	97	169	1985-1989	64.1	68.8	66.8

OBSERVED AND RELATIVE SURVIVAL (%) BY AGE (number of cases in parentheses)

	AGE CLASS										ALL	
	15-44		45-54		55-64		65-74		75-99			
	obs	rel	obs	rel	obs	rel	obs	rel	obs	rel	obs	rel
Males	(1)		(14)		(19)		(28)		(10)		(72)	
1 year	100	100	86	86	79	80	57	60	30	34	65	68
3 years	100	100	50	51	47	50	32	37	20	29	39	44
5 years	100	100	50	52	47	52	20	26	10	21	32	40
Females	(1)		(13)		(19)		(26)		(38)		(97)	
1 year	0	0	77	77	74	74	58	59	47	51	59	61
3 years	0	0	62	62	47	49	38	41	13	17	33	37
5 years	0	0	46	46	33	35	25	28	7	11	22	27
Overall	(2)		(27)		(38)		(54)		(48)		(169)	
1 year	50	50	81	82	76	77	57	59	44	48	62	64
3 years	50	50	56	56	47	49	35	39	15	19	36	40
5 years	50	51	47	49	40	43	22	27	8	13	26	33

ICELAND

AREA	NUMBER OF CASES			PERIOD	MEAN AGE		
	Males	Females	All		Males	Females	All
Iceland	28	29	57	1985-1989	66.3	68.1	67.2

OBSERVED AND RELATIVE SURVIVAL (%) BY AGE (number of cases in parentheses)

	AGE CLASS										ALL	
	15-44		45-54		55-64		65-74		75-99			
	obs	rel	obs	rel	obs	rel	obs	rel	obs	rel	obs	rel
Males	(1)		(3)		(7)		(11)		(6)		(28)	
1 year	100	100	33	34	86	87	64	66	67	73	68	70
3 years	100	100	33	34	86	89	36	40	17	22	46	52
5 years	0	0	33	34	71	76	27	32	17	27	36	43
Females	(0)		(4)		(8)		(9)		(8)		(29)	
1 year	-	-	75	75	75	75	78	79	75	82	76	78
3 years	-	-	75	76	38	38	44	47	25	33	41	46
5 years	-	-	75	76	38	39	33	38	25	41	38	45
Overall	(1)		(7)		(15)		(20)		(14)		(57)	
1 year	100	100	57	57	80	81	70	72	71	78	72	74
3 years	100	100	57	58	60	62	40	43	21	28	44	49
5 years	0	0	57	58	53	56	30	35	21	35	37	44

MULTIPLE MYELOMA (ICD-9 203)

ITALY

AREA	NUMBER OF CASES			PERIOD	MEAN AGE			5-YR RELATIVE SURVIVAL (%)	
	Males	Females	All		Males	Females	All	Males	Females
Florence	184	159	343	1985-1989	68.8	70.6	69.7		
Genoa	83	58	141	1986-1988	70.7	70.3	70.5		
Latina	17	12	29	1985-1987	66.5	67.7	67.0		
Modena	46	38	84	1988-1989	68.8	70.7	69.7		
Parma	36	42	78	1985-1987	70.9	72.1	71.6		
Ragusa	38	31	69	1985-1989	69.1	70.2	69.6		
Romagna	50	32	82	1986-1988	69.7	69.7	69.7		
Turin	44	59	103	1985-1987	66.2	68.8	67.7		
Varese	74	92	166	1985-1989	65.9	69.6	67.9		
Italian Registries	572	523	1095		68.7	70.2	69.4		

OBSERVED AND RELATIVE SURVIVAL (%) BY AGE (number of cases in parentheses)

	AGE CLASS										ALL	
	15-44		45-54		55-64		65-74		75-99			
	obs	rel	obs	rel	obs	rel	obs	rel	obs	rel	obs	rel
Males	(10)		(46)		(138)		(185)		(193)		(572)	
1 year	80	80	76	76	73	74	67	69	51	56	64	67
3 years	50	50	37	38	42	44	42	47	24	32	36	41
5 years	20	20	35	36	30	33	29	36	13	22	24	31
Females	(8)		(39)		(109)		(154)		(213)		(523)	
1 year	75	75	87	87	80	80	73	75	54	58	68	70
3 years	50	50	64	65	54	55	47	49	26	32	41	46
5 years	50	50	38	39	39	41	31	34	12	18	26	31
Overall	(18)		(85)		(247)		(339)		(406)		(1095)	
1 year	78	78	81	81	76	77	70	72	52	57	66	69
3 years	50	50	49	50	47	49	44	48	25	32	38	43
5 years	33	34	36	37	34	36	30	35	12	20	25	31

NETHERLANDS

AREA	NUMBER OF CASES			PERIOD	MEAN AGE		
	Males	Females	All		Males	Females	All
Eindhoven	72	80	152	1985-1989	67.0	68.5	67.8

OBSERVED AND RELATIVE SURVIVAL (%) BY AGE (number of cases in parentheses)

	AGE CLASS										ALL	
	15-44		45-54		55-64		65-74		75-99			
	obs	rel	obs	rel	obs	rel	obs	rel	obs	rel	obs	rel
Males	(2)		(6)		(20)		(24)		(20)		(72)	
1 year	100	100	50	50	70	71	88	91	55	61	71	74
3 years	100	100	33	34	45	47	54	61	20	28	42	48
5 years	100	100	17	17	20	22	25	32	10	18	21	27
Females	(3)		(6)		(17)		(23)		(31)		(80)	
1 year	100	100	83	84	88	89	57	58	74	78	74	76
3 years	33	33	67	67	65	66	39	42	34	41	44	49
5 years	33	34	50	51	47	49	17	18	16	23	26	31
Overall	(5)		(12)		(37)		(47)		(51)		(152)	
1 year	100	100	67	67	78	79	72	74	66	72	72	75
3 years	60	60	50	51	54	56	47	51	28	36	43	48
5 years	60	61	33	34	32	34	21	25	13	21	24	29

MULTIPLE MYELOMA (ICD-9 203)

POLAND

AREA	NUMBER OF CASES			PERIOD	MEAN AGE			5-YR RELATIVE SURVIVAL (%)	
	Males	Females	All		Males	Females	All	Males	Females
Cracow	40	38	78	1985-1989	64.8	64.5	64.7		
Warsaw	36	44	80	1988-1989	66.3	68.3	67.4		
Polish Registries	76	82	158		65.6	66.6	66.1		

OBSERVED AND RELATIVE SURVIVAL (%) BY AGE (number of cases in parentheses)

	AGE CLASS										ALL	
	15-44		45-54		55-64		65-74		75-99			
	obs	rel	obs	rel	obs	rel	obs	rel	obs	rel	obs	rel
Males	(0)		(10)		(24)		(27)		(15)		(76)	
1 year	-	-	50	51	54	56	41	43	40	45	46	48
3 years	-	-	30	31	42	45	15	18	25	36	27	32
5 years	-	-	20	22	17	20	4	5	17	31	12	16
Females	(1)		(6)		(28)		(25)		(22)		(82)	
1 year	100	100	67	67	81	82	38	39	27	29	52	54
3 years	100	100	67	68	27	28	21	23	9	11	24	26
5 years	100	100	0	0	12	12	4	5	5	7	8	10
Overall	(1)		(16)		(52)		(52)		(37)		(158)	
1 year	100	100	56	57	68	70	40	41	32	35	49	51
3 years	100	100	44	45	34	36	18	20	16	20	26	29
5 years	100	100	18	19	14	16	4	5	9	15	10	13

SCOTLAND

AREA	NUMBER OF CASES			PERIOD	MEAN AGE		
	Males	Females	All		Males	Females	All
Scotland	580	612	1192	1985-1989	68.7	71.5	70.1

OBSERVED AND RELATIVE SURVIVAL (%) BY AGE (number of cases in parentheses)

	AGE CLASS										ALL	
	15-44		45-54		55-64		65-74		75-99			
	obs	rel	obs	rel	obs	rel	obs	rel	obs	rel	obs	rel
Males	(13)		(44)		(133)		(199)		(191)		(580)	
1 year	85	85	66	66	56	58	47	49	34	38	47	50
3 years	62	62	39	40	33	35	21	25	13	18	23	28
5 years	46	47	20	21	20	22	11	14	6	11	13	17
Females	(8)		(42)		(101)		(192)		(269)		(612)	
1 year	88	88	74	74	69	70	51	53	41	44	51	54
3 years	38	38	40	41	47	48	31	34	19	25	29	34
5 years	25	25	33	34	37	39	16	19	8	14	17	23
Overall	(21)		(86)		(234)		(391)		(460)		(1192)	
1 year	86	86	70	70	62	63	49	51	38	42	49	52
3 years	52	53	40	40	39	41	26	29	16	22	26	31
5 years	38	39	27	28	27	30	13	16	7	13	15	20

MULTIPLE MYELOMA (ICD-9 203)

SLOVAKIA

AREA	NUMBER OF CASES			PERIOD	MEAN AGE		
	Males	Females	All		Males	Females	All
Slovakia	345	341	686	1985-1989	64.3	66.3	65.3

OBSERVED AND RELATIVE SURVIVAL (%) BY AGE (number of cases in parentheses)

	AGE CLASS										ALL	
	15-44		45-54		55-64		65-74		75-99			
	obs	rel	obs	rel	obs	rel	obs	rel	obs	rel	obs	rel
Males	(19)		(46)		(95)		(116)		(69)		(345)	
1 year	84	85	83	84	61	63	54	57	43	49	59	62
3 years	63	64	52	54	35	38	33	39	23	34	36	42
5 years	34	35	33	35	25	30	23	31	16	31	24	32
Females	(16)		(31)		(95)		(115)		(84)		(341)	
1 year	75	75	84	84	71	71	64	66	51	56	65	67
3 years	56	57	68	69	48	50	42	46	30	40	44	49
5 years	50	50	50	51	40	43	33	39	22	38	35	42
Overall	(35)		(77)		(190)		(231)		(153)		(686)	
1 year	80	80	83	84	66	67	59	62	48	53	62	65
3 years	60	61	58	60	42	44	37	43	27	37	40	45
5 years	41	42	40	42	33	36	28	35	19	35	29	37

SLOVENIA

AREA	NUMBER OF CASES			PERIOD	MEAN AGE		
	Males	Females	All		Males	Females	All
Slovenia	113	109	222	1985-1989	62.7	65.0	63.8

OBSERVED AND RELATIVE SURVIVAL (%) BY AGE (number of cases in parentheses)

	AGE CLASS										ALL	
	15-44		45-54		55-64		65-74		75-99			
	obs	rel	obs	rel	obs	rel	obs	rel	obs	rel	obs	rel
Males	(5)		(17)		(45)		(27)		(19)		(113)	
1 year	100	100	82	83	62	64	44	47	53	58	61	63
3 years	80	81	59	61	29	31	19	22	21	29	32	36
5 years	80	81	29	31	20	23	15	20	16	29	22	27
Females	(4)		(13)		(32)		(39)		(21)		(109)	
1 year	100	100	85	85	78	79	69	71	43	47	70	72
3 years	100	100	62	62	50	52	31	33	10	13	39	42
5 years	75	76	53	55	25	26	18	21	10	16	25	29
Overall	(9)		(30)		(77)		(66)		(40)		(222)	
1 year	100	100	83	84	69	70	59	61	48	52	65	68
3 years	89	90	60	61	38	40	26	29	15	20	35	39
5 years	78	79	39	41	22	24	17	20	13	22	23	28

MULTIPLE MYELOMA (ICD-9 203)

SPAIN

AREA	NUMBER OF CASES			PERIOD	MEAN AGE			5-YR RELATIVE SURVIVAL (%)	
	Males	Females	All		Males	Females	All	Males	Females
Basque Country	79	102	181	1986-1988	65.6	68.7	67.3		
Mallorca	23	24	47	1988-1989	64.4	70.0	67.3		
Navarra	41	34	75	1985-1989	65.5	67.9	66.6		
Tarragona	58	47	105	1985-1989	67.0	70.2	68.4		
Spanish Registries	201	207	408		65.8	69.1	67.5		

OBSERVED AND RELATIVE SURVIVAL (%) BY AGE (number of cases in parentheses)

	AGE CLASS										ALL	
	15-44		45-54		55-64		65-74		75-99			
	obs	rel	obs	rel	obs	rel	obs	rel	obs	rel	obs	rel
Males	(13)		(23)		(43)		(76)		(46)		(201)	
1 year	92	93	83	83	81	82	66	68	72	80	74	77
3 years	69	70	43	44	56	58	41	45	50	71	48	55
5 years	59	60	37	38	36	39	23	28	28	52	31	38
Females	(7)		(12)		(47)		(69)		(72)		(207)	
1 year	100	100	92	92	60	60	75	77	53	56	66	68
3 years	71	72	58	59	45	45	48	50	21	25	39	43
5 years	71	72	30	30	38	39	30	33	15	22	28	33
Overall	(20)		(35)		(90)		(145)		(118)		(408)	
1 year	95	95	86	86	70	71	70	72	60	65	70	72
3 years	70	70	49	49	50	51	44	48	32	42	44	48
5 years	64	65	36	37	37	39	26	30	20	32	30	36

SWEDEN

AREA	NUMBER OF CASES			PERIOD	MEAN AGE		
	Males	Females	All		Males	Females	All
South Sweden	257	196	453	1985-1989	70.1	72.6	71.2

OBSERVED AND RELATIVE SURVIVAL (%) BY AGE (number of cases in parentheses)

	AGE CLASS										ALL	
	15-44		45-54		55-64		65-74		75-99			
	obs	rel	obs	rel	obs	rel	obs	rel	obs	rel	obs	rel
Males	(4)		(18)		(54)		(82)		(99)		(257)	
1 year	100	100	94	95	76	77	78	81	61	68	72	77
3 years	100	100	50	51	43	44	50	56	29	42	41	49
5 years	75	76	22	23	30	32	27	33	17	33	24	33
Females	(2)		(9)		(24)		(67)		(94)		(196)	
1 year	100	100	89	89	79	80	85	87	63	67	74	77
3 years	100	100	56	56	71	72	48	51	29	36	42	48
5 years	0	0	56	57	67	69	33	36	16	24	30	37
Overall	(6)		(27)		(78)		(149)		(193)		(453)	
1 year	100	100	93	93	77	78	81	83	62	67	73	77
3 years	100	100	52	53	51	53	49	53	29	39	42	49
5 years	50	50	33	34	41	44	30	34	17	28	26	34

MULTIPLE MYELOMA (ICD-9 203)

SWITZERLAND

AREA	NUMBER OF CASES			PERIOD	MEAN AGE			5-YR RELATIVE SURVIVAL (%)	
	Males	Females	All		Males	Females	All	Males	Females
Basel	23	31	54	1985-1988	67.0	71.4	69.5		
Geneva	41	41	82	1985-1989	66.8	71.3	69.1		
Swiss Registries	64	72	136		66.9	71.4	69.3		

5-YR RELATIVE SURVIVAL (%)

Males: 100 80 60 40 20 0   Females: 0 20 40 60 80 100

Basel
Geneva

OBSERVED AND RELATIVE SURVIVAL (%) BY AGE (number of cases in parentheses)

	15-44		45-54		55-64		65-74		75-99		ALL	
	obs	rel	obs	rel	obs	rel	obs	rel	obs	rel	obs	rel
Males	(2)		(9)		(15)		(19)		(19)		(64)	
1 year	50	50	100	100	93	95	84	87	79	87	86	90
3 years	50	50	78	79	67	70	37	41	32	43	48	55
5 years	50	50	56	57	38	41	19	24	11	18	27	34
Females	(3)		(7)		(7)		(15)		(40)		(72)	
1 year	100	100	86	86	100	100	87	88	50	53	68	71
3 years	67	67	51	52	86	87	47	49	27	34	41	47
5 years	33	34	34	35	71	74	33	36	11	16	25	31
Overall	(5)		(16)		(22)		(34)		(59)		(136)	
1 year	80	80	94	94	95	96	85	88	59	64	76	80
3 years	60	60	67	68	73	75	41	45	29	37	45	51
5 years	40	40	47	48	49	52	26	30	11	17	26	33

MULTIPLE MYELOMA (ICD-9 203)

EUROPE, 1985-89
Weighted analyses

COUNTRY	% COVERAGE WITH C.R.s	YEARLY NO. OF CASES (Mean No. of cases recorded)			RELATIVE SURVIVAL (%) (Age-standardized)
		Males	Females	All	
AUSTRIA	8	10	11	21	
DENMARK	100	131	117	248	
ENGLAND	50	593	551	1144	
ESTONIA	100	12	16	28	
FINLAND	100	109	125	234	
FRANCE	4	31	38	69	
GERMANY	2	14	19	33	
ICELAND	100	6	6	12	
ITALY	10	159	143	302	
NETHERLANDS	6	14	16	30	
POLAND	6	26	30	56	
SCOTLAND	100	116	122	238	
SLOVAKIA	100	69	68	137	
SLOVENIA	100	23	22	45	
SPAIN	10	58	62	120	
SWEDEN	17	51	39	90	
SWITZERLAND	11	14	16	30	

□ 1 year ■ 5 years

OBSERVED AND RELATIVE SURVIVAL (%) BY AGE

	AGE CLASS										ALL	
	15-44		45-54		55-64		65-74		75-99			
	obs	rel	obs	rel	obs	rel	obs	rel	obs	rel	obs	rel
Males												
1 year	86	86	78	78	71	72	64	66	46	51	63	66
3 years	65	65	47	48	45	47	36	41	22	31	36	42
5 years	51	51	37	39	31	34	22	28	12	22	24	31
Females												
1 year	70	70	76	77	78	78	64	65	50	54	63	65
3 years	53	53	58	59	51	52	39	41	22	27	36	41
5 years	46	46	36	37	36	38	25	28	10	16	23	28
Overall												
1 year	78	78	77	77	75	75	64	66	48	53	63	66
3 years	59	59	53	54	48	50	37	41	22	29	36	41
5 years	48	49	37	38	34	36	24	28	11	19	23	29

AGE STANDARDIZED RELATIVE SURVIVAL(%)

COUNTRY	MALES		FEMALES	
	1-year (95% C.I.)	5-years (95% C.I.)	1-year (95% C.I.)	5-years (95% C.I.)
AUSTRIA	59.5 (53.4 - 66.3)	35.6 (22.7 - 55.8)	73.8 (56.7 - 96.0)	29.2 (16.7 - 51.3)
DENMARK	59.9 (56.2 - 64.0)	22.6 (19.0 - 26.8)	62.2 (58.5 - 66.3)	22.1 (18.6 - 26.1)
ENGLAND	54.4 (52.6 - 56.3)	19.4 (17.8 - 21.2)	57.6 (55.7 - 59.5)	21.6 (20.0 - 23.4)
ESTONIA	38.0 (30.0 - 48.2)	14.3 (8.4 - 24.5)	57.5 (46.3 - 71.4)	21.1 (12.8 - 35.0)
FINLAND	67.4 (63.2 - 71.8)	28.6 (24.4 - 33.6)	70.9 (67.3 - 74.6)	30.8 (27.0 - 35.0)
FRANCE	67.6 (60.1 - 76.1)	-	69.3 (62.8 - 76.5)	29.8 (23.1 - 38.5)
GERMANY	57.9 (45.8 - 73.2)	33.6 (20.9 - 54.3)	59.4 (50.3 - 70.2)	24.4 (16.2 - 36.8)
ICELAND	70.9 (54.3 - 92.4)	39.2 (22.4 - 68.6)	-	-
ITALY	66.4 (62.4 - 70.6)	29.7 (25.6 - 34.6)	70.8 (66.9 - 74.9)	30.4 (26.4 - 35.1)
NETHERLANDS	73.2 (62.9 - 85.2)	25.4 (15.6 - 41.4)	74.7 (65.4 - 85.2)	29.4 (20.3 - 42.5)
POLAND	-	-	48.5 (39.0 - 60.4)	9.2 (4.6 - 18.1)
SCOTLAND	49.2 (45.2 - 53.6)	16.2 (13.0 - 20.3)	56.0 (52.1 - 60.1)	22.6 (19.2 - 26.8)
SLOVAKIA	58.2 (52.5 - 64.7)	31.4 (24.5 - 40.1)	65.4 (60.0 - 71.2)	40.8 (34.1 - 48.9)
SLOVENIA	58.6 (48.2 - 71.3)	26.0 (16.0 - 42.2)	65.8 (56.5 - 76.8)	24.3 (16.3 - 36.2)
SPAIN	77.2 (70.6 - 84.4)	40.5 (31.2 - 52.6)	67.6 (61.5 - 74.3)	31.1 (24.5 - 39.6)
SWEDEN	77.0 (71.6 - 82.7)	32.9 (26.4 - 40.9)	78.8 (72.9 - 85.0)	39.7 (32.8 - 47.9)
SWITZERLAND	88.8 (79.6 - 98.9)	28.8 (18.2 - 45.5)	78.4 (70.4 - 87.3)	37.0 (26.1 - 52.4)
EUROPE, 1985-89	63.6 (61.1 - 66.2)	28.7 (25.8 - 31.8)	65.0 (62.7 - 67.4)	26.8 (24.5 - 29.3)

ACUTE LYMPHATIC LEUKAEMIA (ICD-9 204.0)

AUSTRIA

AREA	NUMBER OF CASES			PERIOD	MEAN AGE		
	Males	Females	All		Males	Females	All
Tirol	6	4	10	1988-1989	38.2	54.8	44.9

OBSERVED AND RELATIVE SURVIVAL (%) BY AGE (number of cases in parentheses)

	AGE CLASS										ALL	
	15-44		45-54		55-64		65-74		75-99			
	obs	rel	obs	rel	obs	rel	obs	rel	obs	rel	obs	rel
Males	(4)		(0)		(1)		(0)		(1)		(6)	
1 year	75	75	-	-	0	0	-	-	0	0	50	51
3 years	50	50	-	-	0	0	-	-	0	0	33	35
5 years	50	50	-	-	0	0	-	-	0	0	33	36
Females	(1)		(1)		(0)		(1)		(1)		(4)	
1 year	100	100	100	100	-	-	0	0	0	0	50	51
3 years	100	100	100	100	-	-	0	0	0	0	50	54
5 years	100	100	100	100	-	-	0	0	0	0	50	58
Overall	(5)		(1)		(1)		(1)		(2)		(10)	
1 year	80	80	100	100	0	0	0	0	0	0	50	51
3 years	60	60	100	100	0	0	0	0	0	0	40	42
5 years	60	60	100	100	0	0	0	0	0	0	40	44

DENMARK

AREA	NUMBER OF CASES			PERIOD	MEAN AGE		
	Males	Females	All		Males	Females	All
Denmark	78	64	142	1985-1989	45.8	55.1	50.0

OBSERVED AND RELATIVE SURVIVAL (%) BY AGE (number of cases in parentheses)

	AGE CLASS										ALL	
	15-44		45-54		55-64		65-74		75-99			
	obs	rel	obs	rel	obs	rel	obs	rel	obs	rel	obs	rel
Males	(40)		(3)		(10)		(11)		(14)		(78)	
1 year	78	78	100	100	30	31	36	38	0	0	53	54
3 years	40	40	33	34	10	11	27	31	0	0	27	29
5 years	35	35	33	34	0	0	27	35	0	0	23	27
Females	(20)		(5)		(12)		(15)		(12)		(64)	
1 year	75	75	0	0	42	42	27	27	8	9	39	40
3 years	35	35	0	0	8	9	20	21	0	0	17	18
5 years	20	20	0	0	8	9	13	15	0	0	11	12
Overall	(60)		(8)		(22)		(26)		(26)		(142)	
1 year	77	77	38	38	36	37	31	32	4	4	46	48
3 years	38	38	13	13	9	10	23	25	0	0	23	24
5 years	30	30	13	13	5	5	19	23	0	0	18	20

ACUTE LYMPHATIC LEUKAEMIA   (ICD-9 204.0)

ENGLAND

AREA	NUMBER OF CASES			PERIOD	MEAN AGE			5-YR RELATIVE SURVIVAL (%)	
	Males	Females	All		Males	Females	All	Males	Females
East Anglia	23	18	41	1985-1989	46.3	52.0	48.9		
Mersey	29	27	56	1985-1989	47.8	44.1	46.0		
Oxford	31	30	61	1985-1989	35.8	47.3	41.5		
South Thames	78	49	127	1985-1989	42.8	52.0	46.4		
Wessex	77	34	111	1985-1989	43.2	50.6	45.5		
West Midlands	95	56	151	1985-1989	44.7	51.9	47.4		
Yorkshire	48	32	80	1985-1989	40.8	46.1	42.9		
English Registries	381	246	627		43.1	49.6	45.7		

OBSERVED AND RELATIVE SURVIVAL (%) BY AGE (number of cases in parentheses)

	AGE CLASS										ALL	
	15-44		45-54		55-64		65-74		75-99			
	obs	rel	obs	rel	obs	rel	obs	rel	obs	rel	obs	rel
Males	(215)		(29)		(32)		(56)		(49)		(381)	
1 year	71	71	52	52	50	51	16	17	6	7	51	52
3 years	43	43	38	39	22	23	4	4	2	3	29	32
5 years	35	35	14	14	16	17	2	2	2	4	23	25
Females	(109)		(19)		(37)		(36)		(45)		(246)	
1 year	70	70	58	58	46	46	47	48	11	12	51	52
3 years	50	51	42	43	16	17	25	27	7	9	33	35
5 years	40	40	37	37	11	11	14	16	7	11	26	29
Overall	(324)		(48)		(69)		(92)		(94)		(627)	
1 year	70	70	54	54	48	48	28	29	9	9	51	52
3 years	45	45	40	40	19	20	12	13	4	6	31	33
5 years	37	37	23	24	13	14	7	8	4	7	24	27

ESTONIA

AREA	NUMBER OF CASES			PERIOD	MEAN AGE		
	Males	Females	All		Males	Females	All
Estonia	13	9	22	1985-1989	45.5	67.3	54.5

OBSERVED AND RELATIVE SURVIVAL (%) BY AGE (number of cases in parentheses)

	AGE CLASS										ALL	
	15-44		45-54		55-64		65-74		75-99			
	obs	rel	obs	rel	obs	rel	obs	rel	obs	rel	obs	rel
Males	(7)		(2)		(1)		(2)		(1)		(13)	
1 year	57	57	0	0	100	100	0	0	100	100	46	48
3 years	43	43	0	0	100	100	0	0	0	0	31	34
5 years	29	29	0	0	0	0	0	0	0	0	15	18
Females	(0)		(1)		(3)		(2)		(3)		(9)	
1 year	-	-	0	0	33	34	0	0	33	36	22	23
3 years	-	-	0	0	0	0	0	0	0	0	0	0
5 years	-	-	0	0	0	0	0	0	0	0	0	0
Overall	(7)		(3)		(4)		(4)		(4)		(22)	
1 year	57	57	0	0	50	51	0	0	50	57	36	38
3 years	43	43	0	0	25	26	0	0	0	0	18	20
5 years	29	29	0	0	0	0	0	0	0	0	9	11

ACUTE LYMPHATIC LEUKAEMIA (ICD-9 204.0)

FINLAND

AREA	NUMBER OF CASES			PERIOD	MEAN AGE		
	Males	Females	All		Males	Females	All
Finland	93	74	167	1985-1989	42.1	49.4	45.4

OBSERVED AND RELATIVE SURVIVAL (%) BY AGE (number of cases in parentheses)

	AGE CLASS										ALL	
	15-44		45-54		55-64		65-74		75-99			
	obs	rel	obs	rel	obs	rel	obs	rel	obs	rel	obs	rel
Males	(58)		(6)		(8)		(13)		(8)		(93)	
1 year	71	71	50	50	25	25	8	8	0	0	51	51
3 years	40	40	0	0	25	26	8	9	0	0	28	29
5 years	26	26	0	0	0	0	8	9	0	0	17	19
Females	(29)		(11)		(15)		(14)		(5)		(74)	
1 year	66	66	64	64	67	67	21	22	0	0	53	53
3 years	38	38	36	37	47	48	7	8	0	0	31	32
5 years	34	35	9	9	40	42	7	8	0	0	24	26
Overall	(87)		(17)		(23)		(27)		(13)		(167)	
1 year	69	69	59	59	52	53	15	15	0	0	51	52
3 years	39	39	24	24	39	40	7	8	0	0	29	31
5 years	29	29	6	6	26	28	7	9	0	0	20	22

FRANCE

AREA	NUMBER OF CASES			PERIOD	MEAN AGE			5-YR RELATIVE SURVIVAL (%)	
	Males	Females	All		Males	Females	All	Males	Females
Somme	6	7	13	1985-1989	40.3	60.0	51.0		
Calvados	11	7	18	1985-1989	56.9	62.4	59.1		
Côte d'Or	4	6	10	1985-1989	22.3	46.8	37.1		
Doubs	11	3	14	1985-1989	31.5	46.7	34.9		
French Registries	32	23	55		40.9	55.7	47.1		

5-YR RELATIVE SURVIVAL (%) chart — Males scale: 100 80 60 40 20 0; Females scale: 0 20 40 60 80 100. Bars labelled Somme, Calvad, Côte d.

OBSERVED AND RELATIVE SURVIVAL (%) BY AGE (number of cases in parentheses)

	AGE CLASS										ALL	
	15-44		45-54		55-64		65-74		75-99			
	obs	rel	obs	rel	obs	rel	obs	rel	obs	rel	obs	rel
Males	(20)		(0)		(4)		(3)		(5)		(32)	
1 year	70	70	-	-	75	76	67	68	60	65	69	70
3 years	36	36	-	-	50	53	33	37	40	52	38	41
5 years	36	36	-	-	25	28	0	0	20	33	26	28
Females	(6)		(2)		(7)		(5)		(3)		(23)	
1 year	82	82	50	50	43	43	100	100	100	100	74	75
3 years	61	61	50	50	29	29	80	84	33	47	51	54
5 years	20	21	50	51	29	30	60	66	33	61	34	38
Overall	(26)		(2)		(11)		(8)		(8)		(55)	
1 year	73	73	50	50	55	55	88	89	75	82	71	72
3 years	42	42	50	50	36	38	63	67	38	50	44	47
5 years	30	30	50	51	26	28	38	42	25	43	30	33

ACUTE LYMPHATIC LEUKAEMIA   (ICD-9 204.0)

GERMANY

AREA	NUMBER OF CASES			PERIOD	MEAN AGE		
	Males	Females	All		Males	Females	All
Saarland	17	20	37	1985-1989	41.6	51.5	47.0

OBSERVED AND RELATIVE SURVIVAL (%) BY AGE (number of cases in parentheses)

	AGE CLASS										ALL	
	15-44		45-54		55-64		65-74		75-99			
	obs	rel	obs	rel	obs	rel	obs	rel	obs	rel	obs	rel
Males	(10)		(1)		(4)		(1)		(1)		(17)	
1 year	80	80	0	0	50	51	100	100	0	0	65	66
3 years	40	40	0	0	50	53	0	0	0	0	35	37
5 years	40	40	0	0	50	56	0	0	0	0	35	38
Females	(6)		(2)		(5)		(5)		(2)		(20)	
1 year	67	67	100	100	40	40	20	20	0	0	45	46
3 years	67	67	100	100	20	20	0	0	0	0	35	37
5 years	67	67	-	-	20	21	0	0	0	0	35	38
Overall	(16)		(3)		(9)		(6)		(3)		(37)	
1 year	75	75	67	67	44	45	33	34	0	0	54	55
3 years	50	50	67	68	33	35	0	0	0	0	35	37
5 years	50	50	-	-	33	36	0	0	0	0	35	38

ICELAND

AREA	NUMBER OF CASES			PERIOD	MEAN AGE		
	Males	Females	All		Males	Females	All
Iceland	3	3	6	1985-1989	19.3	48.7	34.2

OBSERVED AND RELATIVE SURVIVAL (%) BY AGE (number of cases in parentheses)

	AGE CLASS										ALL	
	15-44		45-54		55-64		65-74		75-99			
	obs	rel	obs	rel	obs	rel	obs	rel	obs	rel	obs	rel
Males	(3)		(0)		(0)		(0)		(0)		(3)	
1 year	67	67	-	-	-	-	-	-	-	-	67	67
3 years	33	33	-	-	-	-	-	-	-	-	33	33
5 years	0	0	-	-	-	-	-	-	-	-	0	0
Females	(1)		(1)		(0)		(1)		(0)		(3)	
1 year	100	100	0	0	-	-	100	100	-	-	67	67
3 years	100	100	0	0	-	-	100	100	-	-	67	68
5 years	0	0	0	0	-	-	100	100	-	-	33	34
Overall	(4)		(1)		(0)		(1)		(0)		(6)	
1 year	75	75	0	0	-	-	100	100	-	-	67	67
3 years	50	50	0	0	-	-	100	100	-	-	50	50
5 years	0	0	0	0	-	-	100	100	-	-	17	17

ACUTE LYMPHATIC LEUKAEMIA (ICD-9 204.0)

ITALY

AREA	Males	Females	All	PERIOD	Males	Females	All
	NUMBER OF CASES				MEAN AGE		
Florence	21	18	39	1985-1989	41.4	49.2	45.1
Genoa	7	12	19	1986-1988	59.4	59.2	59.3
Latina	9	2	11	1985-1987	56.7	30.5	52.0
Modena	1	1	2	1988-1989	29.0	65.0	47.5
Parma	6	4	10	1985-1987	51.5	55.5	53.2
Ragusa	8	6	14	1985-1989	53.9	44.8	50.1
Romagna	3	7	10	1986-1988	43.0	58.1	53.7
Turin	11	7	18	1985-1987	49.1	61.0	53.8
Varese	14	14	28	1985-1989	27.6	59.7	43.7
Italian Registries	80	71	151		45.4	54.8	49.8

5-YR RELATIVE SURVIVAL (%)

OBSERVED AND RELATIVE SURVIVAL (%) BY AGE (number of cases in parentheses)

	AGE CLASS										ALL	
	15-44		45-54		55-64		65-74		75-99			
	obs	rel	obs	rel	obs	rel	obs	rel	obs	rel	obs	rel
Males	(39)		(9)		(10)		(8)		(14)		(80)	
1 year	67	67	22	22	40	41	0	0	36	39	46	47
3 years	38	39	11	11	20	21	0	0	21	30	26	28
5 years	31	31	11	11	20	22	0	0	7	13	20	22
Females	(25)		(6)		(11)		(11)		(18)		(71)	
1 year	67	67	50	50	36	37	36	37	11	12	42	43
3 years	34	34	33	34	9	9	27	29	6	7	22	23
5 years	29	29	33	34	9	9	9	10	6	9	17	20
Overall	(64)		(15)		(21)		(19)		(32)		(151)	
1 year	67	67	33	33	38	38	21	22	22	24	44	45
3 years	37	37	20	20	14	15	16	17	13	17	24	26
5 years	30	30	20	20	14	15	5	6	6	10	19	21

NETHERLANDS

AREA	Males	Females	All	PERIOD	Males	Females	All
	NUMBER OF CASES				MEAN AGE		
Eindhoven	13	11	24	1985-1989	34.2	49.2	41.1

OBSERVED AND RELATIVE SURVIVAL (%) BY AGE (number of cases in parentheses)

	AGE CLASS										ALL	
	15-44		45-54		55-64		65-74		75-99			
	obs	rel	obs	rel	obs	rel	obs	rel	obs	rel	obs	rel
Males	(9)		(1)		(3)		(0)		(0)		(13)	
1 year	78	78	100	100	33	34	-	-	-	-	69	70
3 years	44	45	100	100	0	0	-	-	-	-	38	39
5 years	44	45	100	100	0	0	-	-	-	-	38	40
Females	(4)		(1)		(1)		(3)		(2)		(11)	
1 year	50	50	0	0	0	0	0	0	0	0	18	18
3 years	50	50	0	0	0	0	0	0	0	0	18	19
5 years	50	50	0	0	0	0	0	0	0	0	18	20
Overall	(13)		(2)		(4)		(3)		(2)		(24)	
1 year	69	69	50	50	25	25	0	0	0	0	46	46
3 years	46	46	50	51	0	0	0	0	0	0	29	30
5 years	46	46	50	51	0	0	0	0	0	0	29	31

ACUTE LYMPHATIC LEUKAEMIA   (ICD-9 204.0)

POLAND

AREA	NUMBER OF CASES			PERIOD	MEAN AGE			5-YR RELATIVE SURVIVAL (%)	
	Males	Females	All		Males	Females	All	Males	Females
Cracow	12	6	18	1985-1989	47.8	56.3	50.7		
Warsaw	7	5	12	1988-1989	51.3	56.6	53.6		
Polish Registries	19	11	30		49.2	56.6	51.9		

OBSERVED AND RELATIVE SURVIVAL (%) BY AGE (number of cases in parentheses)

	AGE CLASS										ALL	
	15-44		45-54		55-64		65-74		75-99			
	obs	rel	obs	rel	obs	rel	obs	rel	obs	rel	obs	rel
Males	(7)		(3)		(5)		(1)		(3)		(19)	
1 year	14	14	0	0	60	62	0	0	0	0	21	22
3 years	14	14	0	0	20	22	0	0	0	0	11	12
5 years	14	14	0	0	20	23	0	0	0	0	11	12
Females	(2)		(2)		(4)		(0)		(3)		(11)	
1 year	0	0	50	50	0	0	-	-	67	71	27	28
3 years	0	0	0	0	0	0	-	-	67	81	18	19
5 years	0	0	0	0	0	0	-	-	33	48	9	10
Overall	(9)		(5)		(9)		(1)		(6)		(30)	
1 year	11	11	20	20	33	34	0	0	33	37	23	24
3 years	11	11	0	0	11	12	0	0	33	45	13	15
5 years	11	11	0	0	11	12	0	0	17	28	10	12

SCOTLAND

AREA	NUMBER OF CASES			PERIOD	MEAN AGE		
	Males	Females	All		Males	Females	All
Scotland	70	49	119	1985-1989	38.9	54.0	45.1

OBSERVED AND RELATIVE SURVIVAL (%) BY AGE (number of cases in parentheses)

	AGE CLASS										ALL	
	15-44		45-54		55-64		65-74		75-99			
	obs	rel	obs	rel	obs	rel	obs	rel	obs	rel	obs	rel
Males	(46)		(5)		(4)		(8)		(7)		(70)	
1 year	72	72	60	60	50	51	38	39	0	0	59	60
3 years	54	55	40	41	0	0	25	29	0	0	41	44
5 years	43	44	20	21	0	0	13	16	0	0	31	34
Females	(17)		(4)		(5)		(12)		(11)		(49)	
1 year	82	82	25	25	0	0	17	17	27	29	41	42
3 years	65	65	0	0	0	0	0	0	0	0	22	24
5 years	59	59	0	0	0	0	0	0	0	0	20	24
Overall	(63)		(9)		(9)		(20)		(18)		(119)	
1 year	75	75	44	45	22	23	25	26	17	18	51	52
3 years	57	57	22	23	0	0	10	11	0	0	34	36
5 years	48	48	11	11	0	0	5	6	0	0	27	30

ACUTE LYMPHATIC LEUKAEMIA   (ICD-9 204.0)

SLOVAKIA

AREA	NUMBER OF CASES			PERIOD	MEAN AGE		
	Males	Females	All		Males	Females	All
Slovakia	60	59	119	1985-1989	49.7	46.8	48.3

OBSERVED AND RELATIVE SURVIVAL (%) BY AGE (number of cases in parentheses)

	AGE CLASS										ALL	
	15-44		45-54		55-64		65-74		75-99			
	obs	rel	obs	rel	obs	rel	obs	rel	obs	rel	obs	rel
Males	(23)		(7)		(11)		(12)		(7)		(60)	
1 year	70	70	71	72	27	28	25	26	0	0	45	46
3 years	35	35	57	59	9	10	8	10	0	0	23	26
5 years	28	28	57	61	-	-	-	-	0	0	20	24
Females	(26)		(5)		(13)		(9)		(6)		(59)	
1 year	73	73	20	20	31	31	11	11	17	18	44	45
3 years	42	42	0	0	15	16	11	12	17	22	25	27
5 years	42	42	0	0	15	16	0	0	-	-	23	25
Overall	(49)		(12)		(24)		(21)		(13)		(119)	
1 year	71	72	50	50	29	30	19	20	8	9	45	46
3 years	39	39	33	34	13	13	10	11	8	11	24	26
5 years	36	36	33	35	13	14	-	-	-	-	22	25

SLOVENIA

AREA	NUMBER OF CASES			PERIOD	MEAN AGE		
	Males	Females	All		Males	Females	All
Slovenia	26	30	56	1985-1989	43.0	45.1	44.2

OBSERVED AND RELATIVE SURVIVAL (%) BY AGE (number of cases in parentheses)

	AGE CLASS										ALL	
	15-44		45-54		55-64		65-74		75-99			
	obs	rel	obs	rel	obs	rel	obs	rel	obs	rel	obs	rel
Males	(14)		(5)		(2)		(3)		(2)		(26)	
1 year	57	57	20	20	100	100	67	70	0	0	50	51
3 years	36	36	20	21	50	54	33	39	0	0	31	32
5 years	29	29	20	21	0	0	0	0	0	0	19	21
Females	(19)		(0)		(6)		(3)		(2)		(30)	
1 year	47	47	-	-	17	17	0	0	0	0	33	34
3 years	37	37	-	-	0	0	0	0	0	0	23	24
5 years	26	26	-	-	0	0	0	0	0	0	17	18
Overall	(33)		(5)		(8)		(6)		(4)		(56)	
1 year	52	52	20	20	38	38	33	35	0	0	41	42
3 years	36	37	20	21	13	13	17	19	0	0	27	28
5 years	27	27	20	21	0	0	0	0	0	0	18	19

ACUTE LYMPHATIC LEUKAEMIA (ICD-9 204.0)

SPAIN

AREA	NUMBER OF CASES			PERIOD	MEAN AGE			5-YR RELATIVE SURVIVAL (%)	
	Males	Females	All		Males	Females	All	Males	Females
Basque Country	23	15	38	1986-1988	45.8	45.4	45.7		
Mallorca	3	1	4	1988-1989	53.0	30.0	47.5		
Navarra	4	4	8	1985-1989	37.8	51.3	44.6		
Tarragona	11	6	17	1985-1989	48.5	50.7	49.4		
Spanish Registries	41	26	67		46.4	47.1	46.7		

OBSERVED AND RELATIVE SURVIVAL (%) BY AGE (number of cases in parentheses)

	AGE CLASS										ALL	
	15-44		45-54		55-64		65-74		75-99			
	obs	rel	obs	rel	obs	rel	obs	rel	obs	rel	obs	rel
Males	(22)		(1)		(4)		(8)		(6)		(41)	
1 year	64	64	100	100	50	51	25	26	0	0	46	48
3 years	41	41	0	0	25	26	13	14	0	0	27	29
5 years	36	36	0	0	25	27	13	15	0	0	24	28
Females	(12)		(1)		(8)		(2)		(3)		(26)	
1 year	83	83	0	0	50	50	0	0	33	35	58	58
3 years	33	33	0	0	38	38	0	0	33	39	31	32
5 years	33	33	0	0	38	38	0	0	33	46	31	32
Overall	(34)		(2)		(12)		(10)		(9)		(67)	
1 year	71	71	50	50	50	50	20	21	11	12	51	52
3 years	38	38	0	0	33	34	10	11	11	15	28	30
5 years	35	35	0	0	33	35	10	12	11	19	27	30

SWEDEN

AREA	NUMBER OF CASES			PERIOD	MEAN AGE		
	Males	Females	All		Males	Females	All
South Sweden	30	18	48	1985-1989	42.1	54.3	46.7

OBSERVED AND RELATIVE SURVIVAL (%) BY AGE (number of cases in parentheses)

	AGE CLASS										ALL	
	15-44		45-54		55-64		65-74		75-99			
	obs	rel	obs	rel	obs	rel	obs	rel	obs	rel	obs	rel
Males	(17)		(4)		(3)		(2)		(4)		(30)	
1 year	82	82	50	50	33	34	50	52	0	0	60	61
3 years	65	65	50	51	33	35	0	0	0	0	47	49
5 years	65	65	25	26	0	0	0	0	0	0	40	44
Females	(7)		(2)		(2)		(3)		(4)		(18)	
1 year	86	86	100	100	50	50	100	100	0	0	67	68
3 years	43	43	50	51	50	51	33	35	0	0	33	36
5 years	43	43	50	51	50	52	0	0	0	0	28	31
Overall	(24)		(6)		(5)		(5)		(8)		(48)	
1 year	83	83	67	67	40	40	80	82	0	0	63	64
3 years	58	59	50	51	40	42	20	22	0	0	42	44
5 years	58	59	33	34	20	21	0	0	0	0	35	39

ACUTE LYMPHATIC LEUKAEMIA (ICD-9 204.0)

SWITZERLAND

AREA	NUMBER OF CASES			PERIOD	MEAN AGE			5-YR RELATIVE SURVIVAL (%)	
	Males	Females	All		Males	Females	All	Males	Females
Basel	7	4	11	1985-1988	38.4	47.3	41.7		
Geneva	7	7	14	1985-1989	52.7	57.7	55.3		
Swiss Registries	14	11	25		45.7	54.1	49.4		

OBSERVED AND RELATIVE SURVIVAL (%) BY AGE (number of cases in parentheses)

	AGE CLASS										ALL	
	15-44		45-54		55-64		65-74		75-99			
	obs	rel	obs	rel	obs	rel	obs	rel	obs	rel	obs	rel
Males	(7)		(2)		(2)		(1)		(2)		(14)	
1 year	57	57	100	100	0	0	100	100	0	0	50	51
3 years	14	14	50	51	0	0	-	-	0	0	19	20
5 years	0	0	50	51	0	0	-	-	0	0	10	11
Females	(5)		(1)		(1)		(1)		(3)		(11)	
1 year	60	60	100	100	100	100	100	100	0	0	55	57
3 years	40	40	100	100	0	0	0	0	0	0	27	31
5 years	40	40	0	0	0	0	0	0	0	0	18	22
Overall	(12)		(3)		(3)		(2)		(5)		(25)	
1 year	58	58	100	100	33	34	100	100	0	0	52	53
3 years	25	25	67	67	0	0	-	-	0	0	23	25
5 years	17	17	33	34	0	0	-	-	0	0	14	16

ACUTE LYMPHATIC LEUKAEMIA (ICD-9 204.0)

EUROPE, 1985-89
Weighted analyses

COUNTRY	% COVERAGE WITH C.R.s	YEARLY NO. OF CASES (Mean No. of cases recorded)			RELATIVE SURVIVAL (%) (Age-standardized)
		Males	Females	All	Males / Females
AUSTRIA	8	3	2	5	
DENMARK	100	16	13	29	
ENGLAND	50	76	49	125	
ESTONIA	100	3	2	5	
FINLAND	100	19	15	34	
FRANCE	4	7	5	12	
GERMANY	2	3	4	7	
ICELAND	100	1	1	2	
ITALY	10	22	19	41	
NETHERLANDS	6	3	2	5	
POLAND	6	6	4	10	
SCOTLAND	100	14	10	24	
SLOVAKIA	100	12	12	24	
SLOVENIA	100	5	6	11	
SPAIN	10	12	8	20	
SWEDEN	17	6	4	10	
SWITZERLAND	11	3	2	5	

□ 1 year ■ 5 years

OBSERVED AND RELATIVE SURVIVAL (%) BY AGE

	AGE CLASS										ALL	
	15-44		45-54		55-64		65-74		75-99			
	obs	rel	obs	rel	obs	rel	obs	rel	obs	rel	obs	rel
Males												
1 year	67	67	40	40	48	49	40	41	17	19	53	54
3 years	38	38	18	19	29	30	9	10	11	14	30	32
5 years	34	35	13	14	22	25	2	3	5	8	25	28
Females												
1 year	67	67	60	60	38	39	39	40	25	26	49	50
3 years	49	49	50	50	18	18	22	24	14	18	32	34
5 years	40	41	29	29	17	18	13	14	11	18	27	30
Overall												
1 year	67	67	49	49	44	44	40	40	21	22	51	52
3 years	43	43	32	33	24	25	15	16	12	16	31	33
5 years	37	37	20	21	20	22	7	8	8	13	26	29

AGE STANDARDIZED RELATIVE SURVIVAL(%)

COUNTRY	MALES		FEMALES	
	1-year (95% C.I.)	5-years (95% C.I.)	1-year (95% C.I.)	5-years (95% C.I.)
AUSTRIA	-	-	-	-
DENMARK	55.9 (47.9 - 65.2)	25.2 (17.0 - 37.3)	47.7 (37.9 - 59.9)	13.2 (6.5 - 26.8)
ENGLAND	49.2 (44.9 - 53.9)	21.6 (17.9 - 26.0)	54.1 (48.5 - 60.3)	28.4 (23.2 - 34.7)
ESTONIA	56.1 (40.8 - 77.2)	14.2 (4.4 - 45.8)	-	-
FINLAND	43.4 (35.9 - 52.3)	14.1 (9.1 - 21.8)	49.7 (40.7 - 60.7)	24.5 (16.6 - 36.2)
FRANCE	-	-	79.2 (63.5 - 98.8)	36.8 (18.8 - 71.8)
GERMANY	60.8 (48.3 - 76.4)	27.2 (14.8 - 50.2)	49.3 (32.9 - 74.0)	-
ICELAND	-	-	-	-
ITALY	45.6 (37.0 - 56.2)	20.8 (13.6 - 31.9)	49.0 (38.8 - 62.1)	21.2 (12.9 - 34.7)
NETHERLANDS	-	-	24.3 (9.1 - 64.9)	24.4 (9.1 - 65.0)
POLAND	15.4 (6.2 - 38.3)	10.3 (2.6 - 40.0)	-	-
SCOTLAND	52.8 (42.6 - 65.4)	25.4 (18.0 - 36.0)	49.0 (39.3 - 61.2)	28.7 (19.3 - 42.8)
SLOVAKIA	47.7 (37.9 - 60.0)	-	45.9 (36.1 - 58.3)	-
SLOVENIA	53.7 (40.3 - 71.5)	15.8 (7.4 - 33.9)	-	-
SPAIN	50.1 (38.8 - 64.7)	23.8 (14.0 - 40.2)	52.5 (40.3 - 68.5)	28.2 (15.2 - 52.5)
SWEDEN	56.6 (42.5 - 75.3)	33.8 (23.9 - 47.8)	71.8 (57.6 - 89.5)	32.3 (16.7 - 62.5)
SWITZERLAND	51.0 (35.9 - 72.4)	-	66.1 (48.1 - 90.7)	19.6 (6.7 - 57.2)
EUROPE, 1985-89	51.3 (46.3 - 56.9)	23.0 (17.9 - 29.6)	52.7 (46.2 - 60.0)	29.4 (22.3 - 38.9)

CHRONIC LYMPHATIC LEUKAEMIA   (ICD-9 204.1)

AUSTRIA

AREA	NUMBER OF CASES			PERIOD	MEAN AGE		
	Males	Females	All		Males	Females	All
Tirol	28	17	45	1988-1989	69.9	69.6	69.8

OBSERVED AND RELATIVE SURVIVAL (%) BY AGE (number of cases in parentheses)

	AGE CLASS										ALL	
	15-44		45-54		55-64		65-74		75-99			
	obs	rel	obs	rel	obs	rel	obs	rel	obs	rel	obs	rel
Males	(1)		(1)		(7)		(7)		(12)		(28)	
1 year	100	100	100	100	86	87	86	88	83	92	86	90
3 years	100	100	0	0	86	89	71	78	25	34	54	63
5 years	100	100	0	0	71	76	57	67	25	44	46	61
Females	(1)		(2)		(4)		(2)		(8)		(17)	
1 year	100	100	100	100	100	100	100	100	75	82	88	92
3 years	100	100	100	100	100	100	100	100	50	66	76	87
5 years	100	100	100	100	100	100	50	54	50	82	71	88
Overall	(2)		(3)		(11)		(9)		(20)		(45)	
1 year	100	100	100	100	91	92	89	91	80	88	87	91
3 years	100	100	67	67	91	93	78	84	35	47	62	72
5 years	100	100	67	68	82	86	56	64	35	59	56	71

DENMARK

AREA	NUMBER OF CASES			PERIOD	MEAN AGE		
	Males	Females	All		Males	Females	All
Denmark	800	471	1271	1985-1989	70.1	73.4	71.3

OBSERVED AND RELATIVE SURVIVAL (%) BY AGE (number of cases in parentheses)

	AGE CLASS										ALL	
	15-44		45-54		55-64		65-74		75-99			
	obs	rel	obs	rel	obs	rel	obs	rel	obs	rel	obs	rel
Males	(23)		(53)		(143)		(281)		(300)		(800)	
1 year	96	96	91	91	83	85	79	82	55	62	72	77
3 years	91	92	75	77	62	65	54	62	32	47	50	60
5 years	83	84	60	63	46	51	33	42	19	38	34	47
Females	(8)		(15)		(68)		(141)		(239)		(471)	
1 year	100	100	100	100	84	85	82	84	72	78	78	82
3 years	100	100	93	95	74	76	67	72	38	51	55	64
5 years	88	88	80	82	59	63	52	61	18	29	37	50
Overall	(31)		(68)		(211)		(422)		(539)		(1271)	
1 year	97	97	93	93	83	85	80	83	63	69	74	79
3 years	94	94	79	81	65	69	58	65	35	49	51	62
5 years	84	85	65	67	50	55	40	49	19	34	35	48

CHRONIC LYMPHATIC LEUKAEMIA   (ICD-9 204.1)

ENGLAND

AREA	NUMBER OF CASES			PERIOD	MEAN AGE			5-YR RELATIVE SURVIVAL (%)	
	Males	Females	All		Males	Females	All	Males	Females
East Anglia	195	105	300	1985-1989	70.0	74.5	71.6		
Mersey	141	98	239	1985-1989	72.5	73.7	73.0		
Oxford	140	109	249	1985-1989	72.0	77.2	74.3		
South Thames	407	326	733	1985-1989	69.0	73.5	71.0		
Wessex	266	246	512	1985-1989	71.5	75.7	73.5		
West Midlands	434	265	699	1985-1989	69.6	72.9	70.9		
Yorkshire	364	274	638	1985-1989	69.0	73.4	70.9		
English Registries	1947	1423	3370		70.1	74.1	71.8		

OBSERVED AND RELATIVE SURVIVAL (%) BY AGE (number of cases in parentheses)

	AGE CLASS										ALL	
	15-44		45-54		55-64		65-74		75-99			
	obs	rel	obs	rel	obs	rel	obs	rel	obs	rel	obs	rel
Males	(31)		(125)		(403)		(658)		(730)		(1947)	
1 year	100	100	93	93	87	89	77	81	57	64	73	78
3 years	90	91	79	81	74	79	58	66	37	53	55	67
5 years	84	85	63	65	60	66	40	51	19	37	39	53
Females	(12)		(72)		(183)		(406)		(750)		(1423)	
1 year	92	92	97	98	92	93	81	83	59	65	72	76
3 years	92	92	88	89	84	86	65	70	36	49	53	64
5 years	92	92	79	81	70	74	52	59	24	41	41	56
Overall	(43)		(197)		(586)		(1064)		(1480)		(3370)	
1 year	98	98	94	95	89	90	79	81	58	64	73	77
3 years	91	91	82	84	77	81	61	68	36	51	55	65
5 years	86	87	69	71	63	69	45	54	22	39	40	54

ESTONIA

AREA	NUMBER OF CASES			PERIOD	MEAN AGE		
	Males	Females	All		Males	Females	All
Estonia	172	129	301	1985-1989	64.6	64.8	64.7

OBSERVED AND RELATIVE SURVIVAL (%) BY AGE (number of cases in parentheses)

	AGE CLASS										ALL	
	15-44		45-54		55-64		65-74		75-99			
	obs	rel	obs	rel	obs	rel	obs	rel	obs	rel	obs	rel
Males	(7)		(18)		(58)		(53)		(36)		(172)	
1 year	71	72	100	100	91	94	79	83	61	69	81	86
3 years	71	73	89	93	81	88	53	62	47	69	66	77
5 years	57	59	65	71	62	73	40	54	28	55	48	64
Females	(4)		(21)		(35)		(46)		(23)		(129)	
1 year	100	100	90	91	89	89	93	96	61	66	86	89
3 years	75	75	86	87	83	86	78	87	43	57	74	82
5 years	75	76	76	78	71	76	54	66	39	63	60	71
Overall	(11)		(39)		(93)		(99)		(59)		(301)	
1 year	82	82	95	96	90	92	86	90	61	68	83	87
3 years	73	74	87	90	82	87	65	74	46	64	69	79
5 years	64	65	71	75	66	74	46	60	32	59	53	67

CHRONIC LYMPHATIC LEUKAEMIA   (ICD-9 204.1)

FINLAND

AREA	NUMBER OF CASES			PERIOD	MEAN AGE		
	Males	Females	All		Males	Females	All
Finland	362	259	621	1985-1989	67.7	71.6	69.3

OBSERVED AND RELATIVE SURVIVAL (%) BY AGE (number of cases in parentheses)

	AGE CLASS										ALL	
	15-44		45-54		55-64		65-74		75-99			
	obs	rel	obs	rel	obs	rel	obs	rel	obs	rel	obs	rel
Males	(14)		(37)		(79)		(120)		(112)		(362)	
1 year	93	93	95	95	92	94	77	80	69	78	80	85
3 years	86	87	81	83	78	83	53	61	40	59	59	70
5 years	71	72	65	68	59	66	38	49	21	42	42	56
Females	(4)		(15)		(39)		(80)		(121)		(259)	
1 year	100	100	93	94	87	88	86	88	75	82	82	86
3 years	100	100	93	94	85	87	70	75	53	69	66	76
5 years	75	76	60	61	67	69	58	65	32	51	47	61
Overall	(18)		(52)		(118)		(200)		(233)		(621)	
1 year	94	95	94	95	91	92	81	83	72	80	81	85
3 years	89	90	85	86	81	85	60	67	47	64	62	72
5 years	72	73	63	66	62	67	46	56	27	47	44	58

FRANCE

AREA	NUMBER OF CASES			PERIOD	MEAN AGE			5-YR RELATIVE SURVIVAL (%)	
	Males	Females	All		Males	Females	All	Males	Females
Somme	75	62	137	1985-1989	67.8	69.7	68.7		
Calvados	43	20	63	1985-1989	64.9	65.7	65.2		
Côte d'Or	73	54	127	1985-1989	70.7	70.5	70.7		
Doubs	37	28	65	1985-1989	64.2	71.4	67.3		
French Registries	228	164	392		67.6	69.8	68.5		

OBSERVED AND RELATIVE SURVIVAL (%) BY AGE (number of cases in parentheses)

	AGE CLASS										ALL	
	15-44		45-54		55-64		65-74		75-99			
	obs	rel	obs	rel	obs	rel	obs	rel	obs	rel	obs	rel
Males	(6)		(17)		(66)		(73)		(66)		(228)	
1 year	83	84	94	95	91	93	93	96	72	80	86	90
3 years	83	84	87	90	83	88	74	83	52	72	72	83
5 years	83	85	87	92	71	79	64	79	39	70	62	79
Females	(4)		(13)		(33)		(50)		(64)		(164)	
1 year	100	100	100	100	100	100	96	97	90	97	95	98
3 years	100	100	92	93	97	99	87	91	66	83	82	91
5 years	100	100	84	85	89	92	76	84	49	76	70	84
Overall	(10)		(30)		(99)		(123)		(130)		(392)	
1 year	90	90	97	97	94	95	94	97	81	89	90	94
3 years	90	91	89	91	88	92	79	87	59	78	76	86
5 years	90	91	86	89	77	83	69	81	44	73	65	81

CHRONIC LYMPHATIC LEUKAEMIA   (ICD-9 204.1)

GERMANY

AREA	NUMBER OF CASES			PERIOD	MEAN AGE		
	Males	Females	All		Males	Females	All
Saarland	84	67	151	1985-1989	65.4	68.7	66.9

OBSERVED AND RELATIVE SURVIVAL (%) BY AGE (number of cases in parentheses)

	AGE CLASS										ALL	
	15-44		45-54		55-64		65-74		75-99			
	obs	rel	obs	rel	obs	rel	obs	rel	obs	rel	obs	rel
Males	(4)		(11)		(21)		(29)		(19)		(84)	
1 year	100	100	91	91	86	87	83	87	58	65	80	83
3 years	100	100	64	65	76	81	62	72	42	61	63	73
5 years	100	100	64	66	62	69	55	72	42	84	57	74
Females	(1)		(7)		(13)		(22)		(24)		(67)	
1 year	100	100	100	100	100	100	95	98	58	63	84	87
3 years	100	100	86	86	100	100	73	78	38	48	67	75
5 years	100	100	86	87	89	94	52	59	33	53	56	69
Overall	(5)		(18)		(34)		(51)		(43)		(151)	
1 year	100	100	94	95	91	92	88	91	58	64	81	85
3 years	100	100	72	73	85	89	67	75	40	53	65	74
5 years	100	100	72	74	74	80	53	66	37	65	57	72

ICELAND

AREA	NUMBER OF CASES			PERIOD	MEAN AGE		
	Males	Females	All		Males	Females	All
Iceland	11	11	22	1985-1989	72.7	76.6	74.7

OBSERVED AND RELATIVE SURVIVAL (%) BY AGE (number of cases in parentheses)

	AGE CLASS										ALL	
	15-44		45-54		55-64		65-74		75-99			
	obs	rel	obs	rel	obs	rel	obs	rel	obs	rel	obs	rel
Males	(0)		(0)		(1)		(6)		(4)		(11)	
1 year	-	-	-	-	100	100	100	100	50	57	82	87
3 years	-	-	-	-	100	100	100	100	50	74	82	98
5 years	-	-	-	-	100	100	67	79	0	0	45	62
Females	(1)		(1)		(0)		(2)		(7)		(11)	
1 year	100	100	100	100	-	-	50	51	43	51	55	61
3 years	100	100	100	100	-	-	50	54	43	71	55	74
5 years	0	0	100	100	-	-	0	0	14	33	18	29
Overall	(1)		(1)		(1)		(8)		(11)		(22)	
1 year	100	100	100	100	100	100	88	90	45	53	68	74
3 years	100	100	100	100	100	100	88	95	45	72	68	87
5 years	0	0	100	100	100	100	50	59	9	20	32	47

CHRONIC LYMPHATIC LEUKAEMIA (ICD-9 204.1)

ITALY

AREA	NUMBER OF CASES			PERIOD	MEAN AGE			5-YR RELATIVE SURVIVAL (%)	
	Males	Females	All		Males	Females	All	Males	Females
Florence	106	83	189	1985-1989	70.2	72.6	71.3		
Genoa	40	41	81	1986-1988	68.8	72.1	70.5		
Latina	20	12	32	1985-1987	63.9	66.7	65.0		
Modena	32	24	56	1988-1989	69.7	67.1	68.6		
Parma	23	13	36	1985-1987	72.4	77.5	74.3		
Ragusa	11	7	18	1985-1989	75.7	75.9	75.8		
Romagna	42	24	66	1986-1988	67.5	72.7	69.4		
Turin	20	19	39	1985-1987	66.1	75.9	70.9		
Varese	61	58	119	1985-1989	65.3	73.5	69.3		
Italian Registries	355	281	636		68.6	72.6	70.3		

OBSERVED AND RELATIVE SURVIVAL (%) BY AGE (number of cases in parentheses)

	AGE CLASS										ALL	
	15-44		45-54		55-64		65-74		75-99			
	obs	rel	obs	rel	obs	rel	obs	rel	obs	rel	obs	rel
Males	(9)		(30)		(80)		(121)		(115)		(355)	
1 year	100	100	90	90	84	85	79	82	60	67	76	79
3 years	100	100	80	81	65	68	54	60	35	48	53	62
5 years	100	100	73	76	57	62	37	46	20	36	41	53
Females	(4)		(12)		(51)		(73)		(141)		(281)	
1 year	75	75	100	100	98	99	85	86	67	73	79	83
3 years	50	50	100	100	86	88	74	79	43	55	62	70
5 years	50	50	92	93	78	81	60	67	30	47	50	63
Overall	(13)		(42)		(131)		(194)		(256)		(636)	
1 year	92	92	93	93	89	90	81	84	64	70	77	81
3 years	85	85	86	87	73	76	61	67	39	52	57	66
5 years	85	85	79	81	65	69	46	54	26	42	45	57

NETHERLANDS

AREA	NUMBER OF CASES			PERIOD	MEAN AGE		
	Males	Females	All		Males	Females	All
Eindhoven	59	33	92	1985-1989	65.4	66.5	65.8

OBSERVED AND RELATIVE SURVIVAL (%) BY AGE (number of cases in parentheses)

	AGE CLASS										ALL	
	15-44		45-54		55-64		65-74		75-99			
	obs	rel	obs	rel	obs	rel	obs	rel	obs	rel	obs	rel
Males	(2)		(9)		(15)		(20)		(13)		(59)	
1 year	100	100	100	100	93	95	75	78	69	78	83	87
3 years	100	100	100	100	73	77	60	68	35	51	66	75
5 years	100	100	89	92	40	44	60	75	35	67	55	69
Females	(1)		(4)		(10)		(9)		(9)		(33)	
1 year	100	100	100	100	100	100	100	100	78	84	94	97
3 years	100	100	100	100	80	81	89	95	67	85	82	89
5 years	100	100	100	100	47	48	89	100	56	87	69	81
Overall	(3)		(13)		(25)		(29)		(22)		(92)	
1 year	100	100	100	100	96	97	83	85	73	80	87	90
3 years	100	100	100	100	76	79	69	77	48	67	72	80
5 years	100	100	92	95	42	45	69	83	44	77	60	73

CHRONIC LYMPHATIC LEUKAEMIA (ICD-9 204.1)

POLAND

AREA	NUMBER OF CASES			PERIOD	MEAN AGE			5-YR RELATIVE SURVIVAL (%)	
	Males	Females	All		Males	Females	All	Males	Females
Cracow	29	18	47	1985-1989	68.6	69.3	68.9		
Warsaw	27	12	39	1988-1989	66.8	70.3	67.9		
Polish Registries	56	30	86		67.8	69.7	68.5		

OBSERVED AND RELATIVE SURVIVAL (%) BY AGE (number of cases in parentheses)

	AGE CLASS										ALL	
	15-44		45-54		55-64		65-74		75-99			
	obs	rel	obs	rel	obs	rel	obs	rel	obs	rel	obs	rel
Males	(1)		(8)		(11)		(18)		(18)		(56)	
1 year	100	100	100	100	64	65	56	58	22	26	54	57
3 years	100	100	63	65	55	59	33	39	22	35	39	48
5 years	100	100	38	40	36	42	28	37	11	24	27	38
Females	(0)		(3)		(8)		(6)		(13)		(30)	
1 year	-	-	67	67	63	63	67	69	31	33	50	52
3 years	-	-	67	68	38	39	67	76	23	29	40	46
5 years	-	-	33	34	25	27	33	42	8	12	20	25
Overall	(1)		(11)		(19)		(24)		(31)		(86)	
1 year	100	100	91	92	63	64	58	61	26	29	52	56
3 years	100	100	64	66	47	50	42	49	23	32	40	47
5 years	100	100	36	38	32	35	29	38	10	18	24	33

SCOTLAND

AREA	NUMBER OF CASES			PERIOD	MEAN AGE		
	Males	Females	All		Males	Females	All
Scotland	432	291	723	1985-1989	68.5	74.1	70.8

OBSERVED AND RELATIVE SURVIVAL (%) BY AGE (number of cases in parentheses)

	AGE CLASS										ALL	
	15-44		45-54		55-64		65-74		75-99			
	obs	rel	obs	rel	obs	rel	obs	rel	obs	rel	obs	rel
Males	(10)		(35)		(105)		(142)		(140)		(432)	
1 year	90	90	91	92	87	88	77	81	56	64	74	79
3 years	80	81	83	85	74	79	61	71	31	46	56	68
5 years	60	61	74	78	55	62	37	50	19	37	39	54
Females	(1)		(13)		(39)		(90)		(148)		(291)	
1 year	100	100	92	93	87	88	89	92	60	67	74	79
3 years	100	100	92	94	69	72	68	75	37	52	54	66
5 years	100	100	85	87	46	49	50	60	22	41	37	52
Overall	(11)		(48)		(144)		(232)		(288)		(723)	
1 year	91	91	92	92	87	88	81	85	58	66	74	79
3 years	82	82	85	87	73	77	63	73	34	49	55	67
5 years	64	64	77	80	53	59	42	54	20	39	38	53

CHRONIC LYMPHATIC LEUKAEMIA (ICD-9 204.1)

SLOVAKIA

AREA	NUMBER OF CASES			PERIOD	MEAN AGE		
	Males	Females	All		Males	Females	All
Slovakia	489	322	811	1985-1989	66.6	68.6	67.4

OBSERVED AND RELATIVE SURVIVAL (%) BY AGE (number of cases in parentheses)

	AGE CLASS										ALL	
	15-44		45-54		55-64		65-74		75-99			
	obs	rel	obs	rel	obs	rel	obs	rel	obs	rel	obs	rel
Males	(16)		(47)		(124)		(173)		(129)		(489)	
1 year	81	82	87	88	81	84	72	76	50	57	71	75
3 years	75	76	79	82	56	62	51	61	33	49	51	62
5 years	75	77	69	74	45	53	39	53	25	49	41	56
Females	(4)		(33)		(77)		(90)		(118)		(322)	
1 year	75	75	97	97	88	89	79	81	65	71	78	81
3 years	75	75	91	92	65	67	58	64	47	62	59	68
5 years	45	45	68	70	49	53	41	49	32	54	43	54
Overall	(20)		(80)		(201)		(263)		(247)		(811)	
1 year	80	80	91	92	84	86	74	78	57	64	73	77
3 years	75	76	84	86	60	64	54	62	40	56	54	64
5 years	69	70	69	73	47	53	40	52	28	51	41	55

SLOVENIA

AREA	NUMBER OF CASES			PERIOD	MEAN AGE		
	Males	Females	All		Males	Females	All
Slovenia	161	160	321	1985-1989	66.3	70.3	68.3

OBSERVED AND RELATIVE SURVIVAL (%) BY AGE (number of cases in parentheses)

	AGE CLASS										ALL	
	15-44		45-54		55-64		65-74		75-99			
	obs	rel	obs	rel	obs	rel	obs	rel	obs	rel	obs	rel
Males	(6)		(25)		(40)		(40)		(50)		(161)	
1 year	100	100	88	89	77	79	72	76	54	62	71	76
3 years	83	84	80	83	51	55	57	66	26	40	50	60
5 years	83	85	48	51	44	49	41	55	8	17	34	46
Females	(4)		(10)		(33)		(48)		(65)		(160)	
1 year	100	100	90	90	94	95	79	81	57	62	74	78
3 years	75	75	90	91	78	80	60	66	35	48	56	65
5 years	75	76	70	72	68	72	52	62	26	45	46	60
Overall	(10)		(35)		(73)		(88)		(115)		(321)	
1 year	100	100	89	89	84	86	76	79	56	62	73	77
3 years	80	81	83	85	63	66	59	66	31	44	53	63
5 years	80	81	54	57	54	60	47	59	18	34	40	53

CHRONIC LYMPHATIC LEUKAEMIA (ICD-9 204.1)

SPAIN

AREA	NUMBER OF CASES			PERIOD	MEAN AGE			5-YR RELATIVE SURVIVAL (%)	
	Males	Females	All		Males	Females	All	Males	Females
Basque Country	69	50	119	1986-1988	68.7	73.8	70.8		
Mallorca	17	8	25	1988-1989	68.8	73.4	70.3		
Navarra	42	30	72	1985-1989	69.1	67.5	68.4		
Tarragona	53	23	76	1985-1989	68.2	69.4	68.6		
Spanish Registries	181	111	292		68.7	71.2	69.6		

OBSERVED AND RELATIVE SURVIVAL (%) BY AGE (number of cases in parentheses)

	AGE CLASS										ALL	
	15-44		45-54		55-64		65-74		75-99			
	obs	rel	obs	rel	obs	rel	obs	rel	obs	rel	obs	rel
Males	(5)		(14)		(48)		(51)		(63)		(181)	
1 year	100	100	86	86	94	95	84	87	79	89	86	90
3 years	100	100	71	73	79	82	71	78	57	82	69	81
5 years	80	81	51	53	72	77	56	68	33	61	53	69
Females	(1)		(5)		(23)		(34)		(48)		(111)	
1 year	100	100	80	80	100	100	94	96	83	89	90	93
3 years	100	100	80	81	91	93	76	80	63	78	74	82
5 years	100	100	80	81	82	85	61	67	44	66	60	72
Overall	(6)		(19)		(71)		(85)		(111)		(292)	
1 year	100	100	84	85	96	97	88	90	81	89	87	91
3 years	100	100	74	75	83	86	73	79	59	80	71	81
5 years	83	84	60	62	75	80	58	67	38	63	55	70

SWEDEN

AREA	NUMBER OF CASES			PERIOD	MEAN AGE		
	Males	Females	All		Males	Females	All
South Sweden	216	115	331	1985-1989	69.8	74.3	71.3

OBSERVED AND RELATIVE SURVIVAL (%) BY AGE (number of cases in parentheses)

	AGE CLASS										ALL	
	15-44		45-54		55-64		65-74		75-99			
	obs	rel	obs	rel	obs	rel	obs	rel	obs	rel	obs	rel
Males	(4)		(17)		(42)		(69)		(84)		(216)	
1 year	100	100	100	100	86	87	77	79	71	79	79	83
3 years	100	100	88	90	76	79	59	66	40	56	58	69
5 years	100	100	65	67	48	51	48	58	20	36	39	52
Females	(0)		(6)		(10)		(40)		(59)		(115)	
1 year	-	-	100	100	90	91	93	94	75	81	83	88
3 years	-	-	83	84	90	92	80	85	66	87	74	87
5 years	-	-	83	85	70	73	63	70	41	67	53	70
Overall	(4)		(23)		(52)		(109)		(143)		(331)	
1 year	100	100	100	100	87	88	83	85	73	80	80	85
3 years	100	100	87	88	79	82	67	73	51	69	64	75
5 years	100	100	70	71	52	56	53	63	29	49	44	58

CHRONIC LYMPHATIC LEUKAEMIA   (ICD-9 204.1)

SWITZERLAND

AREA	NUMBER OF CASES			PERIOD	MEAN AGE			5-YR RELATIVE SURVIVAL (%)	
	Males	Females	All		Males	Females	All	Males	Females
Basel	47	23	70	1985-1988	68.2	67.9	68.1		
Geneva	39	23	62	1985-1989	71.7	72.7	72.1		
Swiss Registries	86	46	132		69.8	70.3	70.0		

OBSERVED AND RELATIVE SURVIVAL (%) BY AGE (number of cases in parentheses)

	AGE CLASS										ALL	
	15-44		45-54		55-64		65-74		75-99			
	obs	rel	obs	rel	obs	rel	obs	rel	obs	rel	obs	rel
Males	(3)		(8)		(12)		(31)		(32)		(86)	
1 year	100	100	88	88	92	93	87	90	84	93	87	92
3 years	100	100	88	89	67	70	71	80	53	74	66	78
5 years	33	34	88	91	67	72	61	77	31	56	52	70
Females	(3)		(1)		(12)		(12)		(18)		(46)	
1 year	100	100	100	100	92	92	92	93	72	79	85	88
3 years	100	100	100	100	73	75	92	97	56	75	74	84
5 years	100	100	100	100	64	67	75	83	39	67	60	75
Overall	(6)		(9)		(24)		(43)		(50)		(132)	
1 year	100	100	89	89	92	93	88	91	80	88	86	91
3 years	100	100	89	91	70	72	77	85	54	74	69	80
5 years	67	67	89	92	65	69	65	79	34	60	55	72

CHRONIC LYMPHATIC LEUKAEMIA   (ICD-9 204.1)

EUROPE, 1985-89

Weighted analyses

COUNTRY	% COVERAGE WITH C.R.s	YEARLY NO. OF CASES (Mean No. of cases recorded)		
		Males	Females	All
AUSTRIA	8	14	9	23
DENMARK	100	160	94	254
ENGLAND	50	389	285	674
ESTONIA	100	34	26	60
FINLAND	100	72	52	124
FRANCE	4	46	33	79
GERMANY	2	17	13	30
ICELAND	100	2	2	4
ITALY	10	100	78	178
NETHERLANDS	6	12	7	19
POLAND	6	19	10	29
SCOTLAND	100	86	58	144
SLOVAKIA	100	98	64	162
SLOVENIA	100	32	32	64
SPAIN	10	51	31	82
SWEDEN	17	43	23	66
SWITZERLAND	11	20	10	30

RELATIVE SURVIVAL (%) (Age-standardized)

□ 1 year ■ 5 years

OBSERVED AND RELATIVE SURVIVAL (%) BY AGE

	AGE CLASS										ALL	
	15-44		45-54		55-64		65-74		75-99			
	obs	rel	obs	rel	obs	rel	obs	rel	obs	rel	obs	rel
Males												
1 year	96	96	92	93	87	88	81	85	63	71	79	83
3 years	94	94	76	77	74	78	62	70	41	59	60	71
5 years	89	90	67	70	60	67	49	62	29	54	48	63
Females												
1 year	93	93	97	97	96	96	90	91	70	76	83	86
3 years	88	88	90	91	88	90	76	81	48	62	67	76
5 years	87	87	83	85	77	80	60	67	36	56	54	68
Overall												
1 year	95	95	94	94	90	91	85	87	66	73	80	84
3 years	92	92	82	83	80	83	68	74	44	60	63	73
5 years	88	89	74	76	67	72	54	64	32	55	51	65

AGE STANDARDIZED RELATIVE SURVIVAL(%)

COUNTRY	MALES		FEMALES	
	1-year (95% C.I.)	5-years (95% C.I.)	1-year (95% C.I.)	5-years (95% C.I.)
AUSTRIA	90.3 (77.8 -104.8)	55.4 (36.7 - 83.5)	93.0 (80.9 -106.8)	78.3 (51.6 -118.9)
DENMARK	75.8 (72.6 - 79.1)	44.6 (40.2 - 49.4)	83.2 (79.6 - 86.9)	50.8 (45.8 - 56.4)
ENGLAND	76.9 (74.9 - 79.0)	49.9 (47.1 - 52.9)	79.1 (76.9 - 81.2)	57.3 (54.3 - 60.6)
ESTONIA	80.7 (73.0 - 89.2)	59.3 (47.5 - 74.0)	82.8 (74.1 - 92.4)	68.1 (55.2 - 84.0)
FINLAND	83.2 (78.6 - 88.1)	51.3 (44.5 - 59.2)	86.1 (81.5 - 90.9)	60.6 (53.5 - 68.5)
FRANCE	88.8 (83.6 - 94.4)	76.4 (66.4 - 87.8)	98.1 (94.6 -101.8)	82.8 (73.5 - 93.2)
GERMANY	78.7 (68.2 - 90.8)	76.2 (58.8 - 98.7)	84.5 (76.2 - 93.8)	66.2 (52.9 - 82.9)
ICELAND	-	-	-	-
ITALY	77.7 (72.9 - 82.8)	48.4 (42.1 - 55.6)	84.2 (79.9 - 88.7)	63.3 (56.9 - 70.5)
NETHERLANDS	83.2 (71.2 - 97.3)	67.4 (47.9 - 94.9)	93.7 (82.9 -106.1)	84.6 (65.0 -110.1)
POLAND	50.7 (39.3 - 65.5)	34.6 (21.3 - 56.3)	-	-
SCOTLAND	76.7 (72.2 - 81.4)	49.6 (43.4 - 56.6)	81.5 (77.0 - 86.3)	53.0 (46.3 - 60.7)
SLOVAKIA	71.0 (66.5 - 75.9)	53.3 (46.5 - 61.2)	79.9 (75.1 - 84.9)	53.3 (46.0 - 61.6)
SLOVENIA	72.2 (64.4 - 81.0)	39.2 (30.5 - 50.4)	77.5 (71.1 - 84.6)	58.2 (49.1 - 68.9)
SPAIN	89.6 (84.0 - 95.6)	66.0 (55.3 - 78.7)	92.9 (87.4 - 98.8)	71.6 (60.9 - 84.1)
SWEDEN	82.7 (77.2 - 88.6)	49.7 (42.0 - 58.9)	-	-
SWITZERLAND	92.0 (84.8 - 99.9)	67.7 (54.6 - 83.9)	88.1 (78.0 - 99.4)	74.9 (58.6 - 95.7)
EUROPE, 1985-89	80.6 (78.1 - 83.2)	60.9 (56.6 - 65.4)	86.5 (84.3 - 88.7)	67.1 (63.2 - 71.2)

ACUTE MYELOID LEUKAEMIA (ICD-9 205.0)

AUSTRIA

AREA	NUMBER OF CASES			PERIOD	MEAN AGE		
	Males	Females	All		Males	Females	All
Tirol	14	15	29	1988-1989	46.1	55.9	51.2

OBSERVED AND RELATIVE SURVIVAL (%) BY AGE (number of cases in parentheses)

	AGE CLASS										ALL	
	15-44		45-54		55-64		65-74		75-99			
	obs	rel	obs	rel	obs	rel	obs	rel	obs	rel	obs	rel
Males	(5)		(3)		(3)		(3)		(0)		(14)	
1 year	60	60	33	33	0	0	33	34	-	-	36	36
3 years	60	60	33	34	0	0	0	0	-	-	29	29
5 years	60	60	33	34	0	0	0	0	-	-	29	30
Females	(3)		(3)		(6)		(2)		(1)		(15)	
1 year	67	67	33	33	67	67	0	0	0	0	47	47
3 years	33	33	33	34	50	51	0	0	0	0	33	34
5 years	33	34	0	0	33	34	0	0	0	0	20	21
Overall	(8)		(6)		(9)		(5)		(1)		(29)	
1 year	63	63	33	33	44	45	20	20	0	0	41	42
3 years	50	50	33	34	33	34	0	0	0	0	31	32
5 years	50	50	17	17	22	23	0	0	0	0	24	25

DENMARK

AREA	NUMBER OF CASES			PERIOD	MEAN AGE		
	Males	Females	All		Males	Females	All
Denmark	489	456	945	1985-1989	64.0	63.0	63.5

OBSERVED AND RELATIVE SURVIVAL (%) BY AGE (number of cases in parentheses)

	AGE CLASS										ALL	
	15-44		45-54		55-64		65-74		75-99			
	obs	rel	obs	rel	obs	rel	obs	rel	obs	rel	obs	rel
Males	(65)		(38)		(114)		(135)		(137)		(489)	
1 year	63	63	34	34	33	34	24	25	7	7	27	29
3 years	34	34	24	24	16	17	7	8	0	0	12	14
5 years	29	30	18	19	10	11	4	6	0	0	9	11
Females	(75)		(46)		(73)		(135)		(127)		(456)	
1 year	59	59	46	46	36	36	23	23	13	14	30	31
3 years	37	37	13	13	21	21	5	6	2	2	13	14
5 years	32	32	11	11	11	12	3	3	2	2	9	11
Overall	(140)		(84)		(187)		(270)		(264)		(945)	
1 year	61	61	40	41	34	35	24	24	9	10	29	30
3 years	36	36	18	18	18	19	6	7	1	1	12	14
5 years	31	31	14	15	10	11	4	4	1	1	9	11

ACUTE MYELOID LEUKAEMIA (ICD-9 205.0)

ENGLAND

AREA	NUMBER OF CASES			PERIOD	MEAN AGE			5-YR RELATIVE SURVIVAL (%)	
	Males	Females	All		Males	Females	All	Males	Females
East Anglia	150	131	281	1985-1989	64.3	65.4	64.8		
Mersey	142	131	273	1985-1989	62.6	61.8	62.2		
Oxford	134	164	298	1985-1989	65.3	67.0	66.3		
South Thames	310	292	602	1985-1989	61.8	62.6	62.2		
Wessex	230	196	426	1985-1989	62.9	66.4	64.5		
West Midlands	299	306	605	1985-1989	61.5	63.2	62.3		
Yorkshire	200	205	405	1985-1989	62.4	65.1	63.8		
English Registries	1465	1425	2890		62.6	64.3	63.5		

OBSERVED AND RELATIVE SURVIVAL (%) BY AGE (number of cases in parentheses)

	AGE CLASS										ALL	
	15-44		45-54		55-64		65-74		75-99			
	obs	rel	obs	rel	obs	rel	obs	rel	obs	rel	obs	rel
Males	(231)		(144)		(278)		(424)		(388)		(1465)	
1 year	53	53	53	54	36	37	22	23	10	11	29	31
3 years	26	26	22	22	14	15	4	5	4	5	11	13
5 years	23	23	16	17	10	11	2	3	3	5	9	11
Females	(236)		(128)		(221)		(334)		(506)		(1425)	
1 year	61	61	48	48	35	36	22	22	8	9	28	29
3 years	34	34	19	19	12	13	6	6	2	3	11	12
5 years	30	30	13	14	9	9	5	5	1	2	9	11
Overall	(467)		(272)		(499)		(758)		(894)		(2890)	
1 year	57	57	51	51	36	36	22	22	9	10	29	30
3 years	30	30	20	21	13	14	5	5	3	4	11	13
5 years	26	27	15	15	9	10	3	4	2	3	9	11

ESTONIA

AREA	NUMBER OF CASES			PERIOD	MEAN AGE		
	Males	Females	All		Males	Females	All
Estonia	48	40	88	1985-1989	54.0	60.3	56.9

OBSERVED AND RELATIVE SURVIVAL (%) BY AGE (number of cases in parentheses)

	AGE CLASS										ALL	
	15-44		45-54		55-64		65-74		75-99			
	obs	rel	obs	rel	obs	rel	obs	rel	obs	rel	obs	rel
Males	(17)		(7)		(7)		(7)		(10)		(48)	
1 year	24	24	14	14	0	0	14	15	20	22	17	17
3 years	12	12	0	0	0	0	0	0	10	14	6	7
5 years	12	12	0	0	0	0	0	0	10	19	6	8
Females	(7)		(2)		(13)		(13)		(5)		(40)	
1 year	57	57	0	0	23	23	23	24	0	0	25	26
3 years	29	29	0	0	8	8	15	17	0	0	13	13
5 years	29	29	0	0	8	8	8	9	0	0	10	11
Overall	(24)		(9)		(20)		(20)		(15)		(88)	
1 year	33	33	11	11	15	15	20	21	13	15	20	21
3 years	17	17	0	0	5	5	10	11	7	9	9	10
5 years	17	17	0	0	5	6	5	6	7	11	8	9

ACUTE MYELOID LEUKAEMIA (ICD-9 205.0)

FINLAND

AREA	NUMBER OF CASES			PERIOD	MEAN AGE		
	Males	Females	All		Males	Females	All
Finland	246	269	515	1985-1989	58.6	63.0	60.9

OBSERVED AND RELATIVE SURVIVAL (%) BY AGE (number of cases in parentheses)

	15-44		45-54		55-64		65-74		75-99		ALL	
	obs	rel	obs	rel	obs	rel	obs	rel	obs	rel	obs	rel
Males	(63)		(33)		(40)		(58)		(52)		(246)	
1 year	71	72	58	58	30	31	31	32	12	13	41	42
3 years	46	46	27	28	23	24	9	10	2	3	22	24
5 years	37	37	21	22	15	17	3	4	2	4	16	19
Females	(40)		(30)		(52)		(64)		(83)		(269)	
1 year	58	58	50	50	40	41	16	16	11	12	29	30
3 years	30	30	23	24	19	20	3	3	2	3	12	13
5 years	28	28	17	17	10	10	2	2	1	2	9	10
Overall	(103)		(63)		(92)		(122)		(135)		(515)	
1 year	66	66	54	54	36	36	23	24	11	12	35	36
3 years	40	40	25	26	21	21	6	6	2	3	17	19
5 years	33	33	19	20	12	13	2	3	1	3	12	14

FRANCE

AREA	NUMBER OF CASES			PERIOD	MEAN AGE			5-YR RELATIVE SURVIVAL (%)	
	Males	Females	All		Males	Females	All	Males	Females
Somme	29	27	56	1985-1989	57.5	58.1	57.8		
Calvados	9	13	22	1985-1989	44.2	64.0	56.0		
Côte d'Or	48	43	91	1985-1989	69.0	59.8	64.6		
Doubs	28	37	65	1985-1989	60.7	59.6	60.1		
French Registries	114	120	234		62.1	59.9	61.0		

OBSERVED AND RELATIVE SURVIVAL (%) BY AGE (number of cases in parentheses)

	15-44		45-54		55-64		65-74		75-99		ALL	
	obs	rel	obs	rel	obs	rel	obs	rel	obs	rel	obs	rel
Males	(21)		(10)		(19)		(30)		(34)		(114)	
1 year	65	66	30	30	32	32	28	29	13	14	31	32
3 years	44	44	20	21	9	10	11	12	0	0	15	17
5 years	44	45	20	21	9	10	11	13	0	0	15	19
Females	(33)		(9)		(16)		(21)		(41)		(120)	
1 year	67	67	44	45	31	31	29	29	17	18	37	38
3 years	23	23	33	34	19	19	14	15	0	0	15	16
5 years	23	23	33	34	19	19	14	16	0	0	15	18
Overall	(54)		(19)		(35)		(51)		(75)		(234)	
1 year	66	66	37	37	31	32	28	29	15	16	34	35
3 years	31	31	25	26	14	14	12	13	0	0	15	17
5 years	31	31	25	26	14	14	12	14	0	0	15	18

ACUTE MYELOID LEUKAEMIA (ICD-9 205.0)

GERMANY

AREA	NUMBER OF CASES			PERIOD	MEAN AGE		
	Males	Females	All		Males	Females	All
Saarland	53	43	96	1985-1989	60.8	62.8	61.7

OBSERVED AND RELATIVE SURVIVAL (%) BY AGE (number of cases in parentheses)

	AGE CLASS										ALL	
	15-44		45-54		55-64		65-74		75-99			
	obs	rel	obs	rel	obs	rel	obs	rel	obs	rel	obs	rel
Males	(7)		(8)		(15)		(14)		(9)		(53)	
1 year	86	86	25	25	53	54	0	0	22	25	34	35
3 years	57	58	13	13	13	14	0	0	0	0	13	15
5 years	38	39	-	-	-	-	0	0	0	0	9	11
Females	(5)		(5)		(11)		(7)		(15)		(43)	
1 year	20	20	40	40	36	37	0	0	7	7	19	19
3 years	20	20	20	20	36	37	0	0	0	0	14	15
5 years	-	-	-	-	36	38	0	0	0	0	14	16
Overall	(12)		(13)		(26)		(21)		(24)		(96)	
1 year	58	58	31	31	46	47	0	0	13	13	27	28
3 years	42	42	15	16	23	24	0	0	0	0	14	15
5 years	28	28	-	-	19	21	0	0	0	0	11	13

ICELAND

AREA	NUMBER OF CASES			PERIOD	MEAN AGE		
	Males	Females	All		Males	Females	All
Iceland	11	12	23	1985-1989	52.2	67.6	60.3

OBSERVED AND RELATIVE SURVIVAL (%) BY AGE (number of cases in parentheses)

	AGE CLASS										ALL	
	15-44		45-54		55-64		65-74		75-99			
	obs	rel	obs	rel	obs	rel	obs	rel	obs	rel	obs	rel
Males	(5)		(1)		(2)		(0)		(3)		(11)	
1 year	40	40	0	0	50	50	-	-	0	0	27	28
3 years	0	0	0	0	0	0	-	-	0	0	0	0
5 years	0	0	0	0	0	0	-	-	0	0	0	0
Females	(2)		(0)		(3)		(1)		(6)		(12)	
1 year	50	50	-	-	67	67	0	0	17	18	33	34
3 years	50	50	-	-	0	0	0	0	0	0	8	9
5 years	50	50	-	-	0	0	0	0	0	0	8	10
Overall	(7)		(1)		(5)		(1)		(9)		(23)	
1 year	43	43	0	0	60	61	0	0	11	12	30	31
3 years	14	14	0	0	0	0	0	0	0	0	4	5
5 years	14	14	0	0	0	0	0	0	0	0	4	5

ACUTE MYELOID LEUKAEMIA (ICD-9 205.0)

ITALY

AREA	NUMBER OF CASES			PERIOD	MEAN AGE			5-YR RELATIVE SURVIVAL (%)	
	Males	Females	All		Males	Females	All	Males	Females
Florence	77	48	125	1985-1989	58.7	59.8	59.1		
Genoa	31	28	59	1986-1988	59.3	60.7	60.0		
Latina	19	16	35	1985-1987	58.0	47.2	53.1		
Modena	16	7	23	1988-1989	63.5	58.9	62.1		
Parma	25	20	45	1985-1987	63.5	60.8	62.3		
Ragusa	14	12	26	1985-1989	62.3	61.1	61.8		
Romagna	21	15	36	1986-1988	59.0	67.7	62.6		
Turin	42	25	67	1985-1987	55.6	65.4	59.3		
Varese	57	52	109	1985-1989	61.3	62.0	61.6		
Italian Registries	302	223	525		59.6	60.8	60.2		

OBSERVED AND RELATIVE SURVIVAL (%) BY AGE (number of cases in parentheses)

	AGE CLASS										ALL	
	15-44		45-54		55-64		65-74		75-99			
	obs	rel	obs	rel	obs	rel	obs	rel	obs	rel	obs	rel
Males	(53)		(43)		(69)		(71)		(66)		(302)	
1 year	45	45	28	28	16	16	20	20	8	8	22	23
3 years	23	23	14	14	7	8	7	8	0	0	9	10
5 years	21	21	12	12	4	5	4	5	0	0	7	9
Females	(37)		(32)		(47)		(53)		(54)		(223)	
1 year	49	49	38	38	34	34	21	21	9	10	28	28
3 years	30	30	16	16	17	17	2	2	4	5	12	13
5 years	27	27	16	16	9	9	2	2	2	3	9	11
Overall	(90)		(75)		(116)		(124)		(120)		(525)	
1 year	47	47	32	32	23	24	20	21	8	9	24	25
3 years	26	26	15	15	11	12	5	5	2	2	10	11
5 years	23	23	13	14	6	6	3	4	1	1	8	9

NETHERLANDS

AREA	NUMBER OF CASES			PERIOD	MEAN AGE		
	Males	Females	All		Males	Females	All
Eindhoven	42	37	79	1985-1989	61.0	62.8	61.8

OBSERVED AND RELATIVE SURVIVAL (%) BY AGE (number of cases in parentheses)

	AGE CLASS										ALL	
	15-44		45-54		55-64		65-74		75-99			
	obs	rel	obs	rel	obs	rel	obs	rel	obs	rel	obs	rel
Males	(8)		(8)		(4)		(12)		(10)		(42)	
1 year	38	38	38	38	0	0	8	9	10	11	19	20
3 years	25	25	25	25	0	0	8	9	0	0	12	13
5 years	-	-	0	0	0	0	0	0	0	0	0	0
Females	(8)		(4)		(4)		(8)		(13)		(37)	
1 year	50	50	50	50	25	25	13	13	15	16	27	28
3 years	50	50	25	25	25	25	0	0	0	0	16	18
5 years	38	38	0	0	25	26	0	0	0	0	11	13
Overall	(16)		(12)		(8)		(20)		(23)		(79)	
1 year	44	44	42	42	13	13	10	10	13	14	23	24
3 years	38	38	25	25	13	13	5	6	0	0	14	16
5 years	25	25	0	0	13	13	0	0	0	0	7	9

ACUTE MYELOID LEUKAEMIA   (ICD-9 205.0)

POLAND

AREA	NUMBER OF CASES			PERIOD	MEAN AGE			5-YR RELATIVE SURVIVAL (%)	
	Males	Females	All		Males	Females	All	Males	Females
Cracow	17	19	36	1985-1989	50.6	53.3	52.0		
Warsaw	23	24	47	1988-1989	64.7	59.5	62.1		
Polish Registries	40	43	83		58.7	56.8	57.7		

OBSERVED AND RELATIVE SURVIVAL (%) BY AGE (number of cases in parentheses)

	AGE CLASS										ALL	
	15-44		45-54		55-64		65-74		75-99			
	obs	rel	obs	rel	obs	rel	obs	rel	obs	rel	obs	rel
Males	(9)		(5)		(9)		(9)		(8)		(40)	
1 year	67	67	20	20	11	11	0	0	0	0	20	21
3 years	11	11	0	0	11	12	0	0	0	0	5	6
5 years	0	0	0	0	0	0	0	0	0	0	0	0
Females	(11)		(7)		(8)		(10)		(7)		(43)	
1 year	55	55	29	29	0	0	10	10	0	0	21	21
3 years	9	9	0	0	0	0	0	0	0	0	2	3
5 years	9	9	0	0	0	0	0	0	0	0	2	3
Overall	(20)		(12)		(17)		(19)		(15)		(83)	
1 year	60	60	25	25	6	6	5	5	0	0	20	21
3 years	10	10	0	0	6	6	0	0	0	0	4	4
5 years	5	5	0	0	0	0	0	0	0	0	1	1

SCOTLAND

AREA	NUMBER OF CASES			PERIOD	MEAN AGE		
	Males	Females	All		Males	Females	All
Scotland	303	341	644	1985-1989	63.2	62.4	62.8

OBSERVED AND RELATIVE SURVIVAL (%) BY AGE (number of cases in parentheses)

	AGE CLASS										ALL	
	15-44		45-54		55-64		65-74		75-99			
	obs	rel	obs	rel	obs	rel	obs	rel	obs	rel	obs	rel
Males	(44)		(34)		(54)		(79)		(92)		(303)	
1 year	55	55	24	24	24	25	15	16	5	6	20	22
3 years	27	27	6	6	13	14	3	3	1	2	8	9
5 years	20	21	3	3	9	10	0	0	0	0	5	6
Females	(67)		(38)		(47)		(86)		(103)		(341)	
1 year	43	43	29	29	34	34	19	19	7	8	23	24
3 years	24	24	16	16	9	9	3	4	1	1	9	10
5 years	24	24	16	16	6	7	3	4	1	2	9	10
Overall	(111)		(72)		(101)		(165)		(195)		(644)	
1 year	48	48	26	27	29	29	17	18	6	7	22	23
3 years	25	25	11	11	11	12	3	3	1	1	8	10
5 years	23	23	10	10	8	9	2	2	1	1	7	9

ACUTE MYELOID LEUKAEMIA (ICD-9 205.0)

SLOVAKIA

AREA	NUMBER OF CASES			PERIOD	MEAN AGE		
	Males	Females	All		Males	Females	All
Slovakia	182	186	368	1985-1989	56.7	54.6	55.7

OBSERVED AND RELATIVE SURVIVAL (%) BY AGE (number of cases in parentheses)

	15-44 obs rel		45-54 obs rel		55-64 obs rel		65-74 obs rel		75-99 obs rel		ALL obs rel	
Males	(44)		(22)		(41)		(45)		(30)		(182)	
1 year	32	32	14	14	10	10	18	19	3	4	16	17
3 years	14	14	5	5	2	3	9	10	3	5	7	8
5 years	9	9	0	0	-	-	9	12	3	7	5	7
Females	(50)		(31)		(42)		(43)		(20)		(186)	
1 year	50	50	35	36	19	19	12	12	10	11	27	28
3 years	14	14	13	13	2	2	5	5	0	0	8	8
5 years	8	8	10	10	-	-	5	6	0	0	5	6
Overall	(94)		(53)		(83)		(88)		(50)		(368)	
1 year	41	42	26	27	14	15	15	15	6	7	22	23
3 years	14	14	9	10	2	3	7	8	2	3	7	8
5 years	8	8	6	6	-	-	7	9	2	4	5	6

SLOVENIA

AREA	NUMBER OF CASES			PERIOD	MEAN AGE		
	Males	Females	All		Males	Females	All
Slovenia	64	72	136	1985-1989	55.8	58.6	57.3

OBSERVED AND RELATIVE SURVIVAL (%) BY AGE (number of cases in parentheses)

	15-44 obs rel		45-54 obs rel		55-64 obs rel		65-74 obs rel		75-99 obs rel		ALL obs rel	
Males	(14)		(14)		(16)		(9)		(11)		(64)	
1 year	50	50	50	50	13	13	11	12	0	0	27	28
3 years	14	14	7	7	0	0	0	0	0	0	5	5
5 years	14	14	7	8	0	0	0	0	0	0	5	6
Females	(18)		(10)		(11)		(11)		(22)		(72)	
1 year	44	44	30	30	45	46	9	9	18	20	29	30
3 years	28	28	0	0	18	19	0	0	0	0	10	11
5 years	28	28	0	0	0	0	0	0	0	0	7	8
Overall	(32)		(24)		(27)		(20)		(33)		(136)	
1 year	47	47	42	42	26	26	10	10	12	13	28	29
3 years	22	22	4	4	7	8	0	0	0	0	7	8
5 years	22	22	4	4	0	0	0	0	0	0	6	7

ACUTE MYELOID LEUKAEMIA (ICD-9 205.0)

SPAIN

AREA	NUMBER OF CASES			PERIOD	MEAN AGE			5-YR RELATIVE SURVIVAL (%)	
	Males	Females	All		Males	Females	All	Males	Females
Basque Country	43	19	62	1986-1988	54.8	49.8	53.3		
Mallorca	12	16	28	1988-1989	50.0	55.8	53.4		
Navarra	15	17	32	1985-1989	55.1	66.1	61.0		
Tarragona	22	17	39	1985-1989	61.2	64.1	62.5		
Spanish Registries	92	69	161		55.8	58.8	57.1		

5-YR RELATIVE SURVIVAL (%) scale — Males: 100 80 60 40 20 0; Females: 0 20 40 60 80 100

Bars labelled: Basque, Mallor, Navarr, Tarrag

OBSERVED AND RELATIVE SURVIVAL (%) BY AGE (number of cases in parentheses)

	AGE CLASS										ALL	
	15-44		45-54		55-64		65-74		75-99			
	obs	rel	obs	rel	obs	rel	obs	rel	obs	rel	obs	rel
Males	(24)		(11)		(18)		(25)		(14)		(92)	
1 year	58	58	27	27	33	34	8	8	7	8	28	29
3 years	33	34	18	18	11	12	4	4	7	10	15	17
5 years	33	34	18	19	11	12	4	5	7	13	15	18
Females	(16)		(8)		(14)		(19)		(12)		(69)	
1 year	50	50	25	25	36	36	21	21	0	0	28	28
3 years	19	19	13	13	21	22	11	11	0	0	13	14
5 years	19	19	13	13	21	22	0	0	0	0	11	13
Overall	(40)		(19)		(32)		(44)		(26)		(161)	
1 year	55	55	26	26	34	35	14	14	4	4	28	29
3 years	28	28	16	16	16	16	7	7	4	5	14	15
5 years	28	28	16	16	16	17	3	4	4	7	14	15

SWEDEN

AREA	NUMBER OF CASES			PERIOD	MEAN AGE		
	Males	Females	All		Males	Females	All
South Sweden	98	94	192	1985-1989	65.4	65.4	65.4

OBSERVED AND RELATIVE SURVIVAL (%) BY AGE (number of cases in parentheses)

	AGE CLASS										ALL	
	15-44		45-54		55-64		65-74		75-99			
	obs	rel	obs	rel	obs	rel	obs	rel	obs	rel	obs	rel
Males	(12)		(7)		(15)		(38)		(26)		(98)	
1 year	75	75	57	57	40	41	26	27	0	0	30	31
3 years	33	33	14	15	13	14	5	6	0	0	9	11
5 years	25	25	14	15	7	7	3	3	0	0	6	8
Females	(15)		(4)		(19)		(28)		(28)		(94)	
1 year	60	60	75	75	58	58	21	22	11	12	34	35
3 years	47	47	25	25	21	22	7	8	0	0	15	17
5 years	33	33	0	0	16	16	4	4	0	0	10	11
Overall	(27)		(11)		(34)		(66)		(54)		(192)	
1 year	67	67	64	64	50	50	24	25	6	6	32	33
3 years	41	41	18	18	18	18	6	7	0	0	12	14
5 years	30	30	9	9	12	12	3	4	0	0	8	10

ACUTE MYELOID LEUKAEMIA   (ICD-9 205.0)

SWITZERLAND

AREA	NUMBER OF CASES			PERIOD	MEAN AGE			5-YR RELATIVE SURVIVAL (%)	
	Males	Females	All		Males	Females	All	Males	Females
Basel	21	21	42	1985-1988	58.7	67.0	62.9		
Geneva	18	22	40	1985-1989	62.1	61.6	61.9		
Swiss Registries	39	43	82		60.3	64.3	62.4		

OBSERVED AND RELATIVE SURVIVAL (%) BY AGE (number of cases in parentheses)

	AGE CLASS										ALL	
	15-44		45-54		55-64		65-74		75-99			
	obs	rel	obs	rel	obs	rel	obs	rel	obs	rel	obs	rel
Males	(9)		(3)		(6)		(11)		(10)		(39)	
1 year	67	67	100	100	33	34	9	9	30	33	38	40
3 years	56	56	0	0	17	17	0	0	10	13	18	20
5 years	56	56	0	0	0	0	0	0	10	17	15	19
Females	(11)		(2)		(7)		(5)		(18)		(43)	
1 year	36	36	0	0	43	43	40	41	11	12	26	27
3 years	18	18	0	0	0	0	0	0	6	8	7	8
5 years	18	18	0	0	0	0	0	0	6	10	7	9
Overall	(20)		(5)		(13)		(16)		(28)		(82)	
1 year	50	50	60	60	38	39	19	19	18	20	32	33
3 years	35	35	0	0	8	8	0	0	7	10	12	14
5 years	35	35	0	0	0	0	0	0	7	12	11	13

ACUTE MYELOID LEUKAEMIA (ICD-9 205.0)

EUROPE, 1985-89

Weighted analyses

COUNTRY	% COVERAGE WITH C.R.s	YEARLY NO. OF CASES (Mean No. of cases recorded)		
		Males	Females	All
AUSTRIA	8	7	8	15
DENMARK	100	98	91	189
ENGLAND	50	293	285	578
ESTONIA	100	10	8	18
FINLAND	100	49	54	103
FRANCE	4	23	24	47
GERMANY	2	11	9	20
ICELAND	100	2	2	4
ITALY	10	84	61	145
NETHERLANDS	6	8	7	15
POLAND	6	15	16	31
SCOTLAND	100	61	68	129
SLOVAKIA	100	36	37	73
SLOVENIA	100	13	14	27
SPAIN	10	28	21	49
SWEDEN	17	20	19	39
SWITZERLAND	11	9	10	19

RELATIVE SURVIVAL (%) (Age-standardized)

□ 1 year ■ 5 years

OBSERVED AND RELATIVE SURVIVAL (%) BY AGE

	AGE CLASS										ALL	
	15-44		45-54		55-64		65-74		75-99			
	obs	rel	obs	rel	obs	rel	obs	rel	obs	rel	obs	rel
Males												
1 year	61	61	34	35	29	30	16	17	11	12	28	29
3 years	35	35	16	16	10	11	5	6	1	2	12	14
5 years	29	30	14	14	7	7	4	4	1	2	9	11
Females												
1 year	51	51	40	40	33	34	18	18	9	10	28	29
3 years	27	27	19	19	19	20	5	5	1	2	13	14
5 years	25	25	15	15	16	17	4	4	1	1	11	13
Overall												
1 year	56	56	37	37	31	32	17	17	10	11	28	29
3 years	31	31	18	18	15	15	5	5	1	2	12	14
5 years	27	28	14	15	11	12	4	4	1	2	10	12

AGE STANDARDIZED RELATIVE SURVIVAL(%)

COUNTRY	MALES		FEMALES	
	1-year (95% C.I.)	5-years (95% C.I.)	1-year (95% C.I.)	5-years (95% C.I.)
AUSTRIA	-	-	27.8 (17.3 - 44.5)	12.3 (4.6 - 32.5)
DENMARK	29.7 (26.1 - 33.8)	10.7 (8.2 - 14.1)	31.7 (27.9 - 36.1)	10.6 (8.1 - 13.9)
ENGLAND	30.6 (28.5 - 33.0)	10.1 (8.6 - 11.9)	30.8 (28.5 - 33.1)	10.3 (8.8 - 12.0)
ESTONIA	15.8 (7.7 - 32.4)	7.5 (1.9 - 29.6)	20.6 (12.7 - 33.2)	9.0 (3.7 - 21.9)
FINLAND	36.4 (31.2 - 42.5)	14.2 (10.5 - 19.3)	30.4 (25.6 - 36.0)	9.5 (6.6 - 13.8)
FRANCE	32.1 (24.7 - 41.6)	15.4 (10.0 - 23.6)	34.8 (27.1 - 44.7)	15.2 (9.6 - 24.1)
GERMANY	34.7 (25.3 - 47.8)	-	16.5 (9.0 - 30.4)	-
ICELAND	-	-	-	-
ITALY	21.6 (17.5 - 26.5)	7.2 (4.8 - 10.7)	27.1 (22.1 - 33.3)	9.4 (6.3 - 14.0)
NETHERLANDS	16.0 (8.6 - 29.8)	-	26.7 (15.8 - 45.1)	11.5 (4.8 - 27.5)
POLAND	16.2 (10.0 - 26.1)	0.0 (0.0 - 0.0)	15.4 (9.2 - 25.9)	1.6 (0.2 - 10.8)
SCOTLAND	22.5 (18.4 - 27.5)	5.9 (3.7 - 9.5)	24.1 (20.0 - 29.0)	8.8 (6.2 - 12.4)
SLOVAKIA	14.8 (10.6 - 20.7)	-	22.3 (17.0 - 29.2)	-
SLOVENIA	19.6 (12.8 - 30.0)	3.4 (1.1 - 10.0)	27.4 (19.0 - 39.3)	5.0 (2.4 - 10.5)
SPAIN	23.8 (17.1 - 33.1)	14.9 (8.3 - 26.6)	23.6 (16.4 - 34.0)	8.8 (4.5 - 17.2)
SWEDEN	33.9 (26.5 - 43.3)	8.2 (3.9 - 17.1)	38.2 (30.0 - 48.6)	10.0 (5.7 - 17.6)
SWITZERLAND	40.2 (28.9 - 55.8)	14.8 (7.2 - 30.6)	28.2 (16.8 - 47.5)	5.9 (2.0 - 17.8)
EUROPE, 1985-89	27.5 (24.8 - 30.6)	9.9 (7.3 - 13.3)	26.9 (24.2 - 30.0)	10.6 (8.4 - 13.3)

<h1 style="text-align:center">CHRONIC MYELOID LEUKAEMIA   (ICD-9 205.1)</h1>

AUSTRIA

AREA	NUMBER OF CASES			PERIOD	MEAN AGE		
	Males	Females	All		Males	Females	All
Tirol	9	6	15	1988-1989	53.7	62.3	57.2

OBSERVED AND RELATIVE SURVIVAL (%) BY AGE (number of cases in parentheses)

	AGE CLASS										ALL	
	15-44		45-54		55-64		65-74		75-99			
	obs	rel	obs	rel	obs	rel	obs	rel	obs	rel	obs	rel
Males	(3)		(1)		(1)		(2)		(2)		(9)	
1 year	100	100	100	100	0	0	100	100	100	100	89	91
3 years	67	67	100	100	0	0	100	100	50	59	67	71
5 years	67	67	100	100	0	0	50	58	0	0	44	50
Females	(1)		(1)		(1)		(1)		(2)		(6)	
1 year	100	100	100	100	100	100	100	100	0	0	67	68
3 years	100	100	100	100	0	0	0	0	0	0	33	36
5 years	100	100	0	0	0	0	0	0	0	0	17	19
Overall	(4)		(2)		(2)		(3)		(4)		(15)	
1 year	100	100	100	100	50	50	100	100	50	53	80	82
3 years	75	75	100	100	0	0	67	72	25	30	53	57
5 years	75	75	50	51	0	0	33	39	0	0	33	37

DENMARK

AREA	NUMBER OF CASES			PERIOD	MEAN AGE		
	Males	Females	All		Males	Females	All
Denmark	191	145	336	1985-1989	64.5	64.1	64.3

OBSERVED AND RELATIVE SURVIVAL (%) BY AGE (number of cases in parentheses)

	AGE CLASS										ALL	
	15-44		45-54		55-64		65-74		75-99			
	obs	rel	obs	rel	obs	rel	obs	rel	obs	rel	obs	rel
Males	(33)		(15)		(26)		(51)		(66)		(191)	
1 year	82	82	60	60	81	82	61	63	29	32	56	59
3 years	48	49	40	41	31	33	22	25	8	11	24	28
5 years	45	46	13	14	15	17	8	10	2	3	14	18
Females	(26)		(14)		(21)		(30)		(54)		(145)	
1 year	96	96	93	93	86	87	60	61	43	46	67	69
3 years	54	54	64	65	48	49	43	47	13	17	37	41
5 years	46	46	43	44	38	40	20	23	4	6	23	29
Overall	(59)		(29)		(47)		(81)		(120)		(336)	
1 year	88	88	76	76	83	84	60	63	35	39	61	64
3 years	51	51	52	53	38	40	30	33	10	14	29	34
5 years	46	46	28	29	26	28	12	15	3	4	18	23

CHRONIC MYELOID LEUKAEMIA (ICD-9 205.1)

ENGLAND

AREA	NUMBER OF CASES			PERIOD	MEAN AGE			5-YR RELATIVE SURVIVAL (%)	
	Males	Females	All		Males	Females	All	Males	Females
East Anglia	80	49	129	1985-1989	68.4	70.5	69.2		
Mersey	67	59	126	1985-1989	60.7	69.6	64.8		
Oxford	101	77	178	1985-1989	64.6	69.7	66.8		
South Thames	140	148	288	1985-1989	66.4	66.9	66.6		
Wessex	160	128	288	1985-1989	66.4	70.9	68.4		
West Midlands	180	140	320	1985-1989	63.2	64.6	63.8		
Yorkshire	135	115	250	1985-1989	63.8	69.7	66.5		
English Registries	863	716	1579		64.9	68.4	66.5		

OBSERVED AND RELATIVE SURVIVAL (%) BY AGE (number of cases in parentheses)

	15-44		45-54		55-64		65-74		75-99		ALL	
	obs	rel	obs	rel	obs	rel	obs	rel	obs	rel	obs	rel
Males	(135)		(77)		(138)		(219)		(294)		(863)	
1 year	81	82	73	73	72	74	57	60	40	46	59	62
3 years	50	50	39	40	41	43	26	30	17	25	30	36
5 years	33	33	21	22	25	28	15	19	7	14	17	23
Females	(81)		(61)		(107)		(129)		(338)		(716)	
1 year	88	88	72	72	72	73	63	64	43	48	59	62
3 years	59	59	51	51	49	50	33	35	20	28	34	39
5 years	47	47	34	35	25	26	16	18	11	19	20	26
Overall	(216)		(138)		(245)		(348)		(632)		(1579)	
1 year	84	84	72	73	72	73	59	61	42	47	59	62
3 years	53	53	44	45	44	46	29	32	19	26	32	37
5 years	38	39	27	28	25	27	15	19	9	17	19	24

ESTONIA

AREA	NUMBER OF CASES			PERIOD	MEAN AGE		
	Males	Females	All		Males	Females	All
Estonia	37	41	78	1985-1989	57.5	56.9	57.2

OBSERVED AND RELATIVE SURVIVAL (%) BY AGE (number of cases in parentheses)

	15-44		45-54		55-64		65-74		75-99		ALL	
	obs	rel	obs	rel	obs	rel	obs	rel	obs	rel	obs	rel
Males	(9)		(3)		(12)		(8)		(5)		(37)	
1 year	78	78	67	68	75	77	25	26	100	100	68	70
3 years	56	56	67	70	50	55	13	15	40	55	43	48
5 years	33	34	33	36	25	29	0	0	20	36	22	26
Females	(11)		(3)		(12)		(10)		(5)		(41)	
1 year	82	82	33	33	83	84	40	41	40	45	63	65
3 years	73	73	0	0	58	60	20	22	0	0	41	45
5 years	55	55	0	0	33	36	20	24	0	0	29	33
Overall	(20)		(6)		(24)		(18)		(10)		(78)	
1 year	80	80	50	50	79	81	33	35	70	78	65	67
3 years	65	66	33	34	54	58	17	19	20	28	42	46
5 years	45	46	17	18	29	33	11	14	10	18	26	30

CHRONIC MYELOID LEUKAEMIA (ICD-9 205.1)

FINLAND

AREA	NUMBER OF CASES			PERIOD	MEAN AGE		
	Males	Females	All		Males	Females	All
Finland	112	95	207	1985-1989	58.8	58.7	58.7

OBSERVED AND RELATIVE SURVIVAL (%) BY AGE (number of cases in parentheses)

	AGE CLASS										ALL	
	15-44		45-54		55-64		65-74		75-99			
	obs	rel	obs	rel	obs	rel	obs	rel	obs	rel	obs	rel
Males	(28)		(16)		(17)		(27)		(24)		(112)	
1 year	82	82	75	76	82	84	48	51	38	43	63	66
3 years	54	54	38	38	59	62	22	26	17	25	37	42
5 years	36	36	38	39	35	39	4	5	13	26	23	29
Females	(19)		(22)		(12)		(19)		(23)		(95)	
1 year	100	100	86	87	75	75	89	91	48	53	79	81
3 years	68	69	77	78	50	51	53	56	22	29	54	58
5 years	53	53	55	55	42	43	26	30	13	22	37	42
Overall	(47)		(38)		(29)		(46)		(47)		(207)	
1 year	89	90	82	82	79	80	65	68	43	48	71	73
3 years	60	60	61	61	55	57	35	39	19	27	44	49
5 years	43	43	47	49	38	40	13	16	13	24	29	35

FRANCE

AREA	NUMBER OF CASES			PERIOD	MEAN AGE			5-YR RELATIVE SURVIVAL (%)	
	Males	Females	All		Males	Females	All	Males	Females
Somme	28	13	41	1985-1989	59.3	56.6	58.5		
Calvados	20	14	34	1985-1989	56.5	47.4	52.8		
Côte d'Or	74	44	118	1985-1989	71.5	67.5	70.0		
Doubs	11	15	26	1985-1989	61.1	58.8	59.8		
French Registries	133	86	219		65.9	61.1	64.0		

OBSERVED AND RELATIVE SURVIVAL (%) BY AGE (number of cases in parentheses)

	AGE CLASS										ALL	
	15-44		45-54		55-64		65-74		75-99			
	obs	rel	obs	rel	obs	rel	obs	rel	obs	rel	obs	rel
Males	(16)		(13)		(22)		(38)		(44)		(133)	
1 year	88	88	92	93	70	72	74	76	61	69	73	77
3 years	56	57	75	77	54	58	47	53	23	33	44	52
5 years	41	42	50	52	54	60	23	29	9	18	27	36
Females	(19)		(11)		(15)		(17)		(24)		(86)	
1 year	89	90	100	100	93	94	76	78	50	59	78	82
3 years	79	79	78	78	86	88	57	60	40	62	65	73
5 years	51	51	78	79	47	49	22	23	24	46	40	48
Overall	(35)		(24)		(37)		(55)		(68)		(219)	
1 year	89	89	96	96	80	81	74	77	58	66	75	79
3 years	68	69	77	78	68	71	50	55	28	42	52	60
5 years	46	46	62	64	49	52	23	27	13	26	32	41

CHRONIC MYELOID LEUKAEMIA   (ICD-9 205.1)

GERMANY

AREA	NUMBER OF CASES			PERIOD	MEAN AGE		
	Males	Females	All		Males	Females	All
Saarland	56	36	92	1985-1989	52.5	65.0	57.4

OBSERVED AND RELATIVE SURVIVAL (%) BY AGE (number of cases in parentheses)

	AGE CLASS										ALL	
	15-44		45-54		55-64		65-74		75-99			
	obs	rel	obs	rel	obs	rel	obs	rel	obs	rel	obs	rel
Males	(21)		(7)		(11)		(10)		(7)		(56)	
1 year	81	81	86	86	91	92	60	62	57	66	77	79
3 years	52	53	71	73	55	58	30	34	43	68	50	54
5 years	43	43	-	-	22	24	10	13	29	67	29	33
Females	(2)		(6)		(6)		(10)		(12)		(36)	
1 year	100	100	83	84	83	84	60	62	42	44	64	66
3 years	100	100	83	84	67	69	50	54	33	40	56	61
5 years	100	100	67	68	29	30	30	35	6	8	30	35
Overall	(23)		(13)		(17)		(20)		(19)		(92)	
1 year	83	83	85	85	88	89	60	62	47	52	72	74
3 years	57	57	77	78	59	61	40	44	37	49	52	57
5 years	48	48	48	49	24	26	19	24	14	23	29	34

ICELAND

AREA	NUMBER OF CASES			PERIOD	MEAN AGE		
	Males	Females	All		Males	Females	All
Iceland	9	1	10	1985-1989	62.3	64.0	62.6

OBSERVED AND RELATIVE SURVIVAL (%) BY AGE (number of cases in parentheses)

	AGE CLASS										ALL	
	15-44		45-54		55-64		65-74		75-99			
	obs	rel	obs	rel	obs	rel	obs	rel	obs	rel	obs	rel
Males	(3)		(0)		(0)		(3)		(3)		(9)	
1 year	67	67	-	-	-	-	67	69	67	71	67	69
3 years	33	33	-	-	-	-	33	37	0	0	22	25
5 years	0	0	-	-	-	-	33	40	0	0	11	13
Females	(0)		(0)		(0)		(1)		(0)		(1)	
1 year	-	-	-	-	-	-	100	100	-	-	100	100
3 years	-	-	-	-	-	-	0	0	-	-	0	0
5 years	-	-	-	-	-	-	0	0	-	-	0	0
Overall	(3)		(0)		(0)		(4)		(3)		(10)	
1 year	67	67	-	-	-	-	75	77	67	71	70	72
3 years	33	33	-	-	-	-	25	27	0	0	20	22
5 years	0	0	-	-	-	-	25	29	0	0	10	12

CHRONIC MYELOID LEUKAEMIA (ICD-9 205.1)

ITALY

AREA	NUMBER OF CASES			PERIOD	MEAN AGE			5-YR RELATIVE SURVIVAL (%)	
	Males	Females	All		Males	Females	All	Males	Females
Florence	63	36	99	1985-1989	57.0	59.4	57.9		
Genoa	27	16	43	1986-1988	68.2	74.3	70.5		
Latina	7	7	14	1985-1987	59.3	41.1	50.3		
Modena	13	10	23	1988-1989	60.9	75.3	67.2		
Parma	10	10	20	1985-1987	70.3	71.2	70.8		
Ragusa	12	8	20	1985-1989	63.3	65.5	64.2		
Romagna	18	13	31	1986-1988	63.9	62.9	63.5		
Turin	18	18	36	1985-1987	63.1	67.4	65.3		
Varese	49	34	83	1985-1989	62.1	62.2	62.2		
Italian Registries	217	152	369		61.9	64.2	62.9		

OBSERVED AND RELATIVE SURVIVAL (%) BY AGE (number of cases in parentheses)

	AGE CLASS										ALL	
	15-44		45-54		55-64		65-74		75-99			
	obs	rel	obs	rel	obs	rel	obs	rel	obs	rel	obs	rel
Males	(32)		(33)		(40)		(53)		(59)		(217)	
1 year	72	72	64	64	70	71	62	64	47	52	61	64
3 years	53	53	42	43	48	50	30	34	12	16	34	38
5 years	41	41	24	25	30	33	15	18	7	11	21	25
Females	(19)		(18)		(33)		(27)		(55)		(152)	
1 year	84	84	94	95	67	67	70	72	60	65	70	73
3 years	47	47	77	77	55	56	41	43	27	35	44	48
5 years	32	32	53	54	36	38	11	12	15	22	25	30
Overall	(51)		(51)		(73)		(80)		(114)		(369)	
1 year	76	77	74	74	68	69	65	67	54	58	65	67
3 years	51	51	54	55	51	52	34	37	19	25	38	42
5 years	37	37	34	35	33	35	14	16	11	17	23	27

NETHERLANDS

AREA	NUMBER OF CASES			PERIOD	MEAN AGE		
	Males	Females	All		Males	Females	All
Eindhoven	30	15	45	1985-1989	64.0	66.2	64.8

OBSERVED AND RELATIVE SURVIVAL (%) BY AGE (number of cases in parentheses)

	AGE CLASS										ALL	
	15-44		45-54		55-64		65-74		75-99			
	obs	rel	obs	rel	obs	rel	obs	rel	obs	rel	obs	rel
Males	(5)		(2)		(4)		(11)		(8)		(30)	
1 year	80	80	100	100	75	76	27	28	13	14	43	46
3 years	80	80	50	51	75	79	0	0	13	19	30	35
5 years	80	80	0	0	25	28	0	0	0	0	16	21
Females	(3)		(0)		(4)		(1)		(7)		(15)	
1 year	100	100	-	-	100	100	0	0	43	47	67	70
3 years	67	67	-	-	75	77	0	0	29	37	47	53
5 years	67	67	-	-	50	52	0	0	14	22	33	41
Overall	(8)		(2)		(8)		(12)		(15)		(45)	
1 year	88	88	100	100	88	89	25	26	27	30	51	54
3 years	75	75	50	51	75	78	0	0	20	28	36	41
5 years	75	75	0	0	38	40	0	0	7	12	22	28

CHRONIC MYELOID LEUKAEMIA (ICD-9 205.1)

POLAND

AREA	NUMBER OF CASES			PERIOD	MEAN AGE			5-YR RELATIVE SURVIVAL (%)	
	Males	Females	All		Males	Females	All	Males	Females
Cracow	10	11	21	1985-1989	50.8	59.0	55.1		
Warsaw	12	15	27	1988-1989	58.6	67.1	63.3		
Polish Registries	22	26	48		55.1	63.7	59.8		

5-YR RELATIVE SURVIVAL (%) chart: Males scale 100 80 60 40 20 0, Females scale 0 20 40 60 80 100; Cracow, Warsaw

OBSERVED AND RELATIVE SURVIVAL (%) BY AGE (number of cases in parentheses)

	AGE CLASS										ALL	
	15-44		45-54		55-64		65-74		75-99			
	obs	rel	obs	rel	obs	rel	obs	rel	obs	rel	obs	rel
Males	(6)		(2)		(7)		(3)		(4)		(22)	
1 year	67	67	50	51	29	29	0	0	25	29	36	38
3 years	33	34	50	52	29	31	0	0	0	0	23	26
5 years	17	17	0	0	0	0	0	0	0	0	5	6
Females	(3)		(1)		(9)		(5)		(8)		(26)	
1 year	33	33	100	100	44	45	40	41	38	40	42	44
3 years	0	0	100	100	33	34	20	22	13	15	23	25
5 years	0	0	100	100	11	12	0	0	0	0	8	9
Overall	(9)		(3)		(16)		(8)		(12)		(48)	
1 year	56	56	67	67	38	38	25	26	33	37	40	41
3 years	22	22	67	68	31	33	13	14	8	11	23	25
5 years	11	11	33	35	6	7	0	0	0	0	6	7

SCOTLAND

AREA	NUMBER OF CASES			PERIOD	MEAN AGE		
	Males	Females	All		Males	Females	All
Scotland	141	123	264	1985-1989	61.5	62.7	62.1

OBSERVED AND RELATIVE SURVIVAL (%) BY AGE (number of cases in parentheses)

	AGE CLASS										ALL	
	15-44		45-54		55-64		65-74		75-99			
	obs	rel	obs	rel	obs	rel	obs	rel	obs	rel	obs	rel
Males	(29)		(19)		(17)		(36)		(40)		(141)	
1 year	76	76	79	80	82	84	39	41	33	37	55	58
3 years	48	49	53	54	47	50	22	26	15	23	33	38
5 years	34	35	21	22	24	26	17	22	10	21	20	26
Females	(20)		(15)		(28)		(21)		(39)		(123)	
1 year	100	100	93	94	75	76	52	54	31	34	63	66
3 years	70	70	67	68	39	41	29	31	8	10	36	40
5 years	35	35	33	34	25	27	10	11	3	4	18	22
Overall	(49)		(34)		(45)		(57)		(79)		(264)	
1 year	86	86	85	86	78	79	44	46	32	35	59	62
3 years	57	57	59	60	42	44	25	28	11	16	34	39
5 years	35	35	26	27	24	27	14	18	6	12	19	24

CHRONIC MYELOID LEUKAEMIA (ICD-9 205.1)

SLOVAKIA

AREA	NUMBER OF CASES			PERIOD	MEAN AGE		
	Males	Females	All		Males	Females	All
Slovakia	190	141	331	1985-1989	57.0	57.1	57.1

OBSERVED AND RELATIVE SURVIVAL (%) BY AGE (number of cases in parentheses)

	AGE CLASS										ALL	
	15-44		45-54		55-64		65-74		75-99			
	obs	rel	obs	rel	obs	rel	obs	rel	obs	rel	obs	rel
Males	(45)		(31)		(40)		(38)		(36)		(190)	
1 year	89	89	81	82	73	74	55	58	31	35	66	69
3 years	56	56	52	54	43	46	21	25	25	38	39	45
5 years	33	34	35	37	31	37	9	12	17	35	25	31
Females	(31)		(19)		(37)		(30)		(24)		(141)	
1 year	90	90	79	79	59	60	63	65	33	37	65	67
3 years	61	61	53	53	46	48	47	51	21	28	46	50
5 years	54	55	40	41	26	28	43	50	14	24	36	41
Overall	(76)		(50)		(77)		(68)		(60)		(331)	
1 year	89	90	80	81	66	67	59	61	32	36	66	68
3 years	58	58	52	54	44	47	32	37	23	34	42	47
5 years	41	42	37	39	29	33	24	30	16	30	30	35

SLOVENIA

AREA	NUMBER OF CASES			PERIOD	MEAN AGE		
	Males	Females	All		Males	Females	All
Slovenia	61	60	121	1985-1989	60.1	60.0	60.1

OBSERVED AND RELATIVE SURVIVAL (%) BY AGE (number of cases in parentheses)

	AGE CLASS										ALL	
	15-44		45-54		55-64		65-74		75-99			
	obs	rel	obs	rel	obs	rel	obs	rel	obs	rel	obs	rel
Males	(14)		(6)		(9)		(16)		(16)		(61)	
1 year	77	77	67	67	78	80	75	79	31	35	63	66
3 years	54	54	33	35	44	48	25	29	13	18	32	36
5 years	39	39	33	36	0	0	25	33	13	23	21	27
Females	(12)		(8)		(17)		(11)		(12)		(60)	
1 year	100	100	88	88	65	65	55	56	42	46	68	70
3 years	67	67	15	15	53	54	36	40	17	23	41	45
5 years	25	25	0	0	29	31	27	32	8	15	20	24
Overall	(26)		(14)		(26)		(27)		(28)		(121)	
1 year	88	88	79	79	69	70	67	69	36	40	66	68
3 years	60	60	22	23	50	52	30	34	14	20	36	41
5 years	32	32	11	12	19	21	26	33	11	20	21	25

CHRONIC MYELOID LEUKAEMIA   (ICD-9 205.1)

SPAIN

AREA	NUMBER OF CASES			PERIOD	MEAN AGE			5-YR RELATIVE SURVIVAL (%)	
	Males	Females	All		Males	Females	All	Males	Females
Basque Country	30	17	47	1986-1988	59.1	57.5	58.5		
Mallorca	7	6	13	1988-1989	76.1	54.5	66.2		
Navarra	18	8	26	1985-1989	61.7	56.9	60.2		
Tarragona	29	10	39	1985-1989	64.9	55.4	62.5		
Spanish Registries	84	41	125		63.1	56.5	60.9		

5-YR RELATIVE SURVIVAL (%) chart — Males scale: 100 80 60 40 20 0; Females scale: 0 20 40 60 80 100. Bars labelled: Basque, Mallor, Navarr, Tarrag.

OBSERVED AND RELATIVE SURVIVAL (%) BY AGE (number of cases in parentheses)

	AGE CLASS										ALL	
	15-44		45-54		55-64		65-74		75-99			
	obs	rel	obs	rel	obs	rel	obs	rel	obs	rel	obs	rel
Males	(12)		(5)		(21)		(24)		(22)		(84)	
1 year	83	83	80	80	81	82	58	60	32	35	62	64
3 years	58	59	80	81	57	59	17	19	18	24	37	41
5 years	58	59	80	83	36	39	13	15	18	30	30	37
Females	(9)		(9)		(11)		(8)		(4)		(41)	
1 year	100	100	67	67	55	55	100	100	25	27	73	74
3 years	67	67	44	45	45	46	50	52	25	31	49	50
5 years	67	67	44	45	7	7	25	27	25	37	32	35
Overall	(21)		(14)		(32)		(32)		(26)		(125)	
1 year	90	91	71	72	72	73	69	71	31	33	66	67
3 years	62	62	57	58	53	55	25	27	19	25	41	44
5 years	62	62	57	58	25	26	16	19	19	31	31	36

SWEDEN

AREA	NUMBER OF CASES			PERIOD	MEAN AGE		
	Males	Females	All		Males	Females	All
South Sweden	41	36	77	1985-1989	53.4	66.5	59.5

OBSERVED AND RELATIVE SURVIVAL (%) BY AGE (number of cases in parentheses)

	AGE CLASS										ALL	
	15-44		45-54		55-64		65-74		75-99			
	obs	rel	obs	rel	obs	rel	obs	rel	obs	rel	obs	rel
Males	(15)		(8)		(3)		(8)		(7)		(41)	
1 year	80	80	88	88	100	100	75	77	29	31	73	75
3 years	33	33	63	63	67	70	13	14	14	19	34	37
5 years	27	27	50	51	33	36	13	15	14	24	27	30
Females	(7)		(2)		(4)		(7)		(16)		(36)	
1 year	100	100	100	100	75	76	71	73	50	55	69	73
3 years	43	43	50	50	50	51	29	30	19	26	31	35
5 years	43	43	0	0	25	26	14	16	13	22	19	25
Overall	(22)		(10)		(7)		(15)		(23)		(77)	
1 year	86	86	90	90	86	87	73	75	43	48	71	74
3 years	36	37	60	61	57	59	20	22	17	24	32	36
5 years	32	32	40	41	29	30	13	15	13	23	23	28

CHRONIC MYELOID LEUKAEMIA (ICD-9 205.1)

SWITZERLAND

AREA	NUMBER OF CASES			PERIOD	MEAN AGE			5-YR RELATIVE SURVIVAL (%)	
	Males	Females	All		Males	Females	All	Males	Females
Basel	12	11	23	1985-1988	63.5	62.3	63.0		
Geneva	27	15	42	1985-1989	68.1	73.7	70.2		
Swiss Registries	39	26	65		66.8	69.0	67.6		

OBSERVED AND RELATIVE SURVIVAL (%) BY AGE (number of cases in parentheses)

	AGE CLASS										ALL	
	15-44		45-54		55-64		65-74		75-99			
	obs	rel	obs	rel	obs	rel	obs	rel	obs	rel	obs	rel
Males	(5)		(1)		(7)		(8)		(18)		(39)	
1 year	100	100	100	100	100	100	88	91	72	79	85	89
3 years	60	60	100	100	100	100	50	56	28	36	51	60
5 years	60	60	100	100	29	31	25	31	6	9	23	30
Females	(4)		(0)		(6)		(1)		(15)		(26)	
1 year	100	100	-	-	100	100	100	100	33	35	62	64
3 years	75	75	-	-	33	34	100	100	27	33	38	43
5 years	25	25	-	-	17	17	100	100	20	29	23	29
Overall	(9)		(1)		(13)		(9)		(33)		(65)	
1 year	100	100	100	100	100	100	89	92	55	59	75	79
3 years	67	67	100	100	69	71	56	62	27	35	46	53
5 years	44	45	100	100	23	24	33	41	12	19	23	30

CHRONIC MYELOID LEUKAEMIA (ICD-9 205.1)

EUROPE, 1985-89

Weighted analyses

COUNTRY	% COVERAGE WITH C.R.s	YEARLY NO. OF CASES (Mean No. of cases recorded) Males	Females	All
AUSTRIA	8	5	3	8
DENMARK	100	38	29	67
ENGLAND	50	173	143	316
ESTONIA	100	7	8	15
FINLAND	100	22	19	41
FRANCE	4	27	17	44
GERMANY	2	11	7	18
ICELAND	100	2	0	2
ITALY	10	58	42	100
NETHERLANDS	6	6	3	9
POLAND	6	8	10	18
SCOTLAND	100	28	25	53
SLOVAKIA	100	38	28	66
SLOVENIA	100	12	12	24
SPAIN	10	23	12	35
SWEDEN	17	8	7	15
SWITZERLAND	11	8	6	14

RELATIVE SURVIVAL (%) (Age-standardized) Males / Females

□ 1 year ■ 5 years

OBSERVED AND RELATIVE SURVIVAL (%) BY AGE

	AGE CLASS										ALL	
	15-44 obs rel		45-54 obs rel		55-64 obs rel		65-74 obs rel		75-99 obs rel		obs rel	
Males												
1 year	81	81	80	81	74	76	61	63	49	55	67	69
3 years	54	54	62	63	51	54	31	35	23	34	40	45
5 years	43	43	39	40	31	34	15	19	13	26	24	30
Females												
1 year	88	88	89	89	77	77	67	68	45	49	67	69
3 years	66	67	73	74	59	60	43	46	28	37	47	53
5 years	54	54	58	59	31	32	20	22	13	22	28	33
Overall												
1 year	84	84	84	84	75	76	63	65	48	53	67	69
3 years	59	59	67	68	54	57	36	40	25	35	43	48
5 years	47	47	47	48	31	33	17	20	13	25	26	31

AGE STANDARDIZED RELATIVE SURVIVAL(%)

COUNTRY	MALES 1-year (95% C.I.)	5-years (95% C.I.)	FEMALES 1-year (95% C.I.)	5-years (95% C.I.)
AUSTRIA	82.5 (82.3 - 82.6)	35.1 (19.8 - 62.3)	67.5 (67.2 - 67.8)	17.0 (16.6 - 17.5)
DENMARK	59.4 (53.1 - 66.5)	15.5 (11.1 - 21.7)	70.2 (63.6 - 77.5)	26.8 (20.3 - 35.2)
ENGLAND	62.7 (59.5 - 66.1)	21.6 (18.7 - 25.1)	65.1 (61.7 - 68.8)	26.5 (23.1 - 30.4)
ESTONIA	72.4 (62.1 - 84.5)	26.6 (11.3 - 62.2)	56.1 (40.0 - 78.6)	21.0 (13.2 - 33.4)
FINLAND	62.0 (53.1 - 72.4)	26.5 (17.6 - 39.8)	76.9 (68.3 - 86.6)	36.4 (26.6 - 49.6)
FRANCE	76.9 (69.5 - 85.1)	35.6 (26.9 - 47.0)	78.7 (69.6 - 89.0)	45.8 (31.9 - 65.5)
GERMANY	74.4 (59.9 - 92.5)	-	68.7 (56.6 - 83.4)	39.9 (29.0 - 55.1)
ICELAND	-	-	-	-
ITALY	62.8 (56.3 - 69.9)	23.1 (17.7 - 30.1)	73.2 (66.3 - 80.8)	27.7 (21.0 - 36.5)
NETHERLANDS	48.7 (36.4 - 65.2)	18.5 (10.7 - 32.1)	-	-
POLAND	31.4 (16.7 - 59.0)	2.9 (0.5 - 17.4)	46.4 (31.1 - 69.3)	12.8 (9.5 - 17.3)
SCOTLAND	57.4 (49.9 - 66.0)	24.6 (17.1 - 35.5)	63.3 (56.0 - 71.5)	18.3 (12.5 - 26.6)
SLOVAKIA	61.2 (54.2 - 69.2)	30.4 (21.5 - 42.9)	60.8 (52.7 - 70.1)	37.7 (28.1 - 50.4)
SLOVENIA	63.1 (52.1 - 76.5)	25.4 (15.1 - 42.7)	65.3 (53.6 - 79.6)	21.7 (12.0 - 39.0)
SPAIN	61.9 (52.5 - 73.0)	38.8 (28.5 - 53.0)	64.7 (50.6 - 82.7)	35.6 (18.8 - 67.4)
SWEDEN	68.0 (55.0 - 84.1)	27.7 (13.8 - 55.8)	75.1 (62.5 - 90.3)	22.6 (11.6 - 43.9)
SWITZERLAND	91.0 (82.4 -100.5)	36.2 (24.7 - 53.2)	-	-
EUROPE, 1985-89	67.7 (63.5 - 72.2)	30.3 (24.1 - 38.3)	69.3 (65.4 - 73.5)	33.4 (28.6 - 39.0)

LEUKAEMIA   (ICD-9 204-208)

AUSTRIA

AREA	NUMBER OF CASES			PERIOD	MEAN AGE		
	Males	Females	All		Males	Females	All
Tirol	64	48	112	1988-1989	59.6	62.9	61.0

OBSERVED AND RELATIVE SURVIVAL (%) BY AGE (number of cases in parentheses)

	AGE CLASS										ALL	
	15-44		45-54		55-64		65-74		75-99			
	obs	rel	obs	rel	obs	rel	obs	rel	obs	rel	obs	rel
Males	(14)		(5)		(13)		(13)		(19)		(64)	
1 year	71	72	60	60	54	54	77	79	63	69	66	68
3 years	57	57	40	41	54	56	62	67	21	28	45	50
5 years	57	57	40	41	46	49	46	54	16	27	39	47
Females	(7)		(7)		(12)		(8)		(14)		(48)	
1 year	71	71	71	72	83	84	38	38	50	54	63	64
3 years	57	57	71	72	67	68	25	26	36	46	50	54
5 years	57	57	43	43	58	60	13	14	29	45	40	45
Overall	(21)		(12)		(25)		(21)		(33)		(112)	
1 year	71	72	67	67	68	69	62	63	58	63	64	66
3 years	57	57	58	59	60	62	48	51	27	36	47	52
5 years	57	57	42	42	52	54	33	38	21	34	39	46

DENMARK

AREA	NUMBER OF CASES			PERIOD	MEAN AGE		
	Males	Females	All		Males	Females	All
Denmark	1645	1227	2872	1985-1989	66.5	67.5	66.9

OBSERVED AND RELATIVE SURVIVAL (%) BY AGE (number of cases in parentheses)

	AGE CLASS										ALL	
	15-44		45-54		55-64		65-74		75-99			
	obs	rel	obs	rel	obs	rel	obs	rel	obs	rel	obs	rel
Males	(167)		(112)		(303)		(503)		(560)		(1645)	
1 year	74	74	66	67	60	61	59	62	36	40	53	56
3 years	46	46	50	51	39	41	35	41	18	27	32	38
5 years	41	42	38	39	27	30	21	28	11	20	22	29
Females	(135)		(86)		(185)		(336)		(485)		(1227)	
1 year	70	70	59	60	61	61	51	52	45	49	53	55
3 years	43	43	35	35	42	44	35	38	21	28	32	36
5 years	36	36	27	27	32	34	26	30	10	16	22	27
Overall	(302)		(198)		(488)		(839)		(1045)		(2872)	
1 year	72	72	63	63	60	61	56	58	40	44	53	56
3 years	45	45	43	44	40	42	35	39	20	27	32	37
5 years	39	39	33	34	29	32	23	29	10	18	22	28

LEUKAEMIA   (ICD-9 204-208)

ENGLAND

AREA	NUMBER OF CASES			PERIOD	MEAN AGE			5-YR RELATIVE SURVIVAL (%)	
	Males	Females	All		Males	Females	All	Males	Females
East Anglia	487	349	836	1985-1989	66.8	68.6	67.6		
Mersey	438	381	819	1985-1989	65.3	66.8	66.0		
Oxford	490	453	943	1985-1989	65.7	69.3	67.5		
South Thames	1071	940	2011	1985-1989	64.5	67.7	66.0		
Wessex	814	681	1495	1985-1989	65.4	70.7	67.8		
West Midlands	1160	869	2029	1985-1989	64.0	66.8	65.2		
Yorkshire	822	677	1499	1985-1989	65.1	69.0	66.8		
English Registries	5282	4350	9632		65.0	68.3	66.5		

OBSERVED AND RELATIVE SURVIVAL (%) BY AGE (number of cases in parentheses)

	AGE CLASS										ALL	
	15-44		45-54		55-64		65-74		75-99			
	obs	rel	obs	rel	obs	rel	obs	rel	obs	rel	obs	rel
Males	(665)		(411)		(955)		(1526)		(1724)		(5281)	
1 year	66	66	69	69	64	65	51	54	36	41	52	55
3 years	39	39	45	46	45	47	32	36	21	30	32	38
5 years	32	32	32	33	34	38	21	27	11	20	22	29
Females	(473)		(308)		(602)		(1035)		(1932)		(4350)	
1 year	67	67	66	66	60	61	51	53	36	40	49	51
3 years	43	43	45	45	42	43	34	37	20	27	31	35
5 years	37	37	37	37	32	34	26	29	13	21	23	29
Overall	(1138)		(719)		(1557)		(2561)		(3656)		(9631)	
1 year	67	67	68	68	62	63	51	53	36	40	50	53
3 years	41	41	45	46	44	46	33	36	20	28	32	37
5 years	34	34	34	35	33	36	23	28	12	21	23	29

ESTONIA

AREA	NUMBER OF CASES			PERIOD	MEAN AGE		
	Males	Females	All		Males	Females	All
Estonia	320	265	585	1985-1989	60.1	60.5	60.3

OBSERVED AND RELATIVE SURVIVAL (%) BY AGE (number of cases in parentheses)

	AGE CLASS										ALL	
	15-44		45-54		55-64		65-74		75-99			
	obs	rel	obs	rel	obs	rel	obs	rel	obs	rel	obs	rel
Males	(49)		(40)		(87)		(87)		(57)		(320)	
1 year	47	47	63	63	79	81	60	63	53	59	62	65
3 years	31	31	50	52	67	73	36	42	35	51	45	52
5 years	22	23	37	40	48	57	25	34	21	42	32	41
Females	(39)		(35)		(69)		(83)		(39)		(265)	
1 year	62	62	66	66	67	67	61	63	44	48	61	62
3 years	41	41	54	55	55	57	49	55	26	34	47	51
5 years	33	34	49	50	45	48	35	42	23	38	37	43
Overall	(88)		(75)		(156)		(170)		(96)		(585)	
1 year	53	54	64	65	74	75	61	63	49	54	62	64
3 years	35	36	52	54	62	66	42	49	31	44	46	51
5 years	27	28	42	45	47	53	30	39	22	40	34	42

LEUKAEMIA (ICD-9 204-208)

FINLAND

AREA	NUMBER OF CASES			PERIOD	MEAN AGE		
	Males	Females	All		Males	Females	All
Finland	920	811	1731	1985-1989	61.3	65.0	63.0

OBSERVED AND RELATIVE SURVIVAL (%) BY AGE (number of cases in parentheses)

	AGE CLASS										ALL	
	15-44		45-54		55-64		65-74		75-99			
	obs	rel	obs	rel	obs	rel	obs	rel	obs	rel	obs	rel
Males	(175)		(108)		(166)		(239)		(232)		(920)	
1 year	75	75	75	76	69	71	54	57	43	48	60	63
3 years	50	50	51	52	57	61	34	39	23	35	40	46
5 years	38	38	43	44	42	47	22	28	14	28	29	37
Females	(102)		(85)		(128)		(213)		(283)		(811)	
1 year	73	73	71	71	65	65	53	54	43	47	56	58
3 years	45	45	54	55	49	50	36	38	27	36	38	42
5 years	39	39	36	37	38	40	27	31	17	27	28	34
Overall	(277)		(193)		(294)		(452)		(515)		(1731)	
1 year	74	74	73	73	67	68	54	55	43	48	58	61
3 years	48	48	52	53	54	56	35	39	25	35	39	45
5 years	38	39	40	41	40	44	25	30	16	28	28	35

FRANCE

AREA	NUMBER OF CASES			PERIOD	MEAN AGE			5-YR RELATIVE SURVIVAL (%)
	Males	Females	All		Males	Females	All	Males / Females
Somme	151	115	266	1985-1989	62.6	65.0	63.6	
Calvados	96	75	171	1985-1989	60.5	62.0	61.2	
Côte d'Or	209	158	367	1985-1989	69.6	65.6	67.9	
Doubs	97	86	183	1985-1989	60.0	63.4	61.6	
French Registries	553	434	987		64.4	64.4	64.4	

OBSERVED AND RELATIVE SURVIVAL (%) BY AGE (number of cases in parentheses)

	AGE CLASS										ALL	
	15-44		45-54		55-64		65-74		75-99			
	obs	rel	obs	rel	obs	rel	obs	rel	obs	rel	obs	rel
Males	(67)		(44)		(121)		(156)		(165)		(553)	
1 year	71	71	74	75	75	76	71	73	51	57	66	69
3 years	45	45	62	64	60	64	50	56	29	41	47	54
5 years	40	41	53	56	52	58	39	48	19	34	37	48
Females	(66)		(37)		(79)		(105)		(147)		(434)	
1 year	77	77	84	84	73	74	72	73	61	66	70	73
3 years	49	49	66	67	66	67	57	60	42	55	53	59
5 years	38	38	63	64	54	56	44	49	30	49	42	50
Overall	(133)		(81)		(200)		(261)		(312)		(987)	
1 year	74	74	79	79	74	75	71	73	56	62	68	71
3 years	47	47	64	65	62	65	53	58	35	47	49	56
5 years	39	39	58	60	53	57	41	48	24	42	40	49

LEUKAEMIA   (ICD-9 204-208)

GERMANY

AREA	NUMBER OF CASES			PERIOD	MEAN AGE		
	Males	Females	All		Males	Females	All
Saarland	252	203	455	1985-1989	59.7	65.4	62.3

OBSERVED AND RELATIVE SURVIVAL (%) BY AGE (number of cases in parentheses)

	AGE CLASS										ALL	
	15-44		45-54		55-64		65-74		75-99			
	obs	rel	obs	rel	obs	rel	obs	rel	obs	rel	obs	rel
Males	(47)		(30)		(64)		(65)		(46)		(252)	
1 year	79	79	67	67	69	70	48	50	39	44	60	62
3 years	51	51	43	44	45	48	32	38	24	35	39	44
5 years	44	45	34	35	33	36	26	34	21	43	31	39
Females	(15)		(21)		(42)		(56)		(69)		(203)	
1 year	60	60	81	81	67	67	57	58	36	39	55	56
3 years	53	53	71	72	62	63	43	46	20	25	43	47
5 years	53	54	65	66	52	55	31	35	14	21	34	41
Overall	(62)		(51)		(106)		(121)		(115)		(455)	
1 year	74	74	73	73	68	69	52	54	37	41	57	59
3 years	52	52	55	56	52	54	37	42	22	29	41	45
5 years	46	47	47	48	41	44	28	35	17	28	33	40

ICELAND

AREA	NUMBER OF CASES			PERIOD	MEAN AGE		
	Males	Females	All		Males	Females	All
Iceland	42	33	75	1985-1989	59.8	66.7	62.8

OBSERVED AND RELATIVE SURVIVAL (%) BY AGE (number of cases in parentheses)

	AGE CLASS										ALL	
	15-44		45-54		55-64		65-74		75-99			
	obs	rel	obs	rel	obs	rel	obs	rel	obs	rel	obs	rel
Males	(12)		(3)		(4)		(10)		(13)		(42)	
1 year	50	50	0	0	75	76	80	83	38	43	52	54
3 years	17	17	0	0	25	26	70	78	23	32	31	35
5 years	0	0	0	0	25	26	50	60	8	13	17	20
Females	(7)		(2)		(3)		(5)		(16)		(33)	
1 year	71	71	50	50	67	67	60	61	31	35	48	51
3 years	57	57	50	50	0	0	40	43	19	26	30	35
5 years	29	29	50	51	0	0	20	22	6	11	15	20
Overall	(19)		(5)		(7)		(15)		(29)		(75)	
1 year	58	58	20	20	71	72	73	75	34	38	51	53
3 years	32	32	20	20	14	15	60	66	21	28	31	35
5 years	11	11	20	20	14	15	40	47	7	12	16	20

LEUKAEMIA (ICD-9 204-208)

ITALY

AREA	NUMBER OF CASES			PERIOD	MEAN AGE			5-YR RELATIVE SURVIVAL (%)	
	Males	Females	All		Males	Females	All	Males	Females
Florence	346	242	588	1985-1989	62.5	65.4	63.7		
Genoa	121	113	234	1986-1988	66.0	67.5	66.7		
Latina	59	41	100	1985-1987	60.1	52.0	56.8		
Modena	69	46	115	1988-1989	65.6	68.2	66.6		
Parma	93	60	153	1985-1987	66.7	68.3	67.3		
Ragusa	60	42	102	1985-1989	65.5	62.2	64.1		
Romagna	93	70	163	1986-1988	62.4	68.1	64.9		
Turin	120	84	204	1985-1987	59.2	67.5	62.7		
Varese	204	176	380	1985-1989	60.4	66.0	63.0		
Italian Registries	1165	874	2039		62.7	65.8	64.0		

(Bar chart, 5-YR RELATIVE SURVIVAL (%) for Males and Females, scale 100 80 60 40 20 0 / 0 20 40 60 80 100, rows: Floren, Genoa, Latina, Modena, Parma, Ragusa, Romagn, Turin, Varese)

OBSERVED AND RELATIVE SURVIVAL (%) BY AGE (number of cases in parentheses)

	AGE CLASS										ALL	
	15-44		45-54		55-64		65-74		75-99			
	obs	rel	obs	rel	obs	rel	obs	rel	obs	rel	obs	rel
Males	(158)		(135)		(233)		(318)		(321)		(1165)	
1 year	59	59	54	54	52	53	51	53	38	42	49	51
3 years	37	37	37	38	36	38	30	34	15	21	29	33
5 years	32	32	30	31	29	31	19	24	9	15	21	26
Females	(99)		(80)		(169)		(197)		(329)		(874)	
1 year	63	63	58	58	59	59	53	54	44	48	53	54
3 years	37	37	43	43	45	46	36	38	24	31	34	38
5 years	31	31	37	37	37	38	25	28	17	25	26	31
Overall	(257)		(215)		(402)		(515)		(650)		(2039)	
1 year	60	61	56	56	55	55	52	54	41	45	51	52
3 years	37	37	39	40	40	41	32	35	20	26	31	35
5 years	31	32	33	33	32	34	21	25	13	21	23	28

NETHERLANDS

AREA	NUMBER OF CASES			PERIOD	MEAN AGE		
	Males	Females	All		Males	Females	All
Eindhoven	169	109	278	1985-1989	62.5	63.6	62.9

OBSERVED AND RELATIVE SURVIVAL (%) BY AGE (number of cases in parentheses)

	AGE CLASS										ALL	
	15-44		45-54		55-64		65-74		75-99			
	obs	rel	obs	rel	obs	rel	obs	rel	obs	rel	obs	rel
Males	(24)		(23)		(31)		(49)		(42)		(169)	
1 year	67	67	70	70	71	72	43	45	29	32	51	54
3 years	50	50	57	58	52	54	27	30	13	19	35	41
5 years	46	46	42	44	26	28	24	31	11	21	27	34
Females	(19)		(9)		(19)		(25)		(37)		(109)	
1 year	58	58	67	67	79	80	52	53	35	38	53	55
3 years	47	47	56	56	63	64	36	38	24	31	40	44
5 years	42	42	44	45	41	42	36	41	16	25	32	38
Overall	(43)		(32)		(50)		(74)		(79)		(278)	
1 year	63	63	69	69	74	75	46	48	32	35	52	54
3 years	49	49	56	57	56	58	30	33	19	25	37	42
5 years	44	44	43	44	31	34	28	35	13	23	29	35

LEUKAEMIA   (ICD-9 204-208)

POLAND

AREA	NUMBER OF CASES			PERIOD	MEAN AGE			5-YR RELATIVE SURVIVAL (%)	
	Males	Females	All		Males	Females	All	Males	Females
Cracow	88	70	158	1985-1989	59.5	62.5	60.8		
Warsaw	82	71	153	1988-1989	64.1	64.5	64.3		
Polish Registries	170	141	311		61.7	63.5	62.5		

OBSERVED AND RELATIVE SURVIVAL (%) BY AGE (number of cases in parentheses)

	AGE CLASS										ALL	
	15-44		45-54		55-64		65-74		75-99			
	obs	rel	obs	rel	obs	rel	obs	rel	obs	rel	obs	rel
Males	(24)		(23)		(40)		(37)		(46)		(170)	
1 year	54	54	43	44	35	36	30	31	13	15	32	34
3 years	21	21	26	27	28	30	19	22	9	13	19	23
5 years	13	13	13	14	15	17	14	18	4	9	11	15
Females	(19)		(16)		(34)		(27)		(45)		(141)	
1 year	37	37	38	38	29	30	37	38	22	24	30	32
3 years	5	5	19	19	21	21	30	33	13	18	18	20
5 years	5	5	13	13	12	13	11	13	4	7	8	10
Overall	(43)		(39)		(74)		(64)		(91)		(311)	
1 year	47	47	41	41	32	33	33	34	18	20	31	33
3 years	14	14	23	24	24	26	23	27	11	15	19	21
5 years	9	9	13	14	14	15	13	16	4	8	10	13

SCOTLAND

AREA	NUMBER OF CASES			PERIOD	MEAN AGE		
	Males	Females	All		Males	Females	All
Scotland	1102	972	2074	1985-1989	64.5	67.4	65.9

OBSERVED AND RELATIVE SURVIVAL (%) BY AGE (number of cases in parentheses)

	AGE CLASS										ALL	
	15-44		45-54		55-64		65-74		75-99			
	obs	rel	obs	rel	obs	rel	obs	rel	obs	rel	obs	rel
Males	(137)		(96)		(213)		(313)		(343)		(1102)	
1 year	66	67	63	63	61	62	49	51	33	38	50	53
3 years	45	45	47	48	47	51	33	39	16	24	33	39
5 years	34	35	35	37	33	38	20	26	9	19	22	30
Females	(113)		(78)		(133)		(253)		(395)		(972)	
1 year	58	58	54	54	60	61	47	49	33	37	45	47
3 years	38	38	38	39	35	36	31	34	18	24	27	32
5 years	31	31	29	30	23	24	22	26	10	18	19	25
Overall	(250)		(174)		(346)		(566)		(738)		(2074)	
1 year	63	63	59	59	61	62	48	50	33	37	48	50
3 years	42	42	43	44	42	45	32	37	17	24	31	36
5 years	33	33	33	34	29	32	21	26	10	19	21	27

LEUKAEMIA   (ICD-9 204-208)

SLOVAKIA

AREA	NUMBER OF CASES			PERIOD	MEAN AGE		
	Males	Females	All		Males	Females	All
Slovakia	976	760	1736	1985-1989	61.6	60.9	61.3

OBSERVED AND RELATIVE SURVIVAL (%) BY AGE (number of cases in parentheses)

	15-44		45-54		55-64		65-74		75-99		ALL	
	obs	rel	obs	rel	obs	rel	obs	rel	obs	rel	obs	rel
Males	(135)		(116)		(223)		(286)		(216)		(976)	
1 year	62	62	66	67	62	64	57	60	36	41	55	58
3 years	39	39	51	53	40	44	37	44	25	36	37	43
5 years	28	29	41	44	32	37	27	37	18	36	28	37
Females	(118)		(98)		(177)		(183)		(184)		(760)	
1 year	69	69	62	63	59	60	52	54	50	55	57	59
3 years	36	36	47	48	40	42	38	42	34	46	38	42
5 years	30	30	36	37	29	31	28	34	24	39	28	34
Overall	(253)		(214)		(400)		(469)		(400)		(1736)	
1 year	65	65	64	65	61	62	55	57	43	47	56	59
3 years	37	37	49	50	40	43	37	43	29	41	37	43
5 years	29	29	39	41	31	35	27	35	20	38	28	35

SLOVENIA

AREA	NUMBER OF CASES			PERIOD	MEAN AGE		
	Males	Females	All		Males	Females	All
Slovenia	337	338	675	1985-1989	61.1	63.4	62.3

OBSERVED AND RELATIVE SURVIVAL (%) BY AGE (number of cases in parentheses)

	15-44		45-54		55-64		65-74		75-99		ALL	
	obs	rel	obs	rel	obs	rel	obs	rel	obs	rel	obs	rel
Males	(52)		(53)		(71)		(75)		(86)		(337)	
1 year	67	67	66	67	62	63	61	64	38	43	57	60
3 years	41	42	45	47	37	40	37	43	17	26	34	39
5 years	35	36	29	31	26	29	27	36	7	14	23	30
Females	(56)		(30)		(68)		(76)		(108)		(338)	
1 year	61	61	67	67	70	71	62	64	43	47	57	60
3 years	41	41	39	39	53	55	45	49	23	31	38	43
5 years	29	29	28	29	40	42	38	45	17	28	29	35
Overall	(108)		(83)		(139)		(151)		(194)		(675)	
1 year	64	64	66	67	66	67	61	64	41	45	57	60
3 years	41	41	43	44	45	47	41	46	21	29	36	41
5 years	32	32	29	30	32	35	33	41	12	23	26	33

LEUKAEMIA (ICD-9 204-208)

SPAIN

AREA	NUMBER OF CASES			PERIOD	MEAN AGE			5-YR RELATIVE SURVIVAL (%)	
	Males	Females	All		Males	Females	All	Males	Females
Basque Country	205	130	335	1986-1988	60.6	62.5	61.3		
Mallorca	43	36	79	1988-1989	63.5	61.6	62.7		
Navarra	98	71	169	1985-1989	62.2	63.2	62.6		
Tarragona	133	62	195	1985-1989	64.9	63.8	64.6		
Spanish Registries	479	299	778		62.4	62.8	62.5		

OBSERVED AND RELATIVE SURVIVAL (%) BY AGE (number of cases in parentheses)

	AGE CLASS										ALL	
	15-44		45-54		55-64		65-74		75-99			
	obs	rel	obs	rel	obs	rel	obs	rel	obs	rel	obs	rel
Males	(75)		(38)		(110)		(132)		(124)		(479)	
1 year	67	67	58	58	70	71	51	52	50	56	58	60
3 years	45	46	47	48	52	54	33	37	35	49	41	46
5 years	43	43	40	41	45	49	26	32	21	38	33	41
Females	(46)		(29)		(65)		(77)		(82)		(299)	
1 year	67	67	52	52	63	63	60	61	56	60	60	61
3 years	33	33	41	42	51	52	43	45	43	53	43	46
5 years	33	33	37	37	41	42	30	33	32	47	34	39
Overall	(121)		(67)		(175)		(209)		(206)		(778)	
1 year	67	67	55	55	67	68	54	55	52	58	59	61
3 years	40	41	45	45	51	53	37	40	38	51	42	46
5 years	39	39	39	39	44	46	28	32	25	42	33	40

SWEDEN

AREA	NUMBER OF CASES			PERIOD	MEAN AGE		
	Males	Females	All		Males	Females	All
South Sweden	446	319	765	1985-1989	65.7	69.3	67.2

OBSERVED AND RELATIVE SURVIVAL (%) BY AGE (number of cases in parentheses)

	AGE CLASS										ALL	
	15-44		45-54		55-64		65-74		75-99			
	obs	rel	obs	rel	obs	rel	obs	rel	obs	rel	obs	rel
Males	(49)		(39)		(71)		(140)		(147)		(446)	
1 year	82	82	79	80	73	74	55	57	44	48	59	62
3 years	51	51	59	60	54	56	33	37	24	33	37	43
5 years	47	47	44	45	32	35	26	32	12	22	26	34
Females	(36)		(16)		(38)		(91)		(138)		(319)	
1 year	69	69	88	88	66	66	58	59	42	46	55	57
3 years	42	42	56	57	42	43	42	44	30	41	38	43
5 years	33	33	38	38	32	33	31	34	19	32	26	34
Overall	(85)		(55)		(109)		(231)		(285)		(765)	
1 year	76	77	82	82	71	71	56	58	43	47	57	60
3 years	47	47	58	59	50	51	36	40	27	37	38	43
5 years	41	41	42	43	32	34	28	33	15	27	26	34

LEUKAEMIA (ICD-9 204-208)

SWITZERLAND

AREA	NUMBER OF CASES			PERIOD	MEAN AGE			5-YR RELATIVE SURVIVAL (%)	
	Males	Females	All		Males	Females	All	Males	Females
Basel	113	81	194	1985-1988	63.9	66.9	65.2		
Geneva	96	75	171	1985-1989	67.5	69.2	68.2		
Swiss Registries	209	156	365		65.6	68.0	66.6		

OBSERVED AND RELATIVE SURVIVAL (%) BY AGE (number of cases in parentheses)

	AGE CLASS										ALL	
	15-44		45-54		55-64		65-74		75-99			
	obs	rel	obs	rel	obs	rel	obs	rel	obs	rel	obs	rel
Males	(26)		(17)		(33)		(59)		(74)		(209)	
1 year	77	77	94	95	73	74	68	70	64	70	70	74
3 years	54	54	65	66	58	60	51	57	34	46	47	55
5 years	42	43	59	61	39	43	42	52	19	33	35	45
Females	(23)		(5)		(32)		(25)		(71)		(156)	
1 year	61	61	40	40	78	78	72	73	31	34	52	54
3 years	43	44	40	40	46	46	56	59	23	30	36	41
5 years	34	34	20	20	39	40	44	49	17	28	28	36
Overall	(49)		(22)		(65)		(84)		(145)		(365)	
1 year	69	69	82	82	75	76	69	71	48	52	62	65
3 years	49	49	59	60	52	53	52	58	28	38	43	49
5 years	38	39	50	51	39	42	43	51	18	31	32	41

LEUKAEMIA   (ICD-9 204-208)

EUROPE, 1985-89
Weighted analyses

COUNTRY	% COVERAGE WITH C.R.s	YEARLY NO. OF CASES (Mean No. of cases recorded) Males	Females	All
AUSTRIA	8	32	24	56
DENMARK	100	329	245	574
ENGLAND	50	1056	870	1926
ESTONIA	100	64	53	117
FINLAND	100	184	162	346
FRANCE	4	111	87	198
GERMANY	2	50	41	91
ICELAND	100	8	7	15
ITALY	10	319	238	557
NETHERLANDS	6	34	22	56
POLAND	6	59	50	109
SCOTLAND	100	220	194	414
SLOVAKIA	100	195	152	347
SLOVENIA	100	67	68	135
SPAIN	10	136	88	224
SWEDEN	17	89	64	153
SWITZERLAND	11	48	35	83

RELATIVE SURVIVAL (%) (Age-standardized)

□ 1 year   ■ 5 years

OBSERVED AND RELATIVE SURVIVAL (%) BY AGE

	AGE CLASS 15-44 obs rel	45-54 obs rel	55-64 obs rel	65-74 obs rel	75-99 obs rel	ALL obs rel
Males						
1 year	68 68	65 65	64 65	54 56	41 46	56 58
3 years	43 43	47 48	47 49	36 40	22 32	37 42
5 years	38 38	37 39	36 39	26 33	15 28	28 35
Females						
1 year	65 65	68 68	64 64	57 58	43 47	55 57
3 years	42 42	53 53	51 52	41 44	27 35	39 43
5 years	37 37	45 46	41 43	30 34	19 29	30 36
Overall						
1 year	67 67	66 66	64 64	55 57	42 46	56 58
3 years	43 43	49 50	49 51	38 42	24 33	38 42
5 years	37 38	41 42	38 41	28 33	16 28	29 35

AGE STANDARDIZED RELATIVE SURVIVAL(%)

COUNTRY	MALES 1-year (95% C.I.)	5-years (95% C.I.)	FEMALES 1-year (95% C.I.)	5-years (95% C.I.)
AUSTRIA	68.6 (57.4 - 82.1)	43.1 (30.8 - 60.4)	58.9 (45.9 - 75.6)	40.6 (27.3 - 60.4)
DENMARK	56.3 (53.9 - 58.9)	28.5 (26.0 - 31.2)	55.7 (52.9 - 58.7)	26.5 (23.8 - 29.4)
ENGLAND	54.3 (52.9 - 55.7)	27.9 (26.5 - 29.4)	52.8 (51.3 - 54.4)	29.2 (27.6 - 30.8)
ESTONIA	63.1 (57.1 - 69.7)	39.9 (32.4 - 49.3)	58.7 (52.0 - 66.3)	41.4 (33.6 - 51.0)
FINLAND	60.4 (57.1 - 64.0)	34.1 (30.3 - 38.3)	57.4 (54.0 - 61.0)	33.0 (29.5 - 36.9)
FRANCE	68.3 (64.3 - 72.7)	44.9 (39.6 - 51.0)	72.5 (68.1 - 77.1)	50.2 (44.3 - 56.8)
GERMANY	56.7 (50.1 - 64.1)	39.0 (30.4 - 49.9)	55.6 (49.0 - 62.9)	38.9 (32.0 - 47.2)
ICELAND	56.4 (43.5 - 73.3)	25.4 (13.8 - 46.5)	53.7 (37.7 - 76.4)	17.7 (7.8 - 40.4)
ITALY	50.0 (47.1 - 53.2)	24.0 (21.3 - 27.0)	54.5 (51.2 - 58.0)	30.0 (26.8 - 33.6)
NETHERLANDS	50.5 (43.3 - 58.8)	30.1 (22.5 - 40.2)	54.5 (46.0 - 64.6)	36.2 (27.3 - 48.0)
POLAND	30.6 (24.4 - 38.4)	13.9 (8.7 - 22.1)	31.7 (24.6 - 40.9)	10.0 (5.6 - 17.8)
SCOTLAND	51.6 (48.6 - 54.7)	27.8 (24.8 - 31.2)	48.6 (45.5 - 52.0)	24.1 (21.2 - 27.5)
SLOVAKIA	55.0 (51.7 - 58.6)	36.3 (32.0 - 41.2)	58.0 (54.3 - 61.9)	34.9 (30.5 - 39.9)
SLOVENIA	57.5 (52.0 - 63.6)	27.0 (21.7 - 33.6)	59.0 (53.8 - 64.7)	35.3 (29.7 - 42.1)
SPAIN	59.2 (54.7 - 64.2)	39.2 (33.5 - 45.9)	61.0 (55.4 - 67.1)	39.8 (33.4 - 47.5)
SWEDEN	62.4 (57.9 - 67.1)	32.2 (27.5 - 37.7)	59.9 (54.7 - 65.7)	33.5 (27.9 - 40.3)
SWITZERLAND	73.8 (67.7 - 80.4)	43.5 (36.1 - 52.5)	56.4 (48.8 - 65.1)	35.9 (27.9 - 46.4)
EUROPE, 1985-89	56.5 (54.8 - 58.3)	33.5 (31.3 - 35.8)	57.1 (55.2 - 59.0)	35.3 (33.2 - 37.4)

513

MALIGNANT NEOPLASMS   (ICD-9 140-208)

AUSTRIA

AREA	NUMBER OF CASES			PERIOD	MEAN AGE		
	Males	Females	All		Males	Females	All
Tirol	2071	2262	4333	1988-1989	65.6	64.1	64.8

OBSERVED AND RELATIVE SURVIVAL (%) BY AGE (number of cases in parentheses)

	AGE CLASS					ALL
	15-44	45-54	55-64	65-74	75-99	
	obs rel	obs rel	obs rel	obs rel	obs rel	obs rel
Males	(172)	(198)	(479)	(584)	(638)	(2071)
1 year	87 87	66 66	63 64	66 68	53 58	63 65
3 years	72 72	53 53	46 48	46 50	32 41	44 49
5 years	70 70	50 51	42 44	35 41	23 37	37 45
Females	(292)	(311)	(385)	(589)	(685)	(2262)
1 year	89 89	78 79	79 80	66 67	54 58	70 71
3 years	84 84	67 68	63 64	52 54	37 45	55 60
5 years	78 78	59 60	58 60	43 47	28 40	48 54
Overall	(464)	(509)	(864)	(1173)	(1323)	(4333)
1 year	89 89	73 74	70 71	66 68	54 58	66 68
3 years	79 80	61 62	54 55	49 52	35 43	50 55
5 years	75 75	56 57	49 51	39 44	26 39	43 50

DENMARK

AREA	NUMBER OF CASES			PERIOD	MEAN AGE		
	Males	Females	All		Males	Females	All
Denmark	49950	54362	104312	1985-1989	66.8	64.9	65.8

OBSERVED AND RELATIVE SURVIVAL (%) BY AGE (number of cases in parentheses)

	AGE CLASS					ALL
	15-44	45-54	55-64	65-74	75-99	
	obs rel	obs rel	obs rel	obs rel	obs rel	obs rel
Males	(3755)	(4026)	(9956)	(16910)	(15303)	(49950)
1 year	81 81	61 61	53 54	51 53	43 48	52 55
3 years	68 69	42 43	33 35	31 35	22 32	32 38
5 years	64 64	37 38	26 29	22 28	14 26	25 32
Females	(5781)	(6916)	(11243)	(14701)	(15721)	(54362)
1 year	90 90	80 80	69 70	61 63	46 50	64 66
3 years	78 78	64 65	52 54	44 48	28 37	48 52
5 years	71 71	58 59	45 48	37 42	20 32	40 47
Overall	(9536)	(10942)	(21199)	(31611)	(31024)	(104312)
1 year	86 86	73 73	62 63	56 58	45 49	58 61
3 years	74 74	56 57	44 46	37 41	25 34	40 46
5 years	68 69	50 52	36 39	29 35	17 29	33 41

MALIGNANT NEOPLASMS   (ICD-9 140-208)

ENGLAND

AREA	NUMBER OF CASES			PERIOD	MEAN AGE			5-YR RELATIVE SURVIVAL (%)	
	Males	Females	All		Males	Females	All	Males	Females
East Anglia	18073	17959	36032	1985-1989	68.8	66.4	67.6		
Mersey	21045	21914	42959	1985-1989	67.0	65.5	66.2		
Oxford	20997	22000	42997	1985-1989	67.4	65.3	66.3		
South Thames	48484	52501	100985	1985-1989	67.6	66.1	66.8		
Wessex	28539	29329	57868	1985-1989	68.5	66.6	67.6		
West Midlands	46586	45324	91910	1985-1989	67.3	65.7	66.5		
Yorkshire	32632	33448	66080	1985-1989	67.6	66.1	66.9		
English Registries	16356	22475	438832		67.7	66.0	67.0		

5-YR RELATIVE SURVIVAL (%): Males scale 100 80 60 40 20 0; Females scale 0 20 40 60 80 100. Bars for E.Angl, Mersey, Oxford, S.Tham, Wessex, W.Midl, Yorksh.

OBSERVED AND RELATIVE SURVIVAL (%) BY AGE (number of cases in parentheses)

	AGE CLASS										ALL	
	15-44		45-54		55-64		65-74		75-99			
	obs	rel	obs	rel	obs	rel	obs	rel	obs	rel	obs	rel
Males	(12179)		(15715)		(44683)		(74398)		(69380)		(216355)	
1 year	78	78	58	59	50	51	45	47	38	43	47	49
3 years	65	65	41	42	33	35	28	32	21	30	30	35
5 years	60	61	35	37	27	30	21	27	14	26	23	31
Females	(22166)		(24716)		(44191)		(59424)		(71978)		(222475)	
1 year	88	88	80	81	68	68	57	58	41	45	60	62
3 years	75	75	65	66	52	53	41	44	25	33	44	49
5 years	69	69	58	59	45	47	34	39	18	30	37	45
Overall	(34345)		(40431)		(88874)		(133822)		(141358)		(438830)	
1 year	84	85	72	72	59	60	50	52	40	44	53	56
3 years	71	72	56	56	42	44	34	37	23	32	37	42
5 years	66	66	49	51	36	39	27	32	16	28	30	38

ESTONIA

AREA	NUMBER OF CASES			PERIOD	MEAN AGE		
	Males	Females	All		Males	Females	All
Estonia	9371	9815	19186	1985-1989	61.7	62.1	61.9

OBSERVED AND RELATIVE SURVIVAL (%) BY AGE (number of cases in parentheses)

	AGE CLASS										ALL	
	15-44		45-54		55-64		65-74		75-99			
	obs	rel	obs	rel	obs	rel	obs	rel	obs	rel	obs	rel
Males	(674)		(1638)		(3166)		(2399)		(1494)		(9371)	
1 year	57	57	49	50	43	44	41	43	34	39	43	45
3 years	39	40	28	29	22	24	22	26	17	25	24	27
5 years	35	36	22	24	17	20	16	21	10	19	18	22
Females	(1107)		(1640)		(2556)		(2430)		(2082)		(9815)	
1 year	81	81	79	79	66	67	54	56	38	42	61	63
3 years	62	63	59	60	48	50	36	40	20	27	43	47
5 years	56	56	53	54	40	43	29	34	14	25	36	42
Overall	(1781)		(3278)		(5722)		(4829)		(3576)		(19186)	
1 year	72	72	64	65	53	54	48	50	37	41	52	54
3 years	54	54	44	45	34	36	29	33	19	26	33	37
5 years	48	48	38	40	27	31	22	28	12	23	27	33

MALIGNANT NEOPLASMS   (ICD-9 140-208)

FINLAND

AREA	NUMBER OF CASES			PERIOD	MEAN AGE		
	Males	Females	All		Males	Females	All
Finland	33791	36589	70380	1985-1989	65.7	64.7	65.1

OBSERVED AND RELATIVE SURVIVAL (%) BY AGE (number of cases in parentheses)

	AGE CLASS										ALL	
	15-44		45-54		55-64		65-74		75-99			
	obs	rel	obs	rel	obs	rel	obs	rel	obs	rel	obs	rel
Males	(2476)		(3106)		(8297)		(10854)		(9058)		(33791)	
1 year	80	80	65	65	60	61	57	60	51	57	59	62
3 years	66	67	47	48	39	41	36	42	29	41	38	44
5 years	61	62	41	42	31	34	27	35	18	34	29	38
Females	(4145)		(4778)		(7350)		(9384)		(10932)		(36589)	
1 year	91	91	88	88	78	78	66	67	48	52	69	71
3 years	81	81	76	76	62	64	48	52	29	39	53	58
5 years	74	75	69	70	55	58	40	46	21	34	45	54
Overall	(6621)		(7884)		(15647)		(20238)		(19990)		(70380)	
1 year	87	87	79	79	68	69	61	63	49	54	64	66
3 years	75	76	64	65	50	52	42	46	29	40	46	52
5 years	69	70	58	59	42	46	33	40	20	34	38	46

FRANCE

AREA	NUMBER OF CASES			PERIOD	MEAN AGE			5-YR RELATIVE SURVIVAL (%)	
	Males	Females	All		Males	Females	All	Males	Females
Somme	5297	3542	8839	1985-1989	64.2	63.4	63.9		
Calvados	5576	4056	9632	1985-1989	63.8	63.1	63.5		
Doubs	3910	2938	6848	1985-1989	64.0	62.7	63.4		
French Registries	14783	10536	25319		64.0	63.1	63.6		

OBSERVED AND RELATIVE SURVIVAL (%) BY AGE (number of cases in parentheses)

	AGE CLASS										ALL	
	15-44		45-54		55-64		65-74		75-99			
	obs	rel	obs	rel	obs	rel	obs	rel	obs	rel	obs	rel
Males	(1143)		(1927)		(4265)		(3979)		(3469)		(14783)	
1 year	78	78	65	66	62	63	62	64	54	60	62	64
3 years	58	58	40	41	37	39	40	45	31	43	38	43
5 years	51	52	33	35	30	33	31	38	21	38	30	37
Females	(1466)		(1481)		(2382)		(2320)		(2887)		(10536)	
1 year	91	91	88	88	83	83	74	76	60	65	76	79
3 years	79	79	72	73	65	66	56	59	38	49	59	64
5 years	73	73	67	68	58	60	49	54	28	45	51	59
Overall	(2609)		(3408)		(6647)		(6299)		(6356)		(25319)	
1 year	85	85	75	75	69	70	66	68	57	62	68	70
3 years	70	70	54	55	47	49	46	50	34	46	47	52
5 years	63	64	48	49	40	43	37	44	24	41	39	47

MALIGNANT NEOPLASMS   (ICD-9 140-208)

GERMANY

AREA	NUMBER OF CASES			PERIOD	MEAN AGE		
	Males	Females	All		Males	Females	All
Saarland	9837	9981	19818	1985-1989	64.0	65.5	64.7

OBSERVED AND RELATIVE SURVIVAL (%) BY AGE (number of cases in parentheses)

	AGE CLASS										ALL	
	15-44		45-54		55-64		65-74		75-99			
	obs	rel	obs	rel	obs	rel	obs	rel	obs	rel	obs	rel
Males	(731)		(1410)		(2660)		(2665)		(2371)		(9837)	
1 year	81	81	63	64	59	60	56	59	45	51	57	60
3 years	65	66	43	44	39	42	37	43	25	37	38	44
5 years	61	62	37	39	32	35	30	39	18	36	31	40
Females	(828)		(1309)		(2143)		(2611)		(3090)		(9981)	
1 year	90	90	84	85	74	75	66	67	49	53	67	69
3 years	78	78	69	70	59	60	50	54	31	41	51	56
5 years	71	71	62	63	52	55	42	48	23	38	43	52
Overall	(1559)		(2719)		(4803)		(5276)		(5461)		(19818)	
1 year	86	86	73	74	66	67	61	63	47	52	62	64
3 years	72	72	56	57	48	50	44	49	29	39	45	50
5 years	66	67	49	51	41	44	36	44	21	37	37	46

ICELAND

AREA	NUMBER OF CASES			PERIOD	MEAN AGE		
	Males	Females	All		Males	Females	All
Iceland	1787	1738	3525	1985-1989	66.9	63.2	65.1

OBSERVED AND RELATIVE SURVIVAL (%) BY AGE (number of cases in parentheses)

	AGE CLASS										ALL	
	15-44		45-54		55-64		65-74		75-99			
	obs	rel	obs	rel	obs	rel	obs	rel	obs	rel	obs	rel
Males	(160)		(128)		(378)		(529)		(592)		(1787)	
1 year	83	83	70	70	71	72	63	65	54	60	64	67
3 years	72	72	51	52	54	56	45	50	32	45	46	52
5 years	66	66	46	47	46	49	37	44	22	39	37	47
Females	(232)		(247)		(394)		(401)		(464)		(1738)	
1 year	95	95	83	83	75	76	67	69	50	54	70	72
3 years	85	86	69	70	58	60	53	56	34	45	56	61
5 years	78	78	62	63	53	55	44	50	25	40	48	56
Overall	(392)		(375)		(772)		(930)		(1056)		(3525)	
1 year	90	90	78	79	73	74	65	66	52	57	67	70
3 years	80	80	63	64	56	58	48	52	33	45	51	57
5 years	73	73	56	57	50	52	40	47	23	39	43	51

MALIGNANT NEOPLASMS　　(ICD-9 140-208)

ITALY

AREA	NUMBER OF CASES			PERIOD	MEAN AGE			5-YR RELATIVE SURVIVAL (%)	
	Males	Females	All		Males	Females	All	Males	Females
Florence	14593	12369	26962	1985-1989	66.6	65.7	66.2		
Genoa	5391	4740	10131	1986-1988	66.3	66.0	66.2		
Latina	1616	1348	2964	1985-1987	64.0	60.4	62.3		
Modena	3111	2553	5664	1988-1989	66.0	65.8	65.9		
Parma	3003	2622	5625	1985-1987	66.9	65.9	66.4		
Ragusa	1852	1625	3477	1985-1989	66.9	63.5	65.3		
Romagna	3422	2851	6273	1986-1988	66.3	65.0	65.7		
Turin	6041	5551	11592	1985-1987	64.5	64.3	64.4		
Varese	8169	7308	15477	1985-1989	64.5	64.7	64.6		
Italian Registries	47198	40967	88166		65.8	65.1	65.5		

OBSERVED AND RELATIVE SURVIVAL (%) BY AGE (number of cases in parentheses)

	AGE CLASS										ALL	
	15-44		45-54		55-64		65-74		75-99			
	obs	rel	obs	rel	obs	rel	obs	rel	obs	rel	obs	rel
Males	(2470)		(4990)		(12703)		(14671)		(12364)		(47198)	
1 year	77	77	63	64	57	58	53	55	44	49	54	56
3 years	62	63	44	45	38	39	33	37	23	32	35	39
5 years	57	58	39	40	32	35	26	31	15	27	28	34
Females	(3774)		(5663)		(8880)		(10304)		(12346)		(40967)	
1 year	89	89	86	86	77	77	66	68	49	52	68	70
3 years	77	77	72	73	60	62	50	53	30	38	52	56
5 years	71	71	65	66	53	55	42	47	22	34	45	52
Overall	(6244)		(10653)		(21583)		(24975)		(24710)		(88165)	
1 year	84	84	75	76	65	66	59	60	46	51	61	63
3 years	71	72	59	60	47	49	40	44	27	35	43	47
5 years	66	66	53	54	41	43	32	38	19	31	36	43

NETHERLANDS

AREA	NUMBER OF CASES			PERIOD	MEAN AGE		
	Males	Females	All		Males	Females	All
Eindhoven	6963	6158	13121	1985-1989	65.3	62.2	63.9

OBSERVED AND RELATIVE SURVIVAL (%) BY AGE (number of cases in parentheses)

	AGE CLASS										ALL	
	15-44		45-54		55-64		65-74		75-99			
	obs	rel	obs	rel	obs	rel	obs	rel	obs	rel	obs	rel
Males	(474)		(732)		(1728)		(2309)		(1720)		(6963)	
1 year	78	78	62	63	60	60	54	56	48	54	57	59
3 years	65	65	43	44	38	40	33	38	25	36	36	41
5 years	60	61	37	38	31	34	24	31	16	30	28	35
Females	(851)		(997)		(1358)		(1453)		(1499)		(6158)	
1 year	89	90	86	86	76	77	69	70	52	56	72	74
3 years	78	78	73	74	60	61	51	55	33	42	56	60
5 years	71	71	66	67	52	54	43	48	25	39	48	55
Overall	(1325)		(1729)		(3086)		(3762)		(3219)		(13121)	
1 year	85	86	76	76	67	68	60	62	50	55	64	66
3 years	73	74	61	61	48	49	40	45	29	39	45	50
5 years	67	68	54	55	40	43	32	38	20	34	37	45

MALIGNANT NEOPLASMS   (ICD-9 140-208)

POLAND

AREA	NUMBER OF CASES			PERIOD	MEAN AGE			5-YR RELATIVE SURVIVAL (%)	
	Males	Females	All		Males	Females	All	Males	Females
Cracow	4071	4473	8544	1985-1989	61.7	61.1	61.4		
Warsaw	3929	4649	8578	1988-1989	63.0	62.9	62.9		
Polish Registries	8000	9122	17122		62.3	62.0	62.2		

Males: 100 80 60 40 20 0   Females: 0 20 40 60 80 100   Cracow   Warsaw

OBSERVED AND RELATIVE SURVIVAL (%) BY AGE (number of cases in parentheses)

	AGE CLASS										ALL	
	15-44		45-54		55-64		65-74		75-99			
	obs	rel	obs	rel	obs	rel	obs	rel	obs	rel	obs	rel
Males	(666)		(1114)		(2739)		(2047)		(1434)		(8000)	
1 year	67	67	44	45	41	42	36	38	25	28	40	41
3 years	48	49	25	26	22	24	19	23	11	16	22	25
5 years	44	45	19	21	17	19	13	18	7	12	16	21
Females	(1162)		(1458)		(2473)		(1953)		(2076)		(9122)	
1 year	80	80	76	76	61	62	48	50	30	33	56	58
3 years	63	63	57	58	43	45	30	33	17	22	39	43
5 years	57	57	50	51	36	39	24	29	11	17	33	38
Overall	(1828)		(2572)		(5212)		(4000)		(3510)		(17122)	
1 year	75	75	62	62	51	52	42	44	28	31	48	50
3 years	57	58	43	44	32	34	24	28	14	20	31	35
5 years	52	53	37	38	26	29	18	24	9	16	25	31

SCOTLAND

AREA	NUMBER OF CASES			PERIOD	MEAN AGE		
	Males	Females	All		Males	Females	All
Scotland	49800	51664	101464	1985-1989	67.1	66.2	66.6

OBSERVED AND RELATIVE SURVIVAL (%) BY AGE (number of cases in parentheses)

	AGE CLASS										ALL	
	15-44		45-54		55-64		65-74		75-99			
	obs	rel	obs	rel	obs	rel	obs	rel	obs	rel	obs	rel
Males	(2763)		(3913)		(11246)		(17195)		(14683)		(49800)	
1 year	77	77	56	56	47	48	44	46	35	39	45	47
3 years	64	65	39	39	30	32	26	31	18	27	28	33
5 years	60	61	33	35	24	27	19	25	11	22	21	29
Females	(4658)		(5795)		(10604)		(13946)		(16661)		(51664)	
1 year	87	87	77	77	63	63	52	53	38	41	55	58
3 years	74	74	61	62	46	47	35	39	22	30	40	45
5 years	67	68	55	56	39	41	29	34	15	26	33	41
Overall	(7421)		(9708)		(21850)		(31141)		(31344)		(101464)	
1 year	83	83	69	69	55	56	47	49	36	40	50	53
3 years	70	71	52	53	37	39	30	34	20	29	34	39
5 years	64	65	46	47	31	34	23	29	13	24	27	35

MALIGNANT NEOPLASMS   (ICD-9 140-208)

SLOVAKIA

AREA	NUMBER OF CASES			PERIOD	MEAN AGE		
	Males	Females	All		Males	Females	All
Slovakia	36363	27926	64289	1985-1989	62.2	61.1	61.7

OBSERVED AND RELATIVE SURVIVAL (%) BY AGE (number of cases in parentheses)

	15-44		45-54		55-64		65-74		75-99		ALL	
	obs	rel	obs	rel	obs	rel	obs	rel	obs	rel	obs	rel
Males	(3372)		(5553)		(11052)		(9589)		(6797)		(36363)	
1 year	65	66	52	53	48	49	44	47	39	44	48	50
3 years	47	48	31	32	27	30	27	32	23	35	29	33
5 years	42	43	26	28	23	26	21	29	18	36	24	31
Females	(4049)		(4481)		(7129)		(6481)		(5786)		(27926)	
1 year	84	84	77	78	66	67	54	56	40	44	62	64
3 years	67	67	60	61	49	51	37	41	24	33	45	50
5 years	60	60	54	55	42	45	31	37	19	33	39	46
Overall	(7421)		(10034)		(18181)		(16070)		(12583)		(64289)	
1 year	76	76	64	64	55	56	48	50	40	44	54	56
3 years	58	59	44	45	36	38	31	36	24	34	36	41
5 years	52	53	38	40	30	34	25	33	18	35	30	38

SLOVENIA

AREA	NUMBER OF CASES			PERIOD	MEAN AGE		
	Males	Females	All		Males	Females	All
Slovenia	12900	12200	25100	1985-1989	62.1	62.0	62.1

OBSERVED AND RELATIVE SURVIVAL (%) BY AGE (number of cases in parentheses)

	15-44		45-54		55-64		65-74		75-99		ALL	
	obs	rel	obs	rel	obs	rel	obs	rel	obs	rel	obs	rel
Males	(1104)		(2124)		(4010)		(3102)		(2560)		(12900)	
1 year	69	69	51	51	46	47	43	46	36	40	46	48
3 years	52	53	30	31	24	26	23	27	17	25	26	29
5 years	47	48	24	25	18	20	16	21	11	21	19	24
Females	(1576)		(1897)		(3154)		(2777)		(2796)		(12200)	
1 year	85	85	80	81	69	70	56	57	38	42	63	65
3 years	70	70	63	63	51	52	39	42	23	31	46	50
5 years	62	63	54	55	43	46	31	36	16	28	38	45
Overall	(2680)		(4021)		(7164)		(5879)		(5356)		(25100)	
1 year	78	78	65	65	56	57	49	51	37	41	54	56
3 years	63	63	46	47	36	38	30	34	20	28	36	40
5 years	56	57	38	40	29	32	23	28	14	25	29	35

MALIGNANT NEOPLASMS   (ICD-9 140-208)

SPAIN

AREA	NUMBER OF CASES			PERIOD	MEAN AGE			5-YR RELATIVE SURVIVAL (%)	
	Males	Females	All		Males	Females	All	Males	Females
Basque Country	10186	6582	16768	1986-1988	63.1	62.6	62.9		
Navarra	4332	3097	7429	1985-1989	65.1	63.4	64.4		
Tarragona	4076	3134	7210	1985-1989	65.8	63.8	65.0		
Spanish Registries	18594	12813	31407		64.2	63.1	63.7		

5-YR RELATIVE SURVIVAL (%) bar chart: Males (scale 100 80 60 40 20 0), Females (scale 0 20 40 60 80 100), with bars labelled Basque, Navarr, Tarrag.

OBSERVED AND RELATIVE SURVIVAL (%) BY AGE (number of cases in parentheses)

	AGE CLASS										ALL	
	15-44		45-54		55-64		65-74		75-99			
	obs	rel	obs	rel	obs	rel	obs	rel	obs	rel	obs	rel
Males	(1444)		(2298)		(5015)		(5624)		(4213)		(18594)	
1 year	75	75	63	64	60	60	55	56	48	53	57	59
3 years	58	59	45	46	42	43	36	40	30	40	39	44
5 years	55	56	40	41	36	39	29	36	22	38	33	40
Females	(1636)		(1803)		(2867)		(3252)		(3255)		(12813)	
1 year	89	89	84	85	75	76	64	65	48	52	69	70
3 years	76	77	68	69	60	61	49	51	31	39	53	57
5 years	69	69	61	61	54	55	42	46	25	38	46	52
Overall	(3080)		(4101)		(7882)		(8876)		(7468)		(31407)	
1 year	82	82	73	73	65	66	58	60	48	53	62	64
3 years	68	68	55	56	48	50	41	44	30	40	45	49
5 years	63	63	49	50	42	45	34	39	24	38	38	45

SWEDEN

AREA	NUMBER OF CASES			PERIOD	MEAN AGE		
	Males	Females	All		Males	Females	All
South Sweden	14959	14559	29518	1985-1989	68.3	65.5	66.9

OBSERVED AND RELATIVE SURVIVAL (%) BY AGE (number of cases in parentheses)

	AGE CLASS										ALL	
	15-44		45-54		55-64		65-74		75-99			
	obs	rel	obs	rel	obs	rel	obs	rel	obs	rel	obs	rel
Males	(855)		(974)		(2736)		(5227)		(5167)		(14959)	
1 year	88	88	73	73	68	69	65	67	58	64	65	68
3 years	74	75	56	57	51	53	46	52	36	50	46	53
5 years	71	71	50	51	43	46	37	45	24	43	36	47
Females	(1538)		(1783)		(2736)		(3965)		(4537)		(14559)	
1 year	91	91	85	86	80	81	71	73	56	61	72	74
3 years	81	81	73	74	66	68	56	60	38	49	57	63
5 years	77	77	68	69	60	62	49	55	28	44	50	59
Overall	(2393)		(2757)		(5472)		(9192)		(9704)		(29518)	
1 year	90	90	81	81	74	75	68	70	57	62	68	71
3 years	79	79	67	68	58	60	51	55	37	49	51	58
5 years	75	75	62	63	51	54	42	50	26	43	43	53

MALIGNANT NEOPLASMS   (ICD-9 140-208)

SWITZERLAND

AREA	NUMBER OF CASES			PERIOD	MEAN AGE			5-YR RELATIVE SURVIVAL (%)	
	Males	Females	All		Males	Females	All	Males	Females
Basel	2976	2868	5844	1985-1988	66.2	65.6	65.9		
Geneva	3422	3449	6871	1985-1989	65.4	65.2	65.3		
Swiss Registries	6398	6317	12715		65.8	65.4	65.6		

OBSERVED AND RELATIVE SURVIVAL (%) BY AGE (number of cases in parentheses)

	AGE CLASS										ALL	
	15-44		45-54		55-64		65-74		75-99			
	obs	rel	obs	rel	obs	rel	obs	rel	obs	rel	obs	rel
Males	(514)		(693)		(1452)		(1808)		(1931)		(6398)	
1 year	86	87	72	72	66	67	62	64	53	58	63	66
3 years	72	73	50	51	45	47	42	47	32	45	43	49
5 years	67	68	44	45	36	39	32	39	22	39	34	43
Females	(689)		(878)		(1262)		(1388)		(2100)		(6317)	
1 year	94	94	89	89	82	83	71	72	55	60	73	75
3 years	82	82	74	75	67	68	53	56	37	48	57	62
5 years	75	76	66	67	59	61	46	51	27	43	48	57
Overall	(1203)		(1571)		(2714)		(3196)		(4031)		(12715)	
1 year	91	91	81	82	74	75	66	68	54	59	68	71
3 years	78	78	64	64	55	57	47	51	35	46	50	56
5 years	72	72	56	58	47	50	38	45	25	41	41	50

MALIGNANT NEOPLASMS (ICD-9 140-208)

EUROPE, 1985-89

Weighted analyses

COUNTRY	% COVERAGE WITH C.R.s	YEARLY NO. OF CASES (Mean No. of cases recorded)		
		Males	Females	All
AUSTRIA	8	1036	1131	2167
DENMARK	100	9990	10872	20862
ENGLAND	50	43271	44495	87766
ESTONIA	100	1874	1963	3837
FINLAND	100	6758	7318	14076
FRANCE	4	2957	2107	5064
GERMANY	2	1967	1996	3963
ICELAND	100	357	348	705
ITALY	10	12036	10475	22511
NETHERLANDS	6	1393	1232	2625
POLAND	6	2779	3219	5998
SCOTLAND	100	9960	10333	20293
SLOVAKIA	100	7273	5585	12858
SLOVENIA	100	2580	2440	5020
SPAIN	10	5077	3440	8517
SWEDEN	17	2992	2912	5904
SWITZERLAND	11	1428	1407	2835

RELATIVE SURVIVAL (%) (Age-standardized)

□ 1 year ■ 5 years

OBSERVED AND RELATIVE SURVIVAL (%) BY AGE

	AGE CLASS										ALL	
	15-44		45-54		55-64		65-74		75-99			
	obs	rel	obs	rel	obs	rel	obs	rel	obs	rel	obs	rel
Males												
1 year	78	78	61	62	56	57	53	55	44	49	54	57
3 years	62	62	42	43	37	39	34	38	25	35	35	40
5 years	57	58	36	38	30	33	26	33	17	31	28	35
Females												
1 year	89	89	83	84	73	74	63	65	47	51	66	68
3 years	76	76	68	69	57	59	47	50	30	38	50	55
5 years	70	70	61	62	50	53	40	45	22	35	43	50
Overall												
1 year	83	83	72	72	65	65	58	60	46	50	60	62
3 years	69	69	55	55	47	48	40	44	27	36	42	47
5 years	63	64	48	50	40	43	33	38	19	33	35	43

AGE STANDARDIZED RELATIVE SURVIVAL(%)

COUNTRY	MALES		FEMALES	
	1-year (95% C.I.)	5-years (95% C.I.)	1-year (95% C.I.)	5-years (95% C.I.)
AUSTRIA	65.4 (63.3 - 67.6)	44.3 (41.8 - 46.8)	70.4 (68.5 - 72.4)	51.9 (49.7 - 54.3)
DENMARK	55.3 (54.8 - 55.7)	31.8 (31.3 - 32.3)	64.9 (64.5 - 65.3)	44.8 (44.3 - 45.3)
ENGLAND	50.7 (50.5 - 50.9)	31.1 (30.8 - 31.3)	61.5 (61.3 - 61.7)	42.7 (42.5 - 43.0)
ESTONIA	44.1 (42.9 - 45.2)	22.0 (20.9 - 23.2)	59.0 (58.0 - 60.1)	37.5 (36.4 - 38.7)
FINLAND	61.7 (61.1 - 62.2)	37.7 (37.0 - 38.3)	69.5 (69.1 - 70.0)	50.1 (49.6 - 50.7)
FRANCE	64.0 (63.2 - 64.9)	37.7 (36.6 - 38.9)	76.7 (75.8 - 77.6)	55.7 (54.5 - 57.0)
GERMANY	59.1 (58.1 - 60.2)	39.2 (37.9 - 40.5)	68.6 (67.7 - 69.5)	50.1 (48.9 - 51.3)
ICELAND	67.3 (65.0 - 69.6)	45.8 (43.1 - 48.6)	69.8 (67.5 - 72.1)	52.1 (49.3 - 55.0)
ITALY	56.7 (56.2 - 57.1)	33.9 (33.4 - 34.4)	69.2 (68.7 - 69.7)	49.2 (48.7 - 49.8)
NETHERLANDS	59.2 (58.0 - 60.5)	34.7 (33.3 - 36.1)	71.0 (69.8 - 72.2)	50.7 (49.2 - 52.3)
POLAND	39.2 (38.1 - 40.4)	19.2 (18.1 - 20.3)	53.1 (52.0 - 54.1)	32.7 (31.6 - 33.8)
SCOTLAND	48.2 (47.7 - 48.7)	28.8 (28.4 - 29.3)	57.5 (57.1 - 58.0)	38.5 (38.1 - 39.0)
SLOVAKIA	48.9 (48.3 - 49.4)	31.7 (31.0 - 32.4)	59.5 (58.8 - 60.1)	41.6 (40.9 - 42.4)
SLOVENIA	46.9 (46.0 - 47.9)	23.5 (22.6 - 24.5)	60.6 (59.7 - 61.6)	40.0 (38.9 - 41.0)
SPAIN	58.7 (58.0 - 59.5)	39.4 (38.5 - 40.3)	67.8 (67.0 - 68.6)	49.2 (48.2 - 50.3)
SWEDEN	69.1 (68.4 - 69.9)	47.6 (46.6 - 48.6)	73.8 (73.1 - 74.6)	56.7 (55.7 - 57.6)
SWITZERLAND	66.0 (64.8 - 67.3)	42.2 (40.8 - 43.8)	74.6 (73.5 - 75.7)	54.9 (53.5 - 56.4)
EUROPE, 1985-89	56.7 (56.4 - 57.0)	35.0 (34.7 - 35.4)	66.9 (66.6 - 67.2)	47.5 (47.2 - 47.9)

Chapter 5

Overview of the EUROCARE-2 results on survival of cancer patients diagnosed in 1985–89

M. Sant and the EUROCARE Working Group

Introduction

The results from the first EUROCARE study, published in 1995, showed substantial differences in the survival of cancer patients in different European countries (Berrino *et al.*, 1995). The study included patients diagnosed between 1978 and 1985, and followed for 5–10 years. Systematic centralized data checking and uniform methods of statistical analysis ensured an unprecedented level of reliability. One of the main aims of the second EUROCARE project was to update the database by adding data for more recently diagnosed patients. This chapter provides an overview of the results of that project, for adult patients diagnosed between 1985 and 1989. A major aim of the forthcoming EUROCARE-3 project will be to explain the reasons for the marked differences in survival which have emerged from the basic analyses.

The first EUROCARE publication excluded certain tumours for which there were problems regarding standardization of data collection, diagnostic criteria or classification, which might have hindered meaningful comparison. The experience gained during EUROCARE-1, together with the increasing standardization between registries, made it possible to include practically all tumours in this second survey. In addition, new registries and new countries have been added to the project and the database, so that the present survey is based on about 1 300 000 cases involving 45 cancer sites, from 47 registries in 17 countries. EUROCARE-2 therefore provides a wider and more reliable picture of cancer survival in Europe, not only by including more countries from eastern and northern Europe, but also because countries such as France, Italy and Spain are better represented than before as a result of the inclusion of additional registries.

Where cancer registration is not nationwide, it is possible that survival in the registry areas may not be representative of survival in the country as a whole, since areas where registries are established may be better equipped than others in terms of oncological care. This potential bias is more likely to occur if the registries cover only a small fraction of the population.

In the present monograph, intercountry comparisons performed on the European pool of cancer cases show the 95% confidence intervals of the age-standardized figures. The numbers of cases included in the analyses by registry and country are given in the country-specific pages of Chapter 4. These indicators give an idea of the statistical variability.

A major advantage of multicentric studies is that they provide an opportunity to study rare tumours on a population basis, rather than from selected clinical series. The EUROCARE database includes a large number of rare tumours. Country-specific survival figures for such tumours, for example bone, soft tissue, testis, head and neck subsites, and specific types of leukaemia, are often based on few cases, so that random variability may have a relatively large effect on survival estimates, whereas the whole set of cases is able to give a reliable picture of the European situation.

An additional point is that this study reflects the prognoses of patients who were diagnosed with cancer approximately ten years ago. Analysis of time trends in survival, presented in Chapter 6, reveals a general increase in cancer survival over the entire period covered by the EUROCARE study and it is likely that this improvement has continued subsequently. Improvements in curative treatments affect mainly newly diagnosed patients, but surviving patients diagnosed some years ago will also benefit from recent improvements in supportive care, in the treatment of relapses and in palliative care (Verdecchia *et al.*, 1998). The present picture for European cancer patients is therefore probably better than that given by this survey.

This chapter gives an overview of the main results of the EUROCARE-2 survival analysis, presenting:

- the prognostic rank by tumour, based on the estimated average relative survival for the whole of Europe;
- a survey of intercountry differences in prognosis for some of the most common tumours;
- an analysis of the prognostic roles of sex and age at diagnosis;

- an analysis of the influence of socioeconomic and demographic indicators on survival for some of the most common tumours by means of simple correlation and multiple linear regression procedures.

More extensive presentations of the EUROCARE-2 data for selected tumour sites can be found in a special issue of the *European Journal of Cancer* (Coebergh *et al.*, 1998).

Methods

The data presented in the figures and tables of this chapter were derived from the five-year age-specific and age-adjusted survival data, which are reported separately for males and females in the summary European pages of Chapter 4. The following analyses were carried out on the basic data:

- Computation of age-adjusted relative survival rates for both sexes combined, as weighted means of the age-adjusted sex-specific survival, in order to present concisely both the survival rank by tumour and the range of geographic variability. The weightings used are the yearly mean numbers of cases recorded by country and sex, as reported in the monograph.

- Comparison of prognosis by country, age and sex, also expressed in terms of the risk ratio for death (RR). The RR was defined as the ratio of the logarithm of five-year relative survival of the group of interest to that of a chosen reference group.

- Calculation of Pearson correlation coefficients between certain country-specific socio-economic indicators and the five-year age-adjusted relative survival for some tumours. The aim here was to explore the influence on survival of socio-economic level in different countries. Country-specific indicators were taken from the OECD database (OECD, 1998). Multiple linear regression analysis with a stepwise method using the SAS system was carried out with socioeconomic indicators as independent variables and country-specific five-year age-standardized relative survival as dependent variable. The eastern European countries (Estonia, Poland, Slovakia and Slovenia) were excluded from this analysis, since the required socioeconomic data were not available in full from these countries for the period analysed.

Results

Tumour site and survival

Figure 1 shows the mean age-standardized five-year relative survival for Europe as a whole by tumour site, ranked from highest to lowest, for both sexes combined. To provide an indication of variability in survival between countries, excluding extremes, the figures for the countries with the second highest and second lowest survival are also given, as the white and black bars, respectively.

The survival rank reflects the natural history of the tumours and the efficacy of therapy. For tumours of high rank, some respond well to treatment (e.g., testicular cancer, Hodgkin's disease), others have a relatively good prognosis, particularly when treated appropriately (e.g., breast cancer, melanoma). Highly aggressive tumours for which therapy has little or no effect rank lowest (e.g., lung and pancreatic cancer).

In addition to the variation in tumour prognosis, Figure 1 highlights considerable intercountry differences in survival for several cancers. This variation is no surprise, as the first EUROCARE study already revealed large intercountry differences, particularly for tumours where stage at diagnosis is an important prognostic factor, such as stomach, colon, rectum and breast cancers.

Tumours with very poor prognosis are a challenge to clinical and pharmacological research, but from a public health perspective, it is important to focus on malignancies that can be cured, or for which survival can be prolonged, if effective treatment is given. In such cases, longer survival reflects the ability of a nation's health system to effectively manage the disease, whereas poor survival is likely to indicate that the necessary diagnostic and therapeutic facilities are generally unavailable. By contrast, the prognosis for low-survival tumours is probably related more to biological factors that are largely unmodified even by the best available treatment and early diagnosis modalities; this is the case for malignancies of the oesophagus, pancreas and pleura. For tumours of the lung, the slightly higher survival figures probably reflect the proportion of patients who are operated, since chemotherapy has little effect (Janssen-Heijnen *et al.*, 1998). The most effective approach to lung cancer remains prevention. For testicular cancer and Hodgkin's disease, survival is high, reflecting the fact that effective chemotherapy protocols have been in place since the 1970s (van Basten *et al.*, 1997). However, even for these malignancies, some variation is evident, with the lowest survival seen in eastern European countries. It is likely that this

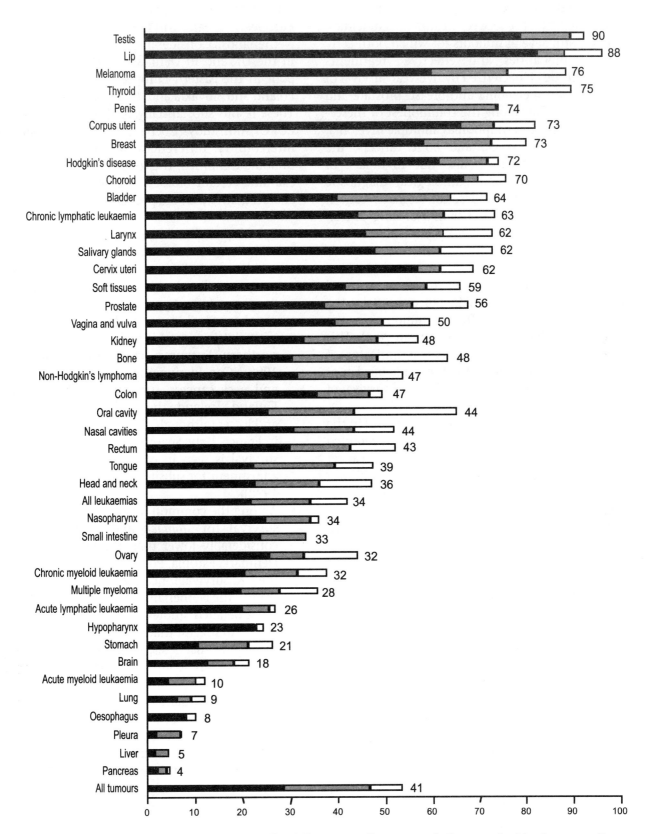

Figure 1. Comparison of mean age-standardized European five-year relative survival by tumour site, 1985–89. Mean weighted survival of males and females (except for sex-specific tumours).

Black = 2nd last value; grey and numbers = mean European survival; white = 2nd highest value.

variation reflects differences between countries in the availability of effective treatment guidelines, drugs or both. Several tumours for which both early diagnosis modalities and effective treatments are available are characterized by five-year survival of over 50%: skin melanoma and breast, prostate and thyroid cancer are among the commonest of these.

For non-Hodgkin's lymphomas, multiple myeloma, bladder, head and neck, and bone cancers, the variability of prognosis is also due to a lack of standardized clinical and pathological diagnostic criteria and registration rules. For stomach cancer, the lowest survival approaches that of lung cancer, but there is a wide difference between the lowest and highest survival, suggesting that there is room to improve care for this cancer.

The five-year survival for all tumours combined (excluding non-melanoma skin cancers) reflects the varying frequencies of different tumours in the countries contributing to the European pool. This figure must not be taken as a real indicator of prognosis, but represents the entire crude burden of cancer in Europe, and expresses the mean survival of all patients.

The ranking of survival by cancer site found in the present EUROCARE study is similar to that reported by the other major systematic survey of cancer survival, that of the SEER project in the USA (Ries *et al.*, 1991). However, for most sites, survival is lower in Europe, with a few exceptions, notably cancer of the stomach, although the European countries with highest survival have figures which approach those in the USA.

Geographical differences in survival

Figure 2 provides an overview of the variation in cancer survival between countries for some of the most common tumours, for both sexes combined. For each tumour site, the country-specific RR was calculated, using mean European survival for that tumour as reference category. The grey dots indicate an RR in the range 0.85–1.15, corresponding to survival levels similar to the European mean; the black dots indicate an RR > 1.15 and the white dots an RR < 0.85, i.e., lower and higher survival, respectively, than the European mean. Dots are absent for countries for which it was not possible to calculate age-standardized survival, due to lack of cases in one or more age classes. Note also that the figures for Austria, the Netherlands and Spain (and also Iceland for certain tumours) should be regarded with caution, due to the small number of cases.

Iceland, Sweden and Switzerland had the highest survival for many of the commonest tumours. For

some common tumours, survival was also above the European mean in Finland, France and the Netherlands. Considerably lower survival was seen in the UK and in Denmark. Survival was generally poor in the eastern European countries of Estonia, Poland and Slovakia and, to a lesser extent, Slovenia. These results substantially confirm those of the first EUROCARE study (Coebergh, 1995). This pattern of intercountry differences was consistent for all tumours examined; the following comments briefly examine certain biological, clinical and occurrence characteristics that are peculiar to each site.

- For *head and neck cancers*, the between-country variation in survival reflects the pattern of incidence of different subsites, which differ in prognosis. The incidence of tumours with poor prognosis (e.g., hypopharyngeal compared with oropharyngeal cancer; supraglottic compared with glottic cancer) is higher in southern than in northern European countries (Berrino *et al.*, 1998). Considering the entire category of head and neck cancers, survival is higher in Austria, Finland, Iceland, the Netherlands and Sweden, and lower (although close to the European mean) in France, Italy, Spain and Switzerland; the lowest survival is seen in eastern countries, even after adjustment for subsite distribution (Berrino *et al.*, 1998).

- Among the common *tumours of the digestive tract*, survival for *stomach* and *colorectal cancer* is considerably lower than the European mean in Denmark, Estonia, Poland, Slovakia, Slovenia and the UK. Survival for colorectal cancer is highest in France, the Netherlands, Sweden and Switzerland. More detailed studies (Sant *et al.*, 1995; Gatta *et al.*, 1996) suggest that these differences are related to stage at diagnosis, which was generally more advanced in countries with poor survival. Advanced stage contraindicates radical surgery, which is the main form of treatment for these cancers. The uneven distribution of diagnostic procedures such as endoscopy and occult blood detection in faeces may be assumed to have influenced survival for rectal and distal colon cancers during the study period: countries of more advanced socioeconomic level are more likely to have implemented these procedures, with a favourable effect on survival. It is also notable that Finland, Sweden and Switzerland, which generally are characterized by high survival, are among the lowest for tumours of the *pancreas*; in contrast, Slovakia, where cancer survival is generally low, has higher survival than

Figure 5.2. Death risk ratio of each country versus the mean age-adjusted five-year relative survival of the European pool of cancer patients. Both sexes (weighted mean)

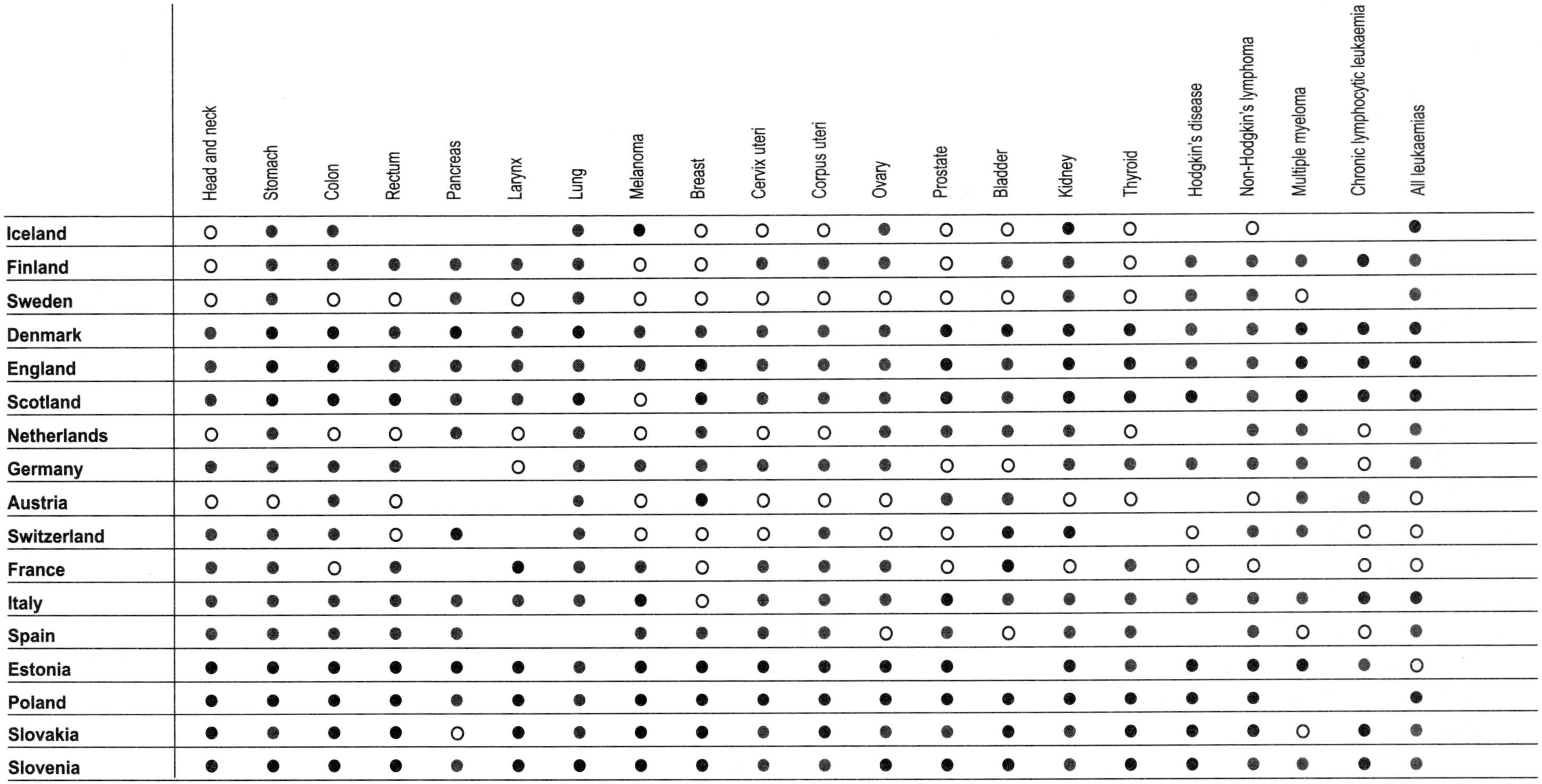

Cancer sites (columns): Head and neck, Stomach, Colon, Rectum, Pancreas, Larynx, Lung, Melanoma, Breast, Cervix uteri, Corpus uteri, Ovary, Prostate, Bladder, Kidney, Thyroid, Hodgkin's disease, Non-Hodgkin's lymphoma, Multiple myeloma, Chronic lymphocytic leukaemia, All leukaemias

Countries (rows): Iceland, Finland, Sweden, Denmark, England, Scotland, Netherlands, Germany, Austria, Switzerland, France, Italy, Spain, Estonia, Poland, Slovakia, Slovenia

● RR > 1.15
● RR = 0.85–1.15
○ RR < 0.85

Dots are absent for countries where it was not possible to calculate age-standardized survival, due to lack of cases in one or more age classes the European mean for pancreatic cancer. This finding is probably due to better diagnostic specificity in the wealthier and technologically better-equipped countries over the study period, rather than to genuinely better prognosis in Slovakia.

- Common cancers other than colorectal cancers for which early diagnosis is the main factor influencing survival are those of breast, cervix uteri, prostate and skin melanoma. For *skin melanoma*, the high survival in northern European countries may be related to greater awareness of skin lesions, leading to better diagnosis of early-stage melanomas which can be cured by surgery (Smith *et al.*, 1998). The low survival for melanoma in Italy is mainly confined to male patients, whereas for females survival is close to the European mean. Low survival in Italian melanoma cancer patients also emerged in another study (Balzi *et al.*, 1998). For *prostate cancer*, Finland, France, Germany, Iceland, Sweden and Switzerland have the highest survival; in Denmark, Italy and the UK, as well as in the eastern European countries, survival is below the European mean. This intercountry variation in survival corresponds to differences in the incidence of prostate cancer, which in turn reflect the availability of diagnostic facilities, and possibly also the inclusion of preclinical tumours with better prognosis which are detected within resected adenomas (Post *et al.*, 1998). Swedish counties with high incidence also had high survival, suggesting that increased diagnostic activity is related to survival, and patients with tumours confirmed by biopsy had higher survival than those with cytological and clinical diagnoses (Helgesen *et al.*, 1996). The low survival in Denmark has been explained by a lower level of diagnostic activity (Tretli *et al.*, 1996). The survival of patients with prostate cancer is closely related to stage at diagnosis, and this factor is probably responsible for at least some of the intercountry differences reported here. Since the 1980s, the spread of transurethral prostate resection (TURP) and of assays for prostate-specific antigen (PSA) has led to the improved detection of asymptomatic, early-stage lesions, and it may be assumed that these techniques were used earlier and more extensively in the wealthier countries of Europe. Similar considerations almost certainly apply to *breast cancer*. Over the period of this study, mammographic screening became established throughout Europe. In certain areas organized

screening was carried out, while in others so-called opportunistic screening was widely implemented, resulting in a general improvement in diagnosis. Breast cancer has some of the widest intercountry differences in survival. Survival is low in the eastern European countries, but is also fairly low in the UK and Denmark (although for Denmark the RR estimates in Figure 2 are close to the European mean). The highest survival levels are seen in the northern European countries and in France, Italy and Switzerland.

- Intercountry differences in survival for *tumours of the female genital tract* are less marked than for breast cancer. Survival for cancer of the *corpus and cervix uteri* is consistently high in Iceland, the Netherlands, Sweden and Switzerland, and lowest in Estonia and Poland, with all other countries fairly close to the European mean. Survival for *ovarian cancer*, which is little influenced by early diagnosis, is generally poor, especially in the elderly. Austria, Sweden and Switzerland have higher survival than the European mean for this cancer site.

- The survival of patients with *haematopoietic malignancies* varies markedly between countries. Differing classification criteria, which have varied over time, particularly for *multiple myeloma*, contributed to this variation. However, the large intercountry differences in outcome for *Hodgkin's disease* were unexpected, mainly because effective therapies for this disease have been available for two decades. This variability was already evident in EUROCARE-1, but it appears that the dissemination of effective treatment guide-lines is still a public health priority. France and Switzerland have the best survival for Hodgkin's disease; survival is close to the European mean in the northern European countries, and markedly lower than the mean in Estonia, Poland, Scotland, Slovakia and Spain. Intercountry survival differences are lower for *non-Hodgkin's lymphomas*, a group of malignancies that are commoner and have a worse prognosis than Hodgkin's disease; the best survival is seen in Austria, France and Iceland. For *all leukaemias* (ICD-9 codes 204–208) (World Health Organization, 1977), survival is lowest in Denmark, Iceland, Italy, Poland and the UK, and highest in Austria, Estonia, France and Switzerland. These differences are partly due to differences in case mix within this broad diagnostic category. Thus, *chronic lymphocytic leukaemia*, which has the best prognosis, constituted 51% of all leukaemias in Estonia (where survival is high) and 31% in Italy (where survival is low). However, differences in care must also be considered. Centralization of treatment has been shown to be effective for some haematological malignancies (Karjalainen et al., 1989; Selby et al., 1996). France has high survival for Hodgkin's and non-Hodgkin's lymphomas, all leukaemias combined, and chronic lymphocytic leukaemia. Most French cases derive from the specialized Côte d'Or registry, and it is possible that the existence of this registry is associated with a particularly good level of care for these diseases in that area.

- Intercountry differences in outcome of *tumours of the urinary tract* do not lend themselves to easy interpretation. *Bladder tumours* were excluded from EUROCARE-1 due to lack of standardized inclusion criteria between registries and of diagnostic criteria between pathologists; distinguishing between benign, borderline and invasive tumours in urothelial cells can be difficult. Only a few cancer registries taking part in EUROCARE-2 explicitly stated that they systematically include benign lesions of the bladder in their incidence series (Parkin et al., 1997), but it is likely that most registries do not perform systematic checks to determine lesion invasiveness for bladder cancer, so that benign lesions are also included. It was therefore decided to include all bladder tumours. It is noticeable that Switzerland, which is among the best for survival for most tumours, ranks very low, together with France, for bladder cancer. This is probably due to stricter classification and inclusion criteria rather than to lower-than-normal levels of care in these countries. Denmark and the UK have very poor survival for *kidney cancer*, close to the levels in Estonia and Poland. The main factor influencing survival for these tumours is stage distribution, and the frequency of early-stage tumours is related to the availability of imaging techniques. Histological type also plays a role, since urothelial tumours have better prognosis than renal-cell carcinomas, but since urothelial tumours constitute a small percentage of all renal tumours, stage remains the most important prognostic factor (Damhuis et al., 1998).

- For *thyroid cancer*, survival is above the European mean in Austria, Finland, Iceland, the Netherlands and Sweden, and below the mean in Denmark, Poland, Slovakia, Slovenia and the UK. Variation in the distribution of the two main histotypes, papillary carcinoma (better prognosis)

and follicular carcinoma (worse prognosis), may explain some of this variation. Papillary carcinoma is the most common histotype in western countries, but the ratio between this and follicular carcinoma varies from 4 in Iceland to 0.6 in Estonia (Teppo et al., 1998).

Age differences in survival

Table 1 shows five-year relative survival by age class, for both sexes combined (except for sex-specific tumours), for the entire weighted European pool of cases. Also given are the RRs of patients aged 75+ versus those aged 45–54 years. Figure 3 shows the pattern of five-year relative survival by age at diagnosis for selected tumour sites. Considering all tumours together, patients in the oldest age class have a 60% greater risk of death compared with those aged 45–54 years, even after adjustment for general mortality (i.e., considering relative survival), which is obviously greater in older patients. Prostate cancer is a notable exception to this pattern, in that survival in the youngest age class is lower than in patients aged 55 years and above, with no substantial decrease in survival with increasing age (Figure 3(a)). Breast cancer is also an exception (Figure 3(a)), as also revealed by a more detailed EUROCARE study, which showed lower survival among the youngest and oldest patients, with more favourable prognosis for women aged 40–49 years at diagnosis (Sant et al., 1998). Other studies have noted worse survival in the youngest and oldest breast cancer patients (Yancik et al., 1989; Albain et al., 1994; Quinn et al., 1998).

The most marked decrease in survival with advancing age is for thyroid cancer, where good survival among the youngest patients probably reflects more favourable histotypes (Teppo et al., 1998). A decrease in survival with increasing age at diagnosis is also marked for lymphomas (see Figure 3(b)) and here the explanation is probably the difficulty of administering adequate and complete chemotherapy to the elderly, due to impaired general health and the presence of comorbidity (Satariano et al., 1994; Piccirillo et al., 1996; Carli et al., 1998). For cancers of the cervix and corpus uteri (Figure 3(c)), more advanced stage at diagnosis is the main reason for the poorer survival of older patients, while for cancer of the ovary, the difficulty of administering adequate chemotherapy to elderly patients again plays a role (Kosary, 1994; Gatta et al., 1998).

For testicular cancer, which occurs mainly in younger patients, with relatively few cases in the 75+ age class, decreasing survival with age is evident on passing from the 45–54 to the 55–64 age class. For

Table 1. Five-year relative survival by tumour site and age at diagnosis, with risk ratio for death (RR) for the oldest age class versus those aged 45–54 years. Both sexes. Weighted European pool, 1985–89

Tumour site	Five-year relative survival of patients aged:					RR for 75+ vs 45-54
	15–44	45–54	55–64	65–74	75+	
Lip	97	89	91	88	86	1.3
Tongue	49	38	40	37	40	0.9
Oral cavity	51	53	43	44	30	1.9
Hypopharynx	30	23	26	21	12	1.4
Head and neck	46	39	36	34	31	1.2
Oesophagus	19	10	9	9	6	1.2
Stomach	38	31	25	21	15	1.6
Small intestine	46	43	40	29	27	1.6
Colon	57	53	49	48	42	1.4
Rectum	49	48	45	44	37	1.4
Liver	8	5	5	5	3	1.2
Gallbladder	15	21	12	13	9	1.5
Pancreas	14	6	3	4	3	1.2
Larynx	71	63	63	62	63	1.0
Lung	18	14	11	8	5	1.5
Pleura	19	8	5	9	3	1.4
Bone	56	49	58	42	29	1.7
Soft tissues	65	61	54	54	60	1.0
Melanoma	81	80	76	73	64	2.0
Breast	74	75	73	73	68	1.3
Cervix uteri	75	63	59	51	36	2.2
Corpus uteri	88	86	79	70	55	4.0
Ovary	65	45	34	20	18	2.1
Vagina and vulva	79	56	62	55	39	1.6
Prostate	53	49	58	60	51	0.9
Testis	91	92	85	58	59	6.3
Penis	87	76	67	68	77	1.0
Bladder	87	78	71	63	56	2.3
Kidney	63	59	53	45	36	1.9
Thyroid	97	86	73	55	36	6.8
Brain	45	18	9	4	6	1.6
Hodgkin's disease	84	77	58	39	32	4.4
Non-Hodgkin's lymphoma	63	59	53	42	31	2.2
Multiple myeloma	48	38	36	27	19	1.7
Acute lymphocytic leukaemia	38	20	21	7	11	1.4
Chronic lymphocytic leukaemia	88	75	72	63	54	2.1
Acute myeloid leukaemia	27	14	12	4	2	2.0
Chronic myeloid leukaemia	48	47	32	20	24	1.9
All leukaemias	37	41	40	32	28	1.4
All tumours	**64**	**50**	**43**	**38**	**33**	*1.6*

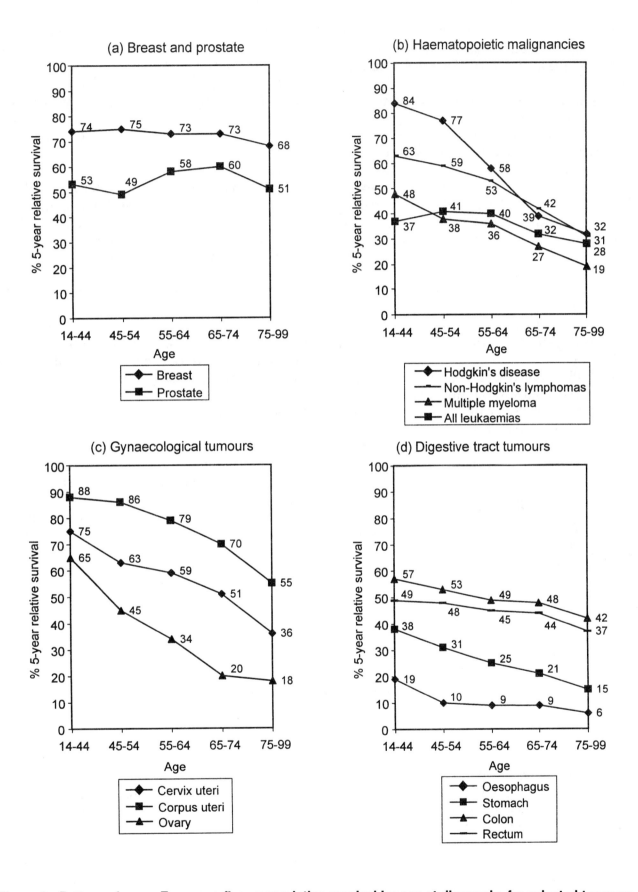

Figure 3. Pattern of mean European five-year relative survival by age at diagnosis, for selected tumours. Weighted European pool, 1985–89, both sexes (except sex-specific tumours)

skin melanoma, the poor survival of the oldest patients could be related to lack of awareness of the disease, resulting in diagnosis at later stages (Smith *et al.*, 1998).

As shown in Figure 3(*d*), digestive tract tumours are also characterized by poorer survival with increasing age at diagnosis. The steepest decrease is for stomach cancer, where the oldest patients have a 60% greater risk of death compared with those aged 45–54 years; for colon and rectal cancers, the excess risk is 40%. For the highly lethal oesophageal, pancreatic and hepatic cancers, the largest survival difference is between the youngest age class and the next class. Since stage at diagnosis and surgical radicality are the main prognostic factors for all digestive tract tumours, it would seem that elderly patients more often present at an advanced stage of disease or with contraindication to extensive surgery than younger patients (Faivre *et al.*, 1998; Gatta *et al.*, 1998).

Poorer prognosis in older patients was also a major finding of the EUROCARE-1 study, and has been confirmed by a detailed analysis carried out on the EUROCARE-2 data (Vercelli *et al.*, 1998). However, the reasons for this phenomenon are not completely clear and contrast somewhat with findings in the USA, where the association between age at diagnosis and cancer survival is much weaker (Wingo *et al.*, 1998).

To further explore this relationship in the present study, we compared survival differences between countries with the second highest and second lowest survival, for young (age class 45–54 years) and old patients (75+ years), for some of the most common tumours. These data are presented in Table 2, which shows, for each cancer site and age class, the RR for the country with low survival versus that with high survival. For many tumours that benefit from curative therapy, the RR is higher for younger than for older patients, indicating that intercountry differences in disease outcome are greater for the former than for the latter. This trend is particularly marked for skin melanoma and cancers of the stomach, corpus uteri, cervix uteri, bladder, kidney and prostate. In contrast, intercountry differences are similar in young and old patients for colon and rectal cancers, while for the most lethal tumours, intercountry differences are greater for the older age class.

Two possible explanations for the general pattern are that the natural history of the disease has more influence than therapy in determining outcome among older patients, or that older patients are treated less frequently and less intensively than younger patients. As noted previously, advanced age

at diagnosis is often associated with late tumour stage and comorbidity, which can contraindicate the application of potentially curative therapy (Bergman *et al.*, 1992; Havlik *et al.*, 1992), leading to less favourable and more homogeneous outcomes in the old. By contrast, younger patients are generally in better health and their disease may be at an earlier stage, so that more aggressive and effective therapies can be applied.

With the most lethal tumours, for which palliative care is usually the only treatment option, the pattern seems to reverse and intercountry survival differences are more marked for older patients. In the absence of effective therapy, factors such as failure of immune response to the disease or impaired general health can also be responsible for the poor prognosis in the elderly. However, outcomes could still be improved in elderly patients by improving diagnostic and treatment protocols, including palliative care, aimed specifically at such patients (Fentiman *et al.*, 1990).

Sex and cancer survival

Considering all tumour sites together, 50% of women and 35% of men were alive five years after diagnosis. This may be at least partially explained by the fact that in Europe common tumours specifically affecting women (breast and corpus uteri) have relatively favourable prognosis, whereas tumours with poor prognosis (lung, pancreas and oesophagus) are more common in men. Table 3 shows five-year relative survival by sex and age (45–54, 75+, all ages) for selected tumour sites. The RRs of death for females versus males are given for each site and age. For all tumours and all ages together, women have a 30% lower risk of dying than men, and for younger age groups, the risk of dying is even lower for women. For the following sites, women have a lower risk of dying than men (all ages combined): head and neck, oesophagus, stomach, thyroid and brain, as well as melanoma and Hodgkin's disease. Women have worse survival than men for tumours of the bladder and for multiple myeloma. For the other tumours in Table 3, there is no major survival difference between the sexes, considering all ages together. From Table 3, it is also evident that for most cancers the survival advantage for women is confined mainly to the young age groups and is reduced or reversed in the oldest group; thyroid tumours and melanoma are exceptions for which the survival advantage for women was more marked in the oldest group. Bladder cancer was the only cancer site for which women had a worse prognosis than men in all age groups.

Table 2. Intercountry variation in survival, illustrated by five-year relative survival in countries with second highest and second lowest survival for age classes 45–54 and 75+ years and risk ratio for death (RR) of the country with low versus country with high survival, 1985–89. Tumours are ranked according to the usual first-line treatment modality

Tumour site	Patients aged 45–54 years			Patients aged 75+ years		
	Second highest rate (H)	Second lowest rate (L)	RR for L vs H	Second highest rate	Second lowest rate	RR for L vs H
Surgery						
Stomach	37 I	13 PL	2.1	23 E	7 SCO	1.8
Colon	60 F S	42 SLO	1.7	53 F	32 EST	1.8
Rectum	57 FIN	37 SK	1.8	49 NL	22 SLO EST	2.1
Melanoma	92 CH	60 E	6.1	86 CH	46 PL	5.1
Corpus uteri	96 NL	81 EST	5.2	63 F	43 ICE	1.8
Bladder	85 I	50 SLO	4.3	64 E	31 SLO	2.6
Kidney	64 E	42 PL DK	2.0	40 I SLO	23 SCO	1.6
Surgery+adjuvant chemo/radiotherapy						
Breast	81 ICE	62 A	2.3	78 F ICE	52 EST	2.6
Ovary	55 CH	37 PL SLO	1.7	32 ICE	7 SLO	2.3
Cervix uteri	55 D	80 S	2.7	48 ICE NL	29 DK	1.7
Prostate	57 CH	17 PI	3.2	65 SK	39 DK	2.2
Chemo/radiotherapy						
Hodgkin's disease [a]	91 NL	75 PL	3.1	54 D	10 E	3.7
Non-Hodgkin's lymphoma [a]	69 NL	46 PL	2.1	40 F	22 NL PL	1.7
Multiple myeloma	58 ICE	28 SCO	2.3	32 E	10 EST	2.0
All leukaemias [a]	47 D	11 ICE	2.9	40 EST	12 ICE	2.3
Palliative therapy						
Liver	10 E	2 DK	1.7	9 E	1 DK I FIN	1.9
Pancreas	10 SK	2 PL EST DK	1.7	9 A	1 CH DK	1.9
Lung	19 S A	9 DK	1.5	12 ICE	3 PL ENG	1.7
Brain [a]	54 D	34 NL	1.8	12 F	1 SCO	2.2

[a] Youngest age class = 15–44 years

A=Austria, D=Germany, DK=Denmark, E=Spain, ENG=England, EST=Estonia, F=France, FIN=Finland, I=Italy, ICE=Iceland, NL=Netherlands, PL=Poland, SCO=Scotland, SK=Slovakia, SLO=Slovenia, S=Sweden, CH=Switzerland.

Longer survival of women was confirmed by a multivariate analysis on the entire EUROCARE dataset, that took account of age at diagnosis, geographical area and cancer site. Several reasons have been suggested for the better survival of women with cancer, among which are greater attention to and awareness of disease symptoms, leading to earlier diagnosis, less comorbidity, and more favourable distribution of subsites (particularly for head and neck, stomach and skin melanoma) and histotypes (thyroid) (Micheli et al., 1998). Furthermore, since differences in care seem to be related to age at diagnosis, and possibly to comorbidity, irrespective of sex, the better prognosis of women compared with men, which is especially marked at younger ages, suggests that biological rather than treatment factors are mainly responsible for the better outcome.

Table 3. Five-year relative survival by sex and age for selected tumours, with risk ratio for death (RR) for females versus males, 1985-89. Weighted European pool									
Tumour site	Patients aged 45–54 years			Patients aged 75+ years			All patients		
	M	F	RR for F vs M	M	F	RR for F vs M	M	F	RR for F vs M
Head and neck	37	48	0.7	30	38	0.8	35	47	0.7
Oesophagus	8	17	0.7	6	7	0.9	8	12	0.8
Stomach	28	35	0.8	14	17	0.9	21	24	0.9
Colon	50	56	0.8	44	41	1.1	47	47	1.0
Rectum	46	50	0.9	38	35	1.1	43	43	1.0
Larynx	62	65	0.9	64	50	1.6	63	63	1.0
Lung	13	15	0.9	5	4	1.1	10	11	1.0
Melanoma	75	84	0.6	52	73	0.5	70	82	0.6
Bladder	80	73	1.4	58	51	1.2	68	60	1.3
Kidney	56	65	0.7	37	33	1.1	49	50	1.0
Brain	18	18	1.0	8	5	1.2	18	20	0.9
Thyroid	80	88	0.6	20	42	0.5	72	80	0.7
Hodgkin's disease	73	82	0.6	38	24	1.5	72	74	0.9
Non-Hodgkin's lymphoma	57	61	0.9	34	28	1.2	48	48	1.0
Multiple myeloma	38	37	1.0	23	16	1.2	30	28	1.1
All leukaemias	38	45	0.8	27	28	1.0	34	35	1.0
All tumours	**38**	**62**	**0.5**	**31**	**35**	**0.9**	**35**	**50**	**0.7**

Socioeconomic factors and survival

Both in the present study and in EUROCARE-1, certain countries consistently show better survival than others for most tumours, while others are characterized by poor survival for most tumours. This suggests that part of the intercountry differences in cancer survival is related to social and economic factors. Other studies have shown that survival for cancer is related to social class (Bassett et al., 1986; Kogevinas et al., 1991, 1997; Schrijvers et al., 1995, 1997). Furthermore, a recent study in the UK, where survival at the national level is mostly below the European mean, revealed marked differences in survival between regions, with survival in some regions and for some tumours reaching and sometimes surpassing the European mean. In addition, for many tumours, patients living in affluent areas within specific regions had higher survival than those living in less affluent areas of the same region (Coleman et al., 1999).

We have therefore investigated the relationship between country-specific demographic and socio-economic factors in western European countries and survival for some of the most common cancers (breast, colon, rectum, stomach, prostate, lung, skin melanoma and non-Hodgkin's lymphomas). Socioeconomic information was taken from the OECD database (OECD, 1998) and pertains to 1990 or the nearest available year.

The first step involved exploring the relationship between numerous socioeconomic indicators and cancer survival by means of Pearson correlation analysis. Table 4 lists the indicators found to correlate with survival in men and women in most countries. It was found that national expenditure on health as a percentage of the gross national product (TEH/GNP), number of hospital beds, and number of computerized tomography (CT) scanners per million people directly correlated with survival, whereas public expenditure as a proportion of total health expenditure was not consistently related to survival. Furthermore, the percentage of unemployment, infant mortality and general mortality correlated inversely with cancer survival, while life expectancy at birth correlated directly with survival.

In general, these indicators correlate with survival for tumours with relatively good prognosis, for which screening is effective and for which there was improvement in diagnostic modalities over the study period (prostate, breast, rectum and, for women, colon). They correlate poorly or not at all with survival for lung and stomach cancers and non-Hodgkin's lymphomas, which have poor prognosis, for which screening has no effect, and for which early diagnosis, at least during the study years, had little or no effect on survival.

In order to explore further the effect of the variables found to correlate with cancer survival, a multiple linear regression analysis was performed using a stepwise procedure. Separate models for each cancer site were run, and included the following set of variables: TEH/GNP, % unemployment, number of hospital beds, number of CT scanners per million population, life expectancy at birth and sex. Table 5 reports the between-country variance in survival explained by the full model (total R^2) and by each variable considered separately (partial R^2). Only values of the variables that were significantly associated with survival at the 0.15 level of statistical significance were left in the final models and are reported in Table 5. A backward procedure provided closely similar results.

It was found that most selected indicators had a significant effect on cancer survival in the multiple regression models. The models were able to explain most (more than 60%) of the variability in survival for tumours of the breast, prostate and rectum. However, for lung cancer, none of the indicators included in the models was statistically significant (not shown in Table 5). This means that a considerable part of the observed variation in survival across Europe can be explained by socioeconomic factors, that are reliable indicators of the different levels of care provided by health systems.

The results of this analysis provide further evidence that the socioeconomic level of a country is an important determinant of survival from cancer on a population basis, at least in the western European countries considered in this analysis, whose health systems are similarly organized. This hypothesis is consistent with the considerably worse survival in eastern European countries, which would be associated with the lower economic level of these areas during the study period. These findings raise issues concerning inequality of access to and availability of health facilities in relation to socioeconomic level, since these are likely to have contributed to the observed intercountry differences in survival. It should be noted that the indicators used in this analysis were national, and do not take into account possible differences within countries, which would have to be addressed by ad-hoc studies.

Conclusions

- EUROCARE-2 has confirmed that different European populations differ considerably in cancer survival. It is of concern that even for cancers for which effective therapies have been available since the 1970s (in particular Hodgkin's disease), there remain large differences in survival across Europe, indicating that in many areas, internationally agreed treatment guidelines are not adhered to, or treatment facilities are inadequate.

- Survival is generally highest in Iceland, Sweden and Switzerland. For certain common tumours, survival is also above the European mean in Finland, the Netherlands and France. Survival is generally close to the European mean in Germany, Austria, Italy and Spain, and generally low in Estonia, Poland, Slovakia and, to a lesser extent, Slovenia. In Denmark and the UK survival is worryingly low for some of the most common tumours (stomach, colon, rectum, breast, prostate, kidney, thyroid and lung).

- Survival is inversely related to age at diagnosis for practically all tumours, in all countries. This is probably attributable in part to advanced stage at diagnosis and comorbidity in elderly patients, so that treatments were less effective or could not be effectively applied. Impaired immune response to cancers in elderly patients and other biological factors may also contribute to age-related survival differences. A cultural bias, with old patients being treated less intensively than young patients, could also contribute to this finding. For most tumours that respond well to therapy, intercountry differences in survival are more marked for young patients, whereas survival in the elderly tends to be more uniform across countries. For tumours with very poor prognosis (oesophagus, pancreas, lung and brain), the extent of intercountry variation is lower, and similar across ages.

- For most tumours, women survive longer than men, and this difference is more marked in younger age groups. Among women, greater bodily awareness and attention to disease symptoms, leading to earlier diagnosis, better general health and occurrence of less aggressive histotypes than in men may contribute to their better prognosis. However, since the survival advantage of women is evident for nearly all tumour sites, and particularly among younger patients, it may be hypothesized that a greater 'biological' or 'natural' ability of women to respond to cancer also plays a role.

Table 4. Pearson correlation coefficients of socioeconomic and health variables[a] with five-year country-specific age-adjusted relative survival for some of the most common tumours in twelve European countries[b], 1985–89

Tumour	Health expenditure as % of GNP	Public health expenditure as % of total health expenditure	% Unemployment	Hospital beds per million population	CT scanners per milion population	Life expectancy at birth	Infant mortality per 1000 live births	Total population mortality rate per 100 000
Males								
Prostate	0.70*	0.40	−0.51*	0.77*	0.59*	0.27	− 0.65*	− 0.37
Colon	0.36	−0.04	− 0.15	0.34	0.33	0.12	− 0.07	− 0.23
Rectum	0.52*	0.18	− 0.46*	0.85*	0.59*	0.31	− 0.57*	− 0.29
Melanoma	− 0.04	−0.18	− 0.47	0.35	0.31	− 0.14	− 0.18	0.17
Stomach	0.37	−0.03	0.12	0.11	0.32	0.03	− 0.02	−0.35
Lung	0.15	−0.13	0.01	0.38	0.31	0.36	0.03	− 0.49
Non-Hodgkin's lymphoma	− 0.22	−0.51*	− 0.11	−0.02	0.25	0.01	0.34	− 0.22
Females								
Breast	0.65*	0.62*	− 0.22	0.60*	0.37	0.64*	− 0.63*	− 0.27
Colon	0.59*	0.52*	− 0.11	0.45*	0.25	0.49*	− 0.39	− 0.59
Rectum	0.21	0.02	− 0.64*	0.72*	0.70*	0.49*	− 0.39	− 0.46
Melanoma	0.18	0.03	− 0.50*	0.57*	0.38	0.19	− 0.34	− 0.48*
Stomach	0.13	− 0.21	− 0.06	−0.22	0.52*	0.48*	0.03	− 0.10
Non-Hodgkin's lymphoma	− 0.12	− 0.09	− 0.58*	0.41	0.59*	0.13	− 0.25	0.03

* $p < 0.1$

[a] From OECD database; the values pertain to year 1990 $\pm$ 1

[b] Countries included in this analysis were Austria, Denmark, England, Finland, France, Germany, Iceland, Italy, Netherlands, Spain, Sweden and Switzerland.

CT, Computerized tomography; GNP = gross national product

Table 5. Multiple regression analysis of selected socioeconomic variables[a] with five-year country-specific age-adjusted relative survival for some of the most common tumours in twelve European countries[b], 1985-89. Both sexes

Tumour	Partial R^2 values for each indicator						Total R^2 variance explained by the full model	P of the full model
	Health expenditure as % of GNP	Sex	% Unemployment	Hospital beds per million population	CT scanners per million population	Life expectancy at birth		
Breast	0.419					0.238	0.657	0.04
Prostate	0.112			0.598			0.709	0.1
Colon	0.213						0.213	0.02
Rectum				0.607			0.607	0.0001
Melanoma		0.304	0.132				0.436	0.04
Stomach			0.212		0.129	0.169	0.510	0.04
Non-Hodgkin's lymphoma	0.089	0.143			0.168		0.401	0.01

[a] From OECD database; values pertain to year 1990 ±1

[b] Countries included in this analysis were Austria, Denmark, England, Finland, France, Germany, Iceland, Italy, Netherlands, Spain, Sweden and Switzerland.

CT, Computerized tomography; GNP = gross national product

- Certain countries have consistently better survival than others for most tumours, while others are characterized by poor survival for most tumours. Multiple regression analysis was able to explain most of this intercountry variation in survival for tumours of the breast, prostate and rectum, and also indicated contributing factors to explain that of colon, melanoma, stomach cancer and non-Hodgkin's lymphomas. The significant variables emerging from this analysis are proportion of GNP spent on health, percentage unemployment, number of hospital beds, number of CT scanners per million population, life expectancy at birth and sex. These findings indicate that inequality of access to and availability of health facilities contribute to intercountry survival differences.

References

Albain, K.S., Allred, D.C. & Clark G.M. (1994) Breast cancer outcome and predictors of outcome: are there age differentials? *Monogr. Natl Cancer Inst.*, **16**, 35–42

Balzi, D., Carli, P., Giannotti, B. & Buiatti, E. (1998). Skin melanoma in Italy: a population-based study on survival and prognostic factors. *Eur. J. Cancer*, **34**, 699–704

Bassett, M.T. & Krieger, N. (1986) Social class and black–white differences in breast cancer survival. *Am. J. Public Health*, **76**, 1400–1403

Bergman, L., Kluck, H.M., van Leeuwen, M.A., Crommelin, M.A., Dekker, G., Hart, A.A.M. & Coebergh, J.W.W. (1992) The influence on treatment choice and survival of elderly breast cancer patients in South-eastern Netherlands: a population-based study. *Eur. J. Cancer*, **28**, 1475–1480

Berrino, F., Sant, M., Verdecchia, A., Capocaccia, R., Hakulinen, T. & Estève, J., eds (1995) *Survival of Cancer Patients in Europe. The EUROCARE Study* (IARC Scientific Publications No. 132), Lyon, IARC

Berrino, F., Gatta, G. and the EUROCARE Working Group (1998) Variation in survival of patients with head and neck cancer in Europe by the site of origin of the tumours. In: Coebergh, J.W.W., Sant, M., Berrino, F. & Verdecchia, A., eds, Special issue: Survival of adult cancer patients in Europe diagnosed from 1978–1989: The EUROCARE II Study. *Eur. J. Cancer*, **34**, 2154–2161

Carli, P.M., Coebergh, J.W.W., Verdecchia, A. and the EUROCARE Working Group. (1998) Variation in survival of adult patients with haematological malignancies in Europe since 1978. In: Coebergh, J.W.W., Sant, M., Berrino, F. & Verdecchia, A., eds, Special issue: Survival of adult cancer patients in Europe diagnosed from 1978–1989: The EUROCARE II Study. *Eur. J. Cancer*, **34**, 2253–2263

Coebergh, J.W.W. (1995) Summary and discussion of results. In: Berrino, F., Sant, M., Verdecchia, A., Capocaccia, R., Hakulinen, T., & Estève, J., eds, *Survival of cancer patients in Europe. The EUROCARE Study* (IARC Scientific Publications No. 132), Lyon, IARC, pp. 447–463

Coebergh, J.W.W., Sant, M., Berrino, F. & Verdecchia, A., eds (1998) Special issue: Survival of adult cancer patients in Europe diagnosed from 1978–1989: The EUROCARE II Study. *Eur. J. Cancer*, **34**, No. 14

Coleman, M.P., Babb, P., Damiecki, P., Grosclaude, P., Honjo, S., Jones, J., Gerhardt, K., Pitard, A., Quinn, M., Sloggett, A., De Stavola B. (1999) *Cancer Survival Trends in England and Wales, 1971–1995: Deprivation and NHS Region* (Studies in Medical and Population Subjects No. 60), London: Stationery Office

Damhuis, R.A.M., Kirkelz, W.J., and the EUROCARE Working Group (1998) Improvement in survival of patients with cancer of the kidney in Europe since 1978 In: Coebergh, J.W.W., Sant, M., Berrino, F. & Verdecchia, A., eds, Special issue: Survival of adult cancer patients in Europe diagnosed from 1978–1989: The EUROCARE II Study. *Eur. J. Cancer*, **34**, 2232–2235

Faivre, J., Forman, D., Estève, J., Gatta, G., and the EUROCARE Working Group. (1998). Survival of patients with oesophageal and gastric cancer in Europe. In: Coebergh, J.W.W., Sant, M., Berrino, F. & Verdecchia A., eds, Special issue: Survival of adult cancer patients in Europe diagnosed from 1978–1989: The EUROCARE II Study. *Eur. J. Cancer*, **34**, 2167–2175

Fentiman, I.F., Tirelli U., Monfardini, S., Schneider, M., Festen, J., Cognetti, F. & Aapro, M.S.(1990) Cancer in the elderly: why so badly treated? *Lancet*, **335**, 1020–1022

Gatta, G., Sant, M., Coebergh, J.W.W., Hakulinen, T. and the EUROCARE Working Group (1996) Substantial variation in therapy for colorectal cancer across Europe: EUROCARE analysis of cancer registry data for 1987. *Eur. J. Cancer*, **32A**, 831–835

Gatta, G., Faivre, J., Capocaccia, R., Ponz de Leon, M., and the EUROCARE Working Group (1998) Survival of colorectal cancer patients in Europe during the period 1978–1989. In: Coebergh, J.W.W., Sant, M., Berrino, F. & Verdecchia A., eds, Special issue: Survival of adult cancer patients in Europe diagnosed from 1978–1989: The EUROCARE II Study. *Eur. J. Cancer*, **34**, 2176–2183

Gatta, G., Lasota, M.B., Verdecchia, A. and the EUROCARE Working Group (1998) Survival of European women with gynaecological tumours, during the period 1978-1989. In: Coebergh, J.W.W., Sant, M., Berrino, F. & Verdecchia A., eds, Special issue: Survival of adult cancer patients in Europe diagnosed from 1978–1989: The EUROCARE II Study. *Eur. J. Cancer*, **34**, 2218–2225

Havlik, R.J., Yancik, R., Long, S., Ries, L. & Edwards B. (1994) The National Institute of Ageing and the National Cancer Institute SEER collaborative study on comorbidity and early diagnosis of cancer in the elderly. *Cancer*, **74**, 2101–2106

Helgesen, F., Holmberg, L., Johansson, J., Bergström, R. & Adami, H.O. (1996). Trends in prostate cancer survival in Sweden, 1960 through 1988: evidence for increasing diagnosis of non lethal tumours. *J. Natl Cancer Inst.*, **88**, 1216–1221

Janssen-Heijnen, M.L.G., Gatta, G., Forman, D., Capocaccia, R., Coebergh, J.W.W. and the EUROCARE Working Group (1998) Variation in survival of patients with lung cancer in Europe In: Coebergh, J.W.W., Sant, M., Berrino, F. & Verdecchia, A., eds, Special issue: Survival of adult cancer patients in Europe diagnosed from 1978–1989: The EUROCARE II Study. *Eur. J. Cancer*, **34**, 2191–2196

Karjalainen, S. & Palva, I. (1989) Do treatment protocols improve end results? A study of survival of patients with multiple myeloma in Finland. *Br. Med. J.*, **299**, 1069–1072.

Kogevinas, M., Marmot, M.G.; Fox, A.J. & Goldblatt, P.O. (1991) Socioeconomic differences in cancer survival *J. Epidemiol. Commun. Health*, **45**, 216–219

Kogevinas, M. & Porta, M. (1997) Socioeconomic differences in cancer survival: a review of the evidence. In: Kogevinas, M., Pearce, N., Susser, M. & Boffetta, P., eds, *Social Inequalities and Cancer* (IARC Scientific Publications, No. 138), Lyon, IARC, pp. 177–206

Kosary, C.L. (1994) FIGO stage, histology, histologic grade, age, and race as prognostic factors in determining survival for cancers of the female gynecological system: an analysis of 1973–97 SEER cases of cancers of the endometrium, cervix, ovary, vulva, and vagina. *Seminars in Surgical Oncology*, **10**, 31–46

Micheli, A., Mariotto, A., Giorgi Rossi, A., Gatta, G., Muti, P. and the EUROCARE Working Group (1998) The prognostic role of gender in survival of adult cancer patients. In: Coebergh, J.W.W., Sant, M., Berrino, F. & Verdecchia, A., eds, Special issue: Survival of adult cancer patients in Europe diagnosed from 1978–1989: The EUROCARE II Study. *Eur. J. Cancer*, **34**, 2271–2278

OECD Health data (1998) *A Comparative Analysis of 29 Countries*, Paris, Organization for Economic Cooperation and Development

Parkin, D.M., Whelan, S.L., Ferlay, J., Raymond, L. & Young, J., eds (1997) *Cancer Incidence in Five Continents*, Vol VII (IARC Scientific Publications No.143), Lyon, IARC

Piccirillo, J.F. & Feinstein, A.R. (1996) Clinical symptoms and comorbidity: significance for the prognostic classification of cancer. *Cancer*, **77**, 834–842

Post, P.N., Damhuis, R.A.M., van der Meyden, A.P.M. and the EUROCARE Working Group (1998) Variation of survival of patients with prostate cancer in Europe since 1978. In: Coebergh, J.W.W., Sant, M., Berrino, F. & Verdecchia, A., eds, Special issue: Survival of adult cancer patients in Europe diagnosed from 1978–1989: The EUROCARE II Study. *Eur. J. Cancer*, **34**, 2226–2231

Quinn, M.J., Martinez-Garcia C., Berrino, F. and the EUROCARE Working Group (1998) Variation in survival from breast cancer in Europe by age and country, 1978–89 In: Coebergh, J.W.W., Sant, M., Berrino, F. & Verdecchia, A., eds, Special issue: Survival of adult cancer patients in Europe diagnosed from 1978–1989: The EUROCARE II Study. *Eur. J. Cancer*, **34**, 2204–2211

Ries, L.A.G., Hankey, B.F., Miller, B.A., Hartman, A.M. & Edwards, B.K. (1991) *Cancer Statistic Review 1973-88* (NIH Pub. No. 91-2789), Bethesda, MD, National Cancer Institute

Sant, M., Capocaccia, R., Verdecchia, A., Gatta, G., Micheli, A., Mariotto, A., Hakulinen, T., Berrino, F. and the EUROCARE Working Group (1995) Comparisons of colon-cancer survival among European countries: The Eurocare Study. *Int. J. Cancer*, **63**, 43–48

Sant, M., Capocaccia, R., Verdecchia, A., Estève, J., Gatta, G., Micheli, A., Coleman, M., Berrino F. and the EUROCARE Working Group (1998) Survival of women with breast cancer in Europe: variation with age, year of diagnosis and country. *Int. J. Cancer*, **77**, 679–683

Satariano, W.A. & Ragland, D.R. (1994) The effect of comorbidity on 3-year survival of women with primary breast cancer. *Ann. Intern. Med.*, **120**, 104–110

Schrijvers, C.T.M., Mackenbach, J.P.,Lutz, J.M., Quinn, M.J. & Coleman, M.P. (1995) Deprivation and survival from breast cancer. *Br. J. Cancer*, **72**, 738–743

Schrijvers, C.T.M., Coebergh, J.W.W. & Mackenbach, J.P. (1997) Socioeconomic status and comorbidity among newly diagnosed cancer patients. *Cancer*, **80**, 1482–1488

Selby, P., Gilles, C. & Haward, R. (1996) Benefits from specialised cancer care. *Lancet*, **348**, 313–318

Smith, J.A.E., Whatley, P.M., Redburn, J.C. and the EUROCARE Working Group (1998) Improving survival of melanoma patients in Europe since 1978. In: Coebergh, J.W.W., Sant, M., Berrino, F. & Verdecchia, A., eds, Special issue: Survival of adult cancer patients in Europe diagnosed from 1978–1989: The EUROCARE II Study. *Eur. J. Cancer*, **34**, 2197–2203

Teppo, L., Hakulinen, T. and the EUROCARE Working Group (1998) Variation in survival of adult patients with thryoid cancer in Europe. In: Coebergh, J.W.W., Sant, M., Berrino, F. & Verdecchia, A., eds, Special issue: Survival of adult cancer patients in Europe diagnosed from 1978–1989: The EUROCARE II Study. *Eur. J. Cancer*, **34**, 2248–2252

Tretli, S., Engeland, A., Haldorsen, T., Hakulinen, T., Hörte, L.G., Luostarinen, T., Schou, G., Sigvaldason, H., Storm, H.H., Tulinius, H. & Vaittinen, P. (1996) Prostate cancer – look to Denmark? *J. Natl Cancer Inst.*, **88**, 128

van Basten, J.P.,Schrafford Koops, H., Sleijfer, D.T., Pras, E., van Driel, M.F. & Hoekstra, H.J. (1997) Current concepts about testicular cancer. *Eur. J. Surg. Oncol.*, **23**, 354–360

Vercelli, M, Quaglia, A., Casella, C., Parodi, S., Capocaccia, R., Martinez-Garcia, C. and the EUROCARE Working Group (1998) Relative survival in elderly cancer patients in Europe. In: Coebergh, J.W.W., Sant, M., Berrino, F. & Verdecchia, A., eds, Special issue: Survival of adult cancer patients in Europe diagnosed from 1978–1989: The EUROCARE II Study. *Eur. J. Cancer*, **34**, 2264–2270

Verdecchia, A., De Angelis, R., Capocaccia, R., Sant, M., Micheli, A., Gatta, G. & Berrino, F. (1998) The cure for colon cancer: results from the EUROCARE study. *Int. J. Cancer*, **77**, 322–329

Wingo, P.A., Gloeckler Ries, L.A., Parker, S.L. & Heath, Jr, C.W. (1998) Long-term cancer patient survival in the United States. *Cancer Epidemiol. Biomarkers Prev.*, **7**, 271–282

World Health Organization (1977) *Manual of the International Statistical Classification of Diseases, Injuries, and Causes of Death*, ninth revision, Geneva

Yancik, R., Ries, L.G. & Yates, J.W. (1989) Breast cancer in aging women. A population-based study of contrast in stage, surgery and survival. *Cancer*, **63**, 976–981

Chapter 6

Trends in cancer survival probability over the period 1978–89

J. Estève, G. De Angelis and A. Verdecchia

Introduction

The publication of data on cancer survival probability in Europe for a more recent period has provided the opportunity to assess progress made over a 10-year time-span. The first EUROCARE report (Berrino *et al.*, 1995) presented data on survival probability of patients with cancer diagnosed between 1978 and 1984. The present volume reports similar information for the period 1985–89. The registries included in the present publication are not the same set as was included in the first report, so that no direct comparison of the published figures is possible, since place and time are strongly confounded. In order to avoid misleading comparisons, we present in this chapter for selected sites of cancer the results of an analysis of time trends in survival for those registries which provided data for the whole period covered by the EUROCARE study (1978–89). The relative survival probability which is presented here is that of a hypothetical population of European patients living in countries for which at least one registry participated in the study and who would experience the survival probability estimated from the data of these registries. Therefore, these survival probabilities should be interpreted as averages made over the participating countries, rather than as the average survival probability of all European cancer patients. Nevertheless, since this hypothetical European population has been the same over the whole period, the changes in survival observed can be interpreted as the average change in survival observed among the participating countries. This is why, except for the change in relative survival probability for the 'European' population, we have focused on the change in relative cancer death rates, comparing the three periods 1981–83, 1984–86 and 1987–89 with the period 1978–80. Readers interested in the absolute levels of survival probability in the various countries of the study should refer to the other chapters, where the complete information from the second EUROCARE study period is available. The choice of the relative cancer death rate as a measure of improvement in survival is explained further in the section on methods below. In the rest of this chapter, the term survival *probability* always refers to five-year relative survival *probability*, unless otherwise stated. Similarly, the relative death *rate* of one period compared with another always refers to the ratio of average *cancer* death *rates* over the two given periods.

Data

The following data were available to assess the trend in survival probability for each cancer site included in this analysis.

- The number of incident cases per year for the cancer site and for each country eligible for the trend study.
- The crude and relative survival probability at one, three and five years by sex, age and period for 'Europe', estimated as the average of the country-specific values weighted by the number of incident cases in that country. These weights were used for all age groups. The values of the survival probabilities were calculated as explained in the first EUROCARE monograph (Verdecchia *et al.*, 1995). The numbers of patients diagnosed and followed up in each stratum were also given in order to obtain a rough idea of the precision.
- The above sex-specific relative survival probability estimates at one and five years, with the confidence interval for each period of diagnosis. These figures were used in this study to obtain the variance of the logarithm of the survival probability (as described in the section on methods below).
- The age-standardized relative survival probability at one and five years, with the confidence interval, by sex, country and period. The standard distribution was taken as the age distribution of the cancer patients recorded in the entire database for this cancer site. Note that this standard distribution is *not* the same as that used in the first EUROCARE study.

Methods

The improvement in relative survival probability over the study period was measured by the relative death rates (RR), comparing the rates of death *from cancer* between the latest three-year periods of diagnosis and the first. A linear trend test based on the weighted regression of the logarithm of the relative death rate against period of diagnosis was performed to assess the significance of the change over the study period. In order to compare improvements in survival probability between sexes, age groups and countries, we used the same regression and tested for the homogeneity of the slopes using the classical analysis of covariance approach. The relative death rates and their variances were obtained for each period using the following formulae:

$$T_i = \log(RR_i) = \frac{\log (S_i)}{\log (S_1)}$$

$$\text{var}(T_i) = \frac{\text{var}[\log (S_i)]}{[\log (S_i)]^2} + \frac{\text{var}[\log (S_1)]}{[\log (S_1)]^2}$$

where S_i is the relative survival probability for the period i. Var$[\log(S_i)]$ was obtained from the confidence intervals of S_i, or from the number of patients in the stratum when the confidence interval was not available (see below).

The quantity $- \log (S_i)$ can be interpreted as the average *cancer* death rate over the five years of follow-up, or equivalently as the death rate of the exponential survival distribution which would give the same relative survival probability at five years since diagnosis. The statistic T_i has several advantages over other indices of improvement. It has greater statistical stability than the survival difference and its exponential RR_i is widely used in many comparative survival studies under the improper name of relative risk. Note that, in using this approach, we have implicitly assumed that the relative survival was the net survival. In other words, we have attributed to cancer the deaths in excess of those expected from the general population life-table. We now describe some aspects of this method of assessment that are relevant to its application to the evaluation of the three factors analysed in the present study.

Sex

Where there is a large difference between the sex-specific relative survival probabilities, sex-specific relative survival probability is plotted as two separate curves with error-bars.

If the survival was similar for the two sexes, we plotted the overall survival for 'persons' as a continuous curve with error bars, leaving the sex-specific values as isolated points at the centre of the relevant periods. The improvement in survival is assessed through the linear trend test described above.

Age

Since the variance of the age-specific relative survival S_a was not in the database, it was estimated using the following approximation:

$$\text{var}[\log(S_a)] = \frac{n}{n_a} \times \frac{S^2}{S_a^2} \times \text{var}[\log(S)]$$

where S is the corresponding all-age relative survival probability and n and n_a are respectively the total and age-specific numbers of patients diagnosed with cancer at this site in the present study. The above formula implies that the age-distribution is the same in all countries (i.e., n/n_a is equal to n_c/n_{ac}).

Since the variances of the T_{ik} are very different in the different age groups k, we used an empirical Bayes approach to estimate the age-specific relative death rates. Their logarithms T_{ik} were calculated as the weighted averages of the age-specific crude estimate and the precision-weighted mean over age groups. The weights were respectively the variance of the crude estimate and the between-age-group variance. The latter was obtained by averaging its period-specific estimates obtained by the method of moments (see below for details). The weighted mean relative death rates and their confidence intervals were then plotted on a continuous curve together with the above age-specific estimates. The standard errors of the weighted means of the T_{ik} over age were estimated as the square root of the inverse of the sum of the weights.

Country

The relative death rates and their variances were obtained, as explained above, from the age-standardized relative survival and the confidence intervals. A weighted regression of the logarithm of the relative rate against period of diagnosis was carried out for each country and for each sex. A measure of the sex- and country-specific overall improvement in the cancer death rate over the study period was then estimated by the predicted value T_j of the logarithm of the relative rate provided by the regression for the last period of diagnosis. This approach has the advantage of taking the entire information into account and is only slightly biased if the trend is strongly non-linear. For each sex, country-specific estimates were obtained together with their variance v_j and used in the classical way to test their homogeneity through the statistics

$$Q_w = \sum_{j=1}^{13} w_j(T_j - \bar{T})^2$$

where $\bar{T}$ is the weighted mean

$$\bar{T} = \frac{\sum\limits_{j=1}^{13} w_j T_j}{\sum\limits_{j=1}^{13} w_j}$$

$w_j = 1/v_j$ and T_j is the estimate of the logarithm of the relative rate for the jth country. If Q_w was less than its expected value (=12) under the hypothesis of homogeneity, we considered, in the absence of other evidence, that the improvement has been identical in all countries. If not, there was at least some information to estimate a specific change in survival in each country of the trend study. We first estimated the between-country variance Δ^2, using a classical non-iterative method (see, for example, Der Simonian & Laird, 1986):

$$\hat{\Delta}^2 = (Q_w - 12)/[\sum w_j - (\sum w_j^2 / \sum w_j)]$$

which is obtained by replacing the population parameters in $E[Q_w]$ by their sample counterparts. An empirical Bayes approach was then used for final estimation of the overall country-specific improvement:

$$\hat{T}_j = \frac{v_j \bar{T} + \hat{\Delta}^2 T_j}{v_j + \hat{\Delta}^2}$$

that is, the weighted average of the weighted mean improvement and the crude country-specific improvement. In other words, for a given deviation from the mean, the stronger the statistical evidence (small v_j compared with the estimate of Δ^2), the further from the mean is the country-specific estimate (the empirical Bayes estimate of the change in survival). The countries of the study were then sorted according to the average of the sex-specific relative rate estimates obtained by this procedure.

Results
All cancers

Survival probability from all cancers improved significantly over the study period, from 45% to 51% in females and from 30 to 35% in males. The relative death rate for patients diagnosed in the period 1987–89 compared with those diagnosed in 1978–80 is slightly better in females than in males (0.81 vs 0.85).

The improvement in survival is strongly dependent on age, being greater in younger and older male patients. However, despite the larger improvement, the five-year relative survival probability is still poorer among old male patients (31% in males and 35% in females).

The average relative death rate in the latest period compared with the first varies from 0.76 in Italy to 0.93 in Denmark. This trend pattern increased the gap in survival probability that existed between European countries in the first study (survival from all cancers is now 17% in Poland versus 41% in Switzerland for males; 33% versus 54% for females)

Stomach, colon, rectum

The survival probability for stomach cancer showed a steady improvement in both sexes over the period of the study but is still very poor (22%). It depends on age at diagnosis and is clearly higher among older women. The relative death rate is 0.86 in both sexes for the whole of Europe, varying from 0.75 in Italy to 0.96 in the Polish registries.

The relative survival for colon cancer increased from 40% to 49% in a short period of time, mainly between 1982 and 1985, when the improvement in one-year survival was reinforced by a similar improvement in survival up to five years of those surviving the first year. The progress has been greater among females, especially among middle-aged women (RR = 0.68). Age is also a significant factor among men, but it is the older patients who had most improvement (RR = 0.76). This pattern contrasts with that observed for rectal cancer, where the progress has been steadier and better in males (RR = 0.70) than among females (RR = 0.79). For both sites, the net result has been more homogeneous survival across sex and age groups.

The relative death rate is significantly heterogeneous among countries. The overall progress is similar for colon (0.82) and rectum (0.83) and slightly better than for stomach. However, the relative death rate ranges from about 0.70 (female colon cancer in French registries and rectal cancer for Italian registries) to more than 0.90 (practically no progress) in some countries.

Larynx, lung

The survival probability for lung cancer is extremely poor, remaining under 10% on average during the study period. Improvement has been almost absent except for the youngest patients in both sexes and for the 65–74-year age group in males. The situation is similar in all countries. The only improvement seen is for countries where the survival probability was particularly poor in the first period.

The number of larynx cancer cases is extremely low in females and the corresponding survival figures are quite unstable. They are reported for the sake of completeness. The survival probability is fair to good in both sexes and increased during the study period, especially among the youngest and the oldest patients. The improvement is, however, not large and the relative rates are close to the mean of 0.94 for all countries. Exceptions are for England, which showed improvement, and for females in Denmark and Finland, for which the outlying values are explained by high survival probability in the first period that was not confirmed subsequently.

Breast, ovary, corpus and cervix uteri

The survival probability for breast cancer increased from 66% to 74% over the study period. The improvement is strongly heterogeneous when examined by age group. The two younger groups showed the poorest and the best progress. It is also heterogeneous when examined by country: starting from a survival probability of 30%, the Polish registries recorded an improvement to almost 60% at the end of the study period, whereas the Italian and French registries reached 80% from a starting value of about 60%. In contrast, Scotland and Germany showed little change at 63% to 66% for the former and 68% to 69% for the latter.

Only about one third of the women diagnosed with ovarian cancer survive their disease for five years after diagnosis. A small improvement occurred during the study period among women aged less than 65 years, but none was seen in older women. The improvement was particularly clear among patients diagnosed in the 45–54-year age group (RR = 0.79). The improvement in the standardized survival rate was small (RR = 0.87), with a significant but weak variation by country (RR = 0.84 in Denmark and the Dutch registries, RR = 0.89 in Finland)

Little overall progress was seen for cervix and corpus uteri, which already had good survival (60% and 74% respectively). The trend was however significantly different in different age groups, showing some improvement in some and deterioration in others, especially for cervix uteri.

There is no heterogeneity for corpus uteri by country, while the improvement differs quite widely between countries for cervix uteri. Starting from a relative survival of 55% in 1979, the English registries reached 62% in 1988, while the French registries recorded stable survival at 65%. Iceland and the Dutch registries reached a relative survival of about 70%.

Prostate and testis

Prostate cancer survival probability has increased only recently, reaching 59% in the EUROCARE study population. This recent improvement was preceded by a small deterioration, most clearly among older patients. It is interesting to note that the five-year survival conditional on one-year survival decreased in the second period before increasing in the last. The greater progress observed in Italy is explained by a low initial survival of 39%, while Sweden, Finland and the French registries recorded survival probabilities of about 65% in the last period.

Testicular cancer survival probability exceeds 90%, having increased from 80% to 93% over the study period. The progress is practically the same in all age groups except for outlying values, which are difficult to explain. The relative death rate is fairly homogeneous across countries, the death rate having halved in all countries. The relative rate is lower in Finland and Scotland, which started from lower survival levels, and is small in Denmark, where the survival probability was already 91% in 1978–81.

Hodgkin's disease and non-Hodgkin's lymphoma

Hodgkin's disease has good survival, that reached 72% at the end of the study period. The excess mortality in males has tended to disappear. When examined by age, the improvement was more homogeneous in male than in female patients. For the latter, where the heterogeneity was of borderline statistical significance, the improvement was consistently greater for patients less than 65 years old.

When standardized relative survival probability is examined by country, the male–female difference is inverted. This is because about 80% of the patients are less than 65 years old, among whom the improvement has been better for females than for males. However, complete interpretation of the country data would require more extensive analysis.

The prognosis of non-Hodgkin's lymphomas is poorer than for Hodgkin's disease, but the survival probability improved from 43% to 50%. The increase was greater among male patients, for whom the progress was about the same in all age groups (RR = 0.77). Among females the improvement was distinctly heterogeneous, with a worsening of the survival among older women.

The standardized relative survival probability improved on average, but with little consistency between the sexes in the improvement observed in the various countries. The relative death rate varied from 0.72 to 0.81 in males and from 0.67 to 0.89 in females.

Leukaemia

The survival probability for acute lymphocytic leukaemia is still poor (about 24%). It improved in males but not in females in the EUROCARE study population. There is no difference with age, for either males or females. The average relative death rates have wide confidence intervals, since country-specific survival probabilities are estimated on few patients. There is no variation in males across countries in the improvement in survival; the average relative death rate is 0.75 whereas it varies from 0.65 to 0.92 in females.

For acute myeloid leukaemia, the survival probability is poorer than for acute lymphocytic leukaemia. It increased from 5 to 11% over the study period. There is no heterogeneity with age in males (RR = 0.93) and a small heterogeneity of borderline statistical significance in females: the improvement has been greater in the first three age groups (RR about 0.50) than in the last two (RR about 0.55). The improvement in relative survival showed some variation in males but almost none in females. The precision of these figures is obviously fairly low.

Among all leukaemias, chronic lymphocytic leukaemia has the best survival probability (66% at the end of the study period). This increased in both sexes and for all age groups. The average relative death rate was estimated at 0.63 in male and 0.69 in female; the difference was not significant and the improvement was similar in all age groups. The improvement in standardized relative survival differed little between countries. The outlying value of Finland is explained by the high survival of 68% observed in the first period.

For chronic myeloid leukaemia, survival probability changed little over the study period. An initial decrease in survival is seen in both sexes and is stronger in the five-year survival conditional on one-year survival than in the one-year survival. The standardized relative survival followed the same non-linear pattern as the crude relative survival. As a consequence, our estimates, based on a linear trend, cannot readily be interpreted. It suggests, however, that the improvement has been heterogeneous in males.

Discussion and conclusions

Few studies have attempted a systematic evaluation of European trends in survival (Adami et al., 1989; Black et al., 1993; Carstensen et al., 1993; Verdecchia et al., 1997; Coleman et al., 1999) and none have been carried out on an international scale. Despite its obvious limitations, our study brings evidence of improvements in survival from cancer at several sites in many European countries. Such improvements are difficult to attribute to one or several of the factors which might have caused them. Comparison of trends between countries is even more difficult. The change in composition of the denominator is one of the main problems. Several examples may be given. Survival probability from 'all cancers' is the most obvious problem of this type since the heterogeneity of the denominator is the largest. It is often cited when comparing cancer survival between sexes, but should also be considered when looking at the change in survival with time: for example, a decreasing proportion of lung cancer with time in a given country would automatically result in an improvement of survival in that country. The poor improvement in breast cancer survival among young women (15–44 years) may be contrasted with the considerable improvement in the 45–74-year groups, in which screening and early diagnosis may have revealed many non-aggressive tumours. Screening for cervical cancer, by decreasing the incidence of invasive tumours, tends to increase the average aggressiveness of the missed tumours and has thus led to an apparent deterioration of survival. The initial increase in the death rate from prostate cancer among older men was not expected, since screening may have included in the pool of patients those with less aggressive tumours. The worst problem of this type is likely to arise in the interpretation of trends in survival from haematological cancer. The difficulties come mainly from the following facts: (a) the prognosis differs greatly for different lymphoma and leukaemia sub-types; (b) the classification of haematological disorders is continually changing, and (c) registry data come from various sources which differ in methods of diagnosis, classification and staging. Moving tumours from one class to another may lead to "Will-Rogers bias": moving tumours with poorer survival from a category with overall fair prognosis to one with bad prognosis will improve the survival of both groups. An opposite bias may also arise. These difficulties may explain some of the surprising features seen here in the changes in survival from haematological cancer. It is thus clear that understanding the relationship between change in survival and progress in therapy is far from simple when information is obtained from an observational study.

The purpose of this chapter was to present the evidence of change in survival over a ten-year period in the most objective way using the same set of population-based registries and the same methodology for all sites examined. Readers who wish for a more detailed discussion of possible explanations for these changes are referred to the special issue of the *European Journal of Cancer*, where these data are evaluated in various ways (Coebergh *et al.*, 1998).

The interpretation of relative cancer death rates must be made with caution. This measure is expected to have high values when there is room for improvement in survival; in other words, if a particular region initially had a survival probability that was far from optimal, the relative rate is expected to be large. In contrast, the relative rate may be low because the survival was already at the best possible level, given present knowledge.

The nature of the various indices of improvement in survival that have been used here need to be clearly understood. The calculated survival probability for our European population is an attempted estimate, even if imperfect, of the average cancer survival in Europe, based on cancer incidence and survival in each country of the study. The average relative cancer death rate over age is a precision-weighted measure of improvement, which is not representative of the survival of any real group of patients, since none has exactly the corresponding age distribution (this is illustrated by the data for Hodgkin's disease). It is, however, the best average measure of progress. Because the less precise measure is often that of the group where the incidence is lowest, it is usually close to the relative rate which could have been obtained directly from the average European survival (compare the graphs in the top and the middle of each site-specific panel). The standardized relative survival probability can be used to compare survival trends between countries. It may, however, be a very poor measure if the country-specific survival probabilities are based on only few patients, as is the case for some countries and/or for rare cancers with poor survival. As a consequence, the chances of detecting the real geographical pattern in the relative death rates are poor for some cancers. This applies especially to leukaemia, where no estimates of standardized relative survival were available for some sex/country/period cells and would have to be replaced by the sex/period European mean with a wide confidence interval (taken here as 5% to 95%).

Choosing to use a specific statistical method is equivalent to taking a particular point of view on a data-set. In using an empirical Bayesian approach, we have eliminated the danger of interpreting outlying imprecise data-points as genuine features of survival from cancer in Europe and we have considerably smoothed the country-specific estimates of change in survival. Unfortunately, this method of smoothing led us to recognize that for some cancer sites there was no information for such a country-specific estimation (e.g., corpus uteri). The choice of regressing the relative rate over time had also some unfortunate consequences due to the special role played by the death rate in the first period (e.g., testis cancer in Denmark). This approach could be replaced by regression of the death rate itself against time, which might give better results.

Finally, it must be emphasized again that the results presented in this chapter constitute the full extent of reliable information on trends in survival probability based on the database at our disposal. Any further conclusions regarding trends based on the figures in the main text of the two Eurocare monographs would not be advisable since the registries participating in the two studies were not the same.

Acknowledgement

The authors acknowledge the help of Mariano Santaquilani in the preparation of the data for the analyses.

References

Adami, H.O., Sparen, P., Bergstrom, R., Holmberg, L., Krusemo, U.B. & Ponten, J. (1989) Increasing survival trend after cancer diagnosis in Sweden: 1960–1984. *J. Natl Cancer Inst.*, **81**, 1640–1647

Berrino, F., Sant, M., Verdecchia, A., Capocaccia, R., Hakulinen, T. & Estève, J., eds (1995) *Survival of Cancer Patients in Europe. The EUROCARE Study* (IARC Scientific Publications No. 132), Lyon, IARC

Black, R.J., Sharp, L. & Kendrick, S.W. (1993) *Trends in Cancer Survival in Scotland 1968–1990*, Edinburgh, Information & Statistics Division, Directorate of Information Services, National Health Service in Scotland

Carstensen, B., Storm, H.H. & Schou, G., eds (1993) Survival of Danish cancer patients 1943–1987. *Acta Pathol. Microbiol. Immunol.* Scand., **101**, Suppl. 33

Coebergh, J.W.W.,Sant, M., Berrino, F. & Verdecchia, A.,eds (1998) Special issue: Survival of adult cancer patients in Europe diagnosed from 1978–1989: The EUROCARE II study *Eur. J. Cancer*, **34**, No. 14

Coleman, M.P., Babb, P., Damiecki, P., Grosclaude, P., Honjo, S., Jones, J., Gerhardt, K., Pitard, A., Quinn, M., Sloggett, A., De Stavola B. (1999) *Cancer Survival Trends in England and Wales, 1971–1995: Deprivation and NHS Region* (Studies in Medical and Population Subjects No. 60), London: The Stationery Office

DerSimonian, R. & Laird, N. (1986) Meta-analysis in clinical trials. *Contr. Clin. Trials*, **7**, 177–188

Verdecchia, A., Capocaccia, R. & Hakulinen, T. (1995) Methods of data analysis. In: Berrino, F., Sant, M., Verdecchia, A., Capocaccia, R., Hakulinen, T. & Estève, J., eds (1995) *Survival of Cancer Patients in Europe. The EUROCARE Study* (IARC Scientific Publications No. 132), Lyon, IARC, pp. 32–37

Verdecchia, A., Micheli, A. & Gatta, G., eds (1997) Special issue: Survival of cancer patients in Italy. The ITACARE study. *Tumori,* **83**

Stomach

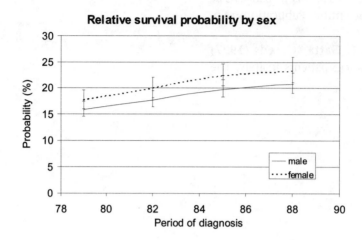

Relative survival probability by sex

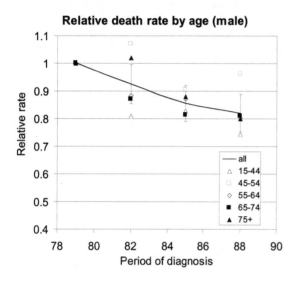

Relative death rate by age (male)

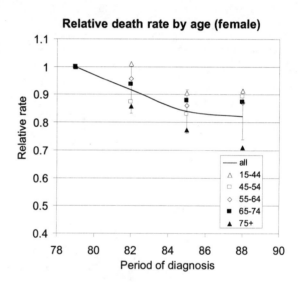

Relative death rate by age (female)

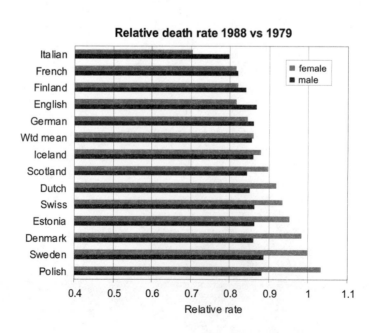

Relative death rate 1988 vs 1979

Colon

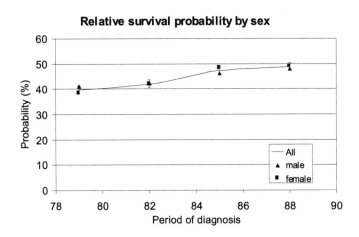

Relative survival probability by sex

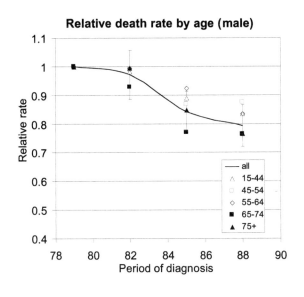

Relative death rate by age (male)

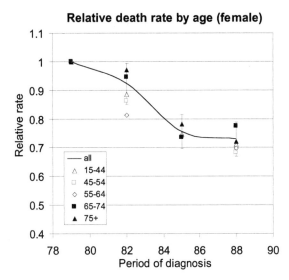

Relative death rate by age (female)

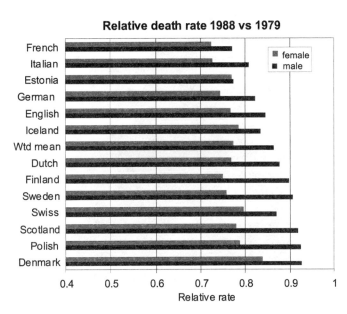

Relative death rate 1988 vs 1979

Rectum

Relative survival probability by sex

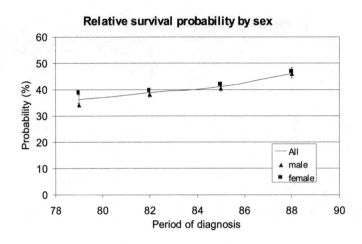

Relative death rate by age (male)

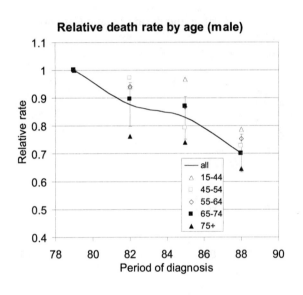

Relative death rate by age (female)

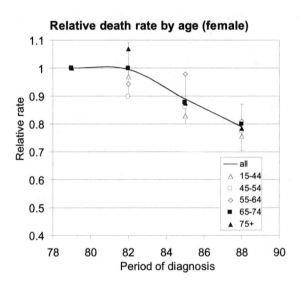

Relative death rate 1988 vs 1979

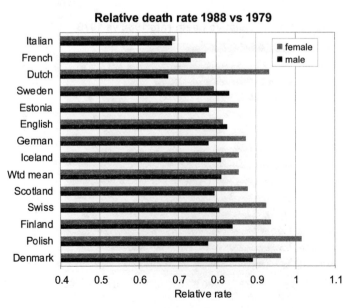

Larynx

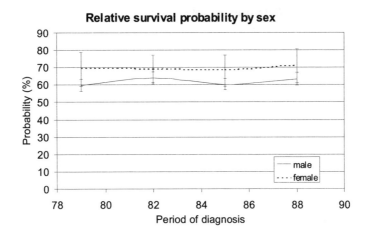

Relative survival probability by sex

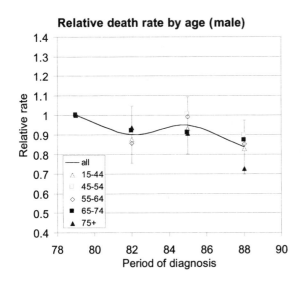

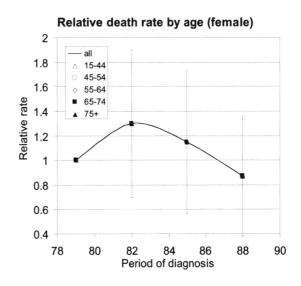

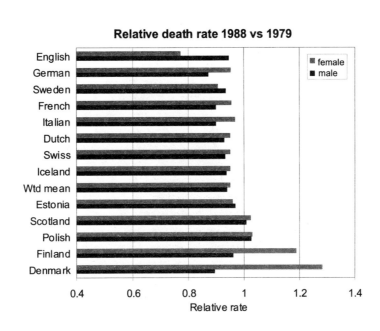

Lung

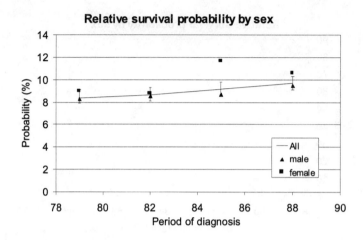

Relative survival probability by sex

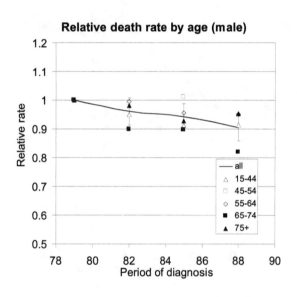

Relative death rate by age (male)

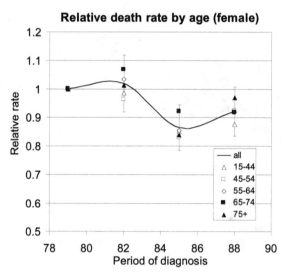

Relative death rate by age (female)

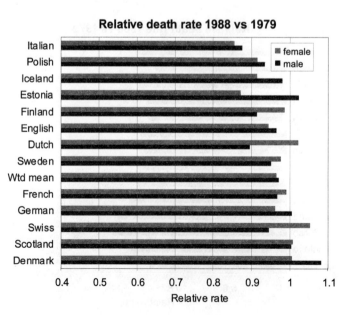

Relative death rate 1988 vs 1979

Breast

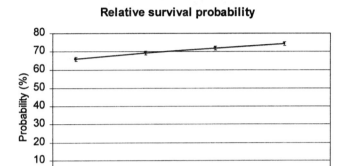

Relative survival probability

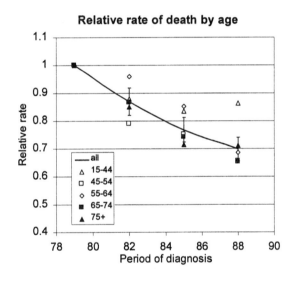

Relative rate of death by age

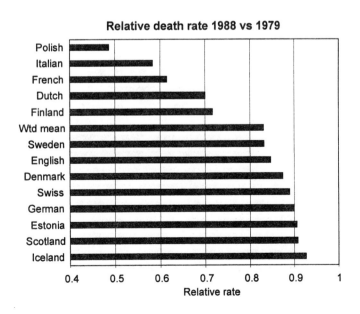

Relative death rate 1988 vs 1979

Cervix uteri

Relative survival probability

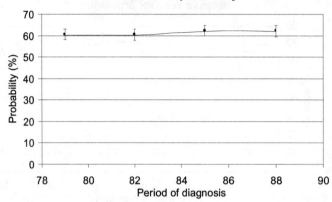

Relative rate of death by age

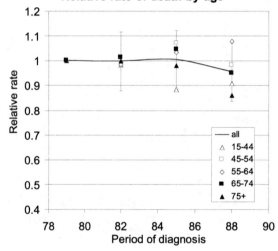

Relative death rate 1988 vs 1979

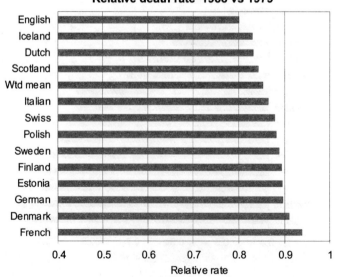

Corpus uteri

Relative survival probability

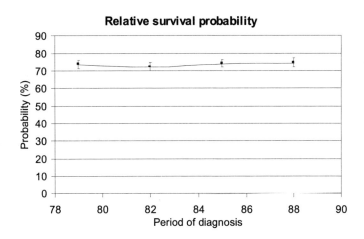

Relative rate of death by age

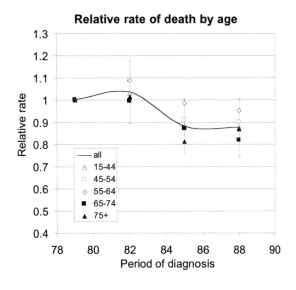

Relative death rate 1988 vs 1979

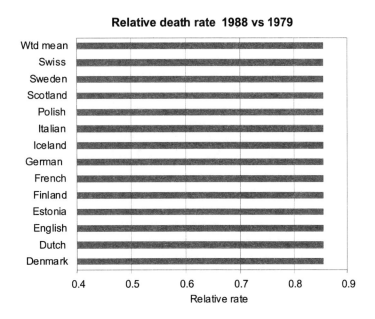

Ovary

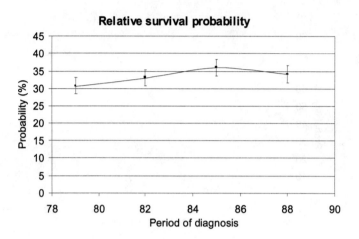

Relative survival probability

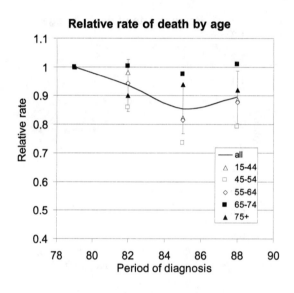

Relative rate of death by age

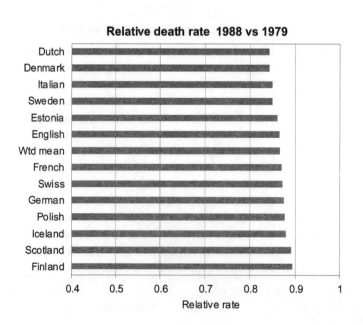

Relative death rate 1988 vs 1979

Prostate

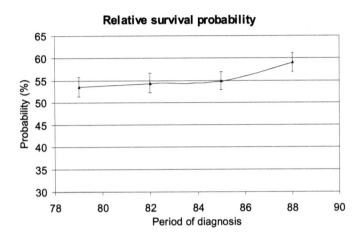

Relative survival probability

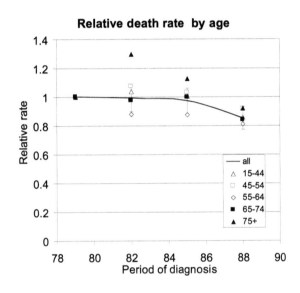

Relative death rate by age

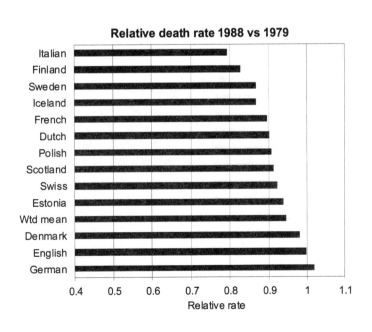

Relative death rate 1988 vs 1979

Testis

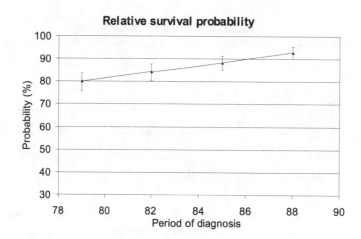

Relative survival probability

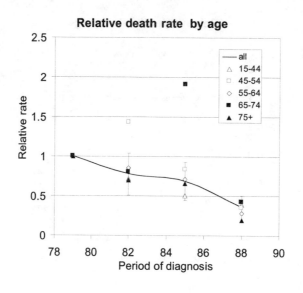

Relative death rate by age

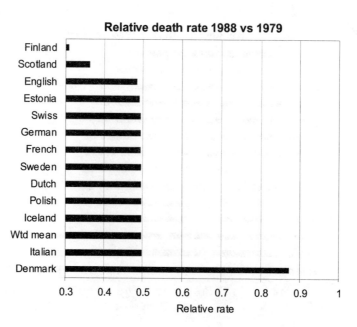

Relative death rate 1988 vs 1979

Non-Hodgkin's lymphomas

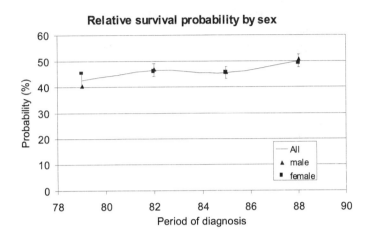

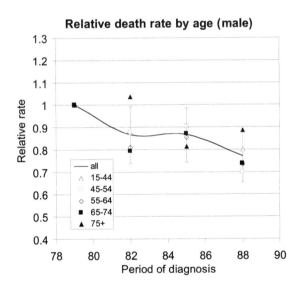

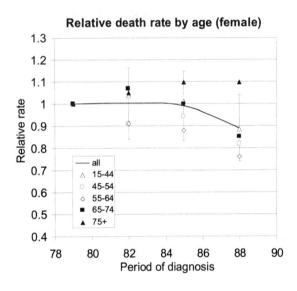

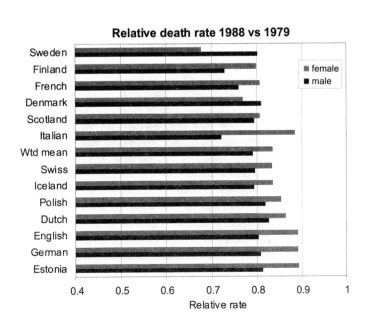

Hodgkin's disease

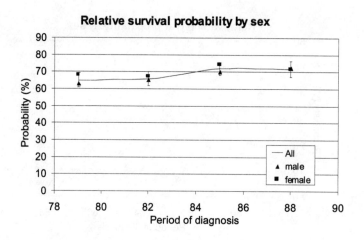

Relative survival probability by sex

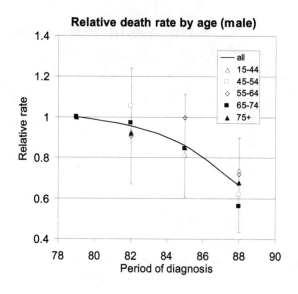

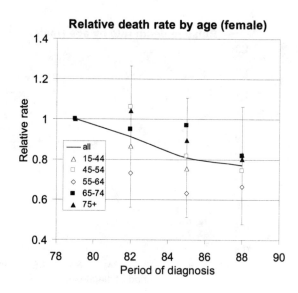

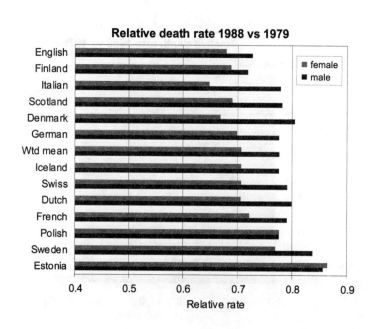

Acute lymphocytic leukaemia

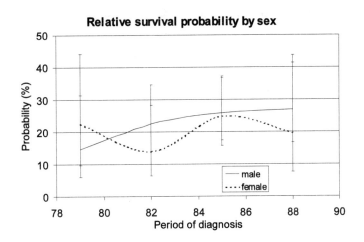

Relative survival probability by sex

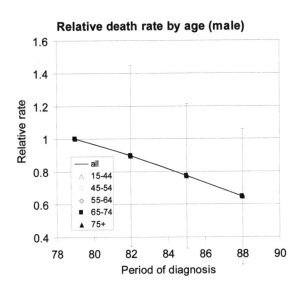

Relative death rate by age (male)

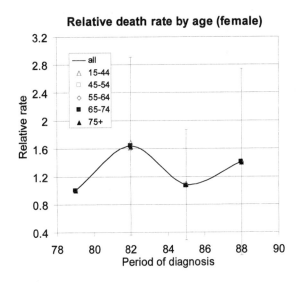

Relative death rate by age (female)

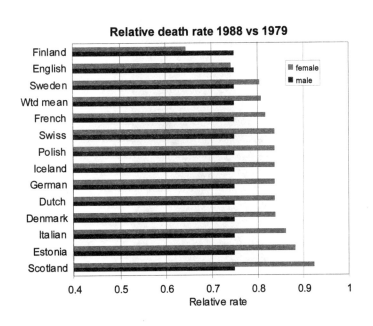

Relative death rate 1988 vs 1979

Chronic lymphocytic leukaemia

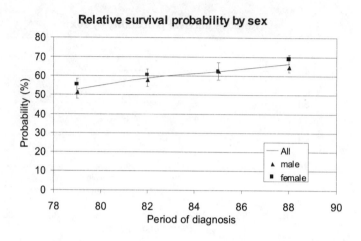

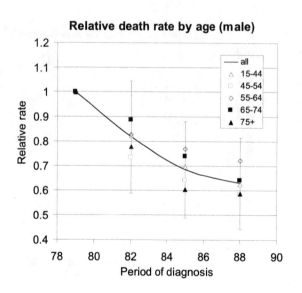

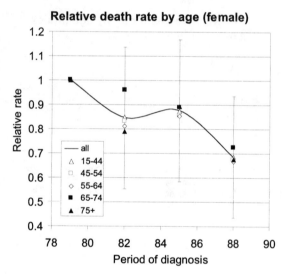

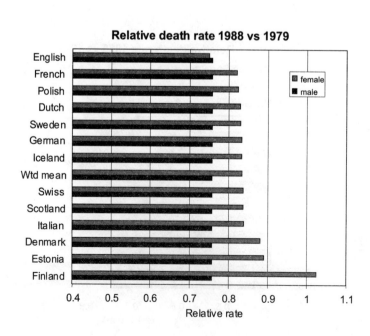

Acute myeloid leukaemia

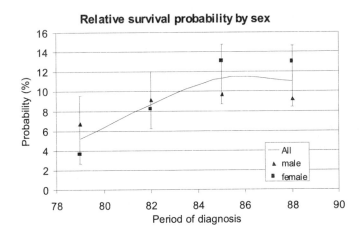

Relative survival probability by sex

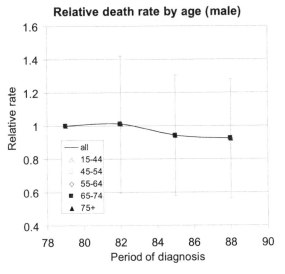

Relative death rate by age (male)

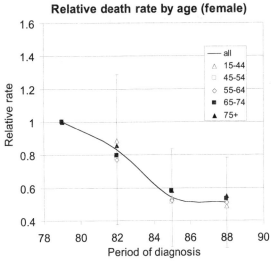

Relative death rate by age (female)

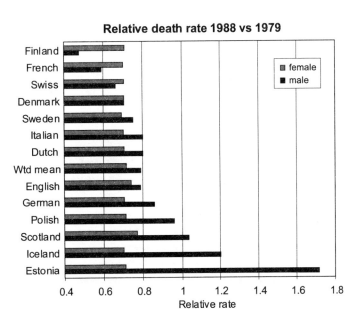

Relative death rate 1988 vs 1979

Chronic myeloid leukaemia

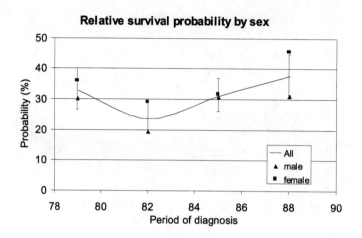

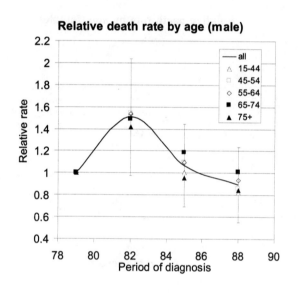

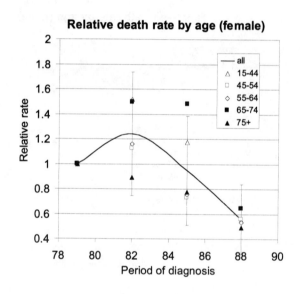

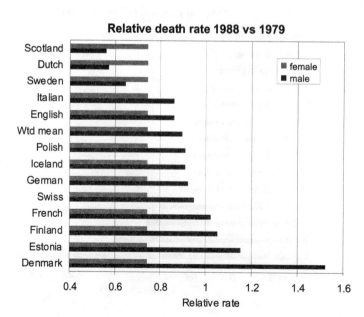

All cancers

Relative survival probability by sex

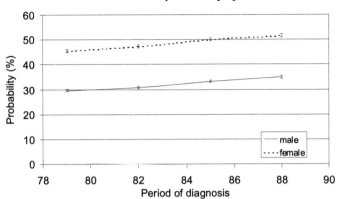

Relative death rate by age (male)

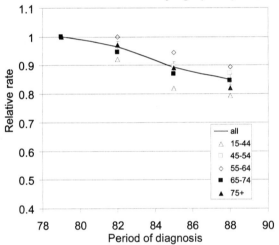

Relative death rate by age (female)

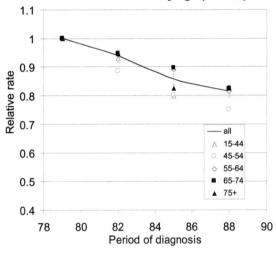

Relative death rate 1988 vs 1979

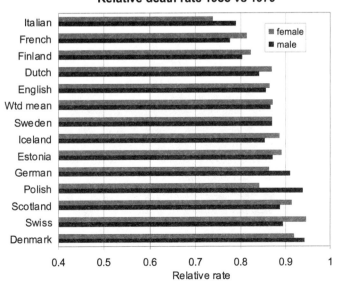

Chapter 7

Organization and use of the EUROCARE-2 compact disk

E. Carrani, P. Roazzi and R. Capocaccia

Introduction

A compact disk (CD) is included with this publication to facilitate use of the EUROCARE database, providing a number of important benefits. Firstly, electronic publication makes a much more extensive set of data available, principally pertaining to survival during the entire period covered by the Eurocare study (1978–89), that could not be included in the printed publication. Secondly, it allows selection and re-organization of cancer survival statistics from the database according to the user's choice. Thirdly, it allows data to be exported in a tabulated form so that further analyses can be carried out using external statistical and graphical software. Furthermore, the disk allows easy consultation of the data at any place where a personal computer is available.

This chapter describes the material on the disk and the software (Access®) used to implement and manipulate it, and provides a brief guide to its use for readers not familiar with this software.

Data accessible

Records of individual patients are not contained on the EUROCARE CD; the survival data and other statistics are available only at the aggregated level. The disk is organized into three sections, which differ in terms of the data accessible and the logic of access.

The **first section** contains survival rates for the incidence period 1985–89, and presents basically the same information as is given in the book. In particular, it contains the following:

- General information (number of cases, incidence period, and mean age) according to cancer site, country, participating registry and sex.
- Numbers of cases considered in the survival analysis, by cancer site (47 sites or combinations of sites), country (17 countries and Europe), sex, and age (five age classes and all ages).
- Observed survival rates at one, three and five years from diagnosis, by cancer site, country, sex and age.
- Relative survival rates at one, three and five years from diagnosis, by cancer site, country, sex and age.

- 95% confidence intervals for the one-year and five-year relative survival rates.
- Age-standardized relative survival one and five years after diagnosis, and corresponding confidence intervals, by cancer site, country and sex. Compared with the printed volume, age-standardized rates for both sexes together have been added.
- A table of weightings used for the calculation of survival rates for the entire European pool of cancer cases.

The **second section** is concerned with time trends of survival; the data are presented for four incidence periods 1978–80, 1981–83, 1984–86, 1987–89, and only for the 21 cancer registries whose data cover all four periods. This part includes the data described above, further stratified by period of diagnosis.

The **third section** allows page views of the main tables in the publication, i.e., pages 74–523, to be displayed (but not the tables pertaining to the text chapters).

Hardware and software requirements

In order to use the EUROCARE CD, the minimum hardware and software requirements are:
- A personal computer with a 486 or higher processor and at least 16 MB of RAM.
- Microsoft Windows® 95 or 98 (or NT 4.0).
- 20 to 80 MB of available hard disk space.
- A CD ROM drive.
- Microsoft Access 97® (a component of Microsoft Office 97®). This is recommended but is not absolutely necessary to access the disk, since a licensed copy of Access 97 runtime is provided on the disk.
- Microsoft Office 97 is required in order to use the data export facilities described below.
- Acrobat Reader 3.0 ® or higher. This product is also loaded on the CD and can be easily installed.

Sections 1 and 2 have been implemented with Microsoft Access 97. Section 3 consists of a set of Postscript files that can be accessed and inspected with Acrobat Reader 3.0, which is available free of charge from numerous sources. This programme is, however, transparent to the user, as individual pages of Section 3 are called up directly from the main menu.

Installing and starting the EUROCARE CD

The installation procedure differs according to whether Microsoft Access 97 and Acrobat Reader 3.01 or 3.02 are already available.

1. If they are already installed, access to the database is obtained simply by double clicking on the **Eurocare.mde** icon on the CD.
2. Otherwise, the SETUP procedure included in the CD INSTALL directory should be executed to make runtime DLLs of ACCESS'97 available, by clicking on the **Setup.exe** icon and following the instructions.
3. If Acrobat reader is already installed in your computer, the product uses the installed version. Otherwise, Acrobat reader 3.02 can be either downloaded free of charge from Adobe Internet site (www.adobe.com, or installed by double clicking on the **AR302.exe** icon and following the instructions.
    IMPORTANT NOTICE. Before installing more recent versions of Acrobat reader, it is strongly recommended to uninstall all previous versions of the product.
4. Once these products are installed, access to the database is obtained by double-clicking the **Eurocare.mde** icon in the Program Files Eurocare-2 directory.
5. To uninstall EUROCARE-2 use the Add/Remove icon from the Windows control panel.
6. To uninstall Acrobat Reader, refer to standard Adobe uninstall procedure.

When the initial (splash) screen appears, click on the picture to continue.

The next screen displays three buttons that give access to the three main sections outlined above, along with two other options.

Accessing 1985–89 survival data (Section 1)

Selecting tables

Several kinds of table can be called up to present or analyse the data for 1985–89. The tables select from the whole data-set, according to the specified cancer site, country, time (years) from diagnosis, sex and age. Not all of these variables are available for all tables. Table 1, below, indicates what selections are available for the different tables.

If a selection is made for a variable not relevant to a particular table, it is ignored. If a given variable is not selected, data for all levels of the variable are presented in the output table.

The type of table required is selected by pressing (clicking on) one of the five buttons on the right-hand side of the screen. Particular variables are selected by clicking on the appropriate row. Standard Windows selection rules apply here. Multiple contiguous rows are selected by holding down the left mouse button and moving the cursor over the rows required. Multiple non-contiguous rows are selected or deselected by holding down the **Ctrl** key while clicking the left mouse button on each desired row. In the **Age Class** selection window, some special age classes are considered for analysing bone and prostate cancers. For bone, the first age class starts at the age of 20 instead of 15. For prostate, analysis has been carried out according to the following age classes: 15–54, 55–64, 65–74, 75–84, 85–99 years. The current selection can be cleared by the **Clear Selection** button. Five different tables are available by clicking the appropriate button:

1. Age trend analysis

This table presents the number of cases in the analysis, the crude relative survival rates at one, three and five years, their 95% confidence limits (at one and five years only), and the corresponding observed survival rates. These data are presented by age class. Values corresponding to the same levels of the other selection variables and to the six age classes are presented on the same row. This kind of

Table 1. Information included in data tables available with the EUROCARE CD					
	Cancer site	Country	Time from diagnosis	Sex	Age class
Age trend analysis	Yes	Yes	Yes	Yes	No
Crude survival rates by age	Yes	Yes	Yes	Yes	Yes
Age-adjusted survival rates	Yes	Yes	Yes	Yes	No
Data description	Yes	Yes	No	Yes	No
Weightings	Yes	Yes	No	Yes	No

presentation is particularly useful for further table construction or graphical analysis. Note that the age classes reported in the table title are the same for all sites, and are therefore not correct for bone and prostate cancers, for which special age classes have been considered (see above).

2. Crude survival rates

This table presents the number of cases in the analysis, the crude observed and relative survival rates and the confidence limits of the relative survival (at one and five years only). In this case, age is treated like the other selection variables. It is possible to present data for just one or for a subset of age classes by clicking on the corresponding rows of the age selection window. It is also possible to obtain the data for all the six age classes *together* by clicking on the **All** row.

3. Age-adjusted survival rates

This table presents the age-standardized relative survival rates for males, females and both sexes at one and five years from diagnosis, and the corresponding 95% confidence limits.

4. Data description

This table corresponds to the first table (at the top of the page) on each standard page of results in the book. These tables present, for each contributing cancer registry, the number of cases, their mean age, and the incidence period. To obtain a global view of all contributing registries, all countries have to be selected manually in the **Country** window.

5. Weightings

This table presents the set of weightings that were used, for each cancer site and by sex, to average the country-specific survival rates in order to estimate survival rates for the entire European pool of cases.

Accessing trend analysis for 1978–89 data (Section 2)

Selecting tables

Five basic kinds of table are available for trend analysis. Data can be selected by cancer site, country, time from diagnosis, sex and age class. The scheme in Table 2 indicates what selections are available for the different tables.

Selections are made on the main menu screen by clicking on one of the five buttons on the right-hand side of the screen in exactly the same way as described previously. The content of the five tables is described below.

1. Time trend analysis

This table presents the number of cases, the crude relative survival rates at one, three, five, eight and ten years, their 95% confidence limits (at one and five years only) and the corresponding observed survival rates. These data are presented separately for the four incidence periods on the same row. Therefore, period of diagnosis is not a selection variable for this table.

2. Crude survival rates

This table presents the number of cases in the analysis, the crude observed and relative survival rates and the confidence limits of the relative survival (at one and five years only). In this case, period is treated like the other variables, and selection according to one or more of the four incidence periods can be made by clicking on the period selection window.

	Cancer site	Country	Time from diagnosis	Sex	Period of diagnosis	Age class
Table 2. Information included in trend tables available with the the Eurocare CD						
Time trend analysis	Yes	Yes	Yes	Yes	No	Yes
Crude survival rates by period	Yes	Yes	Yes	Yes	Yes	Yes
Age-adjusted survival rates	Yes	Yes	Yes	Yes	Yes	No
Data description	Yes	Yes	No	Yes	No	No
Weightings	Yes	Yes	No	Yes	No	No

3. Age-adjusted rates

This table presents the age-standardized relative survival rates in males, females and both sexes, with the corresponding 95% confidence limits, for the four incidence periods (1978–80, 1981–83, 1984–86, 1987–89).

4. Data description

This table presents, for each of the contributing cancer registries, the incidence period for which each contributed data to the analysis, as well as the number and mean age of the cases contributed. To obtain a complete list of contributing registries in Europe, all countries have to be selected manually in the **Countries** window.

5. Weightings

This table presents the set of weightings that were used, for each cancer site and by sex, to average the country-specific survival rates in order to estimate survival rates for the entire European pool of cases.

Operating with tables

Once a table has been selected and displayed, there are two different ways of further displaying the table. These choices are made by clicking on the appropriate button on the tool bar at the top of the screen. The buttons are as follows:

Mask view

This is the default mode, and gives a clear presentation with complete information in column titles on the content of the columns. **Mask view** is particularly indicated for looking at the data and for hard copy printing.

Data-sheet view

This view permits the user to enter the spreadsheet environment, in which all the standard facilities offered by Access are available. For the sophisticated use of Access to manipulate the data and reorganize the tables, the reader should refer to the published manuals of Microsoft Access. However some simple commands are described below.

Commands available

- **Sort**. This command is available in mask and in data-sheet view. Rows in one or more selected columns can be sorted in increasing or decreasing alphanumeric order by selecting the desired columns and clicking on the appropriate button on the tool bar.
- **Filter**. This command is available in mask and in data-sheet view. Filters can be applied by clicking on the appropriate filter button on the tool bar. Particular values in each column then are selected. Further selection rules can be formed using arithmetical operators: $<$, $=$, $>$, connected by the logical operators: *or, and*. When these choices have been made, the **Apply Filter** button on the tool bar is clicked. A defined filter remains active during the whole session.
- **Drag and drop**. This command is available only in data-sheet view. Specific columns can be selected and dragged to any particular position of the table. In this way, it is possible to change the order of the columns.
- **Print**. Available in mask and in data sheet view. This command makes a hard copy print of the current table.

It is not possible to perform arithmetical calculations on the data, nor any other operations which change the data.

Export data

No graphical tool or any software for further statistical analysis is provided on the Eurocare CD. However, the results in the tables can be easily and quickly exported to other software. In the **data sheet** mode, the content of the current table is transferred to the Word or Excel environment by clicking on the corresponding icon on the tool bar. In the new environment, the data can be manipulated with the standard Word or Excel facilities and can be saved as text, Word or Excel files for further processing by appropriate statistical software. The default names for the Word or Excel files carry the initial characters 'ECS' (for 'EuroCare Survival') or 'ECT' (for 'Eurocare Trends') to facilitate their subsequent identification and retrieval. Note that export to Word or Excel does not work correctly in **mask view** mode.

Page view of the monograph tables

This section allows on-screen display of the images of the survival data tables that make up the main body of the Eurocare monograph. The menu page addresses tables by cancer site and country. Once the desired page is obtained, it is possible to browse it, to zoom on it and to print it, but it is not possible to change its content. Page view can be also accessed directly from the tables of Section 1. Clicking on the **Page View** button (at the upper right of the screen), the page referring to the site and country of the current row is displayed.

Achevé d'imprimer sur rotative
par l'Imprimerie Darantiere à Dijon-Quetigny
en septembre 1999

Dépôt légal : 3ᵉ trimestre 1999
N° d'impression : 99-0654